Orthopaedic Knowledge Update

Hip and Knee Reconstruction

American Academy of Orthopaedic Surgeons

Orthopaedic Knowledge Update

Hip and Knee Reconstruction

Edited by
John J. Callaghan, MD
Douglas A. Dennis, MD
Wayne G. Paprosky, MD
Aaron G. Rosenberg, MD

With 120 illustrations

 Developed by the
Hip Society

 and the
Knee Society

 Published by
American Academy of Orthopaedic Surgeons
6300 North River Road   Rosemont, IL 60018

Orthopaedic Knowledge Update: Hip and Knee Reconstruction

American Academy of Orthopaedic Surgeons

The material presented in *Orthopaedic Knowledge Update: Hip and Knee Reconstruction* has been made available by the American Academy of Orthopaedic Surgeons for educational purposes only. This material is not intended to present the only, or necessarily best, methods or procedures for the medical situations discussed, but rather is intended to represent an approach, view, statement, or opinion of the author(s) or producer(s), which may be helpful to others who face similar situations.

Some drugs and medical devices demonstrated in Academy courses or described in Academy print or electronic publications have FDA clearance for use for specific purposes or for use only in restricted settings. The FDA has stated that it is the responsibility of the physician to determine the FDA status of each drug or device he or she wishes to use in clinical practice, and to use the products with appropriate patient consent and in compliance with applicable law.

Furthermore, any statements about commercial products are solely the opinion(s) of the author(s) and do not represent an Academy endorsement or evaluation of these products. These statements may not be used in advertising or for any commercial purpose.

The material contained in this volume was submitted as previously unpublished material, except in the instances in which credit has been given to the source from which some of the illustrative material was derived.

Materials appearing in this book prepared by individuals as part of their official duties as U.S. Government employees are not covered by the above-mentioned copyright.

First Edition
Copyright © 1995 by the
American Academy of Orthopaedic Surgeons

ISBN: 0-89203-117-4

Library of Congress Cataloging-in-Publication Data:
Orthopaedic knowledge update: hip and knee reconstruction/edited by John J. Callaghan...(et al). Developed by the Hip Society and the Knee Society. 1st ed.
 334 p.   Cm.
Includes bibliographical references and index.
ISBN 0-89203-117-4
1. Total hip replacement. 2. Total knee replacement. 3. Hip joint—Surgery. 4. Knee—surgery. I. Callaghan, John J. II. Hip Society (U.S.) II. Knee Society (U.S.)
[DNLM: 1. Hip joint—surgery. 2. Knee joint—surgery. 3. Arthroplasty—methods. WE 860 O77 1995]
RD549.078   1995
617.5'810592—dc20
DNLM/DLC   95-39517
for Library of Congress   CIP

Acknowledgments

American Academy of Orthopaedic Surgeons

Board of Directors, 1995
James W. Strickland, MD, *President*
S. Terry Canale, MD
Charles R. Clark, MD
Paul C. Collins, MD
William C. Collins, MD
Robert D. D'Ambrosia, MD
Kenneth E. DeHaven, MD
Robert N. Hensinger, MD
James H. Herndon, MD
Douglas W. Jackson, MD
Richard F. Kyle, MD
George L. Lucas, MD
David R. Mauerhan, MD
Bernard F. Morrey, MD
Bernard A. Rineberg, MD
D. Eugene Thompson, MD
William W. Tipton, Jr., MD (*ex officio*)

Staff
William W. Tipton, Jr., MD, *Executive Vice-President*
Mark W. Wieting, *Director, Division of Education*
Marilyn L. Fox, PhD, *Director, Department of Publications*
Bruce Davis, *Senior Editor*
Joan Abern, *Associate Senior Editor*
Loraine Edwalds, *Production Manager*
Marcia Biasiello, *Assistant Production Manager*
Sophie Tosta, *Editorial Assistant*
Geraldine Dubberke, *Publications Secretary*
Em Lee Lambos, *Publications Secretary*

The Knee Society Board of Directors
Richard D. Scott, MD
Victor M. Goldberg, MD
W. Norman Scott, MD
James A. Rand, MD
Clifford W. Colwell, Jr., MD
Russell E. Windsor, MD

The Hip Society Board of Directors
Richard B. Welch, MD
Dennis K. Collis, MD
Leo A. Whiteside, MD
John R. Moreland, MD
Robert B. Bourne, MD
Mark G. Lazansky, MD

Contributors

Thomas P. Andriacchi, PhD
Professor and Director of Section of Orthopaedic
  Research
Rush-Presbyterian-St. Luke's Medical Center
Rush Arthritis and Orthopaedics Institute
Department of Orthopaedic Surgery
Chicago, Illinois

Kim C. Bertin, MD
Utah Orthopaedic Specialists
LDS Hospital
Salt Lake City, Utah

James V. Bono, MD
Attending Orthopaedic Surgeon
New England Baptist Hospital
Boston, Massachusetts

Robert Emery Booth, Jr, MD
Co-Chief Orthopaedic Surgery
Rothman Institute
Philadelphia, Pennsylvania

Robert B. Bourne, MD, FRCSC
Professor of Surgery
Division of Orthopaedic Surgery
University of Western Ontario
Chief, Division of Orthopaedic Surgery
University Hospital
London, Ontario, Canada

Michael S. Bradford, MD, FRCSC
Las Vegas, Nevada

Calvin R. Brown, Jr, MD
Assistant Professor of Medicine
Rush-Presbyterian-St. Luke's Medical Center
Chicago, Illinois

John J. Callaghan, MD
Professor, Department of Orthopaedics
University of Iowa College of Medicine
Iowa City, Iowa

Michael J. Chmell, MD
Orthopaedic Surgeon
Rockford Orthopedic Associates
Rockford, Illinois

John P. Collier, DE
Professor of Engineering
Director, Dartmouth Biomedical Engineering Center
Thayer School of Engineering
Dartmouth College
Hanover, New Hampshire

Clifford W. Colwell, Jr, MD
Head, Division of Orthopaedic Surgery
Scripps Clinic and Research Foundation
La Jolla, California

Stephen D. Cook, PhD
Lee C. Schlesinger Professor
Director, Orthopaedic Research
Tulane University School of Medicine
New Orleans, Louisiana

Douglas A. Dennis, MD
Clinical Professor, Colorado School of Mines
Co-Director, Rose Institute for Joint Replacement
Clinical Director, Rose Musculoskeletal Research
  Laboratory
Denver, Colorado

Roger H. Emerson, Jr, MD
Clinical Associate Professor of Orthopaedic Surgery
Southwestern Medical School
Dallas, Texas

John L. Esterhai, Jr, MD
Associate Professor of Orthopaedic Surgery
Veteran's Administration Hospital and Hospital of the
  University of Pennsylvania
University of Pennsylvania School of Medicine
Philadelphia, Pennsylvania

Robert H. Fitzgerald, Jr, MD
Professor and Chairman
Department of Orthopaedic Surgery
University of Pennsylvania
School of Medicine
Philadelphia, Pennsylvania

Andrew H. Glassman, MS, MD
Staff Surgeon
The Anderson Orthopaedic Institute
Chief of Staff
The National Hospital for Orthopaedics and
    Rehabilitation
Arlington, Virginia

Hillary Green, BA
Research Assistant, Department of Orthopaedic Surgery
University of California at San Francisco
San Francisco, California

David A. Heck, MD
Associate Professor, Department of Orthopaedic Surgery
Indiana University School of Medicine
Indianapolis, Indiana

Warren S. Jablonsky, MD
McHenry County Orthopaedics, S.C.
Crystal Lake, Illinois

Murali Jasty, MD
Clinical Associate Professor in Orthopaedic Surgery
Harvard Medical School
Surgeon, Massachusetts General Hospital
Boston, Massachusetts

Brian F. Kavanagh, MD
Clinical Assistant Professor
Department of Orthopaedic Surgery
Yale University, New Haven
Greenwich, Connecticut

Michael A. Kelly, MD
Director
Insall-Scott-Kelly Institute for Orthopaedics and Sports
    Medicine
Beth Israel Hospital North
New York, New York

Kenneth J. Koval, MD
Chief, Fracture Service
Department of Orthopaedics
Hospital for Joint Diseases
New York, New York

Kenneth A. Krackow, MD
Professor, Full Time Faculty
State University of New York at Buffalo
Buffalo, New York

Paul F. Lachiewicz, MD
Associate Professor
Orthopaedic Surgery
University of North Carolina-Chapel Hill
Chapel Hill, North Carolina

William J. Maloney III, MD
Clinical Associate Professor
Stanford University Medical School
Attending Surgeon
Palo Alto Medical Clinic
Palo Alto, California

David A. Mattingly, MD
Director of Education
New England Bone and Joint Institute
New England Baptist Hospital
Boston, Massachusetts

Richard P. Mikosz, PhD
Assistant Professor
Rush-Presbyterian-St. Luke's Medical Center
Rush Arthritis and Orthopaedics Institute
Department of Orthopaedic Surgery
Chicago, Illinois

Sam Nasser, MD
Associate Professor
Department of Orthopaedic Surgery
Wayne State University
School of Medicine
Detroit, Michigan

Philip C. Noble, MD
Director of Orthopaedic Research
Joseph Barnhart Department of Orthopaedic Surgery
Baylor College of Medicine
Houston, Texas

Guy D. Paiement, MD
Associate Professor of Clinical Orthopedics
University of California at San Francisco
San Francisco, California

Wayne G. Paprosky, MD, FACS
Associate Professor, Department of Orthopaedic Surgery
Rush Medical College
Rush-Presbyterian-St. Luke's Medical Center
Chicago, Illinois

James A. Rand, MD
Professor of Orthopaedic Surgery
Mayo Medical School
Consultant in Orthopaedic Surgery
Mayo Clinic, Scottsdale
Scottsdale, Arizona

Merrill A. Ritter, MD
Professor, Orthopaedics
Indiana University School of Medicine
Surgeon-in-Chief
Center for Hip and Knee Surgery
Indianapolis, Indiana

C. H. Rorabeck, MD, FRCSC
Professor and Chairman, Division of Orthopaedic
  Surgery
University Hospital
339 Windermere Road
London, Ontario, Canada

Aaron G. Rosenberg, MD
Associate Professor
Arthritis and Orthopaedic Institute
Rush Medical College
Chicago, Illinois

Harry E. Rubash, MD
Associate Professor and Clinical Vice Chairman
Chief, Division of Adult Reconstructive Surgery
Department of Orthopaedic Surgery
University of Pittsburgh Medical Center
Pittsburgh, Pennsylvania

Richard F. Santore, MD
Clinical Professor of Orthopaedic Surgery
University of California, San Diego
San Diego, California

Richard D. Scott, MD
Associate Clinical Professor of Orthopaedic Surgery
Harvard Medical School
Boston, Massachusetts

Craig D. Silverton, DO
Assistant Professor
Arthritis and Orthopaedic Institute
Rush Medical College
Chicago, Illinois

Bernard N. Stulberg, MD
Director, Cleveland Center for Joint Reconstruction
Cleveland, Ohio

Dale R. Sumner, Jr, MD
Associate Professor
Department of Orthopaedic Surgery
Rush-Presbyterian-St. Luke's Medical Center
Chicago, Illinois

Lauren C. Sutula, MS
Research Engineer
Thayer School of Engineering
Dartmouth College
Hanover, New Hampshire

Bert J. Thomas, MD
Associate Professor of Orthopaedic Surgery
UCLA School of Medicine
Los Angeles, California

Thomas S. Thornhill, MD
Associate Clinical Professor of Orthopaedics
Harvard Medical School
Boston, Massachusetts

Bradley K. Vaughn, MD, FACS
Raleigh Orthopaedic Clinic
Raleigh, North Carolina

Kelly G. Vince, MD, FRCS(C)
Assistant Clinical Professor
University of California, Irvine
Associate Surgeon
Kerlan-Jobe Orthopaedic Clinic
Inglewood, California

Janet Whirlow, MD
Joint Reconstruction Fellow
Department of Orthopaedic Surgery
University of Pittsburgh Medical Center
Pittsburgh, Pennsylvania

Russell E. Windsor, MD
Associate Professor of Surgery (Orthopaedics)
Cornell University Medical College
Associate Attending Orthopaedic Surgeon
The Hospital for Special Surgery
New York, New York

Steven T. Woolson, MD
Clinical Associate Professor of Orthopaedic Surgery
Stanford University Medical School
Menlo Park, California

Timothy W. Wright, PhD
Director, Department of Biomechanics and Biomaterials
The Hospital for Special Surgery
New York, New York

Marguerite Wrona, BS, ME
Project Engineer, Custom Product Service
Johnson & Johnson Professional, Inc.
Raynham, Massachusetts

Joseph D. Zuckerman, MD
Chairman, Department of Orthopaedic Surgery
Hospital for Joint Diseases
New York, New York

Preface

Orthopaedic Knowledge Update: Hip and Knee Reconstruction is one in a series of specialty-oriented OKU volumes that focus on a specific subspecialty of orthopaedics. The purpose is to help the orthopaedic surgeon remain current with information in a selected area of orthopaedics.

The *Orthopaedic Knowledge Update* (OKU) was developed to provide "a useful, comprehensive, and accessible synthesis of the latest information and knowledge available in the literature related to orthopaedic surgery." The OKU Home Study Program is now 11 years old, and each new edition continues to meet the original challenge of emphasizing a learner-centered education.

The *Orthopaedic Knowledge Update: Hip and Knee Reconstruction* is a highly refined and distilled body of knowledge on reconstruction of the adult hip and knee. Every chapter has been critically reviewed, with revision as needed, by a team of physicians with expertise in hip and knee reconstruction. Our goal has been to bring together the most useful up-to-date information. Where relevant, we have included surgical techniques, although usually we have concentrated on providing the basic information needed to make appropriate decisions. This book is designed as a reference and guide to specific problems regarding adult hip and knee reconstruction. In this *Orthopaedic Knowledge Update: Hip and Knee Reconstruction*, we have tried to review general topics related to both hip and knee reconstruction, topics related specifically to hip reconstruction, and topics related specifically to knee reconstruction. General topics include thromboembolic dis-

ease, blood conservation, infection prevention, and the various materials used in arthroplasty procedures (ie, metal, polyethylene, polymethylmethacrylate, and bone graft) as well as the medical treatment of arthritis. The specific hip and knee sections concentrate on issues concerning primary and revision surgery including the complications associated with the procedures and the fixation options for specific conditions and situations.

In addition to the extensive references included in this volume, a broad representation of the literature on the hip and knee can be found in the previous and future *Orthopaedic Knowledge Update* series. The success of this issue is a direct result of the energy and devotion of the individual contributors. A number of people have contributed to making this publication possible. We would especially like to acknowledge the assistance of Marilyn Fox, PhD, in helping us get this project underway, and the superb project management and manuscript editing of Joan Abern, as well as the efforts of members of the Academy's publication production staff.

All of us who have contributed to the completion of this work hope that you, the reader, will find this to be a rich source of information as you seek to update your knowledge of hip and knee reconstruction.

John J. Callaghan, MD
Douglas A. Dennis, MD
Wayne G. Paprosky, MD
Aaron G. Rosenberg, MD

Table of Contents

Section 3: Knee

1

Thromboembolic Disease in Hip and Knee Replacement Patients

Venous thromboembolic disease (TED) is responsible for approximately 200,000 deaths each year in the United States alone, half of which occur in people with an otherwise good prognosis. According to data from a large autopsy series, 13% of all deaths occurring in a general hospital over a period of 40 years were due primarily to pulmonary embolism.

Venous TED remains a major cause of morbidity and mortality for unprotected joint replacement patients. The natural history of the disease in this patient population has not been documented completely, its pathogenesis is not understood totally, and its management remains controversial.

Epidemiology of Venous Thromboembolic Disease in Joint Replacement Patients

The epidemiology of venous TED is difficult to study because the disease consists of a cluster of clinical conditions of variable severity: fatal pulmonary embolism (PE), nonfatal symptomatic PE, asymptomatic PE, proximal deep vein thrombosis (DVT), distal DVT, and postphlebitic syndrome. The true incidence of some of these conditions can only be estimated. The clinical diagnosis of nonfatal symptomatic PE has a specificity of less than 50%, and more than half of the supposedly diagnostic ventilation-perfusion lung scans are read as indeterminate. Furthermore, fewer than 10% of the patients with a hospital discharge diagnosis of PE have undergone pulmonary angiography to confirm the diagnosis. Less than 10% of all patients who die in U.S. general hospitals undergo a postmortem examination.

The epidemiology of venous TED has been studied more extensively in patients who have had hip arthroplasty than in patients who have had knee arthroplasty, but reasonable data are available for both groups (Table 1). It is noteworthy that only 30% of the patients found to have a fatal PE at autopsy had any prior recognized clinical evidence of DVT or PE. So called "typical" clinical findings, such as leg pain, swelling, shortness of breath, and chest pain, generally were absent in these patients. Symptomatic DVT is rare in the community (Table 2). It occurs mainly in hospitalized patients, in whom it complicates another clinical condition or the treatment thereof. Data from large cross-sectional population studies have also indicated an age-adjusted prevalence of postphlebitic sequels between 2.2% and 5.0%.

Table 1. Rate of occurrence of venous thromboembolic disease related conditions in unprotected hip and knee arthroplasty patients

Condition*	Hip Arthroplasty	Knee Arthroplasty
Fatal PE	1.8% to 3.4%	~1%
Symptomatic		
Nonfatal PE	5% to 10%	~5%
Overall DVT	50%	50% to 70%
Proximal DVT	20%	10% to 15%
Postphlebitic syndrome	10% to 20%	

*PE = pulmonary embolism; DVT = deep vein thrombosis

Table 2. Incidence of symptomatic proximal deep vein thrombosis in the community (episodes/1,000 people/year)

Age	Female	Male
	Rural/Urban	Rural/Urban
Under 50 years	0.21/1.10	0.18/0.40
Over 50 years	1.48/3.14	2.25/5.11

Pathogenesis of Venous TED

In 1856 Von Virchow suggested there was a relation between the presence of blood clots in the lower extremity veins and in the pulmonary arteries, with the latter blocking the blood flow to the lungs. Embolization of these clots was hypothesized to prevent oxygenation of the blood and, ultimately, to cause death by anoxia. A triad of factors—stasis, activation of coagulation, and damage to the venous endothelium—was proposed to lead to this situation. To this day, this triad remains the basis of the conceptual understanding of venous TED.

Overview of Hemostasis

The generation of thrombin involves a series of reactions taking place on the surface of relatively stagnant platelets or damaged vessel walls. This generation, ultimately, leads to the formation of fibrin. The exact mechanism by which coagulation is initiated (activation of factor IX) is unclear. Thrombin is at the center of the coagulation process; it activates factors V, VIII, and XIII; cleaves fibrinogen into fibrin; and activates protein C, a fibrinolytic enzyme. It is inactivated mainly by thrombomodulin from the endothelial cells and by antithrombin III. Coagulation is controlled by the inactivation of factors Va and VIIIa, by activated protein C, by dilution of the activated factors in the blood flow and their removal by the liver, and by specific inhibitors of coagulation.

Role of Stasis

A major role for stasis in thrombus formation is supported by the fact that many thrombi originate in valve pockets in which the flow is relatively stagnant. The thrombi are more frequent in old or immobilized patients. Stasis increases the contact time between blood and the irregularities of the vein walls and prevents mixing of the coagulation esterases and their inhibitors. Stagnant blood cells also release adenosine diphosphate (ADP), a potent platelet aggregator.

Hemiparetic stroke patients have a higher frequency of DVT in the paralyzed limb than in the unaffected limb. Hip and knee arthroplasty patients can be considered "temporarily hemiparetic" after their surgery. If only for that reason, adequate pain control and aggressive rehabilitation will bring the operated limb back to normal function and promote venous flow. However, no study statistically supports the value of early aggressive rehabilitation alone in reducing the rate of occurrence of DVT after hip or knee arthroplasty.

Activation of Blood Coagulation

Many of the conditions that predispose to DVT involve both stasis and activation of the coagulation system. In animal models, simple ligation of a vein does not result in DVT; the presence of procoagulants, such as tissue debris, collagen, or fats, is essential. Joint arthroplasty surgery sends large amounts of procoagulants into the blood flow because of the soft-tissue dissection and the rasping of the bone. It has been echographically documented that large amounts of material enter the blood flow when the femoral canal is prepared and the prosthesis is inserted.

Venous Endothelial Wall Damage

Endothelial damage occurs as a result of intraoperative manipulations, such as twisting of the superficial femoral vein, when the hip is dislocated or when retractors are positioned behind the tibial plateaus. It has also been suggested that dislocation of the hip stretches the endothelium intercellular bridges exposing raw collagen and other procoagulants. This damage may contribute to the large number of isolated proximal thrombi seen after hip arthroplasty. Peripheral venodilation often seen with general and regional anesthesia also stretches the endothelium intercellular bridges.

Risk Period for Venous TED

The still-evolving concept of a risk period for postoperative (or postinjury) development of DVT starts at surgery or injury. In unprotected total hip replacement patients, detectable proximal thrombus formation starts about 24 to 48 hours after surgery, peaks around day 5 to 7, and diminishes after day 10, especially if the patient is mobile. However, some preliminary evidence suggests that some patients are at risk for DVT for at least 2 months after their surgery.

Diagnosis of Venous Thromboembolic Disease

The clinical diagnosis of a venous thrombus is difficult, especially in joint replacement patients, because clinical signs, such as edema, pain, Homan's sign, tenderness over the thrombus site, or vein dilation, are nonspecific and often are not present, even in documented cases. Most venous thrombi are still clinically silent when the patient is discharged from the hospital, mostly because the thrombi do not completely obstruct the vein. Clinical examination, even by the most experienced physicians, has a sensitivity of 33% and a specificity of 50% in high-risk patients. DVT of the lower extremity must be assessed by objective methods.

The best method for the diagnosis of DVT of the lower extremities is venography (ascending radiologic phlebography). The use of venography makes it possible to detect both distal thrombi (in the calf veins) and proximal thrombi (in the popliteal, femoral, and iliac veins). Venography has significant side effects, including contrast dye thrombosis of the superficial veins in about 3% of the patients. This rate has not been reduced by the use of iso-osmolar nonionic contrast agents. It is also expensive and cannot be readily repeated, making it a poor choice for patients who need continuous monitoring.

Impedance plethysmography is based on the decreased electric impedance observed when a limb becomes engorged with blood because the venous return is blocked by an obstructive thrombus. It is insensitive in asymptomatic hip arthroplasty patients because a majority of proximal thrombi cause only a partial obstruction at the time of discharge screening.

Duplex scanning (real-time B-mode ultrasonography combined with Doppler flow-detection) provides an interesting alternative because it is noninvasive, repeatable, and relatively inexpensive. However, this technique depends largely on the operator's skills and experience. It is very accurate for the diagnosis of symptomatic proximal thrombi (sensitivity 93%, specificity 98%). This accuracy has not been uniformly reproduced in high-risk asymptomatic populations, such as hip arthroplasty patients. Reported sensitivities in these patients vary from 60% to 98%; however, all series have reported specificities of more than 95%. The small size and the nonocclusive nature of these thrombi at the time of screening and some technical factors may explain these discrepancies. The efficacy of duplex scanning for DVT surveillance in arthroplasty patients needs continued study.

The same remarks apply to the clinical diagnosis of pulmonary embolism in those patients in whom dyspnea, tachypnea, or tachycardia may or may not be present. The current standard modalities for PE diagnosis are ventilation/perfusion scanning and pulmonary angiography. Chest radiograph, electrocardiograph, and arterial blood gases analysis are too insensitive and nonspecific to help diagnose PE.

Treatment of Venous TED

The goal of DVT treatment is to prevent potentially fatal PE, recurrent venous thrombosis, and occlusive thrombus formation, which is closely related to postphlebitic syndrome. The standard protocols and guidelines for treatment of DVT and PE have been developed for symptomatic patients. Treatment of asymptomatic thrombi found on screening before discharge is less clear. Asymptomatic proximal thrombi are usually treated in the same way as symptomatic thrombi: 5 days of heparin therapy followed by 3 months of warfarin. Treatment of symptomatic proximal thrombi with oral anticoagulant alone (without heparin) carries a 20% rate of symptomatic extension or recurrence. Until results of clinical studies on the treatment of asymptomatic proximal thrombi with warfarin alone, with or without serial duplex scanning are published, it is prudent to treat these thrombi as if they were symptomatic.

Venous thrombectomy should be reserved, at this point, for patients in whom the limb is threatened by acute iliofemoral occlusion. Thrombolytic treatment (streptokinase or recombinant tissue plasminogen activator) combined with anticoagulation has been used to dissolve occlusive thrombi in symptomatic patients. The efficacy of this treatment for prevention of postphlebitic syndrome is still debated, and it doubles the risk of bleeding complications without decreasing the rate of PE. Venous thrombectomy should be used with extreme caution and limited to patients with massive occlusive thrombi likely to produce severe postphlebitic syndrome.

The treatment of distal thrombi (symptomatic or not) remains very controversial because there is no consensus as to if and how many of these thrombi will propagate proximally and eventually cause a symptomatic, potentially fatal PE. The rate of proximal extension of distal thrombi has been reported to be from 0 to 40% with the consequent different treatment protocols. Most experts currently recommend 3 months of oral anticoagulation or serial duplex scanning to monitor proximal extension in patients at high risk for bleeding complications.

Prophylaxis

The goal of prophylaxis in joint replacement patients is to prevent DVT and its complications, PE and postphlebitic syndrome. Patients undergoing hip and knee replacement typically have no symptoms and no specific sign of DVT, and the first manifestation of the disease may be a fatal PE or a severe postphlebitic syndrome. All patients undergoing hip and knee replacements are at high risk for DVT, and prevention is far more cost-effective in these patients than treating the condition after it has appeared.

Early Mobilization and Rehabilitation

The postoperative management of joint arthroplasty patients has changed over the last 20 years as surgeons have realized the benefits of early mobilization. Rehabilitation is started earlier and more aggressively than before. There is, however, no controlled study that has specifically looked at this aspect of venous TED prevention. Comparisons with historic control groups do not suggest that early mobilization alone has had a major influence on the venous TED rate in joint replacement patients.

Mechanical Prophylaxis

Lower Extremity Exercises   The influence of various maneuvers on lower extremity venous flow in healthy young subjects has been studied using thermodilution methods. Simple leg raise increases the peak femoral vein flow to more than five times the baseline. Elevation of the foot of the bed on DVT has been shown to significantly lower its rate of occurrence in a small series of hip fracture patients when venography was used as a diagnostic end point.

Active ankle motion doubles the femoral vein peak flow, and passive ankle motion increases it by about 50%. The latter has been proven effective in decreasing DVT in general surgery patients. Both are simple and inexpensive methods with no major side effects or complications and should be used as adjunct measures to an efficacious pharmacologic prophylaxis.

Elastic Stockings   Elastic stockings increase the peak femoral vein flow by about 1.5 times the baseline. They also prevent blood stasis in venous aneurysm enlargements and saccular dilatations present in the deep venous system of older people. Since the early 1950s, elastic compression of the lower extremities has been widely used in hospitalized patients. Effective elastic stockings should provide a gradient of pressure that is greatest at the foot (15 to 18 mm Hg) and decreases to about 5 mm Hg at the proximal thigh, be devoid of garters, and allow an acceptable fit for most patients.

Graded compression elastic stockings have been proven effective in decreasing the rate of DVT occurrence in abdominal surgery patients when used alone or as an adjuvant to low-dose heparin. Above-the-knee stockings have not been found to have any advantage over below-the-knee stockings in this patient population. No published study has looked at the efficacy of elastic stockings alone compared to a placebo in joint replacement patients (using venography as a diagnostic end point), and no cost-effectiveness study is available. Elastic bandages should be abandoned totally because even when they are applied on the most reliable patients by the most expert hands, they displace to create garters, which have a venous tourniquet effect.

Continuous Passive Motion   Continuous passive motion (CPM) has been investigated primarily for its effects on cartilage repair. It is also widely used after knee arthroplasty to help the patient regain motion faster and to control pain. CPM increases the peak femoral vein flow between 2.5 and four times the baseline values, depending on the design of the machines used. At least two large randomized, well-designed studies were *unable* to prove CPM to be of any benefit against DVT in knee arthroplasty patients when venography was used as a diagnostic end point. Similarly, in hip arthroplasty patients, no statistically significant difference, as determined by routine venography, was found between patients on CPM and those simply on leg elevation. There is currently no evidence that suggests that CPM offers any protection against DVT in joint arthroplasty patients.

External Pneumatic Compression External pneumatic compression (EPC) accelerates venous emptying in the lower limb by increasing peak venous flow, and it stimulates the fibrinolytic system locally and systemically. It has the theoretic advantage of leaving the coagulation system undisturbed, thus minimizing the bleeding risks. EPC is especially attractive for neurologic surgery patients and patients with coagulation disorders. EPC prophylaxis is efficacious in reducing the overall DVT rate of occurrence in total hip replacement patients when venography is used as a diagnostic end point. It is not, however, as efficacious as low-dose warfarin in preventing proximal DVT. Improper application of the device and patient compliance are also problems in up to 50% of the patients. These observations should be taken into consideration when selecting a prophylactic measure, especially in hip replacement patients in whom isolated proximal thrombi are frequent.

Venous Interruption Percutaneous insertion of devices such as the Greenfield filter has replaced direct surgical ligation. The use of these devices is indicated mainly for recurring PE in patients on adequate anticoagulation and for prophylaxis in very high risk patients in whom anticoagulation is contraindicated. Venous interruption is rarely used in arthroplasty patients, but caval patency rates up to 95% have been reported from series of studies on multiple trauma patients (head trauma and long bone fractures). Clinical trials and cost-effectiveness analyses are necessary before the identification of arthroplasty patients in whom the prophylactic insertion of these devices should be recommended.

Pharmacologic Prophylaxis

Dextran The antithrombotic properties of dextran have been known for over 30 years. Suggested mechanisms of action include reduction of platelet function, coating of endothelial surfaces, stabilization of red blood cell suspension, plasma volume expansion with subsequent blood viscosity decrease, and weakening of the thrombus structure. Dextran is a branched polysaccharide of bacterial origin, which is available as dextran 70 with an average molecular weight of 70,000 d or dextran 40 with an average molecular weight of 40,000 d. Both preparations are mixtures of polysaccharides with the most recent preparations having a narrower range of molecular weights. As a rule of thumb, there are more complications with higher molecular weight, heterogeneous, highly-branched molecules, and

dextran 40 is generally preferred.

Dextran usually is administered at a dosage of 10 ml/kg during surgery, followed by 7.5 ml/kg on postoperative days 1 and 3. This regimen is effective, and several reliable studies support the efficacy of dextran in reducing the incidence of DVT in hip arthroplasty patients using venography as a diagnostic end-point. Despite its efficacy, however, dextran has not gained wide acceptance as a routine prophylactic agent because of its costs, its side effects (especially bleeding complications and congestive heart failure), and its intravenous administration.

Hydroxychloroquine Hydroxychloroquine sulfate was first used as an antimalarial agent and later as a sludge removal agent in patients with impaired veins. Its exact mechanism of action remains controversial, but hydroxychloroquine reduces the size of experimentally induced thrombi in rabbits and does not affect bleeding time in humans. Evidence of hydroxychloroquine efficacy in joint replacement patients is tenuous. A 0.4% incidence of fatal PE and a 4.2% incidence of symptomatic nonfatal PE were reported in a retrospective series of 1,054 hip arthroplasty patients. These rates were lower than those of historic unprotected controls from the same institution.

Antithrombin III Antithrombin-III (AT-III) is a plasma glycoprotein with a molecular weight of 58,000, which is synthesized by the liver. The vascular endothelium is a possible site of storage and/or synthesis of AT-III. It inhibits thrombin; factors Xa, XIa, and XIIa; and plasmin by forming an inactive complex. This phenomenon is greatly enhanced by heparin. It has been hypothesized that a postoperative decrease of AT-III could be responsible for venous thrombosis after hip arthroplasty, although no statistical correlation has been demonstrated between AT-III level and venous thrombosis. Few studies have been reported, but these data indicate an efficacy and safety comparable to dextran.

Aspirin Aspirin is a household name, is easy to administer, and does not require any monitoring. It affects the platelets by blocking the formation of thromboxane A2, the most potent stimulant of platelet aggregation. The efficacy of aspirin as a prophylactic agent against clot formation in the venous system is controversial because of the paucity of well-designed, large, randomized studies. The data regarding its efficacy are confusing and do not allow any final conclusion. Better studied prophylaxes, which have been proven efficacious, are currently available.

Warfarin Warfarin interferes with vitamin K metabolism in the liver. It prevents the transformation of vitamin K epoxide (inactive) to vitamin K H2 (active) by blocking two enzymes: Vitamin K epoxide reductase and Vitamin K reductase. The active form of Vitamin K is necessary for the synthesis of clotting factors II, VII, IX, and X as well as protein C and protein S, which are important for normal fibrinolysis. In patients receiving warfarin, coagulation factors are missing some gamma-carboxylated glutamyl residues that are essential for the normal Ca^{++}/phospholipid-mediated activation of prothrombin.

Dose response to warfarin is hard to predict because it depends on numerous factors, such as diet, intestinal flora, level of activity, concurrent medications, and so forth. Patients should be carefully evaluated for coagulation and liver problems, and a prothrombin time, partial thromboplastin time, platelet count, and serum glutamic-oxaloacetic transaminase measurement should be obtained. Warfarin can cause fetal damage and should never be used in potentially pregnant women.

The effect of warfarin on the coagulation system is monitored with the one-stage prothrombin-time (PT) test, which is sensitive to the reduction of factors II, VII, and X. This anticoagulant effect is expressed in INR (international normalized ratio) value, which corrects for the variability in sensitivity of the different reagents used to measure the PT. The INR is calculated using the following formula:

$$INR = [Patient\ PT\ /\ Control\ PT\ ]^{ISI}$$

where ISI is the international sensitivity index, which is specific for each reagent. The ISI is determined for every commercial reagent by comparing it with the World Health Organization standard reagent. In a seminal series of hip fracture patients reported in 1959, there was a 10% incidence of fatal PE in unprotected hip fracture patients compared to a 1% incidence in patients protected with warfarin. Many other studies have reported on the efficacy of warfarin in reducing the DVT rate and to a lesser degree the fatal PE rate after hip surgery.

The early North American experience with warfarin in total hip replacement patients included a high rate of major bleeding problems because insensitive reagents were used to measure the PT while using anticoagulation guidelines based on European studies in which more sensitive reagents were used. This overanticoagulation was recognized and corrected in the early 1980s, and warfarin prophylaxis for hip surgery patients was revisited. In a comparative series of hip replacement patients (low-dose warfarin and external pneumatic compression), an increased blood loss or more major bleeds were not found with low-dose warfarin when compared to external pneumatic compression alone.

Warfarin is currently the most commonly used prophylaxis against venous TED in hip and knee replacement patients. The reported rates of overall DVT have been, on average, between 10% and 20%, and of proximal DVT, between 5% and 10%, with a 1% to 3% rate of occurrence for major bleeds and 2% to 5% for minor bleeds. Results of a study of 3,700 patients, although based on clinical end-points, support the efficacy and safety of low-dose warfarin during the hospital stay. During a period of 20 years (1970 to 1990), no fatal PE, 0.57% symptomatic nonfatal PE, and 1.6% major bleeds were reported.

Prolonged routine low-dose warfarin prophylaxis has also been used for 12 weeks postoperatively without screening in a series of 268 patients after elective hip arthroplasty. No fatal PE and no major bleeding complications were reported after discharge. This warfarin regimen is safe, cost effective, and has the advantage of protecting the patient during the postoperative risk period, which is empirically believed to be between 6 and 12 weeks. This regimen is logistically demanding and is best administered through an outpatient anticoagulant clinic.

Heparin Heparin was discovered in 1916 by a Canadian medical student who was looking for coagulant in the liver. In 1939, it was demonstrated that the anticoagulant activity of heparin required a plasma co-factor, which was later named AT-III. In the 1970s, the mechanism of interaction between heparin and AT-III was finally elucidated. More recently, the site on the heparin molecule that binds to the AT-III molecule has been found to be a pentasaccharide sequence. At the molecular level, heparin acts on AT-III by inducing a conformational change that unmasks an arginine center, which in turn inhibits the active serine center of thrombin and other coagulation enzymes. The heparin then dissociates from AT-III and can be reused.

Commercial heparin is a heterogeneous mixture of sulfated polysaccharide chains of molecular weights ranging from 3,000 to 30,000 d (mean 15,000). One third of the heparin, mostly low molecular weight fractions, binds to AT-III and is responsible for most of the anticoagulant activity at therapeutic levels. High molecular weight heparin fractions have a high affinity for, and inhibit the aggregation of, platelets.

Heparin is poorly absorbed by the gastrointestinal tract and has to be administered intravenously or subcutaneously. Once injected intravenously, heparin undergoes a rapid elimination due to equilibration followed by a slower disappearance through saturable processes; therefore, the dose-response relation is not linear. The exact pathway of heparin elimination is not understood. After an intravenous bolus, a variable fraction is eliminated in the urine in a depolymerized and partially desulfated form, which retains about 50% of its original biologic activity. The influence of renal and hepatic disease on heparin metabolism is uncertain. Interaction of heparin with other drugs does not affect its biologic activity, except that recent reports have suggested that concomitant administration of intravenous nitroglycerin may require higher doses of heparin. The pharmacokinetics and the anticoagulant properties of heparin are not affected by its origin (bovine or porcine) or its method of preparation as sodium or calcium salts.

Heparin has been used as a prophylaxis in fixed low doses of 5,000 UI (Unité Internationale) every 8 or 12 hours in various surgical patient populations. The efficacy of heparin, alone or in combination, has been well documented in general and thoracic surgery patients, but its efficacy in joint replacement patients is still debated, especially after hip surgery.

Low-Dose Heparin (mini heparinization, subcutaneous heparin) Low-dose heparin is used to provide a simple protocol, which will lessen the hypercoagulable state caused by the surgical trauma and the subsequent immobilization. It inactivates factors Xa and thrombin while allowing normal clotting to take place. In theory, in order to be effective, low-dose heparin should be started before surgery, when coagulation and fibrinolysis are in balance and low levels of activated factors are present. When started after surgery/trauma, low-dose heparin is less effective because the coagulation cascade has already been initiated, and high levels of factors Xa and thrombin are present.

Randomized clinical trials in elective total hip replacement surgery have shown low-dose heparin prophylaxis to be effective in reducing rate of DVT when radiologic venography is used as the diagnostic end point. A more recent meta-analysis has reported that subcutaneous heparin was effective in reducing DVT and PE in hip surgery patients. This analysis, however, amalgamated clinical trials in which radiologic venography or fibrinogen scanning were used as diagnostic end points. The latter method is notoriously inaccurate in this patient population.

In summary, the protective effect of low-dose heparin against TED and especially DVT in elective total hip replacement patients remains controversial. Given the availability of other prophylactic methods, which are more efficacious and reasonably safe, low-dose heparin should not be the prophylaxis of choice in these patients.

Heparin-Dihydroergotamine (HEP-DHE) Venous stasis is a major factor in venous thrombus formation in surgical patients. This perioperative stasis is partially caused by venodilation, which often is present at some distance from the operative site and which, to a degree, can damage the delicate venous endothelial wall. This endothelial damage occurs mostly near the cusps and the confluence of veins where the intercellular junctions and the basement membrane are weak and the blood flow already is turbulent.

Dihydroergotamine (DHE) directly stimulates venous smooth muscles causing a venoconstriction, and thereby preventing excessive perioperative venous dilation and stasis. It also has an inhibitory effect on platelet function. When used in combination with heparin, it has the theoretical advantage of acting on all three elements of the Virchow triad, with the heparin acting on the hypercoagulability and the DHE on venodilation and endothelial wall damage.

Four studies have been reported that investigated the efficacy of the combination of 5,000 IU of heparin/0.5 mg DHE started 2 hours before surgery and administered every 8 or 12 hours thereafter. Routine radiologic venography was used as a diagnostic end point. HEP/DHE was demonstrated to significantly reduce incidence of both overall and proximal DVT in all four studies. The incidence of bleeding complications was evaluated against a control placebo group in one study and was not found to be statistically different. A worrisome side effect of DHE is ergotism, an arterial vasospasm caused by the medication, which may cause severe ischemia. The European experience has demonstrated a 0.01% annual incidence of ergotism. In any case, the drug has been withdrawn from the American market but it is still available in Europe.

Adjusted-Dose Heparin When it became clear that low-dose heparin did not have the same efficacy in hip arthroplasty patients that it had in general surgery populations, the concept of adjusted-dose heparin resurfaced. This regimen calls for increasing the partial thromboplastin time (PTT) up to, or a few seconds beyond, the upper end of the normal range by monitoring it many times a day and adjusting the subcutaneous heparin dose accordingly. The first series of hip arthroplasty patients protected by adjusted-dose heparin using venography as a diagnostic end point involved a complicated protocol calling for admission of the patient 48 hours before surgery and frequent PTT measurements. The DVT rate in 38 patients was only 14% with a postoperative bleeding rate of 17%. A simplified protocol in which the PTT was measured only on days 1, 3, and 6 after the operation but patients were still admitted 48 hours before surgery was used in a series of 50 patients. An overall DVT rate of 22% and a proximal rate of 16% with a 24% rate of wound hematomas were reported. Adjusted dose heparin is effective in reducing DVT rate, but it is complicated, expensive, and carries a sizable bleeding risk.

Low Molecular Weight Heparins Two observations have prompted the development of low molecular weight heparins (LMWH). First, LMWH produces less bleeding in animal models than standard heparin for the same antithrombotic effect. Second, LMWH does not prolong the PTT but does retain its anti-factor X activity. The theoretical advantages of LMWH compared to unfragmented regular heparin are a greater and more predictable antithrombotic effect, a longer half-life, and a lesser hemorrhagic effect. LMWH, as a class of antithrombotic drugs, are interesting because of their pharmacodynamics, bioavailability, efficacy, safety, and lack of need of monitoring.

LMWH is not a homogenous drug, but a preparation of heparin chains of less than 8,000 d. Commercial preparations have different average molecular weights and proportions of various heparin chains and, therefore, are not interchangeable. Few studies have compared LMWH efficacy with that of DVT in joint replacement patients using venography as a diagnostic end-point.

LMWH is effective in significantly reducing both overall and proximal DVT when compared to a placebo and does not seem to increase bleeding risks. It is at least as efficacious as adjusted-dose heparin or fixed-dose heparin (7,500 IU and 5,000 IU three times a day) and probably causes fewer bleeding complications. Data from studies in which LMWH was compared with low-dose warfarin have indicated similar efficacy and safety in hip arthroplasty patients and, possibly, a better protection in knee arthroplasty patients. Results have not been published of a direct comparison of the only FDA-approved LMWH (as of January 1995), enoxaparin, with low-dose warfarin in hip or knee replacement patients.

Annotated Bibliography

Goldhaber SZ, Morpurgo M: Diagnosis, treatment, and prevention of pulmonary embolism: Report of the WHO/ International Society and Federation of Cardiology Task Force. *JAMA* 1992;268:1727–1733.

This "position" paper addresses pulmonary embolism as the serious public health issue it is. The paper offers a comprehensive approach to the treatment and the prevention of the disease.

Hirsh J: Heparin. *N Engl J Med* 1991;324:1565–1574.

Hirsch J: Oral anticoagulant drugs. *N Engl J Med* 1991;324:1865–1875.

These two papers are review on heparin and oral anticoagulants. Both reviews are comprehensive but concise, eminently practical but with enough basic science to make the reader understand the how and the why of oral anticoagulation.

Paiement GD, Wessinger SJ, Harris WH: Cost-effectiveness of prophylaxis in total hip replacement. *Am J Surg* 1991;161:519–524.

This is a microeconomic study, which supports the cost-effectiveness of efficacious primary prevention of thromboembolic disease in hip arthroplasty patients.

Weinmann EE, Salzman EW: Deep-vein thrombosis. *N Engl J Med* 1994;331:1630–1641.

This recently published review on the topic, by one of the most respected authorities in the field (EW Salzman) covers every aspect of the management of DVT.

2
Blood Conservation in Total Joint Arthroplasty

Total hip and knee arthroplasty procedures involve considerable blood loss because of bleeding from raw cancellous bone surfaces and extensive soft-tissue dissection.

When a tourniquet is used and not released until after wound closure, total knee arthroplasty is a bloodless procedure with an average intraoperative blood loss of less than 100 ml. However, numerous authors have reported that the blood loss from drains after a cemented procedure is 500 to 1,000 ml. When calculations from the preoperative and postoperative hematocrits were used to estimate the blood loss, it was found to be 1,500 ml, or about three times the drain losses. These calculations account for the unevacuated hematoma that remained within the joint and blood that moves into the soft tissues around the knee. Studies have also proven that the blood loss after uncemented knee arthroplasty is significantly greater than after cemented arthroplasty. Bone cement reduces a significant portion of the bone bleeding, which is the major source of postoperative bleeding. Calculated estimates indicate that the total postoperative loss from a unilateral uncemented total knee arthroplasty is as high as 2,000 ml.

Measured loss studies indicate that the intraoperative blood loss during primary cemented or uncemented total hip arthroplasty averages between 500 and 1,000 ml, and the drain losses are 200 to 600 ml for a total blood loss of 700 to 1,600 ml. Revision hip arthroplasty involves more blood loss than a primary procedure, with amount of loss depending on the duration of the procedure. Many revisions of failed cemented arthroplasties, which include changing both components, are associated with as much as 1,500 to 2,000 ml of intraoperative blood loss. Intraoperative blood loss can be reduced to a significant degree, especially during primary total hip procedures, by the use of regional or induced hypotensive anesthesia. As in knee arthroplasty, the use of bone ingrowth implants for hip replacement results in a greater postoperative blood loss than when cement is used.

In summary, the average total blood loss after primary cemented hip or knee arthroplasty is close to 1,500 ml, which represents 30% of the total blood volume of a 70-kg patient who has an average body habitus. Acute anemia and/or hypovolemia produced by this blood loss can produce considerable strain on cardiovascular reserves in some elderly patients, and blood transfusion is routinely needed to prevent serious postoperative complications. Therefore, it is mandatory for every surgeon to plan for perioperative blood transfusion and/or blood salvage for all of these patients, especially those undergoing one-stage bilateral procedures.

Risks of Blood Transfusion

The major risks of homologous blood transfusion are transfusion reactions, bacteremia from contaminated blood, clerical errors resulting in transfusion of the wrong unit of blood, and the transmission of viral and other blood-borne disease. Although the transfusion of ABO incompatible blood or contaminated blood can be fatal, such transfusions are rare occurrences. The most common transfusion reaction is fever related to sensitization to donor white cell antigens. The development of antibodies to red cell antigens is another late problem. The most important of the viral diseases transmitted by transfusions are hepatitis, human immunodeficiency virus (HIV), Epstein-Barr, cytomegalus, and human T-cell leukemia (HTLV-1). The nonviral diseases most often transmitted by blood transfusion are syphilis, malaria, and toxoplasmosis, and these are very rare.

Hepatitis is still the most prevalent serious transfusion-related illness. During the last two decades, the risk of non-A, non-B hepatitis (now recognized as hepatitis C) from homologous transfusion was estimated at 5% to 18%. Hepatitis C is a significant risk because despite treatment, 10% of infected patients develop chronic active hepatitis or cirrhosis. At present, the risk of both hepatitis B and C has been markedly reduced by stringent screening of donors for elevation of alanine aminotransferase, for the antibody to the hepatitis B core antigen, and, more recently, for the antibody to hepatitis C virus. With the use of these screening tests, the current risk of hepatitis C is estimated at 1 per 3,300 units transfused or 0.03%. The risk for hepatitis B is much lower at 1 per 200,000 units. The frequency of human T-cell leukemia is slightly lower than for hepatitis C, or 1 per 50,000 units.

HIV is transmitted by homologous blood approximately 1 per 225,000 screened units or two and one half times less than the risk of death from an earthquake for people living in California. These statistics indicate a significant reduction in the risk of hepatitis and HIV due to stringent donor screening and blood testing; however, a small, but finite, number of false-negative tests will always present a risk.

Many patients who are unable to or who elect not to predonate their own blood have made popular the use of a form of homologous blood donation termed directed-donor blood. These are nearly always patients who fear contracting HIV from random blood donor units and who have the unproven belief that this risk is lowered by the use of blood from relatives or friends. Although there are mixed data, several studies have indicated that the incidence of markers for hepatitis and human-T–cell leukemia is higher in populations of directed donors than in populations of volunteer donors. Because there is a small percentage of false-negative results for all tests for transfusion-transmitted diseases, it is possible that more infectious units will go undetected from directed donor blood, which has a higher prevalence of these positive markers, than from the volunteer donor blood. Because of the increased expense without any measurable benefit, the use of directed donor blood should be discouraged. Surgeons should educate patients that there are only two types of blood, autologous and homologous, and that directed-donor blood is not a separate nor a safer category. However, to convince patients that their children's or sibling's blood is less safe than a random unit from the local blood bank or the Red Cross will be a difficult task.

All surgeons have a responsibility to give adequate informed consent to patients prior to transfusing them with homologous blood because of the above-mentioned risks, especially that of HIV. There are three claims of physician negligence by patients who develop transfusion-related illness, each of which can lead to recovery of damages. The physician may be liable in any of the following three circumstances: (1) negligently determining that a blood transfusion should be given; (2) negligent treatment that creates a necessity for transfusion that is not normally needed; and (3) negligently failing to use available or easily obtainable autologous blood. Some states have laws requiring that patients who undergo elective surgery be informed of their option to predonate autologous blood in order to reduce or eliminate the need for homologous blood. Informed consent prior to homologous transfusion is strongly recommended in order to educate patients of the risks and to protect the surgeon from lawsuits that may result from late complications.

Autotransfusion

The use of autologous blood for total joint arthroplasty occurs in two formats: transfusion of predeposit autologous blood and reinfusion of perioperative salvage autologous blood. Numerous reports concerning predeposit autologous blood for elective orthopaedic surgery have been published since the technique was initially reported in 1968. A large percentage of these reports have dealt with populations of total joint replacement patients. Intraoperative red cell salvage became available for use in 1976 with the introduction of a red cell washing device. More recently, the recovery and reinfusion of shed blood that has not been washed has been a widely used alternative to the washed cell technique.

Predeposit Autologous Blood

This technique involves the preoperative collection from patients of one or more units of blood, which are stored in a liquid or frozen state for perioperative reinfusion. The most common anticoagulant used for liquid blood storage

is adenine citrate-phosphate dextrose (ACD), which allows for a 35-day outdate period. Six weeks of storage is possible for packed red blood cells when additional nutrient solutions (eg, Adsol) are used. Alternatively, red blood cells may be frozen at $-80°C$ after glycerol has been added. Thawing of frozen cells usually requires several hours because the cells must also be washed and resuspended in a balanced electrolyte solution. The cells must then be infused within 24 hours after thawing. Allowing for these inconveniences, frozen red cells may be stored for indefinite time periods and, thereby, allow the greatest latitude for surgical scheduling. However, liquid storage is the preferable means of storing autologous blood in most cases, because the cost of frozen blood is at least twice that of liquid units.

The recommended interval between the donation of each autologous unit is a minimum of 5 to 7 days, and the last donation should be made no less than 3 days prior to surgery. One unit of autologous blood (450 ml) removes approximately 9% of an average patient's total blood volume. Patients weighing less than 50 kg may predonate autologous units that are lower in volume by using collection bags containing proportionately less anticoagulant. All patients who donate predeposit autologous blood should take supplemental oral iron, preferably ferrous sulfate or gluconate, at a dosage of 325 mg, two or three times daily. Many donor-patients who have chronic anemia can benefit from treatment with recombinant human erythropoietin, which can enhance red cell production. This is especially helpful when several units are required. There are no contraindications to autologous donations by patients over 65 years old, because the frequency of donor reactions is no different in this population than in younger donors. Patients who have unstable angina, severe aortic stenosis, or uncontrolled hypertension will require clearance from their medical physician in order to predonate blood. Patients who have an infection, even if they are currently being treated with antibiotics and afebrile, are deferred from donating to avoid contamination of the donated unit(s) from their possible bacteremia. Autologous blood that tests positive for hepatitis will have special handling and warning labels, but is stored and can be reinfused. However, blood banks generally discard autologous blood units from HIV positive donors because of the slight, but fatal risk of infusion to the wrong recipient. Unused autologous and directed-donor blood is discarded. It cannot be crossed over to the general blood bank inventory despite negative screening tests because of the increased risk for disease transmission mentioned earlier.

The use of autologous blood is not problem-free. Some patients attempting to predeposit autologous blood may have difficulties, which include poor venous access and preoperative anemia. The anemia may be chronic (hematocrit < 34), preventing the initial donation, or it may be induced by previous donations if adequate time is not allowed for collection prior to surgery. Postponement of surgery can cause waste of liquid units unless they are frozen before outdating. Aside from these problems, there are only two major risks of autologous transfusion, which also are present for homologous blood: bacterial contamination of the blood during collection and clerical errors resulting in transfusing the wrong unit of blood.

Autologous and directed-donor blood are more costly than homologous blood because of the special handling required. Although predeposit autologous blood is much safer than homologous blood, it is important to understand that the donation of excessive amounts of predeposit blood units is wasteful. Because hospital transfusion committee guidelines recommend against transfusing any blood, even autologous, unless the postoperative hematocrit falls below 30 to 34, a patient who has donated three units of autologous blood before undergoing primary cemented knee arthroplasty may not be "permitted" to receive one or two of these units. This blood cannot be crossed over to the general supply; therefore, the inappropriate ordering of excess autologous blood should be avoided.

The efficacy of predeposit autologous transfusion for total knee arthroplasty was studied in a series of patients who had 110 knee arthroplasties, including 22 one-stage bilateral and 66 unilateral procedures. An average of two units was predonated by 80% of the patients who had bilateral one-stage procedures and an average of 1.3 units by 70% of the patients who had unilateral surgery. Postoperative washed cell salvage was used for 44% of the procedures. The frequency of homologous blood transfusion for patients who predonated blood was 3% compared to 35% for patients who did not predonate autologous blood. Overall, the use of predeposit blood and postoperative salvage reduced the frequency of homologous blood transfusion to 11%. This low frequency occurred not only because a high percentage of the patients predonated blood for surgery, but also because 20% of the patients were discharged with a hematocrit lower than 30. This study suggests that the predonation of one or two units of blood for unilateral procedures and of three or four units for bilateral procedures is the appropriate amount. When cementless knee arthroplasty is planned, the upper limits of these ranges should be collected.

In a study of 154 primary total hip procedures, the incidence of homologous blood transfusion was only 8% in the 133 procedures that were performed with two or three units of predeposited autologous blood. In contrast, the incidence of homologous transfusion after the 21 procedures that were done without predeposit blood was 71%. Washed red cell salvage was done in the operating room and continued in the recovery room for 148 procedures, with an average savings of 400 ml per procedure. Results of other studies also indicate that the risk of homologous blood exposure during primary total hip arthroplasty is low when two or three units of autologous blood are predonated. Revision hip arthroplasty requires an additional amount of predeposited blood (three to four units) because of larger blood losses.

In summary, with adequate preoperative planning a predeposit autologous blood program for primary hip and knee arthroplasty patients should reduce the risk of exposure to homologous blood to less than 15%, without considering perioperative blood salvage.

Perioperative Blood Salvage

Two techniques are available for perioperative salvage: washed or unwashed red cell salvage. Washed red cell salvage involves the aspiration of blood from the wound and/or the drain and anticoagulation of this blood with heparin. This shed blood is washed with saline and centrifuged to concentrate the red cells prior to reinfusion. Unwashed cell salvage entails the postoperative collection of blood from the drain within a sterile plastic container (with or without anticoagulation) and reinfusion without cell washing or concentration. The blood that is salvaged after cell washing has a hematocrit of approximately 50%, which is higher than that of unwashed shed blood (25% to 35%). A blood filter to remove particulate debris is always used when reinfusing either washed or unwashed cells.

There has been considerable controversy on the relative risks and effectiveness of these two forms of blood salvage. The major advantage of cell washing is the removal of a large percentage of the contaminants of the joint drainage fluid including methyl methacrylate monomer, antibiotic from the irrigation fluid, free hemoglobin, fat, and bacteria. Adverse reactions to washed autologous red cells have rarely been reported. However, cell washing is expensive because of the cost of the cell-washing device and the need for a dedicated technician to run it. In addition, a considerable volume of drainage (a minimum of 400 ml) must be available to make cell washing feasible. The collection of blood in a simple sterile reservoir separate from the cell washing device is indicated for procedures in which the blood loss may not be enough to make cell washing cost-effective. This procedure avoids the expense of the cell washing device and technician if the amount of shed blood is insufficient for washing. A cell-washing device has the additional disadvantage of being usable only for a short time postoperatively (while in the recovery room), whereas the unwashed collection devices can be used to collect shed blood for 6 hours.

Washed cell salvage has been shown to save 250 to 500 ml during surgery and in the recovery room after primary total hip replacement. Intraoperative blood salvage is not a practical technique for unilateral total knee arthroplasty because of the use of a tourniquet. Postoperative washed cell salvage is successful in recovering sufficient amounts of blood for reinfusion in only 40% of unilateral knee arthroplasty patients (an average of 200 to 300 ml per procedure) and, therefore, probably should not be used. However, the success rate in patients who had bilateral knee arthroplasty is 90%, because the washed salvage of shed blood from the first joint can be done while the second procedure is proceeding. Washed cell salvage in bilateral knee replacement results in an average savings of 400 to 500 ml of blood during surgery and in the recovery room. Salvage of an average of 1,000 ml is common in revision hip replacement (Table 1).

Unwashed cells are much less expensive than washed cells and unwashed salvage is successful after 80% of unilateral total knee procedures. Studies indicate that between 200 and 400 ml of shed blood may be salvaged for unilateral cemented knee arthroplasty and 800 ml for unilateral uncemented knee procedures. Bilateral knee arthroplasty can yield 500 to 1,100 ml per patient. Primary total hip replacement patients average 400 ml of unwashed cell salvage postoperatively. Most revision hip replacement procedures are performed using intraoperative washed cell salvage, because these procedures are associated with significant intraoperative bleeding. There are no data on the effectiveness of postoperative unwashed cell collection after revision hip surgery (Table 1).

Although there are no major concerns about the safety of washed cells, some surgeons fear that patients will have adverse reactions from reinfusion of unwashed cells. The frequency of febrile responses during reinfusion of unwashed red cells has been reported at 2% to 10%, and this frequency increases if collection and reinfusion is delayed for over 6 hours. Occasional episodes of transient hypotension, which were possibly related to the use of ACD anticoagulant in the collection device, were reported from one series of patients. At the present time, ACD is not recommended for unwashed cell recovery systems, because the blood shed from the hip or knee joint is defibrinated and does not normally clot. Studies have been done to determine the concentrations of methyl methycrylate monomer in shed blood from hip and knee joint drains, and data have shown that these levels are low and do not appear to be a major risk. Although cell washing reduces the concentration of all contaminants, their levels in unwashed shed blood are probably not harmful to the patient unless large volumes are reinfused.

Free fat, which is present in shed blood from all joint arthroplasty procedures, cannot be removed by microaggregate filters. Fat is the most dangerous contaminant of salvaged blood because of its potential to cause pulmonary embolism. Washed salvage reduces the amount of free fat in shed blood by dilution, but does not eliminate it. The best way to avoid the infusion of fat from unwashed blood is to exclude the top layer of drainage fluid, which contains the majority of the fat. Some unwashed cell salvage systems are designed to prevent the supernatant layer of fluid in the collection reservoir from being reinfused, whereas another system has a filter which absorbs fat.

Table 1. Perioperative blood salvage volumes from literature review

Procedure	Washed RBC(ml)*	Unwashed RBC (ml)*
Primary total hip replacement	250–500	400
Revision total hip replacement	1,000	No Data
Primary total knee replacement (40% successful)	200–300	200–400
Bilateral total knee replacement	400–500	500–1,100

*RBC = Red blood cells

Cell washing produces autologous blood that is more concentrated than when collected and is less contaminated. However, if unwashed cell collection is limited to a period of less than 6 hours postoperatively, and if ACD anticoagulant is not used, the risks of this form of autologous blood appear to be minimal. In general, washed cell salvage should be used for all procedures that are likely to have high intraoperative blood losses and unwashed cell salvage should be used for all other procedures when limited predeposit blood is available.

It is difficult to determine how effective the sole use of perioperative blood salvage is in reducing the requirements for homologous transfusion after joint arthroplasty, because all studies of red cell salvage have involved use of predeposit autologous transfusion as well. However, in several studies that compared patients who had postoperative unwashed cell salvage to control groups, there were lower overall transfusion rates (for both homologous and autologous blood) when salvage was used. Because red cell salvage decreases the amount of postoperative blood loss by returning a portion of it to the patient, it seems that salvage should reduce the need for homologous transfusion.

Combined Use of Predeposit Autologous Blood and Perioperative Blood Salvage

Combining the use of predeposit autologous blood and perioperative salvage should have an additive effect in reducing the need for homologous transfusion in joint arthroplasty patients. However, the use of both techniques for all patients is unnecessary and definitely is not cost-effective. An autologous blood program should be tailored to the individual patient and the expected blood loss in order to reduce the risk of homologous blood transfusion and keep expense at a minimum. The following three examples illustrate the appropriate use of predeposit blood and perioperative salvage.

Case Examples

1. Patient with a large blood volume undergoing a procedure associated with a moderate blood loss:

A healthy 45-year-old man weighing 100 kg (estimated total blood volume = 7,500 ml) who has a hematocrit of 45 and is undergoing primary uncemented total hip replacement (average total blood loss = 1,500 to 2,000 ml) should predonate one or two units of predeposit autologous blood and have intraoperative washed cell salvage or predonate three units when perioperative salvage is not planned. His postoperative hematocrit will most likely equilibrate at about 35 with either of these protocols.

2. Patient with a low blood volume undergoing a procedure associated with a large blood loss:

A 60-year-old steroid-dependent female who has rheumatoid disease, weighs 50 kg (estimated total blood volume = 3,750 ml), has a hematocrit of 34, and is scheduled for bilateral knee replacement (average total blood loss = 2,500 ml) should preoperatively donate three or four units and should also have both intraoperative and postoperative salvage. The first predeposit unit should be donated 3 months preoperatively and frozen storage used for the first two or three units. Early use of erythropoietin should be seriously considered to increase the likelihood of obtaining the desired number of donations and also to increase the patient's preoperative hematocrit. The patient will be expected to be discharged with a hematocrit in the low 30's. If the patient is unable to predonate three or four units, it is highly likely that homologous transfusion will be needed, and the patient should be informed of this fact.

3. Patient with a normal blood volume undergoing a procedure associated with moderate blood loss:

A 60-year-old man weighing 70 kg (total blood volume = 5,250 ml) who has a hematocrit of 40 and is scheduled for revision total hip replacement (average total blood loss = 2,000 ml) should predonate three units of blood and have washed cell salvage intraoperatively. This patient would be expected to have a discharge hematocrit of 30 to 35.

Summary

In summary, all total joint replacement patients should be encouraged to predonate autologous blood as the primary means of reducing the need for homologous blood transfusion. Primary total knee replacement requires one to two units, primary total hip and revision total knee two units, and revision total hip three or four units. In procedures associated with a large surgical blood loss, such as revision hip surgery, intraoperative washed cell salvage should always be considered. In procedures expected to have large postoperative blood losses, such as bilateral total knee replacement, postoperative salvage should be considered. Patients having bilateral knee replacements and primary uncemented or revision hip replacements can have either washed or unwashed cell salvage in the operating and recovery rooms. However, until there is evidence that postoperative blood salvage alone is effective in reducing the need for homologous blood transfusion in these patients, predeposit blood should remain the most important technique used to avoid homologous blood transfusion after joint arthroplasty. Perioperative salvage should be considered as an adjunctive technique that is especially helpful for patients who have difficulty in predonating sufficient amounts of predeposit blood and for patients for whom extensive procedures are planned.

General Considerations and Surgical Technique

Preoperative coagulation tests, including a prothrombin time, partial thromboplastin time, and platelet count, should be routine prior to total joint arthroplasty, especially in patients who give a history of excessive bleeding after other surgical procedures. Because nonsteroidal anti-inflammatory medications are known to adversely affect platelet function, thereby prolonging bleeding time, patients should be instructed to discontinue use of these drugs at least a week before surgery to avoid excessive bleeding. A bleeding time should be obtained when there is a concern about platelet function. Preoperative administration of anticoagulants such as heparin or warfarin for thrombosis prophylaxis should be done with caution for the same reason.

There are several controversial aspects of joint arthroplasty that affect the blood loss. These factors are the timing of tourniquet release, the postoperative delay before the initiation of continuous passive motion (CPM) after knee arthroplasty, and whether or not to use a surgical drain.

Tourniquet release prior to total knee wound closure for hemostasis has been advocated in the past by many who felt that this reduces postoperative blood loss. However, data from two randomized studies of patients who had tourniquet release either prior to or after wound closure indicated definitively that intraoperative tourniquet release does not lower the blood loss and actually may increase it. In one study, there was a statistically significant increase in the blood loss after procedures during which the tourniquet was released for hemostasis prior to wound closure when compared to procedures during which the tourniquet was released after the surgery was completed. In a more recent study, researchers found no significant difference in the calculated blood loss of patients randomized to either tourniquet release or no release, when CPM was begun on the second postoperative day. However, there was a significant increase in the blood loss when the tourniquet was released prior to wound closure when the CPM was begun in the recovery room.

If the tourniquet is released after wound closure, hemostatic control of divided geniculate branches of the popliteal artery, especially the superior lateral branch, must not be neglected during the surgical procedure. If there is any question that a geniculate branch may have been divided and not controlled during a lateral retinacular release, the tourniquet should be released and the vessel electrocauterized to avoid substantial postoperative hemorrhage. Tourniquet release prior to 2 hours should be routine to prevent ischemic damage to the leg; if this is done, hemostatic control of arterial bleeders can then be accomplished. However, overall blood losses will be minimized and the surgery expedited by maintaining tourniquet control until wound closure in all uncomplicated procedures.

The use of CPM, which is begun in the recovery room, has been shown in several studies to increase the postoperative blood loss. Because of this increase, some feel that it is prudent to delay the initiation of CPM until the first or second postoperative day.

The ultimate solution for the reduction of all postoperative blood loss after hip and knee arthroplasty is to omit the use of a surgical drain although such omission is contrary to a basic principle of surgery, the prevention of hematoma formation. In a study of a limited number of patients undergoing one-stage bilateral arthroplasty, one side without a drain was compared to the other side, which was drained as a control. There was no difference between the joints of these patients in wound healing, persistent drainage, or other clinical parameters. Nevertheless, most surgeons still worry that omitting a drain will cause prolonged drainage from the incision and from the intra-articular hematoma with a higher incidence of sepsis or joint stiffness. Other well-designed studies on the omission of drains must be done on large series of patients before this technique is widely employed.

Criteria for Transfusing Homologous Blood After Joint Arthroplasty

The criteria that the surgeon uses for ordering transfusions of homologous blood are critically important and may negate all of the techniques for blood conservation that were discussed in this chapter. Guidelines for transfusion of homologous blood in the perioperative period have previously been based on empirical grounds rather than on data from controlled clinical studies. At the present time, most hospital transfusion committee guidelines do not question homologous transfusions given to patients who have a hematocrit below 30. However, there is no scientific evidence indicating that all patients should be transfused at this threshold. The National Institutes of Health held a Consensus Development Conference on Perioperative Red Cell Transfusions in 1988. This conference resulted in the conclusion that mild to moderate anemia does not cause postoperative morbidity, such as poor wound healing or a higher infection rate, nor does it contribute to a longer hospital stay or delayed functional rehabilitation. Therefore, the decision to transfuse homologous blood should be based on other factors, including the patient's age, the potential for further bleeding, and coexisting medical conditions, such as impaired pulmonary function, poor cardiac output, myocardial ischemia, or cerebrovascular insufficiency. The hematocrit should not be the sole criterion for deciding to order homologous blood.

Orthopaedic surgeons performing hip and knee arthroplasty should be aware of these consensus findings and modify their decision-making to limit the number of homologous transfusions in these patients. An effective autologous blood program, which combines predeposit donation and the judicious use of postoperative salvage in selected patients, should lower the risk of exposure to homologous blood to less than 10% of patients. It is very important that an adequate amount of time be allowed for predeposit blood to be collected, because this is the best source of autologous blood. Postoperative blood salvage should be used in all patients at high-risk for homologous transfusions, ie, those with a low blood volume and inadequate amounts of predeposited blood. Finally, the threshold that surgeons use to order homologous blood should be based on the clinical status of each patient and not solely on the hematocrit.

Annotated Bibliography

Anonymous: Perioperative red blood cell transfusion. *JAMA* 1988;260:2700–2703.

The NIH Consensus Development Conference in 1988 outlined the criteria for perioperative red blood cell transfusion, the risks of transfusion, and the morbidity of postoperative anemia. The conclusions were that transfusion is not indicated solely for a low postoperative hematocrit, that there is no evidence that mild to moderate postoperative anemia contributes to morbidity, and that predeposit autologous blood and perioperative blood salvage will minimize the need for homologous transfusion.

Beer KJ, Lombardi AV Jr, Mallory TH, et al: The efficacy of suction drains after routine total joint arthroplasty. *J Bone Joint Surg* 1991;73A:584–587.

In the study of 50 patients who underwent bilateral knee or hip replacements a drain was placed in one joint and not the other. There were no significant differences in the incidence of swelling or drainage, and for knees there were no differences in range of motion.

Gannon DM, Lombardi AV, Mallory TH, et al: An evaluation of the efficacy of postoperative blood salvage after total joint arthroplasty: A prospective randomized trial *J Arthroplasty* 1991;1:109–114.

A randomized study of 239 total hip and knee patients found that postoperative unwashed red cell salvage was quite safe. Hip patients who had postoperative salvage required 80% less homologous blood than those who did not have it, and the patients who predonated blood required the least homologous blood.

Lotke PA, Faralli VJ, Orenstein EM, et al: Blood loss after total knee replacement: Effects of tourniquet release and continuous passive motion. *J Bone Joint Surg* 1991;73A:1037–1040.

The authors found that the mean calculated blood loss for patients undergoing total knee replacement was 1,518 ml and that this directly correlated with the blood loss from the drain, which averaged 511 ml. Intraoperative tourniquet release for hemostasis significantly increased the intraoperative and postoperative blood loss over that of patients who had wound closure prior to tourniquet release in this randomized study.

Martin JW, Whiteside LA, Milliano MT, et al: Postoperative blood retrieval and transfusion in cementless total knee arthroplasty. *J Arthroplasty* 1992;7:205–210.

The authors salvaged an average of 829 ml (59% of total blood loss) from 153 unilateral total knee patients and 1,131 ml (56% of total blood loss) from 44 bilateral knee patients using unwashed red cell collection devices. There were no major complications from perioperative blood salvage in these patients.

Ritter MA, Keating EM, Faris PM: Closed wound drainage in total hip or total knee replacement: A prospective randomized study. *J Bone Joint Surg* 1994; 76A:35–38.

Four hundred and fifteen total hip and total knee replacements were randomized into a group with or without closed wound drainage. There were no differences in patients with excessive postoperative drainage between the two groups, nor differences in postoperative transfusion needs. For the knees there were no differences in postoperative range of motion. A savings of $21,500 would have resulted if drains had not been used at all in this series.

Woolson ST, Pottorff G: Use of preoperatively deposited autologous blood for total knee replacement surgery. *Orthopedics* 1993;16:137–142.

The use of predeposit autologous blood for unilateral or bilateral total knee replacement reduced the frequency of transfusion of homologous blood from 35% to 3% in 88 consecutive procedures. The use of washed red cell salvage (Cell Saver) was not cost-effective in unilateral knee replacement because only 42% of patients had sufficient drainage in the recovery room to allow reinfusion.

Woolson ST, Watt JM: Use of autologous blood in total hip replacement. *J Bone Joint Surg* 1991;73A:76–80.

A prospective study of 154 primary total hip procedures was done to determine the success rate of avoidance of homologous transfusion. Homologous blood was required in only 8% of patients who predonated an average of 2.6 units of autologous blood. Perioperative washed-cell salvage was successful in 148 procedures and resulted in saving an average of 408 ml. Fourteen percent of the patients were discharged with a hematocrit less than 30 and had no problems with delayed rehabilitation or poor healing.

3

Prevention, Diagnosis, and Treatment of Postoperative Wound Infections in Adult Hip and Knee Reconstruction

Introduction

Although scientists and physicians have attempted to diminish the rate of total joint arthroplasty sepsis through modification of the operating room environment and judicious use of perioperative antibiotics, deep joint infection continues to produce morbidity and occasional mortality. Infection can be present subclinically at the arthroplasty site before the replacement surgery, introduced iatrogenically at surgery, or result from subsequent hematogenous spread. Meticulous diagnostic testing and aggressive treatment will improve treatment outcomes. The extent of the nonreimbursed expenses associated with the treatment of these patients is becoming an important issue in their care.

Prevention of Infection

The Operating Room Environment, Skin Preparation, and Equipment

Prevention of infection is crucial. Discipline in the operating room is important. People continuously shed bacteria, the amount varying between individuals. Colonizing bacteria are either indigenous (within the pores and thus cannot be eliminated) or exogenous (acquired by contact and removable with washing). Bacteria have mass, attach to fomites, and settle. An empty operating room has no bacteria in the air, only on the surfaces.

The source of bacteria in the operating room is man. *Staphylococcus aureus* has been cultured from approximately one third of all operating room personnel and *S epidermidis* is cultured almost every time from all operating room personnel. Humans shed between 1,000 and 10,000 organisms per minute. Bathing reduces shedding only temporarily (minutes) before it returns to a level of equilibrium for that individual. The air in an operating room is basically bacteria free if the room has been closed and empty for 4 to 6 hours. The number of bacteria within the environment of an operating room is increased in proportion to the number of people entering the room.

The contamination of operating room surfaces with bacteria remains in a state of constant equilibrium. Disinfecting surfaces has no lasting effect. Compression Rodac plates were used to evaluate the surfaces of the operating room floor before and after surgery, immediately after disinfecting, and 5 minutes after disinfecting. Before surgery there was an average of 43 colonies per plate, after surgery 51, immediately after disinfecting 27, and after conventional use of the room 40. Thus, after reduction, surface contamination rapidly returns to its previous level, making complete asepsis unobtainable.

A conventional operating room has about 10 to 25 air changes per hour compared to approximately 300 air changes per hour for a laminar airflow system. Bacterial sampling demonstrates (Table 1) that horizontal laminar airflow reduces the number of bacteria at the wound, back instrument table, and the periphery of the operating area ($p < 0.005$).

A review of bacterial counts during total hip replacements in which different airflow systems (Table 2) were used demonstrated that horizontal laminar airflow with walls reduced bacterial counts more effectively than either horizontal or vertical airflow without walls. A vertical airflow with walls was not evaluated. It appears that the vertical downflow system without walls brings environmental bacteria from below the wound up toward the wound itself because of the negative pressure that develops when the surgical team leans over the wound. A downflow system with walls (Charnley Greenhouse) helps direct this airflow away from the wound. Laminar airflow not only reduces the number of bacteria at the wound site, it reduces the number of clinically noted postoperative infections as well.

Whereas laminar airflow is used to keep the area about the wound bacteria free, ultraviolet light has been demonstrated to kill the bacteria in the area of the wound. Although it is relatively inexpensive, all operating room per-

Table 1. Comparison of contamination found in conventional versus laminar-airflow operating rooms

Air-Sampling Device	Conventional OR	Laminar-Airflow OR	Reduction (%)	Probability (*P*)
Reyneir*				
Wound	100	7	93	< 0.005
Back-table	74	5	93	< 0.005
Air-settle plates†				
Wound	288	23	92	< 0.005
Back-table	332	9	97	< 0.005
Periphery of the				
operating area	281	111	61	< 0.005

*Colony-forming units/ft³
†Colony-forming units/ft²/hr

Table 2. Colony forming units/ft²/hour for three different laminar airflow alternatives during total hip replacement (THR)

	Horizontal Laminar Air Wall-less	Horizontal Laminar Airflow Walled	Vertical Laminar Airflow Wall-less
Number of THR	189	102	100
Wound	118	16	50
Back-table	5	1	26

Table 3. Percent reduction of environmental contamination with various surgical attires

Attire	% Reduction
Plastic gowns versus scrub clothes	51% ($p < 0.05$)
Body exhaust system versus scrub clothes	69% ($p < 0.01$)
Body exhaust system versus plastic gown	38% ($p < 0.05$)

Table 4. The number of holes in particular gloves and the percent contaminated during 1.5 hour total hip replacement cases

	Number of gloves with holes		Number of gloves contaminated	
Single glove	9/68	13%	21/68	31%
Double gloves				
Outer	33/72	23%	23/72	32%
Inner	7/72	10%	28/72	39%

sonnel and patients need to be protected from the ultraviolet light. The combination of ultraviolet light in addition to a body exhaust unit may be particularly advantageous if any of the operating room personnel are heavy shedders.

The position of the personnel within the laminar flow system appears to be critical. If a team member is standing so as to impede the airflow, a body exhaust system is a must. One report documented an increase in total knee replacement infections in a horizontal laminar airflow environment secondary to placement of the scrubbed personnel between the airflow source and the patient.

The porosity of most cloth scrub clothes measures between 100 and 150 μm. Because bacteria measure 1 μm and fomites carrying bacteria, 20 to 30 μm, it is apparent that the cloth scrub suit offers no barrier. Evaluation of various types of scrub clothes such as dresses, pants, shirts, as well as tucking in the shirt and enclosing the feet reveals basically no difference in environmental contamination.

Comparison of a plastic gown with a cloth hood, face mask, and gloves versus a hooded exhaust gown and of both of these versus scrub clothes found a 51% reduction of environmental bacteria with use of the plastic gown versus scrub clothes, a 69% reduction with use of the body exhaust versus the scrub clothes, and a 38% reduction when comparing the hooded exhaust gown to the plastic wraparound gown (Table 3). To achieve optimal benefit, everyone within the operating room—visitors, circulating nurses, and anesthesiologists must be similarly attired.

The disposable mask has a filter efficiency of greater than 95%. Because bacteria escape around the sides of the mask, evaluation of bacterial reduction within the environment with and without the use of surgical masks by the operating room personnel has shown no effect on the environment. Masks may allow individuals to talk without expelling bacteria directly toward the wound, but they do not reduce environmental bacteria. The type of shoe cover used has no measurable effect on either surface or operating room environmental contamination.

Surgical training emphasizes reducing the number of skin bacteria, both about the area of the wound and on the surgeon's hands, by prepping the patient and scrubbing the surgeon's hands. How is this done best?

There are two microbial populations on the skin, transient and indigenous. The former is acquired by touch and is easily removed with minimal washing. The indigenous population is not so easily affected because it inhabits the glands and ducts of the skin to a depth of 20 cell layers.

The number of bacteria on the skin does not change significantly whether the area is scrubbed for 2 or 10 minutes. Of the compounds used for skin bacterial control, hexachlorophene is bacteriostatic; alcohol, iodine, and chlorhexidine are bactericidal. Studies on the use of Betadine and pHisoHex show no difference in the colony counts obtained from hands scrubbed for 5 minutes versus 10 minutes. With the use of chlorhexidine, this time could be reduced to 2 minutes and to less than 1 minute with use of an alcohol hexachlorophene foam and no scrub. Because operating room personnel are not killing the indigenous bacteria, which regrow from the depths of the sebaceous glands, they only need a few seconds of an alcohol foam loaded with hexachlorophene or chlorhexidine.

Despite the fact that it is possible to decrease the number of bacteria on the hands by greater than 90%, gloves are needed to provide a barrier against the remaining 10%. Bacteria on the gloves appear to come from the environmental contamination of the sterile field, not the hand within the glove. Approximately 30% of all of the gloves, whether they are single, double, inner, or outer become contaminated during a 1.5 hour total hip replacement (Table 4). The hands within the gloves, with or without holes, were not found to be the source of bacterial contamination. The contamination was from another source, the surgical field or the operating room environment.

The bacterial reduction that follows prepping has been shown to be maintained with an adhesive drape. Adhesive drapes have demonstrated no increase in bacteria multiplication, no lateral migration, no drape penetration, and no increase in wound contamination. With the antimicrobial adhesive drapes now available, there appears to be no need for more than alcohol as a prepping agent.

Evaluation of the bacterial contamination of scalpel blades shows that there is no difference in contamination of the skin and deep blades. There is, however, less contamination of both in a laminar airflow versus a conventional setting.

Lastly, suction apparatus which have been used

throughout the procedure may concentrate organisms from the air at their tips, thus contaminating the deepest portions of the wound at the time of closure.

Host Immune Status

Diabetes mellitus, obesity, extreme age, and malnutrition compromise immune status and are important factors in the host's ability to control the bacteria that inevitably settle into the wound during surgery. Rheumatoid arthritis effectively doubles the risk of infection for both total hips and knees. In one series, the infection rate for patients with osteoarthritis was 0.3%; rheumatoid arthritis, 1.2%; psoriasis, 5.5%; postoperative urinary tract infection, 6.2%; and diabetes mellitus, 6.5%. Local factors such as prior surgery can adversely affect the outcome because of the decreased vascularity of scar tissue and the increased time required to perform revision surgery.

Perioperative Antibiotics

Although the above mentioned items are important, the single most important variable influencing the development of postoperative total joint infection is the appropriate use of perioperative antibiotics. Depending upon the host's status and allergies, a first generation cephalosporin or vancomycin are the most frequently used antibiotics. Data suggest that a single dose of antibiotic administered before the start of surgery is as effective as a 48-hour regimen. The overall incidence of sepsis after standard primary total joint replacement procedures has been as low as 0.38% in one series. Late infection is more likely to occur after procedures that involve major bone grafting.

Suction Drainage and Hematomata

The use of suction drainage systems has become controversial. No series reported to date has documented a statistically significant difference in wound drainage, deep infection, or need to return to the operating room whether or not drains were used. The numbers of patients reported with wound drainage have been small so the power to detect differences has been low. It is difficult to draw definitive conclusions. In one study, 35 of 131 total knee arthroplasty patients treated without drains and 30 of 135 treated with drains had significant incisional drainage. Six of 130 total hip arthroplasty patients treated without drains and four of 129 treated with drains had incisional drainage. It is generally agreed that hematoma evacuation should only be accomplished in the operating room.

Diagnostic Evaluation

Delay in either diagnosis or initiation of appropriate treatment may adversely affect outcome. Approximately one third of deep infections occur within 3 months of surgery. The spectrum of symptoms can be variable. Pain, the most frequent symptom, is not always present. Although pain associated with aseptic loosening is frequently of sudden onset, increased with weightbearing, and relieved by rest,

pain due to sepsis can have a more insidious onset. It tends not to be relieved with rest.

Continued unexplained elevation of the erythrocyte sedimentation rate or C-reactive protein remains the most reliable clinical indicator of infection after total hip arthroplasty (Table 5). Eighty-four percent of patients with intraoperative biopsy proven infection had a persistent elevated erythrocyte sedimentation rate. Although the erythrocyte sedimentation rate routinely returns to normal within 1 month of an acute fracture, it may remain elevated for as much as 1 year after routine total hip arthroplasty. A rate that remains greater than 40 mm/hr after 1 year, in the absence of another known inflammatory focus, suggests that the patient has an infection until proven otherwise.

There is no completely reliable study that differentiates a loose, painful prosthesis from one that is also infected. On plain radiographs, periosteal new bone formation and scalloped endosteal resorption are helpful. The latter, however, is also associated with polyethylene and polymethylmethacrylate debris.

In the evaluation of a previously asymptomatic total hip or total knee arthroplasty patient with new onset of periprosthetic pain, the initial history, physical examination, plain radiographs, and laboratory studies should be followed by a technetium scan if the question of possible infection persists. If the technetium scan is negative, infection is unlikely. If a technetium scan reveals increased localized uptake, an indium study should be performed. If the scan shows no increase in uptake, infection is unlikely (Table 6). However, scintigraphy with indium-labeled leukocytes produces both false-positive and false-negative findings. Indium-labeled leukocytes may accumulate in patients with osteosarcoma, pigmented villonodular synovitis, eosinophilia granuloma, Paget's disease, osteolytic carcinoma of the breast, and lymphoma with pathologic fracture.

Material for culture obtained by preoperative aspiration correlates with intraoperative specimens with accuracies ranging from 58% to 96% (Table 7). Meticulous aseptic technique is mandatory to avoid iatrogenic inoculation of a sterile, painful prosthesis. A negative aspiration culture occurs in 15% of patients.

Deep tissue specimens obtained in the operating room provide definitive microorganism identification in 80% to 90% of patients. Histopathology frozen sections may reveal inflammation even in the absence of infection.

Polymerase chain reaction (PCR) will hopefully im-

Table 5. Correlation of erythrocyte sedimentation rate greater than 30 mm/hour with infection

Year of Study	N	Sensitivity (%)	Specificity (%)	Accuracy (%)
1976	8	100	70	73
1982	33	94	73	88
1985	42	73	94	88
1991	33	86	69	73

Table 6. Correlation of indium 111 scintigraphy with infection

Year of Study	N	Sensitivity (%)	Specificity (%)	Accuracy (%)
1984	15	50	100	80
1985	16	86	100	94
1985	19	86	69	79
1986	32	100	66	80
1991	43	60	73	70

Table 7. Correlation of pre-operative aspiration with intra-operative cultures

Year of Study	N	Sensitivity (%)	Specificity (%)	Accuracy (%)
1981	205	69	82	73
1983	136	91	82	83
1984	61	0	80	78
1991	28	50	95	82

prove diagnostic accuracy. Segments of the DNA of aspirated organisms can be replicated, studied, and used for bacterial identification. This technique has the potential to improve the accuracy of presurgical aspiration from the current 80% to above 95%.

Classification System

Three classification systems are in general use. The first describes the infection on the basis of time of presentation from the initial surgery: acute, within 12 weeks; subacute, 12 to 52 weeks; late, after 1 year. The second is based on the complexity of the surgical procedure that becomes infected: group 1, standard primary total hip arthroplasty; group 2, complex primary without extensive autografting; group 3, complex primary with extensive autografting; group 4, revision without major grafting; group 5, revision with major grafting of femur, acetabulum, or both. The third quantitates the level of suspicion of infection to help determine revision strategy.

Treatment

An infection at the site of an arthroplasty should be treated aggressively. Salvage may be possible if the infection is detected early, the components are well fixed, and the organism is sensitive to antibiotics. Infections with *S aureus* and gram-negative organisms do not tend to respond well to debridement and systemic or local antibiotics. The short-term success rate for salvage in situ is less than 50%, and thus it should be reserved for those patients who cannot withstand the rigors of a delayed exchange revision.

Although some investigators, primarily surgeons from Europe, have reported high success rates with one stage re-implantation for infected total joint arthroplasties, the consensus in the United States is that success will be greater if these procedures are performed in stages. In spe-

cial circumstances involving strong medical indications for limiting the treatment to a single surgical procedure and in infections caused by organisms of low virulence with high sensitivity to antimicrobial agents, a one stage re-implantation may be warranted. Published success rates approach 83%.

The use of antibiotic-impregnated cement is appropriate in revision surgery for patients with known previous infections. Cements vary in their ability to release antibiotic. Studies of tensile strength and fatigue testing have revealed that 0.5 g of gentamycin powder/40 g of cement did not significantly change the strength of the cement. The magnitude of the changes equalled that attributable to voids in the cement.

The two-stage exchange has a higher initial cost than the single exchange, but the success rate is closer to 90% (Table 8). The choice of systemic antibiotic used during the interval between surgeries should be made in conjunction with an infectious disease consultant.

If allograft is required at the time of reconstruction, the infection risk is increased. Whether this risk is more likely attributable to the potential for remaining infection, which was not adequately debrided initially secondary to the very extensive nature of the infection, or to the increased biomaterial surface area presented by the allograft has not been determined.

Resection arthroplasty results in decreased function and should be reserved for those patients with immune compromise, inadequate bone stock, abductor mechanism loss, or persistent infection in spite of repeated debridement. Most series report a 15% infection recurrence rate.

Late Infection Prophylactic Antibiotics

The overall incidence of late infections complicating total hip and knee replacements is approximately 0.6%. Every total joint patient should be counseled about the dangers of metastatic, hematogenous infection. The most common origins are soft tissue (46%), dental (15%), and urinary tract (13%). Dental procedures produce a transient bacteremia lasting 5 to 30 minutes after manipulation. Clearly, prophylaxis is warranted for the immunocompromised patient or in the setting of clinical dental sepsis. Although authors differ on their recommendations, one prophylactic regimen would include penicillin V, 2 g 1 hour before and 1 g 6 hours after manipulation or erythromycin, 1 g before and 500 mg after.

Table 8. Comparison of one- and two-stage total hip revisions with antibiotic cement

Year of Study	One-Stage (N)	Success (%)	Two-Stage (N)	Success (%)
1982	101	86	NA	NA
1984	869	77.4	NA	NA
1986	102	91	NA	NA
1988	72	76	30	73.3
1989	72	87	19	100.0

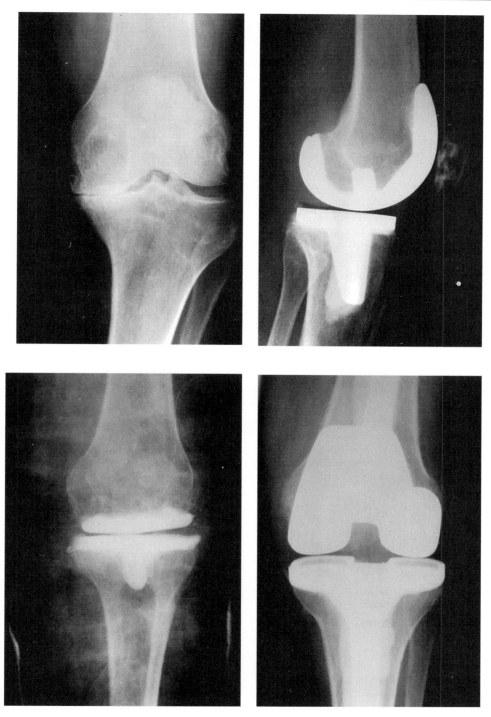

Fig. 1   Top left, Anteroposterior (AP) radiograph of the left knee of a 70-year-old woman with severe medial compartment disease. **Top right,** Lateral radiograph after successful total joint arthroplasty. Unfortunately the patient developed a late hematogenous infection related to surgical treatment of an ipsilateral great toe paronychia. **Bottom left,** The patient underwent removal of the components and cement, 6 weeks of intravenous, organism specific bacteriocidal antibiotics, and the implantation of a vancomycin and tobramycin laden antibiotic spacer. **Bottom right,** AP radiograph after successful, staged, re-implantation procedure. Cultures and histopathologic specimens obtained at the time of that surgery revealed no organisms. Tobramycin and vancomycin were used in the cement. The patient's erythrocyte sedimentation rate and C-reactive protein levels have returned to normal. There has been no suggestion of re-infection at 36-month follow-up.

Total Knee Specifics

Total knee arthroplasty patients at increased risk for infection include those who have rheumatoid arthritis, concurrent skin ulcers, or a history of prior knee surgery. Obesity, intercurrent urinary tract infections, and the use of oral steroids are associated with infection, but not at a statistically significant level. Even more than at the hip, success depends on the choice of incisions and adequate wound care. Areas of skin compromise should be treated aggressively with gastrocnemius or free tissue transfer as required.

Treatment options include antibiotic suppression, debridement with retention of the prosthetic components, debridement and removal of the components, reimplantation, arthrodesis, resection arthroplasty, or amputation. Antibiotic suppression alone is indicated only in those patients who cannot medically tolerate further surgical procedures. Long-term effective suppression depends on a well-fixed prosthesis and low virulence organism sensitive to an oral antibiotic. Suppression may well be required for the remainder of the patient's life. Eradication of the infection should not be anticipated. The risks include the potential for antibiotic toxicity and development of a resistant organism.

Successful salvage of an infected total knee arthroplasty by debridement and retention of the components has been associated with an infection of less than 2 to 4 weeks' duration, sensitive gram-positive organism, lack of a sinus tract, well-fixed components, and good host status. The debridement should be aggressive including an open, complete synovectomy. Multiple debridements may be required. Removal of the components would become necessary if repeated intraoperative cultures remained positive. Again, the patient will most probably require long-term suppression.

Aggressive debridement with removal of all of the prosthetic components and cement followed by a 6-week course of organism-specific intravenous antibiotics prior to a second stage re-implantation remains the most reliable method to restore infection-free function. Many authors favor the use of a cement spacer to maintain knee ligament length and allow for improved interoperative ambulation (Fig. 1).

The results for arthrodesis vary with the type of prosthe-

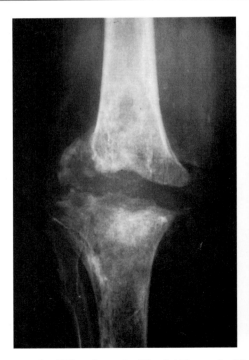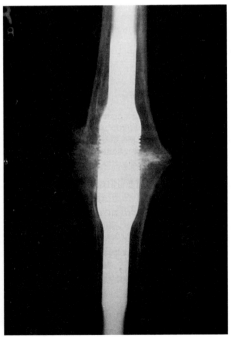

Fig. 2   Left, Anteroposterior (AP) radiograph of the right knee of a 68-year-old woman after resection arthroplasty for a failed, infected constrained prosthesis. The patient's initial knee surgery had been a patellar procedure in 1975, followed by an arthrotomy in 1980, and a total knee replacement in 1981. She underwent a revision arthroplasty in 1982 with a hinged prosthesis. The patient developed a gram-negative late infection. At the time of hardware removal the patient had bone and medial collateral ligament loss and patellar tendon attenuation. All cement and metallic debris was removed. The patient was treated with 6 weeks of intravenous antibiotics in conjunction with long leg cast immobilization. **Right,** AP radiograph after successful intramedullary rod arthrodesis. The patient is comfortable, walking with a 4.0 cm heel and sole lift. Cultures obtained at the time of fusion revealed no organisms. The patient is receiving no long-term suppressive antibiotics.

sis that had been used for the total joint arthroplasty and the fusion technique. Indications include destruction of the extensor mechanism, resistant bacteria, inadequate bone stock or soft tissue, and a young patient in whom the potential for a revision or reinfection is great with reimplantation. Contraindications include contralateral knee arthrodesis or above the knee amputation, severe segmental bone loss, and ipsilateral hip disease. Successful fusion occurs in approximately 80% of patients who had a resurfacing prosthesis but only 55% of those with a constrained device (Fig. 2). Arthrodesis using external fixation has a success rate between 70% and 80%. The most frequent complications are pin tract infections and peroneal nerve

injury. Internal fixation with plates or intramedullary rods has a success rate of 80% to 85%.

Resection arthroplasty, because of the functional limitations imposed, is reserved for severely disabled persons with a sedentary or bedfast lifestyle and those so fragile that they could not tolerate an additional surgery. Postoperative care includes prolonged cylinder cast or brace immobilization during wound healing and subsequent brace use during ambulation.

Amputation is the treatment of choice for elderly, nonambulatory patients and for those with uncontrolled sepsis.

Annotated Bibliography

Operating Room Environment

Berg-Perier M, Cederblad A, Persson U: Ultraviolet radiation and ultra-clean air enclosures in operating rooms: UV-protection, economy, and comfort. *J Arthroplasty* 1992;7:457–463.

The authors discuss the use of 254-nm ultraviolet light to sterilize the air in operating rooms. Bacterial contamination compared favorably with that achieved in laminar flow rooms. They emphasize that ultraviolet light is cost effective.

Bethune DN: Dispersal of Staphylococcus aureus by patients and surgical staff. *Lancet* 1965;1:480–483.

Evaluation of different personnel for type and amount of bacteria was done in controlled isolation chambers. Those that released more than 10,000 viable organisms were "shedders," a problem seen more frequently in males. *Staphylococcus aureus* was present in 30% of operating room personnel.

Fitzgerald RH Jr: Total hip arthroplasty sepsis: Prevention and diagnosis. *Orthop Clin North Am* 1992;23: 259–264.

The author found no significant decrease in deep wound sepsis following total hip arthroplasty in a single center, prospective, randomized study comparing conventional and vertical flow operating rooms.

Lidwell OM, Lowbury EJ, Whyte W, et al: Effect of ultraclean air in operating rooms on deep sepsis in the joint after total hip or knee replacement: A randomized study. *Br Med J* 1982;285:10–14.

The incidence of joint sepsis following total joint replacement was significantly reduced when the surgeries were performed in an ultraclean-air system. Further reduction in infection rates occurred when whole-body exhaust-ventilated suits were worn. The lack of randomization of perioperative antibiotics in this multicenter study has called into question the significance of the results.

Ritter MA, Eitzen H, French ML, et al: The operating room environment as affected by people and the surgical face mask. *Clin Orthop* 1975;111:147–150.

Microbiological counts in operating rooms increased when doors were left open and more significantly when additional people were introduced. The wearing of a face mask had no effect.

Ritter MA, French MLV, Eitzen HE: Bacterial contamination of the surgical knife. *Clin Orthop* 1975;108: 158–160.

No statistical difference was found in contamination frequency between skin and deep surgical knives. However, less knife blade contamination occurred when laminar airflow was used.

Salvati EA, Robinson RP, Zeno SM, et al: Infection rates after 3,175 total hip and total knee replacements performed with and without a horizontal unidirectional filtered air-flow system. *J Bone Joint Surg* 1982;64A:525–535.

The use of a filtered laminar airflow operating room system produced a statistically significant lower infection rate when compared to a conventional operating room during total hip joint arthroplasty.

Operating Room Attire

Alford DJ, Ritter MA, French ML, et al: The operating room gown as a barrier to bacterial shedding. *Am J Surg* 1973;125:589–591.

An evaluation of cloth, paper, and plastic surgical gowns reveals that a plastic, hooded gown reduces microbial contamination more effectively than does either cloth or paper by 71.8% and 57.3%, respectively ($p < 0.005$).

Ritter MA, French ML, Eitzen H: Evaluation of microbial contamination of surgical gloves during actual use. *Clin Orthop* 1976;117:303–306.

Contamination levels on the exterior of surgical gloves were not affected by the use of single or double gloves. Double gloves did reduce the number of holes in gloves. However, contamination was not found to be associated with the holes in gloves. Contamination generally comes from other sources in the operative field.

Ritter MA, Sieber JM, Carlson SR: Street shoes versus surgical footwear in the operating room. *Infect Surg* 1984;3:81–83.

Numerous types of surgical footwear versus street shoes were compared in regard to their bacterial contamination properties in the operating room environment. Both foot movement and airborne bacterial dispersion were also investigated. There was no significant difference in contamination properties among various footwear tested. Airborne bacterial dispersion in association with foot movement also appears to be insignificant.

Surgical Scrub: Hand and Operative Site Skin Preparation

Alexander JW, Aerni S, Plettner JP: Development of a safe and effective one-minute preoperative skin preparation. *Arch Surg* 1985;120:1357–1361.

The use of a polyester antimicrobial incision drape applied to an operative area after a 1-minute skin preparation resulted in wound infection rates comparable to those following a standard 10-minute skin preparation with Betadine.

Eitzen HE, Ritter MA, French ML, et al: A microbiological in-use comparison of surgical hand-washing agents. *J Bone Joint Surg* 1979;61A:403–406.

A hexachlorophene foam compound demonstrated excellent bacteriocidal and bacteriostatic action as compared to a trioclosan compound and iodophors when used as a surgical scrub. It was also less time consuming and easier to use.

Ritter MA, Campbell ED: Retrospective evaluation of an iodophor-incorporated antimicrobial plastic adhesive wound drape. *Clin Orthop* 1988;228:307–308.

Incidence of postoperative wound infection was found to be comparable between the use of an iodophor-incorporated adhesive wound drape and iodine spray as a skin preparation.

Tucci VJ, Stone AM, Thompson C, et al: Studies of the surgical scrub. *Surg Gynecol Obstet* 1977;145:415–416.

A comparison of the efficacy of a 5 minute versus a 10 minute surgical scrub revealed no significant difference between the two. Betadine was a more effective scrubbing agent than pHisoHex.

Zdeblick TA, Lederman MM, Jacobs MR, et al: Preoperative use of povidone-iodine: A prospective, randomized study. *Clin Orthop* 1986;213:211–215.

Povidone-iodine painting alone for presurgical skin preparation was more effective than povidone-iodine scrub and paint in reducing bacteria counts. Preoperative hexachlorophene showers reduced bacterial counts.

Closed Suction Drainage and Hematomata

Beer KJ, Lombardi AV Jr, Mallory TH, et al: The efficacy of suction drains after routine total joint arthroplasty. *J Bone Joint Surg* 1991;73A:584–587.

Ritter MA, Keating EM, Faris PM: Closed wound drainage in total hip or total knee replacement: A prospective, randomized study. *J Bone Joint Surg* 1994;76A:35–38.

Four hundred fifteen patients undergoing either primary total hip or primary total knee arthroplasty were randomized such that 215 received closed suction drainage and 200 did not. All surgeries were performed by the authors. Continuous passive motion was not used. There was no significant difference in the number who had excessive postoperative drainage, the amount of transfused blood, or range of motion. The authors believe that there is no indication for closed wound drainage in primary total joint arthroplasty surgery.

Antibiotics and Delivery Systems

Doyon F, Evrard J, Mazas F, et al: Long-term results of prophylactic cefazolin versus placebo in total hip replacement. *Lancet* 1987;1:860.

Antibiotic prophylaxis, involving 5 days of cefazolin at the time of surgery, significantly reduced early and late infection rates in total hip replacement.

MacMillan M, Petty W, Hendeles L: Effect of irrigation and tourniquet application on aminoglycoside antibiotic concentrations in bone. *J Orthop Res* 1988;6:311–316.

The use of vigorous irrigation in bone preparation had a deleterious effect on the local presence of systemically administered antibiotics. This effect is compounded when the operative site is isolated by the use of a tourniquet. The authors recommend the use of either antibiotic containing irrigant or antibiotic laden polymethylmethacrylate.

Mauerhan DR, Nelson CL, Smith DL, et al: Prophylaxis against infection in total joint arthroplasty: One day of cefuroxime compared with three days of cefazolin. *J Bone Joint Surg* 1994;76A:39–45.

There was no significant difference in the prevalence of wound infection in 1,354 patients treated with either one dose of cefuroxime or nine doses of cefazolin in a randomized, double-blind, multicenter study of primary and revision total hip and total knee arthroplasties. Of the total hip arthroplasty patients, one of 187 treated with cefuroxime and two of 168 treated with cefazolin developed infection. Of the total knee arthroplasty patients, one of 178 treated with cefuroxime and three of 207 treated with cefazolin became infected. No antibiotics were used in the irrigant or bone cement.

Perry CR, Pearson RL: Local antibiotic delivery in the treatment of bone and joint infections. *Clin Orthop* 1991; 263:215–226.

The authors report suppression of infection in 30 of 37 patients with acutely infected total joint arthroplasties, and seven of ten chronically infected arthroplasties treated with an implanted pump that delivered a high concentration of antibiotics to the infected joint through a subcutaneous catheter. There was a 7% pump site infection rate.

Nutrition

Gherini S, Vaughn BK, Lombardi AV Jr, et al: Delayed wound healing and nutritional deficiencies after total knee arthroplasty. *Clin Orthop* 1993;293:188–195.

Patients with nutritional deficiencies were found to have delayed wound healing following total hip arthroplasty.

Jensen JE, Jensen TG, Smith TK, et al: Nutrition in orthopaedic surgery. *J Bone Joint Surg* 1982;64A: 1263–1272.

A significant amount of clinical and subclinical malnutrition was found in orthopaedic surgical patients. Subnormal nutritional indices correlated with the development of complications.

Microbiology

Chang CC, Merritt K: Effect of Staphylococcus epidermidis on adherence of Pseudomonas aeruginosa and Proteus mirabilis to polymethyl methacrylate (PMMA) and gentamicin containing PMMA. *J Orthop Res* 1991;9:284–288.

Biomaterial-centered infections produced by *Staphylococcus epidermidis* are difficult to eradicate, in part, because of the extracellular glycocalyx formed by the organism, which changes the surface charge and surface free energy of the biomaterial and forms a barrier against host defenses. *S epidermidis* biofilms, whether alive or dead, significantly increase the adherence of pseudomonas. Adherence of proteus was greater to dead biofilm than to live biofilm. Adherence of pseudomonas and proteus was found on gentamycin containing polymethylmethacrylate after preincubation with *S epidermidis*. Thus, once adherence of bacteria has begun, adherence of other organisms may be promoted.

Nair S, Song Y, Meghji S, et al: Surface-associated proteins from Staphylococcus aureus demonstrate potent bone resorbing activity. *J Bone Miner Res* 1995;10:726–734.

The surface associated proteins from *Staphylococcus aureus* are extremely potent stimulators of bone resorption. The most active contains a heterodimeric protein of 32 to 36 kd molecular weight.

Stuart GW, McDowell SJ, McDaniel SE, et al: Cross-linked albumin coated surfaces to prevent bacterial adhesion onto titanium plates. *Trans Orthop Res Soc* 1995;20:262.

The "race for the surface" as described by Gristina has not been won to date. The authors present their preliminary data concerning the possibility of precoating biomaterials prior to implantation to inhibit microorganism adhesion.

Webb LX, Holman J, de Araujo B, et al: Antibiotic resistance in staphylococci adherent to cortical bone. *J Orthop Trauma* 1994;8:28–33.

The antibiotic resistance of three staphylococcal subtypes was evaluated for organisms grown in suspension and adherent to bone, polytetrafluoroethylene, and polymethylmethacrylate. Adherent growth on bone was associated with the most antibiotic resistance.

Diagnostic Evaluation

Cuckler JM, Star AM, Alavi A, et al: Diagnosis and management of the infected total joint arthroplasty. *Orthop Clin North Am* 1991;22:523–530.

The authors' review of the literature and personal experience documents the wide variation in value of each of the diagnostic tests commonly used to evaluate the patient for sepsis.

Datz FL, Anderson CE, Ahluwalia R, et al: The efficacy of Indium-III-Polyclonal IgG for the detection of infection and inflammation. *J Nucl Med* 1994;35:74–83.

The polyclonal IgG scan had a sensitivity that was not adversely affected by antibiotics, steroids, anti-inflammatory agents, diabetes, or diminished renal function. Ease of preparation and safety make it an attractive alternative to labeled leukocytes.

Johnson JA, Christie MJ, Sandler MP, et al: Detection of occult infection following total joint arthroplasty using

sequential technetium-99m HDP bone scintigraphy and indium-111 WBC imaging. *J Nucl Med* 1988;29:1347–1353.

In this series, the specificity and accuracy of combined technetium and indium scintigraphy is 95% and 93% respectively in the evaluation of an occult total hip arthroplasty infection.

Unkila-Kallio L, Kallio MJ, Peltola H: The usefulness of C-reactive protein levels in the identification of concurrent septic arthritis in children who have acute hematogenous osteomyelitis: A comparison with the usefulness of the erythrocyte sedimentation rate and the white blood-cell count. *J Bone Joint Surg* 1994;76A:848–853.

C-reactive protein is an acute phase protein synthesized by the liver, mediated by interleukin-6, in response to bacterial infection. It has been a good indicator of complications in recovery from infections, operations, and trauma. The normal value is less than 20 mg/l.

Delayed Infection Prophylactic Antibiotics

Maderazo EG, Judson S, Pasternak H: Late infections of total joint prostheses: A review and recommendations for prevention. *Clin Orthop* 1988;229:131–142.

The authors recommend oral cephalosporins or cefazolin for dental care accompanied by gingival bleeding, head, neck, chest, upper gastrointestinal, and gynecologic surgery with clindamycin, erythromycin, or vancomycin as alternatives.

Nelson JP, Fitzgerald RH Jr, Jaspers MT, et al: Editorial: Prophylactic antimicrobial coverage in arthroplasty patients. *J Bone Joint Surg* 1990;72A:1.

The mortality rate in late infections can approach 18%. This editorial recommends coverage for dental, genitourinary, and gastrointestinal procedures and for such infections as cutaneous abscesses and paronychia.

Treatment

Duncan CP, Masri BA: The role of antibiotic-loaded cement in the treatment of an infection after a hip replacement. *J Bone Joint Surg* 1994;76A:1742–1751.

The authors recommend the use of a temporary, custom, antibiotic laden spacer (2.4 to 3.6 g of tobramycin and 1 to 2 g of vancomycin per 40 g of cement) at the time of initial debridement of an infected total hip arthroplasty. At the subsequent reimplantation they recommend 0.6 to 1.2 g of tobramycin and 0.5 to 1.0 g vancomycin per 40 g of cement.

Nestor BJ, Hanssen AD, Ferrer-Gonzalez R, et al: The use of porous prostheses in delayed reconstruction of total hip replacements that have failed because of infection. *J Bone Joint Surg* 1994;76A:349–359.

Avoiding the use of polymethylmethacrylate cement at the time of revision surgery for infection does not diminish the rate of recurrence. Of 34 patients treated, six (18%) had recurrence of infection, six additional patients had radiographic evidence of loosening. Only 14 (56%) had a satisfactory outcome on the basis of the Mayo Clinic hip score.

Total Knee Specifics

Gerwin M, Rothaus KO, Windsor RE, et al: Gastrocnemius muscle flap coverage of exposed or infected knee prostheses. *Clin Orthop* 1993;286:64–70.

Gastrocnemius muscle flaps provide excellent soft-tissue

coverage, dead space obliteration, improved vascularity, and oxygen delivery.

Windsor RE, Bono JV: Infected total knee replacements. *J Am Acad Orthop Surg* 1994;2:44–53.

Two-stage revision surgery, frequently involving the expertise of the orthopaedist, plastic surgeon, and infectious disease consultant, has provided the most successful functional outcome for this devastating complication. Such a protocol may not be possible, however, if there is extensive bone or soft-tissue loss, a significant risk of antibiotic toxicity, quadriceps necrosis, host medical conditions that preclude additional surgery, or patient preference.

4

Materials Consideration in Total Joint Replacement

Introduction

The human body is a harsh chemical environment for foreign materials. The mechanical and biologic properties of an implanted material can be altered drastically by body fluids. Degradation mechanisms, such as corrosion or leaching, can be accelerated by ion concentrations and pH changes in body fluids. The body's response to an implant can range from a benign to a chronic inflammatory reaction, with the degree of biologic response largely dependent on the implanted material. For optimal performance in physiologic environments, implant materials should have suitable mechanical strength, biocompatibility, and structural biostability.

Biologic classification of implant materials is based on tissue response and on the systemic toxicity effects of the implant. There are three classes of biomaterials: biotolerant, bioinert, and bioactive. Biotolerant materials, such as stainless steel and polymethylmethacrylate (PMMA), are usually characterized by a thin fibrous tissue layer at the bone–implant interface. The fibrous tissue layer develops as a result of irritation of the surrounding tissues by the chemical products from leaching processes. Bioinert materials, such as cobalt alloys, titanium, and aluminum oxide, are characterized by direct bone contact, or osseointegration, at the interface under favorable mechanical conditions. Osseointegration is achieved because the material surface is chemically nonreactive to the surrounding tissues and body fluids. Finally, bioactive materials, such as bioglass and calcium phosphate ceramics, have a bone–implant interface characterized by direct chemical bonding of the implant with surrounding bone. This chemical bond is believed to be caused by the presence of free calcium and phosphate compounds at the implant surface.

Minimization of the local and systemic response to an implanted material through improved biocompatibility is only one engineering concern for reconstructive implant surgery. A prosthetic implant must adequately transfer stress at the bone–implant surface to ensure long-term implant stability. Nonphysiologic stress transfer may cause pressure necrosis and/or resorption at the bone–implant interface or delamination of a polyethylene bearing surface or metal substrate–coating interface. Necrotic and resorbed bone may lead to implant loosening and migration, thus compromising implant longevity. Also, material properties capable of sustaining the cyclic body forces to which the implant will be subjected are essential. For example, if its material properties are not adequate for load sharing, the implant may fail due to fracture. However, if the implant's properties allow stress shielding of the bone to occur, then bone resorption and implant loosening are inevitable.

Implant Materials

The most commonly used biomaterial combinations for orthopaedic implants are metals and their alloys articulating with ultrahigh molecular weight polyethylene (UHMWPE). Stainless steel, an iron-based alloy, was used in Charnley's original hip prosthesis and is the material of choice for internal fixation plates, rods, and screws. Advances in materials science have produced stronger cobalt- and titanium-based alloys. The wear resistance of cobalt-based alloys makes them desirable for applications involving articulating surfaces. Titanium-based alloys, which have a modulus of elasticity closer to that of bone than the other metal alloys, are currently being manufactured as femoral stems to reduce the effects of stress shielding.

Polymers and ceramics are also important classes of materials for orthopaedic implant applications. UHMWPE has a low coefficient of friction, making it ideal for an articulating surface with metals. PMMA has been used as a grouting agent in total joint arthroplasty. Aluminum oxide has gained popularity as a ceramic femoral head due to its high wear resistance and low coefficient of friction. Finally, calcium phosphate ceramics, particularly hydroxyapatite (HA), have been used in monolithic form as an augmentation material for metaphyseal bone defects and as a coating on metal devices for total joint arthroplasty.

Metals

The suitability of a metal component for maintaining longevity of a total joint replacement depends on the design of the implant and the biocompatibility, strength, wear, and corrosion characteristics of the metal. The most important characteristics are yield strength, ultimate tensile strength, and fatigue strength. These properties can be determined from stress-strain and fatigue limit curves. The composition specifications and mechanical characteristics of all metals and their alloys used for orthopaedic implants have been standardized by the American Society for Testing and Materials (ASTM).

Stress, the force a material is subjected to per unit area, and strain, the amount of deformation the material experiences per unit area in response to stress, describe the mechanical characteristics of a material. These characteristics can be determined from a stress-strain curve (Fig. 1),

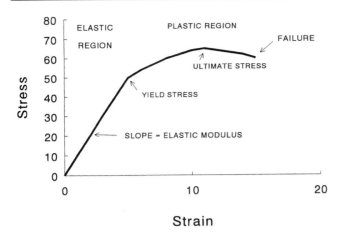

Fig. 1 Stress-strain diagram for a typical material.

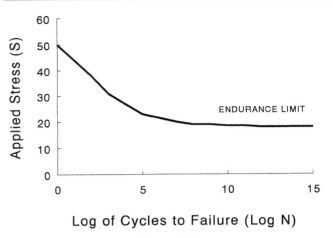

Fig. 2 S-N curve for a typical material.

which is a plot of the effect of a single stress or load to a material. The linear portion of the curve demonstrates the amount of stress a metal can withstand before deforming. The slope of this line is the modulus of elasticity of the metal. A high modulus of elasticity indicates the material is stiff; whereas, a low modulus indicates the metal is more pliable. The modulus of elasticity is an excellent means of comparison among several different materials. However, when making comparisons, it is important to remember that the modulus of elasticity is a property of the material and not of the implant; implant stiffness is a function of both the metal's modulus of elasticity and the implant's design geometry. The yield strength of a metal is the stress at which permanent or plastic deformation begins. The ultimate tensile strength is the stress that a metal can withstand in a single application before fracture. Finally, the ductility of a metal is the amount of plastic deformation it undergoes before failure and is a function of elongation and reduction in total area. A brittle material will fail with little elongation; whereas, a ductile material will fail only after a large amount of elongation.

When subjected to several million cycles in a physiologic environment, a metal may fail at loads well below the ultimate tensile strength. The fatigue or S-N curve (Fig. 2) demonstrates the behavior of a metal during cyclic loading. Generally, as the number of cycles (N) increases, the maximum applied stress (S) the metal can withstand before failure decreases. However, after a large number of cycles, the endurance limit of the metal is reached. Failure will not occur if the applied stress is kept below the endurance limit.

The grain size and the inclusion content (impurities in the metal) or surface porosity influence the strength characteristics of a metal. In general, the larger the grain size, the less tensile strength a metal can endure before fracture. Also, too many inclusions or too large a surface porosity will weaken the metal by acting as stress risers and by pro-

viding areas for crevice corrosion. Manufacturing processes can be used to control these factors. For example, heating metal to approximately its melting point increases the grain size, whereas forging decreases the grain size.

Corrosion is a chemical reaction process that weakens the metal. All metals corrode in the physiologic environment; the severity of corrosion is determined by the chemical composition of the metal. Stainless steel corrodes more readily than either cobalt- or titanium-based alloys. The addition of chromium and molybdenum to both stainless steel and cobalt-based alloys produces a corrosion-resistant surface layer. An oxide passive film layer provides corrosion resistance for titanium-based alloys. The surfaces of all metallic implants are passivated with nitric acid to form an oxide surface layer that increases corrosion resistance. However, scratching or breaking this passive film layer may hasten the corrosion process if the layer cannot passivate itself in vivo.

Three types of corrosion are most prevalent in implant materials: galvanic, crevice, and fatigue. Galvanic corrosion occurs when an electric current is established between two metals that have different chemical compositions. Differences in chemical composition may arise from manufacturing processes, such as in bone plates and screws made of stainless steel, or from two different metals in close contact with each other, such as a titanium alloy femoral stem with a cobalt alloy head. An evaluation of 28 retrieved mixed-metal femoral hip components revealed a 56% incidence of corrosion. Further evaluation determined that corrosion occurred on all components that were implanted for over 40 months. The long-term consequences of corrosion due to femoral component modularity are unknown. However, to avoid catastrophic galvanic corrosion, stainless steels should never be used with either cobalt or titanium alloys. Crevice corrosion generally occurs when the fluid in contact with a metal becomes stagnant, resulting in a local oxygen depletion and a subsequent change in pH. This form of corrosion is most prevalent underneath bone plates at the screw–plate junction. Finally, fatigue corrosion may occur if the passive oxide film on the implant surface has been scratched or cracked. Once corrosion begins, the implant weakens and will fail below the endurance limit of the material.

Iron-Based Alloys There are four major classes of iron-based alloys or stainless steels grouped according to their microstructure. The austenitic or Group III stainless steels (316 and 316L) are used for orthopaedic implants. The ASTM specifications for the chemical composition of these metals are summarized in Table 1. Molybdenum is added to these alloys to increase resistance to pitting corrosion. Corrosion resistance is also increased by lowering the carbon content, as in 316L. Iron-based alloys have a wide range of mechanical properties (Table 2), which make them desirable for implant applications. However, despite

modifications in their composition, stainless steels are susceptible to corrosion inside the body. Therefore, they are most appropriate for temporary devices such as bone plates, bone screws, hip nails, and intramedullary nails.

The most prevalent reason for corrosion of stainless steels is incorrect metal composition. Molybdenum is added to these metals to increase corrosion resistance; however, too much molybdenum can embrittle the alloy. Chromium carbide may form between the grain boundaries and result in grain boundary corrosion. This phenomenon is referred to as sensitization. Another cause of corrosion is mismatch of components, especially bone plates and screws. Implants manufactured by the same company in different lots can corrode because of differences that result from slightly different manufacturing processes. Crevice corrosion may occur at the junction of the screw with the bone plate as a result of local pH and oxygen concentration changes.

Cobalt-Based Alloys The ASTM specifications for the chemical composition of cobalt-based alloys are summarized in Table 3. Molybdenum is added to the alloys to produce finer grains and, consequently, higher strength. Cobalt-based alloys have mechanical properties (Table 2) suitable for load-bearing implant applications. These alloys are characterized by high fatigue and ultimate tensile strength that make them appropriate for applications requiring long service life without fracture. The high wear resistance of these alloys also makes them desirable for load bearing and use at articulating surfaces. However, incidences have been reported in which surface porosities have acted as stress risers and led to premature fatigue failure. Hot isostatic pressing (HIPing), the simultaneous application of heat and pressure to consolidate powder into

Table 1. Chemical composition of stainless steel materials

| Element | Maximum Amount (wt%) | |
	316 ASTM F55–82	316L ASTM F55–82
Carbon	0.08	0.030
Manganese	2.00	2.00
Phosphorus	0.030	0.030
Sulfur	0.030	0.030
Silicon	0.75	0.75
Chromium	17.00 to 19.00	17.00 to 19.00
Nickel	12.00 to 14.00	12.00 to 14.00
Molybdenum	2.00 to 3.00	2.00 to 3.00
Nitrogen	0.10	0.10
Copper	0.50	0.50
Iron	Balance	Balance

Table 2. Minimum mechanical requirements for metal implant materials

Material Type*	Elastic Modulus (GPa)	Ultimate Tensile Strength (MPa)	0.2% Offset Yield Strength (MPa)	Elongation (%)	Reduction of Area (%)
Annealed stainless steel 316 ASTM F55–82	200	515	205	40	—
Annealed stainless steel 316L ASTM F55–82	200	480	170	40	—
Cold-worked stainless steel 316 and 316L ASTM F55–82	200	860	690	12	—
Cast Co-Cr-Mo alloy ASTM F75–87	250	655	450	8	8
Wrought Co-Ni-Cr-Mo alloy ASTM F562–84	240	793–1000	241–448	50	65
Unalloyed titanium ASTM F67–89	105	240–550	170–483	15–24	25–30
Cast Ti-6Al-4V alloy ASTM F1108–88	110	860	858	8	14
Wrought Ti-6Al-4V ELI alloy ASTM F136–84	110	860–896	795–827	10	25

8Co = cobalt; Cr = chromium; Mo = molybdenum; Ni = nickel; Ti = titanium; Al = aluminum; V = vanadium

Table 3. Chemical composition of cobalt-based alloy materials

	Maximum Amount (wt%)	
Element	Cast Co-Cr-Mo ASTM F75–87	Wrought Co-Ni-Cr-Mo ASTM F562–84
Chromium (Cr)	30.00	21.0
Molybdenum (Mo)	7.00	10.5
Nickel (Ni)	1.00	37.0
Iron (Fe)	0.75	1.00
Carbon (C)	0.35	0.025
Silicon (Si)	1.00	0.15
Manganese (Mn)	1.00	0.15
Sulfur (S)	—	0.010
Phosphorus (P)	—	0.015
Titanium (Ti)	—	1.00
Cobalt (Co)	Balance	Balance

Table 4. Chemical composition of titanium and titanium alloy materials

	Maximum Amount (wt%)		
Element	Unalloyed Titanium ASTM F67–89	Wrought Ti6A14V ELI Alloy ASTM F136–84	Cast Ti6Al4V Alloy ASTM F1108–88
Nitrogen (N)	0.05	0.05	0.05
Carbon (C)	0.10	0.08	0.10
Hydrogen (H)	0.015	0.012	0.015
Iron (Fe)	0.50	0.25	0.20
Oxygen (O)	0.40	0.13	0.20
Aluminum (Al)	—	5.5 to 6.5	5.5 to 6.75
Vanadium (Va)	—	3.5 to 4.5	3.5 to 4.5
Titanium (Ti)	Balance	Balance	Balance

a solid form, has been developed to significantly reduce surface porosity. After HIPing, the material must be heat-treated to attain maximum benefit. When performed properly, HIPing increases the fatigue and static strength characteristics and the corrosion resistance of cobalt-based alloys. Sintering beads onto cobalt-based alloys as well as other alloys decreases the strength of the substrate material.

Titanium and Titanium-Based Alloys Commercially pure titanium and titanium-based alloys are low density metals that have chemical properties suitable for implant applications. The ASTM specifications are summarized in Table 4. The high corrosion resistance of titanium is attributed to an oxide surface layer, which also is chemically nonreactive to the surrounding tissues. The mechanical properties of titanium and titanium-based alloys are summarized in Table 2. The modulus of elasticity, approximately 110 GPa, is half of that for iron- or cobalt-based alloys, but is at least five times greater than that of bone. Increasing the impurity content of the metal increases its strength but makes it more brittle. Due to low density, the specific strength (strength per density) of titanium and titanium-based alloys is superior to that of all other metals. However, titanium has poor shear strength and wear resistance, making it unsuitable for articulating surface applications. In addition, titanium is notch sensitive, which limits its potential for porous surface applications. A porous coating cannot be extensively applied to titanium stems without markedly reducing its fatigue strength.

New manufacturing techniques are being developed to improve the wear resistance of titanium-based alloys. Currently, nitrogen ion implantation techniques are being evaluated for this use. The process of ion implantation causes elemental nitrogen ions to become embedded within the surface of the titanium. The presence of these ions causes distortions within the crystal lattice of the metal and results in an increased surface microhardness. This increased surface hardness significantly improved the in vitro wear resistance of the treated implant.

Polymers

Polymers have a wide range of properties that make them suitable for several different implant applications. This range is attributed to variations in the polymers' chemical composition, structure, and manufacturing process. The choice of polymer for a given application is controlled by the effect of the physiologic environment on the stability of the material. Some polymers, such as PMMA, leach toxic substances into the surrounding tissues. Conversely, other polymers absorb fluids from the body, thereby altering mechanical properties. Despite the possible consequences of polymer implantation, the use of polymers as implant materials has been successful.

All polymers are composed of long chains of repeating units, which may form linear, cross-linked, or branched chains. Individual chains may be organized in an orderly crystalline form that has parallel or folded chains, may be amorphous, or may have a mixed crystalline and amorphous structure. The molecular weight, chemical composition, degree of crystallinity, size and polarity of side groups, and degree of cross-linking determine the mechanical properties of the polymer. In general, as the molecular weight and crystallinity increase, the tensile strength and resistance to cracking increase. Crystallinity is decreased by copolymerization, branching of chains, and presence of large side groups.

Ceramics

Ceramics are wear resistant and strong in compression, but are very brittle and susceptible to cracking. Ceramic materials must be chosen carefully for specific implant applications because chemical composition affects the mechanical properties and biologic response of each ceramic. For instance, an alteration in the calcium-to-phosphorus ratio for calcium phosphate ceramics can significantly alter the in vivo dissolution rate of the ceramic. The mechanical properties of ceramics depend on grain size, porosity, density, and crystallinity. Strength is normally improved with increased density, increased crystallinity, and decreased porosity. The design of reliable ceramic implants requires large quantities of material and the avoidance of sharp corners and notches in order to overcome the mechanical weaknesses of the material.

Aluminum Oxide (Al₂O₃) The catastrophic effects of implant loosening resulting from polyethylene wear debris led to interest in using other materials at the articulating surface. Aluminum oxide is a highly biocompatible material with a high resistance to friction. In fact, the coefficient of friction for alumina on alumina articulations is approximately 2.3 times less than that for metal on UHMWPE articulations. Alumina on alumina articulations result in approximately 5,000 times less wear than metal on UHMWPE articulations. Also, any wear debris that does accumulate at the interface is less bioreactive than UHMWPE or PMMA debris. Despite the excellent wear and friction characteristics of aluminum oxide, its fracture resistance is low, which could result in catastrophic breakage and wear. The elastic modulus is approximately 20 times greater than that of cortical bone. However, the modulus can be altered drastically by decreasing crystallinity and increasing porosity and/or grain size. Large grain size has been linked to reported cases of catastrophic wear. Careful regulation of manufacturing processes results in reliable aluminum oxide implants with small grain size, high density, high purity, and adequate strength in the absence of initial manufacturing cracks while ensuring adequate component size.

Hydroxyapatite (HA) Calcium phosphate ceramics, classified as polycrystalline ceramics, have a material structure derived from individual crystals that have become fused at the grain boundaries during high temperature sintering processes. Tribasic calcium phosphate, $[Ca_{10}(PO_4)_6(OH)_2]$, commonly called hydroxyapatite (HA), is a geologic mineral that closely resembles the natural mineral in vertebrate bone tissue. Tribasic calcium phosphate should not be confused with other calcium phosphate ceramics, especially tricalcium phosphate (TCP), $[Ca_3(PO_4)_2]$, which is chemically similar to HA but is not a natural bone mineral.

Bulk HA is manufactured from a starting powder using compression molding techniques and subsequent sintering. Macroporous ceramics can be obtained by mixing the starting mixture with hydrogen peroxide; otherwise, the ceramics will have a dense structure with a small percentage of micropores. Dense HA ceramics have a compressive strength greater than that of cortical bone; however, their tensile strength is approximately 2.5 times less than their compressive strength. Small reductions in density can significantly reduce tensile characteristics of the ceramic. Also, the resistance to fatigue failure is low, as is common with sintered ceramics. Therefore, bulk HA is not suitable for applications requiring mechanical loading. However, bulk HA has been used successfully clinically as a bone graft substitute to fill metaphyseal defects associated with tibial plateau fractures. The development of thin plasma-sprayed HA coatings on metal substrates has provided a composite prosthesis that is able to withstand the physiologic stresses imposed on it while providing an osteoconductive surface to achieve optimal bone apposition and ingrowth.

Summary

The mechanical and chemical properties of metals, such as iron, titanium, and cobalt alloys; ceramics, such as aluminum oxide and calcium phosphate; and polymers, such as UHMWPE and PMMA, make them suitable for implant applications. Several factors affect the biologic response to these implanted materials. The predominate tissue found at the implant interface is affected by implant stability, material biocompatibility, and implant design and placement into the surgical site. The manufacturing processes affect the fatigue, wear, and corrosion properties of the material. Improvements in implant design, surface preparation, and material science may improve implant longevity and fixation for all implant materials. However, the best implant designs cannot overcome inferior implant material properties. Conversely, all materials have mechanical or chemical limitations when placed in the physiologic environment and cannot overcome implant design weaknesses.

Annotated Bibliography

Bucholz RW, Carlton A, Holmes R: Interporous hydroxyapatite as a bone graft substitute in tibial plateau fractures. *Clin Orthop* 1989;240:53–62.

  Metaphyseal defects from tibial plateau fractures in 40 patients were repaired with either cancellous autograft or interporous hydroxyapatite. The interporous hydroxyapatite provided an effective alternative to autogenous bone.

Collier JP, Mayor MB, Surprenant VA, et al: The biomechanical problems of polyethylene as a bearing surface. *Clin Orthop* 1990;261:107–113.

Light and scanning electron microscopy were used to evaluate 85 polyethylene acetabular components for evidence of wear. The investigators express concern that variation in tolerances and mechanical properties of the bulk material may compound the problems of pitting, cracking, and creep deformation.

Cook SD, Renz EA, Barrack RL, et al: Clinical and metallurgical analysis of retrieved internal fixation devices. *Clin Orthop* 1985;194:236–247.

Fifty-one of 82 stainless steel bone plates were retrieved prematurely due to pain, infection, nonunion, and/or malunion. Metallurgical properties of grain size and nonmetallic inclusion content correlated significantly with the degree of surface pitting and screwplate interface crevice and fretting corrosion found on 89% of the implants.

Davies JP, O'Connor DO, Burke DW, et al: Comparison and optimization of three centrifugation systems for reducing porosity of Simplex P bone cement. *J Arthroplasty* 1989;4:15–20.

Simplex P bone cement was spun for 30, 60, and 120 seconds in the I.E.C. HN-SII, I.E.C. Clinical, and Johnson & Johnson centrifuges to determine whether differences among the three systems also produces differences in the fatigue strength of the cement. The I.E.C. HN-SII was determined to be the better suited centrifuge, with two packs of bone cement and a monomer spin time of 30 seconds or 60 seconds for a chilled monomer, which increased the average fatigue life of bone cement from 15,043 cycles to 71,000 cycles.

Georgette FS, Davidson JA: The effect of HIPing on the fatigue and tensile strength of a cast, porous-coated Co-Cr-Mo alloy. *J Biomed Mater Res* 1986;20:1229–1248.

The effectiveness of hot isostatic pressing (HIPing) to eliminate substrate porosity and increase the fatigue strength of sintered porous Co-Cr-Mo alloy was evaluated. The HIPing of sintered materials improved fatigue and tensile properties relative to the "as sintered" condition.

Howie DW: Tissue response in relation to type of wear particles around failed hip arthroplasties. *J Arthroplasty* 1990;5:337–348.

The periprosthetic tissues around 50 hip arthroplasties revised for aseptic loosening of one or more components were examined by light microscopy, transmission electron microscopy, and energy dispersing x-ray microanalysis. Tissues around cementless metal-on-bone and ceramic-on-ceramic prostheses contained few or no prosthetic wear particles, whereas tissues around metal-on-metal and cemented metal-on-polyethylene prostheses contained larger numbers of wear particles and a greater tissue response.

Jarcho M: Calcium phosphate ceramics as hard tissue prosthetics. *Clin Orthop* 1981;157:259–278.

Porous and dense forms of permanent and bioresorbable hard tissue implant materials made of calcium phosphate ceramics are extremely biocompatible and have shown the ability to chemically bond to bone via "natural-appearing bone cementing mechanisms." Animal and clinical study results suggest these materials may be applicable for use as bone graft substitutes or extenders.

Lemons JE: Bioceramics: Is there a difference? *Clin Orthop* 1990;261:153–158.

Three types of bioceramics used in surgical applications (aluminum oxide, hydroxyapatite, and tricalcium phosphate) are quite different from one another, and variations exist within each type. The physical, mechanical, chemical, and biologic properties are specific to each bioceramic, and significantly different tissue responses have been shown among the three types.

McKellop H, Clarke I, Markolf K, et al: Friction and wear properties of polymer, metal, and ceramic prosthetic joint materials evaluated on a multichannel screening device. *J Biomed Mater Res* 1981;15:619–653.

Friction and wear of ultrahigh molecular weight (UHMW) polyethylene was just as low with highly polished, fully dense ceramics as with metals, including 316 stainless steel and cobalt-chromium, multiphase, and titanium 6–4 alloys. Alternate polymers, such as Teflon and polyester, exhibited significantly greater wear rates than UHMW polyethylene.

Willert HG, Bertram H, Buchhorn GH: Osteolysis in alloarthroplasty of the hip: The role of ultra-high molecular weight polyethylene wear particles. *Clin Orthop* 1990;258:95–107.

In a series of eight soft-top hip prostheses with ultrahigh molecular weight polyethylene (UHMWPE) ball heads, all cases showed marked loss of proximal cortical bone combined with osteolysis distal to the femoral shaft and deep into the acetabulum. Large amounts of UHMWPE wear debris found in the joint capsule and surrounding granulomatous tissue together with the near absence or small amounts of metal or polymethylmethacrylate particles indicate that UHMWPE wear particles can cause massive osteolysis by triggering foreign-body granuloma formation at the bone-cement interface.

Wright TM, Bartel DL: The problem of surface damage in polyethylene total knee components. *Clin Orthop* 1986;205:67–74.

Through observation and analytic study, important clinical factors, such as patient weight and the length of implantation time, and design factors were identified as affecting articulating surface damage of total knee components. Design variables that affect the amount of damage are component thickness (more severe in components less than 4 to 6 mm thick), conformity of the articulating surfaces (more severe in relatively flat surfaced tibial components), and the type of polyethylene material used (more severe for carbon-reinforced versus plain polyethylene).

Classic Bibliography

Buchanan RA, Rigney ED Jr, Williams JM: Ion implantation of surgical Ti-6Al-4V for improved resistance to wear-accelerated corrosion. *J Biomed Mater Res* 1987;21:355–366.

Clarke IC, Dorlot JM, Graham J, et al: Biomechanical stability and design: Wear. *Ann NY Acad Sci* 1988;523: 292–296.

Collier JP, Bauer TW, Bloebaum RD, et al: Results of implant retrieval from postmortem specimens in patients with well- functioning, long-term total hip replacement. *Clin Orthop* 1992;274:97–112.

Dorlot JM, Christel P, Sedel L, et al: Examination of retrieved hip-prostheses: Wear of alumina/alumina components, in Christel P, Meunier A, Lee AJC (eds): *Biological and Biomechanical Performance of Biomaterials: Proceedings of the Fifth European Conference on Biomataerials; Paris France, 1985.* Amsterdam, Elsevier Science Publishers, 1986, pp 495–500.

Galante JO, Rostoker W, Doyle JM: Failed femoral stems in total hip prostheses: A report of 6 cases. *J Bone Joint Surg* 1975;57A:230–236.

Geesink RGT, Manley MT (eds): *Hydroxylapatite Coatings in Orthopaedic Surgery.* New York, New York, Raven Press, 1993.

Harris WH, Davies JP: Why cement is weak and how it can be strengthened, in Tullos HS (ed): *Instructional Course Lectures, Volume* XL. Park Ridge, IL, American Academy of Orthopaedic Surgeons, 1990, pp 141–143.

Howie DW, Cornish BL, Vernon-Roberts B: Resurfacing hip arthroplasty: Classification of loosening and the role of prosthesis wear particles. *Clin Orthop* 1990;255:144–159.

Murray DW, Rushton N: Macrophages stimulate bone resorption when they phagocytose particles. *J Bone Joint Surg* 1990;72B:988–992.

Plitz W, Hoss HU: Wear of alumina-ceramic hip joints: Some clinical and tribological aspects, in Winter GD, Gibbons DF, Plenk H (eds): *Biomaterials 1980.* New York, NY, John Wiley & Sons, 1982, pp 187–196.

Rostoker W, Chao EY, Galante JO: Defects in failed stems of hip prostheses. *J Biomed Mater Res* 1978;12:635–651.

5

The Role of Polyethylene Quality in Wear

Wear Damage in Polyethylene

Ultra high molecular weight polyethylene (hereafter referred to as polyethylene) is currently the polymer of choice for bearing surfaces in prosthetic devices. Although polyethylene is well suited for articulation with metal surfaces, clinical data reveal that the material often suffers damage in service (Fig. 1). Observations of fatigue failure and wear damage in polyethylene tibial and acetabular components, and the problems of osteolysis associated with wear debris, have indicated the importance of improving the wear characteristics of the polyethylene components. The requirements are complex; implants are subject to environmental, mechanical, and patient specific demands. In vivo service inevitably initiates polyethylene wear and damage, which are clinically evident to dramatically varying degrees in retrieved components.

Many researchers have hypothesized causes for the wear and damage; these causes include implant and material specific characteristics. Implant specific characteristics include component design and contact stress level, while material specific characteristics include polyethylene molecular weight distribution, presence of fusion defects, and component aging. Some researchers have shown that correlations between damage and patient weight, as well as damage and duration of implantation, indicated that loading was responsible for much damage in knees. The high stresses found subsurface in knee components were logically linked to subsurface delamination and pitting in the tibial trays. However, such studies did not account for variations in wear damage found in polyethylene components with similar designs and service histories. These variations suggest the involvement of other factors in clinical wear. Greater wear in low molecular weight regions has been cited by some. Wear rates have been shown to increase by a factor of up to 30 when molecular weight is reduced. However, examination of two components with the same design—one displaying substantial wear, and the other in fair condition—led to the conclusion that design, contact stress, and molecular weight distribution cannot be solely responsible for wear. This conclusion further supports the idea that undetermined material factors may influence polyethylene wear rates.

In the analyses of polyethylene, studies have been conducted to determine the relationship between material characteristics (ie, consolidation, third body inclusions, oxidation) and implant performance. Studies of retrieved and never implanted polyethylene components have identified in thin sections of polyethylene two distinct characteristics that may be related to the quality and wear resis-

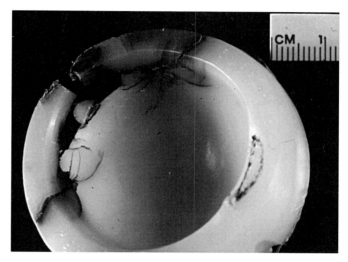

Fig. 1 Clinically retrieved acetabular cup with cracking and delamination.

tance of the material. One phenomenon, termed fusion defects, appears as randomly distributed, often circular, particles. The other phenomenon is a subsurface band, which appears after microtoming as a white line and follows the contour of the component (Fig. 2). Examination of these characteristics indicated that they are the result of polyethylene processing.

Polyethylene Processing

Because wear behaviors may be influenced by the specific properties of the material, information regarding the polyethylene components is becoming more valuable. However, unlike the metal components used in total joint applications, few of the older polyethylene devices are marked with identification numbers. As a result, the history of the components now being analyzed in retrieval studies is extremely difficult to trace back to the raw material from which components were made. The grade of polyethylene powder used, the consolidation processing parameters, the fabrication date, and the sterilization method may all be critical to the subsequent performance of the prosthesis; yet, specific data on any retrieved component are difficult to obtain. It is clear that all polyethylene is not the same and that variations in processing polyethylene may con-

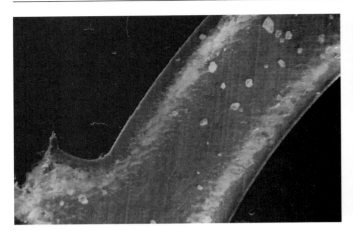

Fig. 2 Thin polyethylene section showing a subsurface band and fusion defects.

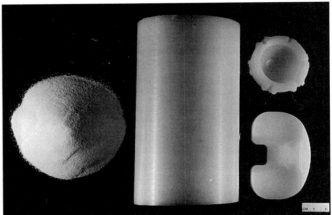

Fig. 3 Polyethylene fabrication stages; resin, stock, and final component.

tribute to the observed differences in fatigue and wear. Motivated by these ideas, several companies are now providing serial numbers on all polyethylene components and carefully recording the origin of the polyethylene and the specifics associated with all of the manufacturing steps. This information will be invaluable in the study of future retrieved components and may yield insight into wear damage and component failures. Figure 3 depicts polyethylene at different processing stages.

Polyethylene Powder Fabrication

There are currently two companies in the United States, Himont (Wilmington, DE) and Hoechst Celanese (Houston, TX), that produce the polyethylene powder from which orthopaedic components are made. Both companies use the same basic technology to form the powder that is provided to companies for resin to stock conversion, followed by commercial use. According to company representatives, the polyethylene powder is produced using titanium chloride and an aluminum alkyl catalyst and a co-catalyst. A different co-catalyst, the identity of which is proprietary information, is used by each company. This difference results in subtle variations in the powder including trace element levels and particle morphology.

The powder resin is generated via a polymerization process whereby ethylene monomers are linked together and transformed into a polymer chain that sustains growth, provided that necessary reactants are supplied. Chains are grown in a reactor using the catalyst, which can be found at the core of every particle. As ethylene gas is bubbled through hexane liquid, monomers diffuse to the surface of the catalyst where outward molecular chain growth begins. According to the manufacturers, the deeply buried catalyst cannot be retrieved from the powder, nor is it thought to

have any effect on the subsequent consolidation process in which the polyethylene stock material is formed. Once the molecular chain growth is completed, the liquid-slurry phase containing the powder and remaining hexane is removed and centrifuged to reduce the hexane content to a few parts per million. The centrifuging and two drying stages are conducted in a nitrogen environment. After a third drying stage in air, the polyethylene powder fabrication is complete.

Physical properties and molecular weight are determined largely by the aforementioned polymerization process. The actual process itself can be affected by conditions including temperature and pressure, and by chemicals including the catalyst. Therefore, it is imperative that the reaction be closely monitored and controlled. The powder must pass the standards indicated in the ASTM Annual Book of Standards. According to one guideline (F648), if the resulting polyethylene powder has a relative solution viscosity of 2.30 or greater and certain trace element levels, it can be used in medical grade applications, such as total joint replacement. The ASTM guidelines (F648), instituted in 1984, also require the amount of the trace elements allowed in the powder to be less than the following: aluminum, 100 ppm; titanium, 300 ppm; calcium, 100 ppm; and chlorine, 120 ppm. Most polyethylene resin fulfills the broad ASTM requirements.

GUR 415

There are three different grades of polyethylene powder typically used in medical grade applications: Hostalen GUR 415 (now labeled GUR 4150HP), Hostalen GUR 412 (Hoechst Celanese and Hoechst Germany), and Himont 1900. GUR 415 is said to have a bulk density of 0.4 g/cm³, an average powder size of 125 μm (range: 60 to 250 μm), and a yield value within the range 0.3 to 0.5

N/mm², 10 min. This yield value is based on the stress required for 600% elongation of the material in 10 minutes. The GUR 415 also contains the additive calcium stearate. This metal stearate is added to the resin (0.05% of the total volume) to act as a lubricant, anticorrosive agent, and whitener. As a lubricant, the calcium stearate is used to reduce friction between polymer particles, thus lowering the melt viscosity and reducing the energy required for processing. Also, it was initially used to lessen corrosion resulting from the residual Cl^- ion from the $TiCl_4$ catalyst used in powder formation. Residual Cl^- ions combine with H^+ from water to form HCl. This problem is no longer of large scale concern due to the reduction of residual Cl^- ions.

GUR 412

Another grade of polyethylene powder, GUR 412, which also contains calcium stearate, is formed by the same method as GUR 415. The differences between GUR 412 and GUR 415 are in the material properties. GUR 412 also has a bulk density of 0.4 g/cm³ and an average powder size of 125 μm (range 60 to 250 μm). However, it has a lower yield value of 0.20 to 0.25 N/mm², 10 min. There is also a difference in the molecular weight of the two powders. GUR 412 typically has a lower molecular weight, which indicates shorter molecular chains in the bulk material. Because the forming process results in a large range of molecular weights of the individual powder particles, some GUR 412 powder particles could have a higher molecular weight than some GUR 415 particles. According to some researchers, the increased chain length of GUR 415 provides increased strength to the bulk material and increased resistance to wear damage, specifically abrasion. Some believe that the decreased molecular weight of GUR 412 may partially explain the differences seen in the wear characteristics of different components.

Himont 1900

The other polyethylene powder used in medical applications is Himont 1900. The differences between Himont 1900 and the GUR powders are in particle morphology, size of the powder, and trace element content. Himont 1900 has an average particle size of 180 to 190 μm with a narrower range. Sources indicate that Himont 1900 typically has a lower molecular weight, but is available in a variety of molecular weights, which can be specified by the purchaser. The levels of trace elements, which are present in the powder as a result of the co-catalyst used by Himont, are said to be slightly higher than those of the GUR resins.

Polyethylene Stock and Component Fabrication

The polyethylene components used in total joint replacement are typically made using one of two processes. Components are either formed by machining or compression molding. In the first case, components are machined directly from either polyethylene sheet or bar stock supplied from a converter (Poly Hi Solidur, Fort Wayne, IN; Westlake Plastics, Lenni, PA; Hoechst, Germany) using one of the powders described above. Compression molded components are made by molding powder directly into the required geometry.

In the fabrication of sheet stock, the powder is press molded into sheets from which components are machined. According to manufacturers, in the press molding process, powder is placed in a 4- by 8-ft mold, leveled with a straightedge, and cold compressed under a pressure of approximately 7 to 10 MPa for 5 to 10 minutes to expel the air trapped in the powder. The press is then heated to approximately 200°C until the powder is plasticated, or fused, throughout. Heating is accomplished using steam heating from pipes within the confines of the plates. Sections adjacent to the steam pipes reach peak temperature before other regions. As a result, the time spent at peak temperature is apparently a function of location. Polyethylene does not flow at its melting point, thus it is unable to transmit uniform pressure. Therefore, compression molded sheet may yield pockets and variations of density. After the powder is completely fused, the mold is cooled under approximately 7 to 10 MPa. Poor quality, initiated by incomplete fusion and porosity, may be apparent if optimum heating, pressurizing, and cooling conditions are not used.

Polyethylene bar stock is formed by ram extrusion. In this process, powder is introduced from a hopper into the cylinder of the ram extruder. The material in the extruder is packed or forced through the die at frequent intervals with a reciprocating ram. The compacted material passes through a heated zone of the die ranging in temperature from 180°C to 200°C in order to become plasticated. The length of this zone is said to depend on the geometry of the final product; it must be long enough for complete fusion of the material. This is important due to the poor melt properties of polyethylene powder.

During the ram extrusion process, a cone of polyethylene material forms in front of the center of the ram, within the die. This cone, opaque in appearance, is made of compacted powder that has not achieved the melt temperature of the powder. Material, which has attained melt temperature and appears as a translucent gel, surrounds the unmelted cone. When the ram moves through the extruder there is a delay in the movement of the extrudate or polyethylene. This delay allows a buildup of pressure that forces the unmelted cone of compacted powder into the gel region surrounding it, where it then melts. Improper pressure and temperature may result in an unfused interface between the gel and cone. Manufacturers agree that care must be taken to avoid the incomplete fusion of the bar stock.

Compression molding directly from polyethylene powder is the other technique used to manufacture components used in total joint replacement. In this process, the polyethylene powder is placed in a die with the desired component geometry and subjected to a heat and pressure cycle to form the final component. The polyethylene components may either be molded directly onto the component's metal backing or may be formed separately and then inserted into the metal.

In both stock formation and direct compression molding, control of the consolidation parameters are necessary to ensure a homogeneous and defect-free material. Due to the characteristics of polyethylene, especially its high melt viscosity, the processing variables must be controlled and specifically adjusted for the die used to avoid material weaknesses, which may give rise to failure. These weaknesses, manifested as a decreased material quality, may be responsible for some of the wear damage noted in retrieved components. By assessing the different parameters and determining the optimal processing conditions, uniform, high quality polyethylene components may be formed. These components may have better fatigue characteristics, thus eliminating several of the recent concerns regarding the wear of polyethylene components, the subsequent generation of wear debris, and the associated tissue and bone necrosis.

Enhanced Polyethylenes

Recently, several companies have introduced "enhanced" polyethylenes, which are so named because of special processing conditions. It is suggested by the manufacturers that these conditions may enhance resistance to wear and oxidation. One such line is the Hylamer product produced by DuPont (Wilmington, DE). Hylamer and Hylamer M are made from GUR 415 bar stock, which has been isostatically compressed to increase the material's crystallinity. It is hypothesized that an increase in crystallinity will enhance the material properties and performance, although stiffness is also increased. Another newly available product is ArCom produced by Biomet (Warsaw, IN). ArCom begins with 1900 resin and is compression molded, in an argon environment, into bar stock from which components can be made. The ArCom products are also packaged and sterilized in an argon environment. ArCom's manufacturer claims that the material has a higher ultimate tensile strength and a lower wear rate than standard polyethylene. However, because each of these materials has only recently been introduced, long-term clinical studies on wear resistance are not yet available.

Component Packaging and Sterilization

Fully fabricated components are packaged in materials selected by the manufacturer, and then they are sterilized. Most polyethylene components are sealed in plastic containers that are nested within an outer plastic container and a box. The protection that the packaging provides

from oxygen infiltration varies depending on the manufacturer.

It is imperative that all prosthetic implants be sterile. Current sterilization techniques employ gamma radiation or ethylene oxide gassing. Gamma irradiation of components is the most common method for sterilization. Components are prepackaged, typically in air, although sometimes in an inert atmosphere such as argon or nitrogen, or in vacuum. The sterilization contractor states that packaged components are placed within a carrier or box, which is conveyed past a cobalt 60 radiation source that emits gamma radiation. Although the beam is assumed to fully penetrate the polyethylene, the amount of radiation absorbed is a function of the location within the carrier. The dose, measured by dosimeters, which change color according to absorbed dosage, typically ranges from 2.5 to 4.5 Mrad. Carrier dosage mappings indicate that there are regions of maximum and minimum absorbance.

The second method for component sterilization is ethylene oxide (EtO) gassing. Currently, two orthopaedic manufacturers state that they are extensively using the EtO method to sterilize components. The entire EtO process comprises a series of interdependent steps. Products to be sterilized are first placed in a vacuum chamber for a pre-humidification or preconditioning stage during which specimens are heated and humidified. This hydrates spores and microbial flora, increasing their susceptibility to the lethal effects of the EtO. The chamber, filled with components, is subsequently charged with EtO gas at specific concentrations. Following exposure, the gas is exhausted in a suitable fashion. The sterilized units are repeatedly flushed with air and finally released from the vacuum chamber upon completion. However, the components must be held in inventory for up to 2 weeks until the outgassing of EtO residuals has reached an acceptable level. Any small deviation from the set parameters may affect the lethality of the gas and render the surface sterilization process ineffective. Although there are some sterility, inventory control, and residual materials concerns associated with EtO, the overall process does not appear to be influential on or detrimental to the polyethylene material, structure, and chemical composition when performed correctly.

Damage Mechanisms

Concerns regarding material consolidation have arisen. Fusion defects have been hypothesized by some as influential in the extent of clinical damage appearing in retrievals. Fusion defects were said to affect crack initiation, crack propagation, and crater formation. Researchers believed that the fusion defects indicated weak bonds between powder particles, predisposing the polyethylene to failure when loaded.

It has been suggested that fusion defects may affect the material behavior of the polyethylene, resulting in great variations in its wear and fatigue resistance. The presence and distribution of these defects, coupled with molecular weight distribution and contact stresses, have been implicated as controlling factors in determining the fatigue resistance of the material. It still appears unclear whether defect-filled material is the result of poorly controlled processing parameters, or if it is, perhaps, due to differences in the polyethylene powder. Whether all of the defects are present at the time of production, or if they emerge with time, has not yet been agreed upon. The production of defect-free material may alleviate the problems in the future; however, current research indicates that the clinical effect of fusion defects remains inconclusive. Other potential wear factors, discussed below, have been discovered.

Another material feature, which consists of fine cracking with the maximum intensity at 1 to 2 mm below a clear zone of material at the surface, was described in literature as a material discontinuity in knees. This phenomenon was more pronounced in worn components. The microcracking was considered to be delamination, and it was attributed to defect-filled material decaying under in vivo stress. This conclusion seemed logical and was supported by the fact that maximum stresses in knees are found at this subsurface location. Others considered the subsurface material cracking to be related to machining or compression molding. However, due to limitations of sample diversity and sample size, there was a lack of conclusive data regarding its cause and effect.

Recent extensive research has revealed that the presence of the subsurface white band has a significant clinical impact and may very well explain excessive wear and fatigue in polyethylene implants. The presence of the band is directly correlated with clinical polyethylene cracking and delamination. An extensive and diverse sample set revealed that the white band clearly did not stem from defects or machining or molding. It was found in defect-free and defect-filled components and in both molded and machined components. Furthermore, the band, which follows the contour of the component, was found in components that were never implanted, indicating that the band was not the result of in vivo stress. The white band was found to be a region of highly oxidized material. The location of the white band corresponded to high, peak levels of oxidation as measured by Fourier Transform Infrared Spectroscopy, a chemical analysis tool. Interestingly, the subsurface white band was found only in components that were gamma sterilized in air, whether they were retrieved or never implanted. Nonsterile and EtO sterilized components studied did not show the white band or the correspondingly high oxidation levels (Fig. 4).

Gamma sterilization has long been recognized as causing chain scission, cross-linking, and oxidation in polymers. The radiation dissociates molecular bonds and generates free radicals in the polymer, which can then bond with oxygen, resulting in oxidation that deteriorates the polyethylene. The process whereby radicals react with oxygen is time dependent and increases with time postirradiation. The subsurface band was seen in components in this

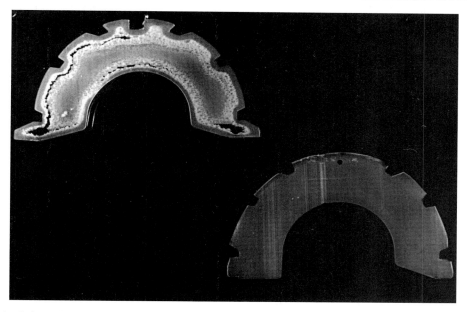

Fig. 4 Nonsterile polyethylene shown with gamma sterilized polyethylene with a subsurface band (same material lot).

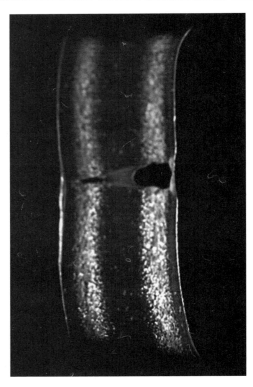

Fig. 5 Tensile sample of polyethylene thin section breaking in subsurface region.

study only when they were near 3 years or more postirradiation.

Further research indicated that the oxidation caused embrittlement and reduction of mechanical properties in the polyethylene. Mechanical testing revealed that components with the white band had dramatically reduced mechanical properties, which thus affect the ability of the component to withstand stress. The ultimate tensile strengths were reduced nearly 50% while the elongation was reduced by an order of magnitude in comparison to polyethylene stock. Thin-section tensile samples from retrievals with a subsurface white band failed almost instantly when loaded in tension, with the crack initiating in the banded region (Fig. 5). Clinical retrievals indicated cracking and delamination, which may be related to the brittleness associated with the presence of the white band.

In support of this, other research on wear testing showed statistically significant differences between polyethylene that was not sterile or recently gamma sterilized when compared to shelf-aged gamma sterilized material. Pin-on disk wear tests on polyethylene samples showed the time dependence of oxidation resulting from gamma irradiation. Shelf-aged, irradiated samples had higher wear rates.

Much of the research on the damage mechanisms of polyethylene comes from retrieved components. The studies presented document the presence of both fusion defects and the gamma-induced, subsurface white band. The presence of the subsurface white band has been verified to be the result of gamma sterilization in air, not only through retrieval studies, but also through laboratory experiments. However, the controlled production of fusion defects is not well documented. These degrading material characteristics require further investigation and understanding so that detrimental stages of material processing can be modified. Modification of material inconsistencies would hopefully lead to higher quality material, with increased wear resistance and increased clinical performance and longevity.

Annotated Bibliography

Bartel DL, Bicknell VL, Wright TM: The effect of conformity, thickness, and material on stresses in ultra-high molecular weight components for total joint replacement. *J Bone Joint Surg* 1986;68A:1041–1051.

Wear debris is thought to contribute to long term problems with prostheses. Knees examined in the study were found to have higher contact stresses than hips. Suggestions for reducing stresses included using more conforming parts and thicker polyethylene.

Ellis JR: EtO: Does it have a future? *Med Device Diagnos Industry* 1990;50–51.

EtO was formerly the most widely used method for sterilization of medical devices. However, radiation has captured much of the market. The paper discusses the safeties and effectiveness of EtO, as well as its chemical reactivity and the need for outgassing.

Fisher J, Hailey JL, Chan KL, et al: The effect of aging following irradiation on the wear of UHMWPE. *Trans Orthop Res Soc* 1995;20:12.

Factors contributing to increased wear rates were identified. Never irradiated material, irradiated material aged for 2 months, and irradiated material at least 5 years old was studied in pin-on disk tests. The wear for the 5-year-old irradiated specimens was three times higher than that for never irradiated components. The differences in these wear rates were statistically significant.

Hastings RS, Woodling T: Polyethylene fatigue performance. *Trans Soc Biomater* 1995;18:341.

Fatigue performance of different polyethylene was investigated. Older material was found to have more unfused particles and higher fatigue failure rates than newer material.

Hoechst Celanese: Hostalen GUR UHMW polymer technical literature. Houston, TX, Hoechst Celanese, 1994.

Material literature contains descriptions of all of the GUR ultrahigh molecular weight polyethylene resin available. The chemical and mechanical properties of each grade are documented along with recommended processing conditions.

Landy MM, Walker PS: Wear of ultra-high-molecular-weight polyethylene components of 90 retrieved knee prostheses. *J Arthroplasty* 1988;3(suppl):S73–S85.

Wear in retrieved knees was investigated. Landy claimed that delamination was only found in material with defects. One material defect was described as a microcracked material zone below a clear zone at the surface. Processing is implicated as affecting the material integrity.

Rimnac CM, Klein RW, Betts F, et al: Post-irradiation aging of ultra high molecular weight polyethylene. *J Bone Joint Surg* 1994;76A:1052–1056.

Oxidative degradation was studied in irradiated shelf-stored samples. Density and infrared spectra were evaluated as a function of depth into the polyethylene. Gamma sterilization and shelf aging supported the hypothesis that oxidative degradation and altered material properties occur. The wear resistance of shelf-stored components was speculated to be poor.

Rose RM, Cimino WR, Ellis E, et al: Exploratory investigations on the structure dependence of the wear resistance of polyethylene. *Wear* 1982;77:89–104.

Wear rates of polyethylene were investigated using hemisphere-on-flat sliding wear testers. The results indicated that wear rates increase by a factor of 30 when molecular weight is decreased. Irradiation at typical doses was said to improve wear resistance, as was having only few material defects present.

Sutula LC, Saum KA, Collier JP, et al: Time dependent oxidation and damage in retrieved and never implanted UHMWPE components. *Trans Orthop Res Soc* 1995;20:118–120.

Gamma sterilization in air was found to produce high subsurface oxidation in many components. The region appeared as a subsurface white band following the component's contour and was not found in never sterilized or EtO sterilized components. The band, which did not appear until several years postirradiation, was highly embrittled and correlated with clinical cracking and delamination.

Sanford WM, Saum KA: Accelerated oxidative aging testing of UHMWPE. *Trans Orthop Res Soc* 1995;20:119.

Accelerated oxidation was used to study oxidative degradation in material sterilized in different fashions and aged for different periods. Oxidation levels increased with aging time. Gamma sterilized components showed high peak levels of oxidation at the subsurface.

Sun DC, Schmidig G, Stark C, et al: On the origins of a subsurface oxidation maximum and its relationship to the performance of UHMWPE implants. *Trans Soc Biomater* 1995;18:362.

This study investigated the subsurface oxidation maximum in polyethylene components. The subsurface location is said to be a function of an oxidation profile and a radiation dose profile. The oxidation is effected by the environment in which it ages.

Trieu HH, Avent RT, Paxson RD: Effect of sterilization on shelf-aged UHMWPE tibial inserts. *Trans Soc Biomater* 1995;18:109.

The effect of different sterilization methods on polyethylene were examined at different poststerilization ages. A highly oxidized subsurface band was seen in aged gamma sterilized in air samples, but not in newly irradiated or EtO samples. Free radicals, availability of oxygen, and sufficient time for oxygen diffusion are all cited as necessary in order for this band to form.

6

Polymethylmethacrylate

The use of polymethylmethacrylate bone cement (PMMA) to anchor total joint prosthetic components to the skeleton has revolutionized the surgical treatment of end-stage arthritis. However, late prosthetic loosening had been a major problem with total joint arthroplasties (TJA) and it was usually due to suboptimal techniques and prosthetic designs resulting in the separation of the interfaces and cement mantle fractures. Improvements in the use of cement, such as plugging the femoral canal, cleaning the bone surfaces, pressurizing the cement with a gun, and maintaining adequate cement mantle thickness around the implants, and improvements in the designs of prosthetic components that protect the cement have markedly reduced the loosening rates. The chemical, physical, and biologic properties of the cement and the recent advances made in use of cement are discussed in this chapter.

Chemical and Physical Properties of PMMA

PMMA is a polymer of methyl methacrylate with the chemical formulation CH_2: $C(CH_2)(COOCH_3)$:CH_2 - - -. Polymerization of methyl methacrylate monomer is usually a highly exothermic and slow process. Industrial polymers of methyl methacrylate such as Plexiglas are made under high pressures and temperatures to yield clear nonporous polymers with high strength. In contrast, the bulk of surgical PMMA is supplied as a powder, which was polymerized in a dispersion medium by a "pearl polymerization" process. The monomer, which is supplied as liquid, fuses the prepolymerized powder particles achieving a rapid cure rate and lower temperatures.

There are subtle differences in the chemical and physical characteristics of the powder and liquid constituents of the different commercial formulations of PMMA, and these can affect the physical properties of the cements. Zimmer Regular (Zimmer, Warsaw, IN), LVC (Zimmer, Warsaw, IN), and CMW (CMW Laboratories Ltd, Exeter, Devon, England) bone cement powders contain polymethylmethacrylate polymer, whereas Simplex P powder contains a mixture of polymethylmethacrylate and methyl methacrylate-styrene copolymer. Barium sulfate is added as a radiopacifier to Zimmer Regular, LVC, CMW, and Simplex P cements, and zirconium oxide is added as a radiopacifier to Palacos (Salzer & Co., GmbH, Wehrheim, Germany). Chlorophyll is used in Palacos to provide a green tint. Hydroquinone is added to PMMA to prevent premature polymerization, and N,N-dimethyl-p-toluidine is added to promote the curing. The powder particle sizes are varied by the manufacturers to obtain different viscosities and working times. By these techniques, low viscosity is obtained for LVC and Zimmer regular bone cements, intermediate viscosity for Simplex P, and high viscosity for Palacos R and CMW bone cements. Chilling the monomer maintains a longer period of low viscosity state for most PMMA formulations. The monomer is sterilized by membrane filtration and the powder is sterilized by gamma irradiation at 2.5 Mrad.

PMMA polymer has an average molecular weight of 200,000. The molecular weight increases by 20% after polymerization. The setting time can vary depending on the brand, batch, ambient temperature, humidity, temperature of the monomer and powder, liquid to powder ratio, and the amount of material polymerized. It is usually about 12 minutes, with a working time of 8 minutes and dough time of 4 minutes. Increase in the ambient temperature is the most usual cause of shorter setting time, and the chilling of the monomer is the most usual cause of longer setting time. It is recommended that PMMA be inserted into the bone in the dough stage (when it does not adhere to the surgical glove). Considerable exothermicity and volumetric changes take place in PMMA during curing. During the initial phase (first 3 to 4 minutes), the monomer molecules form chains leading to polymerization shrinkage of 7% of the mass without temperature rise. During the latter phase (3 to 4 minutes) the temperature rises rapidly (60°C for a 3-mm specimen versus 107°C for a 10-mm specimen), and the cement undergoes thermal expansion while the prosthesis, blood, and bone act as heat sinks. The cement then cools and undergoes thermal contraction. Removal of porosity leads to increased thermal contraction. Volumetric contraction of 3% to 7% has been found between 6 and 40 minutes after mixing (time at which the cement shrinks in the femoral canal). However, the diametric or radial shrinkage, which is a more important parameter for the separation at the interface, is less than 0.5% and is not influenced by porosity reduction.

Mechanical Properties

Once cured, PMMA becomes a brittle glassy polymer with limited plastic deformation prior to failure. Its elastic modulus is approximately 2.3 gigapascals (GPa), between the one GPa of cancellous bone and 16 GPa of cortical bone. Thus, its elasticity is similar to that of bone but ten times lower than that of the metal prostheses. This difference in the elastic modulus between the prosthesis and the cement gives rise to high stresses at the PMMA–prosthesis interface and within the PMMA; it is most pronounced at the most proximal and distal ends of the prosthesis where the stresses are the greatest. Thus, the PMMA is susceptible to debonding from the metal and fracturing, starting at these locations. Prosthetic devices with sharp corners or edges create stress risers in PMMA and can lead to premature fractures of the mantle. The cross-sectional shape, geometric configuration, stem length, and material properties of the femoral components can profoundly influence the stresses in the cement mantle. Femoral components with broad medial borders, large area moments of inertia, and lengths greater than 100 mm are recommended to lower these stresses.

PMMA is stronger in compression than tension. It has a compressive strength of 15,000 psi, tensile strength of 10,000 psi, and flexural strength of 15,000 psi. It is 25% weaker than cortical bone in tension, 50% weaker in compression, and 50% weaker in shear. PMMA should always be supported by bone; unsupported cement tends to fracture. PMMA is also viscoelastic and becomes stiffer and stronger with higher strain rates. It does exhibit creep, but the magnitude of creep under physiologic loads and its significance are not known. PMMA continues to become stronger with time; 90% of the tensile strength is reached by 4 hours and 100% by 24 hours after the start of polymerization. The PMMA does age and absorb fluid in vivo, but the effect of aging on the mechanical strength is minimal.

Loosening of cemented femoral components has been shown to be related to fractures of the cement mantle. Several attempts have been made to improve the strength of PMMA. Modifying the powder phase by techniques such as increasing the degree of polymerization or varying the particle size have thus far been unsuccessful due to the technological limitations and the expenses involved in developing and testing new formulations. Reinforcing fiber additives such as carbon, graphite, Kevlar, titanium, stainless steel fibers, or bioactive glass ceramics also can increase the fatigue strength of PMMA, but they markedly increase the viscosity and limit trabecular bone intrusion. The additives also increase the elastic modulus of PMMA, which may in turn lead to higher cement stresses. Reduction of porosity has shown the most promise. Hand-mixed PMMA contains many large voids from air entrapment during mixing and small voids from evaporation of the volatile monomers; these voids act as stress risers. Mixing the powder and liquid in a vacuum or centrifuging after mixing markedly reduces the porosity and improves the strength of PMMA. Simplex P specimens centrifuged for 30 seconds after mixing at 2,000 rpm showed 50% reduction in porosity, 24% increase in the ultimate tensile strength, 54% increase in the ultimate tensile strain, and 136% increase in fatigue life without a change in the elastic modulus, setting time, or peak temperature. Vacuum mixing also produced a significant reduction in the porosity of Simplex P, increased its fatigue life, and improved the fracture toughness.

The increase in the fatigue strength obtained by reducing the porosity has been related to the mechanical requirements of PMMA. Strains of about 1,000 μS have been measured in PMMA around the femoral components of THA in cadaver femurs under simulated stance. At this strain level, 70% of uncentrifuged PMMA samples failed before 10 million cycles (simulating 10 years of walking), but none of the centrifuged specimens failed reaching what is termed endurance limit (stress below which the material does not fail).

The porosity, fatigue strengths, and the effects of mixing techniques on fatigue strengths vary in the different formulations of PMMA. When mixed according to manufacturer's instructions, the porosity is about 10% for Simplex P, AKZ, and Palacos R; 5% for LVC; and 12% for Zimmer and CMW. The fatigue strengths of the cements range from 879 cycles (Zimmer Regular) to 15,147 cycles (Simplex P). Within each type of cement formulation, the change in porosity by centrifugation correlates with a change in the fatigue strength. Chilling the monomer increases the porosity and reduces fatigue strengths of all cements. Centrifugation for 30 seconds after mixing resulted in significant decrease in porosity and increase in fatigue strengths of Simplex P and Zimmer Regular, but did not substantially improve very low viscosity cements such as LVC or very high viscosity cements such as Palacos. The best fatigue strengths were obtained with Simplex P when it was prepared by mixing with the monomer at 0°C and centrifuging at 2,000 to 4,000 rpm for 60 seconds. This technique provided an excellent low viscosity state and high fatigue strength.

Inclusions and additives may or may not affect the mechanical strength of PMMA. The addition of 10% barium sulfate (to make it radiopaque) was found not to significantly affect the shear strength of PMMA. Inclusions of blood and tissue debris can lead to stress risers and profoundly reduce the strength of cement, although the effect of these substances has not been quantified rigorously. Approximately 20% reduction in compressive strength and 50% to 70% reduction in tensile strength have been reported by the admixture of blood. Laminations in PMMA due to the presence of blood in the femoral canal reduce the tensile strength by half. Thorough cleaning and drying of the canal and maintaining hemostasis either by using hypotensive anesthesia or packing the canal with a sponge soaked in a dilute solution of adrenaline (1:500,000) are recommended to minimize the chances of blood and tissue admixture.

Methylene blue is sometimes added to PMMA to give visual contrast from the surrounding bone if revision becomes necessary. No detrimental effect has been noted by adding 1 cm^3 of methylene blue powder. Irradiation of cement used in the fixation of pathologic fractures has not been found to significantly reduce the mechanical properties of PMMA.

Interface With Bone and Metal

Strong bone support and penetration of PMMA into bone are important for long-term implant fixation. The strongest trabecular bone in the femur is located very near to the cortex, and the cement–bone shear strength can be maximized by curetting the weak trabecular bone up to a millimeter from the cortex and interdigitating the cement with the stronger trabecular bone under pressure. The viscosity and the magnitude of delivery pressures determine the intrusion depth of PMMA into bone. Simplex P injected with a commercially available gun at 20 psi intrudes to a depth of 5 mm in bovine cancellous bone. Low-viscosity cements such as LVC intrude further, but are weaker in fatigue. High-viscosity cements such as Palacos intrude less. Plugging the distal medullary canal and pressurizing cement with a gun improve the PMMA intrusion into bone. Bone, polyethylene, and cement have been used as plugs, but cement plugs and proximal canal seals are more reliable and give greater pressures.

PMMA is more of a grout than an adhesive, and the strength of the cement–metal interface is substantially lower than that of the bulk cement. The cement–metal interface is also degraded by exposure to physiologic fluids. Finite element analysis as well as experimental strain studies suggest that loosening the bond between the metal and cement would cause increased stresses in the cement mantle and lead to fractures and loosening. Radiographic follow-up studies and postmortem studies of patients who have had total hip arthroplasty suggest that separation of the metal–PMMA interface initiates the loosening process. Mechanical interdigitations with rough or textured surfaces improve this bond strength. Electrostatic deposition of a thin film of PMMA onto the prosthesis (precoating) forms an intermolecular adhesion at the surface and markedly improves the shear strength at the cement–metal interface, which is not degraded by saline. The precoated surfaces can also resist tensile strains because of the chemical bonding.

Systemic Effects

PMMA monomer is very volatile and toxic. When injected intravenously in rabbits, a dose of 0.03 ml/kg body weight produces a sudden and transient fall in arterial blood pressure. The fatal dose has been calculated to be 125 mg/l of blood volume. At doses less than this, PMMA monomer has been shown to cause pulmonary congestion, edema, degeneration, and necrosis. It is also very fat soluble. Retrieval studies of the surface of the cement mantle show numerous unpolymerized particles due to loss of monomer in adjacent marrow fat. The major monomer loss occurs during mixing, but small amounts of monomer can enter systemic circulation during injection and curing. The monomer is cleared rapidly by the lung. About 0.2% to 0.5% monomer is retained in PMMA after curing, and this eventually is leached out and excreted by the body. Monomeric PMMA is metabolized to methacrylic acid, which is turned into carbon dioxide via the tricarboxylic acid cycle.

Several instances of cardiac arrest and sudden deaths were attributed to the monomer leaching into the systemic circulation. However, it is not clear that the cause of death is directly related to the toxicity of the monomer, because the hypotension usually precedes the appearance of the monomer in the circulation. The lowering of the blood pressure during cementing the prostheses is related instead to fat, air, or marrow emboli and to release of anaphylaxins. Fat and marrow contents emboli are consistently identified in the pulmonary circulation during autopsies. The embolization of fat and marrow contents precipitates aggregation of platelets and fibrin and releases tissue thromboplastic products into the circulation. It is generally agreed, however, that the hemodynamic instability during cementing can be avoided if the patient is normotensive and normovolemic before the insertion of the cement into the femur. The blood loss should be measured accurately and fluid loss completely replaced before cementing the components to avoid cardiovascular problems.

Allergic reactions to the acrylic cement have been proposed, but there is little evidence to suggest that PMMA induces an allergic response. Transient elevations in liver function tests have also been reported with the use of PMMA, but significant hepatotoxicity has not been shown. Although PMMA has been shown to be mutagenic for bacteria, there is no evidence to suggest that PMMA has a carcinogenic or mutagenic potential in humans.

Long-term Biocompatibility

The initial histologic changes with cementing consist of a small layer of tissue necrosis immediately adjacent to the mantle, followed by a period of repair, which lasts from 3 weeks to 2 years. The PMMA in bulk form, however, is very well tolerated by the skeleton over many years. Postmortem studies of femurs of patients who had received cemented femoral components up to 17 years earlier show the formation of a new layer of bone intimately apposed to the cement mantle (termed neocortex) and osteoporosis of the adjacent cortex. The endosteal expansion does not necessarily lead to prosthetic loosening. An intimate bond exists between PMMA and bone over the long term with rare or no intervening fibrous tissue. The particulate form of PMMA liberated by the mantle fragmentation, however, leads to a foreign-body granulomatous tissue reaction containing numerous macrophages and giant cells in a fibrous tissue stroma. The cells in the tissue have been shown to produce a variety of biochemical products such as interleukin–1, platelet-derived growth factor, tumor necrosis factor, prostaglandin E2, collagenase, and various metalloproteinases, which are implicated in pathologic bone resorption. Cells grown from the tissue have also been shown to resorb bone in vitro. Cell culture studies show that PMMA particles are phagocytosed by macrophages, which leads to their macrophage activation and release of bone resorbing agents. Means to protect the PMMA from fragmentation are expected to improve the longevity of implant fixation by decreasing the particulate debris and the associated adverse biologic reactions.

Adjunctive Applications

Antibiotics are sometimes added to PMMA in the treatment of infected total joint arthroplasties and osteomyelitis to provide high local antibiotic delivery by gradual diffusion into surrounding fluids and tissues. The PMMA is used as beads to fill dead spaces or in the bulk cement during primary or delayed exchange. Most antibiotics remain biologically active in PMMA. Clindamycin was preferred because it was shown to maintain high breakpoint sensitivity concentrations (transition between bacterial killing and resistance) in seroma, granulation tissue, and bone, as well as being effective for *Staphylococcus aureus, S. epidermidis,* nonenterococcal streptococcus, and anaerobes. Tobramycin gives excellent seroma and granulation tissue concentrations and is effective against many Gram negative organisms, but may give low bone concentrations. Elutions of vancomycin, cefazolin, ciprofloxacin, and ticarcillin from PMMA are variable and unreliable.

The role of antibiotic-impregnated PMMA beads in the treatment of chronic osteomyelitis remains controversial. Implantation of gentamicin-impregnated beads into the defects following debridement of an osteomyelitic cavity is as efficacious as conventional treatment, but the beads need to be removed. Future studies may determine if it is superior to conventional treatment.

Addition of antibiotics does weaken PMMA. However, the porosity dominates the fatigue strength of PMMA, and even after adding the antibiotics adequate fatigue strength of PMMA can be maintained by centrifugation or vacuum mixing. Antibiotic addition was highly effective in primary or delayed exchange of infected total joint arthroplasty, but routine use of antibiotics in nonseptic cases may not be justified because they are no more effective than prophylactic antibiotics and laminar flow and have the potential for developing resistant organisms.

PMMA has been very useful in stabilizing pathologic fractures of long bones and spine in conjunction with internal fixation. It allows early mobilization in patients with limited life span. It is also useful in filling defects following curettage of giant cell tumors. In such adjunctive applications, the large mass of PMMA liberates more heat and the surrounding tissues should be cooled.

Annotated Bibliography

Adams K, Couch L, Cierny G, et al: In vitro and in vivo evaluation of antibiotic diffusion from antibiotic-impregnated polymethylmethacrylate beads. *Clin Orthop* 1992;278:244–252.

Cement beads impregnated with clindamycin, vancomycin, and tobramycin exhibited good characteristics and had consistently high levels in bone and granulation tissue.

Ahmed AM, Raab S, Miller JE: Metal/cement interface strength in cemented stem fixation. *J Orthop Res* 1984;2:105–118.

The poor interface shear strength between PMMA and metal is substantially improved and is made resistant to degradation by saline if the metal is precoated with PMMA.

Chan KH, Ahmed AM: Polymethylmethacrylate, in Morrey BF (ed): *Joint Replacement Arthroplasty.* New York, NY, Churchill Livingstone, 1991, pp 23–36.

Large increases in fatigue life of PMMA were obtained either with a small decrease in the applied stress or a small increase in the strength. During different stages of polymerization of PMMA, volumetric changes took place due to polymerization shrinkage, thermal expansion, and thermal contraction.

Crowninshield RD, Brand RA, Johnston RC, et al: An analysis of femoral component stem design in total hip arthroplasty. *J Bone Joint Surg* 1980;62A:68–78.

Femoral components with broad medial borders and large area moments of inertia are useful in lowering the stresses in the cement mantle.

Davies JP, Jasty M, O'Connor DO, et al: The effect of centrifuging bone cement. *J Bone Joint Surg* 1989;71B:39–42.

The porosity and fatigue strength of PMMA vary depending on the commercial formulation and the mixing technique. Centrifugation of Simplex P after mixing provided the highest fatigue strength.

Goldring SR, Jasty M, Roelke M, et al: Biological factors that influence the development of a bone-cement membrane, in Fitzgerald RH Jr (ed): *Non-Cemented Total Hip Arthroplasty.* New York, NY, Raven Press, 1988, pp 35–39.

Bulk cement had excellent biocompatibility, but particulate cement induced a foreign body granulomatous tissue reaction. The cells in the tissue elaborated a variety of biochemical products that could be implicated in periprosthetic bone resorption.

Harris WH (ed): *Advanced Concepts in Total Hip Replacement.* New Jersey, SLACK Inc., 1985.

The techniques in total hip arthroplasty and the proper use of cement are reviewed.

Mulroy RD Jr, Harris WH: The effect of improved cementing techniques on component loosening in total hip replacement: An 11-year radiographic review. *J Bone Joint Surg* 1990;72B:757–760.

Improved cementing techniques including the use of cement plug, cement gun, and cobalt chrome femoral components with rounded contours and collors led to a femoral component loosening rate of only 3% at an average follow-up of 11 years.

Jasty M, Maloney WJ, Bragdon CR, et al: The initiation of failure in cemented femoral components of hip arthroplasties. *J Bone Joint Surg* 1991;73B:551–558.

Postmortem studies on femurs retrieved at autopsy showed that cement–metal interface separation and cement fractures usually initiated femoral component loosening. Adverse biologic responses to nonfragmented cement and endosteal expansion were not found to play a role in loosening.

Lautenschiager EP, Stupp BI, Keller JE: Structure and properties of acrylic bone cement, in Hastings GW, Ducheyne P (eds): *Functional Behavior of Orthopaedic Biomaterials.* Boca Raton, FL, CRC Press, 1984, vol 11, pp 87–119.

The structure and properties of PMMA are reviewed.

Rey RM Jr, Paiement GD, McGann WM, et al: A study of intrusion characteristics of low viscosity cement, Simplex-P and palacos cements in a bovine cancellous bone model. *Clin Orthop* 1987;215:272–278.

The intrusion of PMMA into bovine cancellous bone is enhanced by mixing with chilled monomer and using high pressures.

Saha S, Pal S: Mechanical properties of bone cement: A review. *J Biomed Mater Res* 1984;18:435–462.

Variables that influence the mechanical properties, such as handling characteristics, strain rate, loading modes, additives, porosity, blood inclusion, in vivo environment, and temperature, are reviewed.

Wixson RL, Lautenschiager EP, Novak MA: Vacuum mixing of acrylic bone cement. *J Arthroplasty* 1987;2:141–149.

Mixing PMMA in a vacuum reduced the porosity and improved fatigue strength of PMMA.

Classic Bibliography

Andriacchi TP, Galante JO, Belytschko TB, et al: A stress analysis of the femoral stem in total hip prostheses. *J Bone Joint Surg* 1976;58A:618–624.

Charnley J: *Acrylic Cement in Orthopaedic Surgery.* London, England, ES Livingston, 1970.

Herndon JH, Bechtol CO, Crickenberger DP: Fat embolism during total hip replacement: A prospective study. *J Bone Joint Surg* 1974;56A:1350–1362.

Lee AJ, Ling RS, Vangala SS: Some clinically relevant variables affecting the mechanical behaviour of bone cement. *Acta Orthop Trauma Surg* 1978;92:1–18.

7

Bone Grafts

Introduction

Bone grafting has become an increasingly important part of reconstructive orthopaedic surgery in circumstances of severe bone-stock deficiency. It has a role in fracture care, arthrodeses, cystic defects, congenital conditions, tumor treatment, and most recently, total joint replacement. The basic function of bone grafting is to enhance osteogenesis or to restore structural integrity. The major contribution of the graft to the process of bone repair is in the areas of osteoinduction and osteoconduction. Osteoinduction is the mechanism whereby the host tissue is influenced to form osteogenic elements by a specific stimulus from the graft, for example, bone morphogenetic protein (BMP). Osteoconduction is the process of capillary ingrowth and influx of osteoprogenitor cells in which the graft plays a strictly passive role as a scaffold.

The number of different clinical entities that will benefit from bone grafting are increasing. For example, bone grafting has become an integral part of revision total joint replacement for both the knee and the femur. Experience has shown that failure of the host bone, especially the femur, may limit the longevity of total hip replacement. Particulate debris, stress shielding, and the natural consequences of aging conspire to diminish the quantity of bone around joint prostheses. Also, routine and earlier bone grafting in severe tibial fractures has produced quicker union of these difficult fractures. Just as the number of clinical uses for bone grafting has increased, so has the number of available graft options. However, there is no one universal bone graft material or one surgical graft technique that suits all situations.

Types of Bone Grafts

Bone grafts differ according to the tissue type, cortical versus cancellous bone, and initial viability, that is, whether the graft is vascularized or nonvascularized at surgery. Bone grafts may be fresh, preserved, freeze-dried, or fresh frozen. Some grafts are harvested sterilely and others are harvested cleanly and then subjected to sterilization by boiling, ethylene oxide, or irradiation. Each of these manipulations of the bone tissue has physiologic and mechanical consequences that, in turn, determine the clinical usefulness of the bone. In addition, there are bone graft substitutes, bioactive ceramics, and osteoinductive preparations.

In the past, a general distinction was made between viable transplanted preparations, termed grafts or trans-

plants, which required a vascular anastomosis, and nonviable preparations, termed implants. However, this distinction has become blurred with bone, which can be nonviable but at the same time is biologically active, and with metallic joint replacements covered with porous coatings and bioactive ceramics such as hydroxyapatite.

Autografts (formerly homografts) are tissues transplanted from one place to another in the same individual human or animal. Allografts (allogeneic transplantation), formerly heterografts, are defined as tissues transplanted between members of the same species, who are not genetically identical. Isografts are tissues transplanted between genetically identical individuals: identical twins or inbred laboratory animals. Xenografts are tissues transplanted between different species. These latter grafts are the least well incorporated and, accordingly, have only very limited use in humans at this time.

Biology

Bone healing and remodeling, which is responsible for normal bone homeostasis as well as for fracture repair, is central to an understanding of bone graft biology. This process involves bone resorption carried out by osteoclasts, which are derived from bone-marrow hematopoietic stem cells or macrophage precursors, and bone formation, which occurs with osteoblasts depositing osteoid matrix followed by mineralization with an engulfing of the cells as osteocytes. Normally, bone remodeling is in balance, maintaining a constant bone mass. Resorption and formation are regulated by local factors and systemic influences, including prostaglandins, osteocalcin, bone-derived growth factor, BMP, platelet-derived growth factor, and epidermal growth factor. The soft-tissue bed adjacent to the graft plays an important role. In laboratory models, graft nonunion can be produced when the graft is isolated from the surrounding muscular bed.

Bone repair using cortical and cancellous autografts differs, although histologic findings are the same for each in the first 2 weeks. During the first week, coagulated blood is evident about the graft. There is an inflammatory cellular response with vascular buds infiltrating the graft. In the second week, fibrous granulation tissue becomes dominant, and the number of inflammatory cells decreases. There is osteocytic osteolysis due to anoxia and injury from surgery.

Cortical grafts are penetrated by blood vessels by week one, with osteoclastic resorption and vascular infiltration of Volkmann's and Haversian canals. Most of the resorption of bone matrix is confined to osteons; resorption of the interstitial lamella is unusual. When the resorptive activity has sufficiently enlarged the Haversian canals, osteoblasts appear and refill the area with new bone. Only about 40% to 50% of the cortical graft cross section is repaired. Quantitative studies have shown that the endosteal lining cells in the host marrow stroma produce more than half of the new bone.

In the dog model with a diaphyseal cortical graft, as a result of bone resorption, the grafted cortical bone is weakest at 6 weeks. The weakness persists for about 24 weeks, and strength returns to normal in 48 weeks. New bone formation is present by 6 weeks and stays consistently high for 12 to 48 weeks. The mechanism of repair in human fibula cortical grafts is felt to be the same as that in the dog, except that repair takes twice as long to complete. Humans were not fully back to normal strength until 2 years. The increased porosity of the grafted bone has significant clinical implications because the grafts are weaker and are at risk to fracture during this time in the healing process.

Cancellous repair differs from cortical repair by the rate of revascularization, the completeness of repair, and the mechanism of bone formation, which is creeping substitution rather than osteoclastic cutting. A rapid revascularization from the host precedes a differentiation of primitive mesenchymal cells into osteogenic cells. Both donor and recipient cells may contribute to the new cell lines. Osteogenic cells differentiate into osteoblasts, which line the edges of the dead trabeculae and deposit osteoid on the necrotic graft trabeculae. Radiographically, this process produces an increase in radiodensity. After it is encased in new bone, the necrotic bone is gradually removed. All of the necrotic bone is removed in the cancellous graft repair process.

Autografts

Fresh autogenous bone grafts contain live osteocytes, which make an important contribution to the osteogenesis provided by the graft. This is the most osteogenic graft material. Cancellous grafts are best for small defects, less than 6 cm, that do not require high strength or require specific shapes or an articular surface. This type of graft needs to be handled properly to maximize its potential. The size and shape of the graft are important. If the graft is too small, the cells will be damaged from the surgery, and if it is too large, the diffusion of nutrients may be too slow to ensure survival of graft cells. The ideal graft has been determined to consist of small flat strips or slabs of bone, about 5 mm across. Exposure to antibiotic-containing solutions used to irrigate orthopaedic wounds does not inhibit osteogenesis; however, antibiotic powder is detrimental to osteogenesis.

Cortical autografting is limited, for practical purposes, to the fibula, although strips of tibia have been used in the past in spite of the possibility of late tibial fracture with significant clinical implications. Fibular cortical grafts have been used to reconstruct large defects, in the range of 7.5 to 25 cm, in the humerus, femur, and tibia (using dual grafts) and in the radius and ulna (using single grafts). The time to union for this technique is about 12 months. Stress fractures are a problem in the longer (12 to 25 cm) grafts. These grafts need to be protected for about 2 years.

Electrical stimulation of segmental autogenous cortical bone grafts has been studied in a dog model, using a 2 month and 6 month protocol. No difference could be found in the biomechanical strength, histology, or time to union. Therefore, in the usual circumstance, electrical stimulation is not likely to improve the clinical outcome of the graft.

Vascularized autografts are harvested with a vascular pedicle and are re-anastomosed to the host blood supply at the time of surgery. The only practical sources of autogenous segmental vascularized graft are the fibula, ribs, or iliac crest. In a dog model, these grafts have been shown to have fewer stress fractures and to demonstrate an accelerated repair process, although the process was qualitatively similar to that in the nonvascularized situation. It appears, therefore, that cutting the graft from the host interrupts the intrinsic vascular channels in the bone. The interrupted supply is not fully compensated by the periosteal blood supply, which leads to sufficient bone necrosis to require some cortical repair. However, it would appear that there is less necrotic bone with vascularized allografts, thus allowing the repair process to proceed more quickly.

Several animal studies have shown no difference in the rate of graft union between vascularized and nonvascularized grafts. Other studies have shown that the vascularized grafts healed more quickly. Assessment of the patency of the microvascular anastomosis is difficult. A positive bone scan within the first postoperative week has been shown to correspond with a patent anastomosis, but later bone scanning is invariably positive, even in nonvascularized grafts, because of a surface reaction on the graft.

These grafts are technically demanding and require a period of prolonged immobilization. They should be used only when simpler reconstructive techniques are not available. Because the host tissues must provide the osteoprogenitor cells, vascularized autografts are used primarily in highly traumatized or irradiated tissues in which conventional grafting is less likely to be successful because of vascular insufficiency of the host soft tissues.

Although autografts have some biologic advantages, they also have a number of disadvantages. The supply of available autograft bone is limited, there is no articulating surface, and the material is relatively weak. It is impossible to reconstruct large defects. The patient must sacrifice normal structures and assume the morbidity of a second surgical site. Study of the donor leg after fibulectomy showed that the leg often remained mildly symptomatic and slightly weak. Chronic donor site pain is also a real problem, it has been reported to occur in as many as 31% of patients after spinal surgery. No relationship between the surgical approach used to harvest the graft and chronic pain could be demonstrated in one study.

In another study, an overall minor complication rate of 20.6%, which included superficial infections, minor wound problems, temporary sensory loss, and minimal and resolving pain, occurred at the donor site. If the graft was harvested through the same incision as for the surgical procedure, the complication rate was higher.

Allografts

Allografts address many of the deficiencies of autografts. Allograft bone is both osteoinductive and osteoconductive, although less so than autografts, whereas xenograft has no osteoinductive properties. No separate incision is needed for procurement, decreasing surgical and anesthesia morbidity to the patient, as well as diminishing the risk of tumor spread from resections. It can be stored for long periods of time in the frozen state, theoretically assuring an ample supply of different sizes and shapes. A viable articular cartilage can be maintained with cryopreservation techniques that permit the restoration of articular surfaces. Tendons and ligaments can also be preserved to be used as anchors and stabilizers.

Allografts differ from other organ transplant materials in that they are not vascularized and heal by incorporation. The histologic sequence of events in allograft repair is similar to that in autograft repair, although considerably slowed. Lymphocytes predominate in the initial inflammatory response. Vascular invasion from the periphery is slower, and new bone formation is inferior in quantity, and slower than with autograft repair. By definition, allografts differ from the recipient at major histocompatibility loci, yet the role of the immune system in allograft repair and clinical success has remained elusive.

There are convincing data that immunologic reactions are at work in cases of allograft implantation, but their extent and clinical significance are as yet unknown. The conflicting literature on this subject has been attributed to differences in animal models and assay techniques.

Many of the animal studies in allograft biology have been done using the dog. When a cortical fibula model was used, autografts healed more completely than allografts. Repeating the experiment with either short-term (6 weeks) or long-term (12 weeks) immunosuppression revealed no difference between the allografts and autografts, showing a role for the immune system. When animals with known histocompatibility labels were used in an ulnar model, frozen allografts could not be distinguished from their autograft controls in weak barrier animals; whereas, in animals with strong transplantation barriers, allografts did not heal as rapidly as autograft controls.

The role of immunity in human allograft healing is perplexing and unresolved. It is premature to ascribe all clinical allograft failures to immunologic causes. Anti-HLA (human leukocyte antigen) antibodies have been found in human recipients of freeze-dried and fresh-frozen bone allografts, but follow-up of these individuals has shown no detrimental effect on the clinical outcome of surgery. There is certainly some concern that the nonunions and allograft infections may be a manifestation of low-grade rejection. What stimulates the immune response to an allograft is unknown. Bones are known to be composite tissues consisting of osteogenic, chondrogenic, fibrous, fatty, neural, and hematopoietic cells. Most researchers in this field feel that the marrow elements are the major immunogenic component of allograft bone. There is a small possibility that the bony matrix itself may be somewhat immunogenic. With isolated bone cell preparations, humeral cytotoxicity tests have indicated the presence of histocompatibility antigens. Bone cells, however, do not stimulate allogeneic lymphocytes in vitro, suggesting a low antigen density on their membranes. Previous exposure to bone antigens does not predispose to subsequent graft failure; successful grafting can follow removal of a failed graft. In vitro measurements of immunity have confirmed that fresh bone is significantly immunogenic, whereas preserved preparations are less immunogenic. Bone frozen to $-70°C$ is more immunogenic than is freeze-dried bone, which in turn is more immunogenic than freeze-dried demineralized bone. Freeze-dried bone is weaker than fresh-frozen bone but this weakness does not appear to be clinically significant if the graft is supported by internal fixation or by a joint prosthesis.

Influence of Drugs, Radiation, Sterilization

Bone graft can be treated with or exposed to various physical and pharmacologic measures that affect the function of the graft. High-dose radiation of bone (3.5 to 4 Mrad) has been studied in animal models; it severely damages the bone and marrow, with loss of osteocytes, increased porosity of the bone, and loss of hematopoetic elements of the marrow. Smaller doses repeated over time, as is done in clinical radiation treatments, do not result in such dramatic changes. Radiation of vascularized and nonvascularized autogenous cortical grafts, for a total dose of 48 Gy given over 3 weeks, did not produce significant delay in the rate of healing or torsional strength of the junction, which suggests that radiation can be used with autogenous cortical grafts. Radiation (2.5 Mrad) has also been used to sterilize bone allografts. Irradiation of less than 3 Mrad does not alter the material properties of the bone, but may diminish some of the osteoinductive factors.

Autoclaving has been used to sterilize bone graft. This has a deleterious consequence for the bone. In a rabbit model, autoclaved graft could not bridge a diaphyseal defect. However, in several centers autoclaving has been used successfully for preparation of autogenous segmental bone grafts after low-grade tumor resection. The autoclaved resected specimen was used for the reconstruction.

Ethylene oxide gas has also been used to sterilize bone graft. Care must be taken to remove the toxic by-products of the gas before clinical use. In addition, ethylene oxide exposure causes a dose-dependent decrease in the osteoinductive properties of the graft. In a study of ethylene-oxide sterilized, freeze-dried bone graft in thoracic and lumbar spinal fusions, the pseudarthrosis rate was 76%. Of these, 18% were explored for autogenous grafting, and the finding was for near complete resorption of the ethylene oxide-treated graft. The authors concluded that in this type of surgery, autogenous bone graft was superior to ethylene oxide-treated graft. Chemotherapeutic agents have been shown to negatively affect bone homeostasis. There is a greater effect on osteoblasts than osteoclasts as shown by a reduced volume of osteoid, despite a normal number of osteoblasts and osteoclasts as compared to controls. Other studies have shown that low doses of these drugs have no demonstrable effect on cortical autografts, whereas higher doses lead to decreased new bone formation and an increase in nonunions.

Bone Graft Substitutes

Because the amount of autograft bone is limited, and allograft bone requires complicated tissue banking and, theoretically, has the additional risk of transmitting infectious disease or malignancy, investigators have been pursuing an effective bone graft substitute. Ideally, such a material should have both osteoinductive and osteoconductive properties. These substitutes include demineralized bone matrix, BMP, and such bioactive ceramics as tricalcium phosphate and hydroxyapatite. The literature on this subject has revealed some conflicting observations. A comparison of fresh autogeneic cancellous bone, allogeneic deep-frozen bone, allogeneic decalcified bone matrix, and bone matrix gelatin in a nonunion dog model showed bone healing in all instances only in the autogeneic bone graft group. In a rabbit nonunion model, however, no difference could be found between cancellous autograft and decalcified bone matrix. In a rat model, powdered demineralized bone matrix was more effective than autogenous bone chips at bridging a diaphyseal defect. Porous hydroxyapatite in the form of *Porites goniopora* coral exoskeleton has been shown to duplicate the function of cancellous bone grafts in a dog metaphyseal model. In a clinical series, no difference could be documented between tibial plateau fractures treated with cancellous bone graft and those treated with coral hydroxyapatite. Collagraft (Zimmer, Warsaw, IN) is a commercial bone graft substitute consisting of a mixture of porous beads of 60% hydroxyapatite and 40% tricalcium phosphate and fibrillar collagen. This substance is mixed with the patient's own marrow. When it was compared to autogenous bone graft in a multicenter randomized trial of 267 patients, no difference could be found at 6 and 16 months. Bone marrow by itself is osteogenic, but it can be enhanced when combined with an osteoconductive substance, including xenograft bone.

The bioactive ceramics and coral exoskeleton function by osteoconduction. Demineralized allogeneic bone matrix has been shown to be osteoinductive. However, in a monkey model, demineralized bone implanted in the quadriceps did not change calcium content, whereas, in rats, the implanted matrix showed a 20% increase in new bone suggesting that demineralized bone matrix is a weak bone inductor. Other studies have shown that BMP may be clinically more effective when combined with a carrier substance. Both ceramic and collagen materials have been used in animal models. The active substance in this bone preparation is bone BMP, a glycoprotein with molecular weights from 18,000 to 40,000 daltons. It functions by stimulating the host connective tissue mesenchymal cells to differentiate to osteoprogenitor cells. The material is very potent, with only 50 to 100 ng of BMP needed to produce a response subcutaneously in rats.

Choice of Bone Graft Technique

There is no one best graft and no universal graft material at this time. The clinical circumstance will usually determine the appropriate choice of bone graft. If osteogenic potential is the major requirement, such as for a fracture nonunion, then autograft cancellous bone is the first choice because it is the most osteoinductive. Fracture stability and host soft tissues may also have to be addressed as part of the overall management of the nonunion. In the future, there may be more of a role for the bone inductive substances and bone graft substitutes. The preliminary experience from the literature is quite favorable. Osteoinductive substances such as BMP are not routinely available at this time.

Such osteogenic (inductive) techniques are not capable of providing any structural restoration. In the setting of a bone cyst, in which the graft serves as a filler, cancellous bone would be sufficient, but, depending on the size of the cyst, a large quantity of bone might be required. Ground allograft would be a good choice here, with no limit on the amount available. Clinical studies of unicameral cysts treated with crushed allograft have shown results comparable to those achieved using autograft.

The availability of autograft cortical bone is limited to the fibula, or possibly the ribs and iliac crest. Skeletal defects in the range of 20 cm can be bridged with this technique, with no option to vary the geometry of the graft. With longer defects and situations in which the strength of the graft is especially important or a specific shape is needed, such as part of a joint, the only choice of graft material is allograft. If live articular cartilage is needed, then fresh frozen graft with preserved articular cartilage is the only option.

There are clinical settings in which both autograft and allograft may be equally good choices. In scoliosis surgery, no significant clinical difference could be demonstrated between allograft and autograft bone although there was less blood loss and surgical time where the allograft was used. In a dog revision hip arthroplasty model, autograft and allograft were equivalent in a study of enhancement of fixation of a porous-coated femoral component, and both were superior to a no-graft control. However, in scaphoid nonunions, a total deproteinized commercial bone allograft did not perform as well as autogenous bone. Frozen allograft is stronger than freeze-dried and, therefore, is the graft of choice when mechanical strength is paramount, such as for an acetabular roof or column graft. Frozen graft is also less brittle and can be more easily cut into complex shapes. However, where internal fixation hardware is capable of supporting the allograft, such as on the femoral side of a total hip, or when a graft is providing adjunctive support, such as a strut graft on a deficient femoral tube in the setting of revision total hip arthroplasty, freeze-dried grafts would be a sensible choice because this material is the least immunogenic, and less carpentry of the graft is required.

Promoting Successful Allograft Reconstruction

Major structural allografts continue to have a significant complication rate. This complication rate varies with the clinical setting, differing for tumor patients compared to revision total hip arthroplasty patients. The overall success rate of allografting for bone tumors is 80%, with most failures occurring in the first 3 years as a result of fracture (19%), nonunion (14%), and infection (about 10%). Depending on the tumor, there is variable soft-tissue and host immune compromise that may contribute to postoperative complications. Infection has always been a concern when using large bone grafts. This problem has been investigated in several studies. In one study of 324 grafts from a single bone bank, the incidence of infection was 4% for revision hip surgery and 5% for patients who had treatment of a bone tumor. These rates of infection were felt to be comparable to other cases of similar complexity and time in which a graft was not used. Other studies have shown a higher infection rate of 11.7% in tumor cases, and found that when controlled for anatomic location (distal femur), infection correlated with presence of a nonunion, extent of the tumor dissection, size of allograft segment, skin sloughing, and multiple operations. Gram-positive infections were the most common. Several of the infected cases could be salvaged by removal of the allograft and treatment of the infection, followed by a second allograft.

Improved results of allograft surgery will certainly come with improvement in knowledge of the immune mechanism as it pertains to bone and cartilage. Nevertheless, improving surgical techniques can lead to more uniform and predictable surgery now. Healing of a graft as well as healing of the wound depends on the host soft tissues. Frequently, the addition of a bone allograft adds to the bulk of the surgical construct, putting tension on the wound closure. Part of surgical planning in selected cases is to be prepared for a soft-tissue transfer to assure coverage of the graft with healthy soft tissues.

Predictable allograft host union requires a rigid surgical construct capable of withstanding the forces applied. The geometry of the junction can play a big part in enhancing the stability. Long step-cut junctions in close apposition to the host with plate and screw or intramedullary hardware has been the most successful allograft-host junction in the revision hip arthroplasty setting. In the metaphyseal setting, such as the acetabulum, the grafts must be supported by host bone as much as possible with fixation hardware positioned along the lines of weightbearing force, supplemented by buttress plates if parts of the graft are unsupported. The trabeculae of the graft should be aligned with the weightbearing forces. No piercing instruments should be used on the graft, or extraneous drill holes made. These will be permanent stress risers predisposing to graft fracture. Joint prostheses need to be cemented to the allograft because there is no possibility for biologic fixation to the graft. Safe allografting requires a competently managed bone bank with rigorous standards of procurement and graft processing.

Ideally, both freeze-dried and fresh frozen grafts should be available, along with ground allograft bone. While transmission of viral diseases, both HIV and hepatitis, is possible from these tissues, rigorous screening of bone donors makes this risk negligible. Screening tests for AIDS includes social screening, HIV antigen and antibody, and lymph node biopsy.

Annotated Bibliography

Biology

Friedlaender GE: Bone grafts: The basic science rationale for clinical applications. *J Bone Joint Surg* 1987;69A: 786–790.

This review of bone grafts covers the remodeling cycle and histology of graft incorporation, contrasting allogeneic and autogeneic bone.

Nather A, Balasubramaniam P, Bose K: Healing of non-vascularised diaphyseal bone transplants: An experimental study. *J Bone Joint Surg* 1990;72B:830–834.

In a cat diaphyseal cortical graft model, the authors compared four different circumstances: osteotomized segment with periosteum, segment without periosteum, with medullary canal blocked, and segment separated from host soft tissues. Union occurred at both ends of the graft in 8 to 12 weeks except when the graft was osteotomized from the surrounding soft tissues. The muscle bed, therefore, plays a significant role in the graft repair process.

Poss R: Natural factors that affect the shape and strength of the aging human femur. *Clin Orthop* 1992;274:194–201.

This report describes the age-related and implant-related factors that produce a loss of bone stock to the human femur.

Autografts

Anderson AF, Green NE: Residual functional deficit after partial fibulectomy for bone graft. *Clin Orthop* 1991;267: 137–140.

Ten patients were studied after partial fibulectomy. The donor leg often remained mildly symptomatic and weak. The deficits were not felt to be sufficient to discourage use of the fibula when clinically indicated.

Dell PC, Burchardt H, Glowczewski FP Jr: A roentgenographic, biomechanical, and histological evaluation of vascularized and non-vascularized segmental fibular canine autografts. *J Bone Joint Surg* 1985;67A: 105–112.

In this comparison of vascularized and nonvascularized cortical autografts, the vascularized grafts underwent less resorption and osteonal remodeling. They were stronger than the nonvascularized at 6 weeks, but thereafter there was no difference.

Fernyhough JC, Schimandle JJ, Weigel MC, et al: Chronic donor site pain complicating bone graft harvesting from the posterior iliac crest for spinal fusion. *Spine* 1992;17: 1474–1480.

The incidence of chronic donor site pain varied from 18% to 39%; it was highest in patients with chronic low back pain and lowest after spinal trauma.

Miller GJ, Burchardt H, Enneking WF, et al: Electromagnetic stimulation of canine bone grafts. *J Bone Joint Surg* 1984;66A:693–698.

In a canine model, electrical stimulation demonstrated no enhancement of repair of a cortical autograft.

Nather A, Goh JC, Lee JJ: Biomechanical strength of non-vascularised and vascularised diaphyseal bone transplants: An experimental study. *J Bone Joint Surg* 1990;72B:1031–1035.

In a cat model of vascularized and nonvascularized cortical grafts, there was no difference in the time to graft union, and the grafts were equal in strength at 12 and 16 weeks.

Shaffer JW, Field GA, Goldberg VM, et al: Fate of vascularized and nonvascularized autografts. *Clin Orthop* 1985;197:32–43.

In a canine model, the pattern of bone repair was similar in vascular and nonvascular ulnar grafts. The time intervals in the sequence of events, resorption followed by appositional bone formation, were quicker in the vascularized grafts.

Younger EM, Chapman MW: Morbidity at bone graft donor sites. *J Orthop Trauma* 1989;3:192–195.

In this study of 239 patients with 243 autogenous bone grafts, the overall major complication rate was 8.6% with 2.5% infections, 3.3% hematomas, and 3.8% reoperation.

Allografts

Friedlaender GE, Horowitz MC: Immune responses to osteochondral allografts: Nature and significance. *Orthopedics* 1992;15:1171–1175.

This is a review of the immunologic behavior of allografts. Diminishing the immune response to bone allograft may improve the clinical outcome.

Katoh T, Sato K, Kawamura M, et al: Osteogenesis in sintered bone combined with bovine bone morphogenetic protein. *Clin Orthop* 1993;287:266–275.

In a rabbit model, BMP combined with true bone ceramic produces more new bone formation than the true bone ceramic alone. The combination also produced bone at a faster rate than the ceramic alone. True bone ceramic may be a good carrier for the B<P in future clinical uses.

Mankin HJ, Doppelt S, Tomford W: Clinical experience with allograft implantation: The first ten years. *Clin Orthop* 1983;174:69–86.

This review covers the first 10 years of clinical experience with major segmental allografts.

Pelker RR, Friedlaender GE, Markham TC: Biomechanical properties of bone allografts. *Clin Orthop* 1983;174:54–57.

The biomechanical effects of freezing and low level radiation are minimal. Freeze-drying markedly diminishes the torsional and bending strength of the bone. Irradiation of bone with greater than 3.0 Mrad, especially when combined with freeze-drying, causes a significant reduction in breaking strength.

Ripamonti U: Calvarial regeneration in primates with autolyzed antigen-extracted allogenic bone. *Clin Orthop* 1992;282:293–303.

In a study of cranial clavarial defects, which normally heal very slowly, the defects were grafted with either chemosterilized antigen-extracted autolyzed allogeneic bone matrix (known to retain BMP) on iliac cortico-cancellous autograft bone or left ungrafted. The bone matrix showed superior osteogenesis, which appeared to be primarily due to extensive osteoconductive invasion from adjacent endosteal spaces.

Takaoka U, Koezuka M, Nakahara H: Telopeptide-depleted bovine skin collagen as a carrier for bone morphogenetic protein 1. *J Orthop Res* 1991;9:902–907.

A composite of telopeptide-depleted type 1 collagen and partially purified BMP consistently elicited ectopic bone formation in mice. The authors felt that the collagen permitted a gradual release of the BMP, without causing any interfering immunologic reactions. This fact may have clinical applications in the future.

Drugs and Radiation

Aspenberg P, Johnsson E, Thorngren KG: Dose-dependent reduction of bone inductive properties by ethylene oxide. *J Bone Joint Surg* 1990;72B:1036–1037.

Bone induction properties were studied after varying lengths of exposure to ethylene oxide. The results showed a dose-dependent decrease in bone induction.

De Santis G, Williams JF, Dvir E, et al: Effect of postoperative radiation on the incorporation of tibial bone grafts in the rabbit. *J Bone Joint Surg* 1990;72B:309–311.

Radiation given 2 to 5 weeks after grafting caused no significant delay in the healing of tibial cortical grafts.

Friedlaender GE, Tross RB, Doganis AC, et al: Effects of chemotherapeutic agents on bone: I. Short-term methotrexate and doxorubicin (adriamycin) treatment in a rat model. *J Bone Joint Surg* 1984;66A:602–607

The effect of doxorubicin and methotrexate on normal physiological bone turnover is studied in a rat model. Both drugs diminished bone formation rates by nearly 60%.

Herron LD, Newman MH: The failure of ethylene oxide gas-sterilized freeze-dried bone graft for thoracic and lumbar spinal fusion. *Spine* 1989;14:496–500.

This is a study of 37 patients with a high pseudarthrosis rate when using ethylene oxide-treated graft.

Johnston JO, Harries TJ, Alexander CE, et al: Limb salvage procedure for neoplasms about the knee by spherocentric total knee arthroplasty and autogenous autoclaved bone grafting. *Clin Orthop* 1983;181:137–145.

Nine patients are reported who underwent reconstruction after tumor resection with a total knee and autoclaved resected bone specimen. While there were some implant problems, the bone grafts functioned.

Maeda M, Bryant MH, Yamagata M, et al: Effects of irradiation on cortical bone and their time-related changes: A biomechanical and histomorphological study. *J Bone Joint Surg* 1988;70A:392–399.

The effects of high-dose irradiation (3500 rads) on the biomechanical and morphologic properties of cortical bone in rats were studied. The bone marrow showed reduced hematopoietic elements and increased fat. Decreased cortical area and increased porosity of bone were noted by 14 to 18 weeks. Most of the changes had returned to control levels by 18 weeks.

Oakeshott RD, Morgan DA, Zukor DJ, et al: Revision total hip arthroplasty with osseous allograft reconstruction: A clinical and roentgenographic analysis. *Clin Orthop* 1987;225:37–61.

A series of 72 patients with revision total hip arthroplasty using segmental bone allograft to restore bone deficiencies is reported. The reconstructive objective was achieved 85% of the time with a follow-up of 6 to 72 months.

Smith WS, Struhl S: Replantation of an autoclaved autogenous segment of bone for treatment of chondrosarcoma: Long-term follow-up. *J Bone Joint Surg* 1988;70A:70–75.

Seven patients with a low grade chondrosarcoma underwent resection and reconstruction with the autoclaved resected specimen. At 11 years one patient underwent biopsy, which showed predominantly live bone.

Bone Graft Substitutes

Aspenberg P, Lohmander LS, Thorngren KG: Failure of bone induction by bone matrix in adult monkeys. *J Bone Joint Surg* 1988;70B:625–627.

Extraskeletal bone formation was studied in monkeys with demineralized bone. The monkey implants were harvested in 6 weeks and demonstrated no increased bone formation.

Bolander ME, Balian G: The use of demineralized bone matrix in the repair of segmental defects: Augmentation with extracted matrix proteins and a comparison with autologous grafts. *J Bone Joint Surg* 1986;68A:1264–1274.

Demineralized autologous bone matrix was compared to autologous cancellous bone from the iliac crest in a rabbit ulna model. All of the ulnas healed and the two grafting techniques were substantially equivalent by mechanical testing.

Bucholz RW, Carlton AM: Synthetic porous hydroxyapatite bone graft substitute for the repair of metaphyseal defects in tibial plateau fractures. Presented at the American Academy of Orthopaedic Surgeons 57th Annual Meeting, New Orleans, LA. Rosemont, IL, 1990, p 323.

Synthetic porous hydroxyapatite compared favorably to cancellous autologous bone in 25 patients with tibial plateau fractures.

Buck BE, Malinin TI, Brown MD: Bone transplantation and human immunodeficiency virus: An estimate of risk of acquired immunodeficiency syndrome (AIDS). *Clin Orthop* 1989;240:129–136.

This provides a description of the techniques used to screen for HIV.

Connolly J, Guse R, Lippiello L, et al: Development of an osteogenic bone-marrow preparation. *J Bone Joint Surg* 1989;71A:684–691.

In this study of bone marrow implanted ectopically in chambers in the peritoneal cavities of rabbits and in a delayed union model, simple centrifugation of the marrow increased the osteogenic effect.

Cornell CN, Lane JM, Chapman M, et al: Multicenter trial of collagraft as bone graft substitute. *J Orthop Trauma* 1991;5:1–8.

At the 6 and 12 month follow-up marks in a multicenter randomized trial of Collagraft versus autogenous bone with long bone fractures, no difference could be found between the two graft techniques. Collagraft is a combination of porous beads of 60% hydroxyapatite and 40% tricalcium phosphate and fibrillar collagen with the patient's own marrow.

Gepstein R, Weiss RE, Hallel T: Bridging large defects in bone by demineralized bone matrix in the form of powder: A radiographic, histological, and radioisotope-uptake study in rats. *J Bone Joint Surg* 1987;69A:984–992.

In a rat model, large bone defects were bridged better by demineralized bone powder than by autologous bone chips. It appeared that pulverization of the demineralized matrix to a morsel size of 420 μm enhanced bone induction.

Holmes RE, Bucholz RW, Mooney V: Porous hydroxyapatite as a bone-graft substitute in metaphyseal defects: A histometric study. *J Bone Joint Surg* 1986;68A:904–911.

Interporous hydroxyapatite is as effective as cancellous autograft for the filling of metaphyseal defects associated with tibial plateau fractures.

Salama R: Xenogeneic bone grafting in humans. *Clin Orthop* 1983;174:113–121.

In a series of 89 patients, autologous red bone marrow and xenograft bone were combined as a bone graft material in various bone grafting procedures. These included procedures for bone defects as well as arthrodeses and pseudarthroses. The best results occurred in the defects and arthrodeses.

Schwarz N, Schlag G, Thurnher M, et al: Fresh autogeneic, frozen allogeneic, and decalcified allogeneic bone grafts in dogs. *J Bone Joint Surg* 1991;73B:787–790.

In a dog segmental bone defect model, autograft cancellous bone was superior to allograft deep-frozen cancellous bone, allogenic decalcified bone matrix, and allogenic bone matrix gelatin.

Choice of Bone Graft

Blick SS, Brumback RJ, Lakatos R, et al: Early prophylactic bone grafting of high-energy tibial fractures. *Clin Orthop* 1989;240:21–41.

Compared to matched historical controls, early bone grafting of severe high-energy tibial fractures revealed a mean reduction in the time to union of 11.7 weeks.

Crawford RJ, Gupta A, Risitano G, et al: The use of totally de-proteinized heterologous bone graft in non-union of the scaphoid. *J Hand Surg* 1991;16B:153–155.

In this study of ten patients with deproteinized allograft, the results were inferior to autograft in the same clinical setting.

Dodd CA, Fergusson CM, Freedman L, et al: Allograft versus autograft bone in scoliosis surgery. *J Bone Joint Surg* 1988;70B:431–434.

No difference could be demonstrated between autograft and allograft. Use of the allograft resulted in a marked reduction in operative time and blood loss.

Dorr LD: Bone grafts for bone loss with total knee replacement. *Orthop Clin North Am* 1989;20:179–187.

The use of bone grafts with total knee arthroplasty is described.

Emerson RH Jr, Malinin TI, Cuellar AD, et al: Cortical strut allografts in the reconstruction of the femur in revision total hip arthroplasty: A basic science and clinical study. *Clin Orthop* 1992;285:35–44.

Freeze-dried cortical strut allografts were able to restore lost bone stock in revision total hip surgery such that there was no correlation between the preoperative bone status and the clinical end-result.

Huo MH, Friedlaender GE, Salvati EA: Bone graft and total hip arthroplasty: A review. *J Arthroplasty* 1992;7:109–120.

The use of bone graft with total hip replacement is reviewed.

Lord CF, Gebhardt MC, Tomford WW, et al: Infection in bone allografts: Incidence, nature, and treatment. *J Bone Joint Surg* 1988;70A:369–376.

In a clinical series of massive allograft bone transplants, the rate of infection was 11.7%. Gram-positive organisms were the most common cause of infection. Salvage of the infected allograft can be achieved by staged revision.

Mankin HJ, Springfield DS, Gebhardt MC, et al: Current status of allografting for bone tumors. *Orthopedics* 1992;15:1147–1154.

The 20-year experience of the Massachusetts General Hospital Oncology Unit with massive allograft transplantations is summarized. The overall success rate was 80%.

McDonald DJ, Fitzgerald RH Jr, Chao EY: The enhancement of fixation of a porous-coated femoral component by autograft and allograft in the dog. *J Bone Joint Surg* 1988;70A:728–737.

In a revision femoral component dog model, both allograft and autograft produced enhanced fixation of a porous-coated femoral component compared to bone graft controls.

Tomford WW, Thongphasuk J, Mankin HJ, et al: Frozen musculoskeletal allografts: A study of the clinical incidence and causes of infection associated with their use. *J Bone Joint Surg* 1990;72A:1137–1143.

In a study of allograft infections, contamination of the graft material was not felt to be a factor in the typical infection situation.

8

Bone Ingrowth: Implications for the Establishment and Maintenance of Cementless Porous-Coated Interfaces

Introduction

Enhancement and inhibition of bone ingrowth, bone loss related to both osteolysis and stress shielding, and potential local and systemic consequences are important considerations in cementless fixation with the use of porous coatings. Analyses of components retrieved for cause and at autopsy place a useful framework around the issues discussed in the succeeding sections of this chapter. The basics of bone ingrowth, including some recent studies on the molecular biology of bone repair and factors that enhance or inhibit the process of bone ingrowth, are described. This review ends with a discussion of issues, including osteolysis, adaptive bone remodeling, and biocompatibility, that may affect the long-term efficacy of prostheses fixed by bone ingrowth.

Analysis of Retrieved Components

Analyses of prostheses retrieved from patients indicate that the incidence and amount of bone ingrowth may not be as extensive as is perceived to be necessary to ensure mechanical stability. The reported incidence of bone ingrowth varies from 16% to 100% in the acetabular component, from 27% to 100% in the femoral component of total hip replacement (THR), and from 10% to 100% in the tibial component of total knee replacement (TKR). There are fewer data on the patellar and femoral components of TKR, with reported incidences of 64% and 58%, respectively.

Within each component, two measures have been used to characterize the amount of bone ingrowth: (1) a topographic description of the amount of the porous surface connected to the host skeleton by bony anchorage; and (2) a quantitative description of the amount of bone present within the pores of the coating. The first measure is called the "extent" of bone ingrowth, and typically, is determined by dividing the interface into small units (eg, 1 or 2 mm wide microscopic fields) and calculating the percentage of these fields positive for bone ingrowth. The second measure is called the "volume fraction" or "area density" of bone ingrowth.

Retrieval studies indicate that only occasionally is the extent of bone ingrowth greater than 30%, and the volume fraction is often less than 10%. The volume fraction might not be expected to exceed the local density of the host cancellous bone bed, which often is in the range of 10% to 25%, depending on the anatomic site. However, most authorities would agree that it is preferable to have an extent of bone ingrowth approaching 100%.

Other observations pertinent to the nature of the interface in cementless fixation have been made in these retrieval analyses. The stages of bone ingrowth appear to be similar in humans and in experimental animal models: direct formation of woven bone without a cartilaginous intermediary, followed by lamellar bone remodeling (Fig. 1). Areas within the porous coating not occupied by bone have been described as filled with loose to dense fibrous tissue or fatty marrow. Fibrocartilage has also been found at limited foci, and lymphocytic infiltrates and particulate debris have been noted. Designs that include nonporous-coated areas typically have a fibrous membrane in the uncoated regions (Fig. 2). These membranes occupy the space between the component and a surrounding shell of bone, sometimes called a neocortex. The space between the regions without porous coating and surrounding bone can serve as a pathway for migration of wear debris or corrosion products to the interface.

Although observations from the retrieval studies are relevant to many issues concerning the use of cementless technology, analysis of the response to implants removed for cause should be viewed with caution because these implants may not be representative of clinically successful implants. Emerging information on implants retrieved at autopsy may be a better reflection of the tissue response typical of bone ingrowth type prostheses.

Basic Biology of Bone Ingrowth

The basic principles governing bone ingrowth have been well known for some time. It is generally accepted that porous-coated implants will become attached to the skeleton by bone if (1) there is intimate contact between the porous coating and living host bone; (2) the relative bone implant displacements are sufficiently small to permit osteogenesis (as opposed to development of fibrous tissue); and (3) the porous surface has the appropriate microstructure (interconnecting pores with dimensions in the range of 100 to 400 μm) and is made from a biocompatible material (typically, titanium or one of its alloys or cobalt chrome).

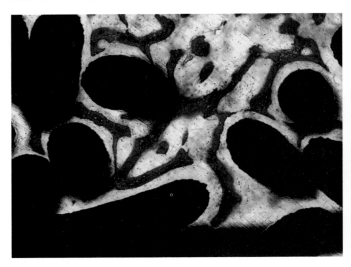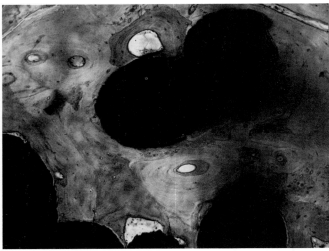

Fig. 1 Photomicrographs of bone ingrowth in autopsy-retrieved acetabular components. **Left,** At 1 month, slender trabeculae of woven bone were present (original magnification × 88). **Right,** Sixty-three months after surgery, mature lamellar bone was present, as evidenced by the presence of Haversian systems within the porous coating (original magnification × 160). (Reproduced with permission from Pidhorz LE, Urban RM, Jacobs JJ, et al: A quantitative study of bone and soft tissues in cementless porous-coated acetabular components retrieved at autopsy. *J Arthroplasty* 1993;8:213–225.)

The process of bone ingrowth depends on the normal healing response to the trauma of surgery. When a hole is drilled within the medullary canal of a long bone, the first part of the response involves formation of a hematoma and development of mesenchymal tissue, which differentiates in the process leading to the formation of woven bone. Lamellar bone is then formed on cores of woven bone, and the marrow is reestablished. Within the diaphysis, osteoclasts eventually remove the newly formed trabeculae. The same processes occur in the presence of implants that are initially mechanically stable. However, in implants, the newly formed bone is not necessarily removed, presumably because of its mechanical role transmitting load from the implant to the host bone. This sequence of events is similar to the development of a medullary callus under conditions of rigid internal fixation. Animal studies and limited data from human retrievals indicate that woven bone begins forming by 1 week and lamellar bone can be found as early as 4 weeks after surgery.

Mesenchymal stem cells residing within the marrow or along the endosteal surface can divide and differentiate into cells with osteoblastic, chondrocytic, or other phenotypes. For reasons not yet understood, injury to the bone or marrow; eg, during surgery, causes some of these cells to differentiate into bone-forming cells. According to an in vivo model in which the marrow of the rat tibial diaphysis is ablated, osteoblast cell density increases rapidly, as does expression of genes for alkaline phosphatase, procollagen α1 (I), and osteopontin (Table 1). Maximal gene expression for osteocalcin occurs slightly later, followed by maximal expression of collagenase (associated with the appearance of osteoclasts). The gene for type II collagen

mRNA does not change, in agreement with histologic observations that indicate there is no cartilaginous phase in this type of bone healing.

An in vitro cell culture system has been used to characterize molecular events associated with differentiation of osteoblasts. Three phases—proliferation, extracellular matrix (ECM) maturation, and mineralization—have been identified, and the transition from one phase to the next is being studied. During proliferation, genes for type I collagen, fibronectin, and transforming growth factor-β (TGF-β) are expressed maximally, and the gene for osteopontin is expressed (not maximally). As proliferation is down-regulated, expression of alkaline phosphatase increases dramatically and then decreases as osteocalcin and osteopontin expression increase during mineralization. It has been hypothesized that maturation of the ECM (associated with expression of alkaline phosphatase) down-regulates cell proliferation and that for differentiation to proceed, the genes for type I collagen, fibronectin, and TGF-β must have been expressed during the proliferative phase.

With use of a cell culture system, it was found that expression of α1 (I) collagen and biglycan was maximal early, osteonectin expression was high throughout, and maximal expression of alkaline phosphatase and osteopontin was somewhat delayed. Mineralization led to down-regulation of many of the genes, with the exception of bone sialoprotein, which increased rapidly after the onset of mineralization. Decorin increased throughout the culture period.

In the rat tibial ablation model, generally similar results were found for expression of procollagen α1 (I), osteopon-

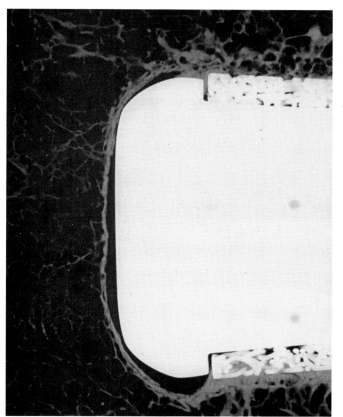 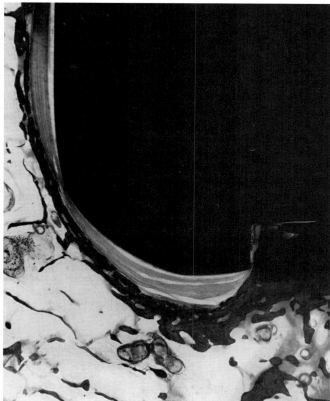

Fig. 2 The uncoated regions of partially porous-coated components often are characterized by the presence of a membrane-filled space. **Left,** This microradiograph of a cross section demonstrates a trabecular shell of bone separated from the implant surface (original magnification × 2.75). **Right,** The corresponding histologic section demonstrates that the space is occupied by a fibrous membrane (original magnification × 5.5). These cavities can serve as conduits for migration of wear debris. (Reproduced with permission from Jacobs JJ, Sumner DR, Urban RM, et al: Retrieval: Successful uncemented implants, in Morrey BF (ed): *Biological, Material and Mechanical Considerations of Joint Replacement.* New York, Raven Press, 1993, pp 185–196.)

tin, alkaline phosphatase, and osteocalcin. In contrast to the in vitro model, however, TGF-β expression, rather than increasing early during the proliferative phase, did not increase until after maximal expression of procollagen α1 (I) and barely exceeded levels found in intact tissue. Insulin-like growth factor-I (IGF-I) was found to increase earlier and to a much greater extent than TGF-β and may have an important trophic role in tissue repair.

Although the understanding of the molecular biology of bone cell differentiation and bone healing is just beginning, some implications for bone ingrowth are already apparent. Factors that stimulate the proliferative phase without inhibiting maturation of the ECM may prove to be potent enhancers of bone ingrowth. However, factors that down-regulate proliferation, ECM maturation, or mineralization would tend to inhibit bone ingrowth.

The osteogenic potential of the implantation site, ie, the presence of appropriate stem cells, is also important. If these cells are not present, bone formation in response to

the surgery cannot be expected. In this case, enhancement of bone ingrowth would depend on recruitment of the appropriate stem cells to the site of implantation, followed, perhaps, by stimulation of the proliferative phase. Failure of prostheses caused by loosening leads to this biologic environment because the normal marrow is replaced by granulation tissue. In addition, the expression of bone related genes following ablation of the tibial marrow is lower in older rats than in younger rats, which indicates that age, itself, may have a negative effect on the osteogenic potential of the marrow.

Initial Interface Gaps

Gaps of various size exist between the implant and host bone immediately after surgery. It has been shown that 1- to 2-mm gaps are routinely created in TKR. The relatively new technique of press-fitting cementless porous-coated

Table 1. Proteins found in bone

Protein*	Type*	Comment*
Procollagen α1	Precursor to mature collagen type I	Predominant organic constituent of bone (by weight) and thought to have mainly a structural role
Alkaline phosphatase	Glycoprotein	Marker of osteoblastic lineage; used as a serum marker of bone formation
Fibronectin	RGD-containing protein	Expressed during early and middle phases of osteogenesis
Biglycan (PG-I)	Cell-surface associated proteoglycan	Binds TGF-β and may regulate its activity
Thrombospondin	RGD-containing protein	Strong binder of Ca^{++}
Decorin (PG-II)	Proteoglycan	Binds to collagen fibrils and TGF-β and may regulate TGF-β activity; regulates collagen fibril growth
Osteonectin	Glycoprotein	High affinity for Ca^{++} and hydroxyapatite; binds collagen and thrombospondin and PDGF; may regulate cell shape and cell cycle progression; characteristically found in growing and healing tissues
Osteopontin	RGD-containing protein	Strong binder of Ca^{++}; expressed during middle and later phases of osteogenesis; aids osteoclast attachment
Bone sialoprotein	RGD- containing protein	Strong binder of Ca^{++}, expressed at time of mineralization, aids osteoclast attachment
Osteocalcin (bone Glaprotein)	Gla-containing protein	Produced late during osteogenesis; may regulate osteoclasts; used as a serum marker of bone formation
Matrix Gla protein	Gla-containing protein	Found in bone and cartilage; specific role not yet determined
Collagenase	Enzyme	Important in breakdown of collagen
TGF-β1-5	Peptide growth factors	Increase cell proliferation and matrix synthesis (but inhibitory at higher doses) (in vitro); stimulate bone formation and bone healing (in vivo)
IGF-I,II	Peptide growth factors	Increase cell proliferation and matrix synthesis (in vitro); bone formation (in vivo)
BMP-2,3,4,5,6,7	Peptide growth factors	Bone cell proliferation and differentiation and maintenance of chondroycte phenotype (in vitro); induce osteogenesis and stimulate bone healing (in vivo)
Basic FGF	Peptide growth factor	Increases cell proliferation (in vitro)
Acidic FGF	Peptide growth factor	Role in bone undetermined
PDGF	Peptide growth factor	Increases cell proliferation (in vitro), may aid bone repair (in vivo)

* RGD = arginine-glycine-aspartic acid; TGF-β = transforming growth factor-beta; PDGF = platelet-derived growth factor; Gla = gamma-carboxyglutamic acid; IGF = insulin-like growth factor; BMP = bone morphogenetic protein; FGF = fibroblast growth factor

acetabular components into beds under-reamed by as much as 4 mm has been shown to create initial gaps of greater than 3 mm adjacent to the dome of the implant. Numerous studies have shown that gaps as small as 0.5 mm can impair bone ingrowth. The presence of interface gaps, besides directly impairing bone ingrowth, may also lead to increased motion at the interface in some circumstances.

Initial Interface Micromotion

The initial mechanical environment at the bone-implant interface is of paramount importance. There has been considerable research in this area. An early review of several experimental studies concluded that bone ingrowth can occur if interface motion is less than 28 μm, but would not occur in the presence of 150 μm or more of interface motion. Tissue response in the range of 28 to 150 μm was not understood at the time of the review and remains poorly understood today.

A number of recent studies have quantitated the initial motion between an implant and the skeleton to determine if the motion at the interface can be reduced by altering the design of the implant. For instance, data from studies of cementless femoral stems indicate that the collar can prevent axial subsidence, and transverse micromotion can be reduced with a tight distal fit, increased stem length, increased metaphyseal fit, or the use of a curved stem. Stability of the femoral stem has been noted to be particularly sensitive to off-axis loading (Fig. 3), and asymmetric (curved) stems tend to have greater initial stability than symmetric (straight) stems.

Motion studies have concentrated on the tibial component in TKR. With eccentrically applied loads varying from less than one to three body weights, vertical displacements as great as 700 μm have been observed at the periphery of the component in in vitro tests of commercially available components. Data have shown that the most effective way to reduce interface motion is to use screws for adjuvant initial fixation.

In animal models with controlled initial bone-implant interface motions of 150 μm or greater, the interface is formed by fibrous tissue. In a canine THR model, three-fold reduction of the initial interface motion occurred after a 4-month period of in vivo service in which bone ingrowth occurred. In another study using a canine THR model, it was shown that the distal uncoated stem was important for initial stability, but after bone ingrowth into a proximal porous coating occurred, the role of the distal

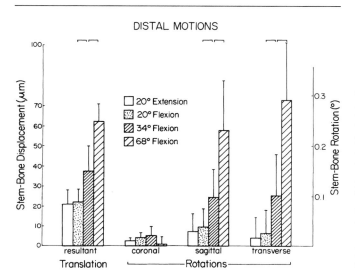

Fig. 3 The initial relative motion between the femoral stem and cortex as determined in tests of proximally porous-coated Ti6Al4V components in cadaver bones in the laboratory. Note that as the femur was placed in a more flexed position and, hence, the degree of off-axis loading increased, the amount of motion increased. The brackets indicate significant differences between adjacent flexion angles. (Reproduced with permission from Berzins A, Sumner DR, Andriacchi TP, et al: Stem curvature and load angle influence the initial relative bone-implant motion of cementless femoral stems. *J Orthop Res* 1993;11:758–769.)

stem was greatly reduced. Eventually these studies should help determine how much interface motion is permissible for bone ingrowth, and the relationship between the quantity of bone ingrowth and the late mechanical stability of the implant.

Enhancement of Bone Ingrowth

Data from retrieval studies suggest that improvements can be made in obtaining fixation by bone ingrowth. Thus, there has been considerable interest in means of enhancing bone ingrowth. Enhancement can be thought of in two ways: (1) developing systems whereby 100% of components will become fixed by bone ingrowth and (2) increasing the extent and volume fraction of bone ingrowth. Although this chapter focuses on biologic approaches to enhancing bone ingrowth, the critical importance of obtaining excellent initial fit—such that interface gaps are eliminated and adequate implant-bone stability is obtained—should not be neglected.

No controlled studies have been reported in which the effectiveness was compared of various bone grafts or graft substitutes for enhancing bone ingrowth in humans. However, various materials have been tested using models that replicate the ideal conditions for bone ingrowth. Data indicate that enhancement of bone ingrowth is usually only modest.

Models have recently been developed to examine enhancement in the presence of excessive bone-implant motion or poor bone-implant contact as might be found in the biologic and mechanical environment associated with aseptic loosening. Treatment of the implant with hydroxyapatite (HA) or hydroxyapatite/tricalcium phosphate (HA/TCP) by plasma flame spraying has been reported to enhance bone ingrowth in the presence of interface gaps. Autogenous bone graft and demineralized allogeneic bone matrix have been shown to be effective enhancing agents when placed into the gap. Presumably, the demineralized bone matrix was effective because of the presence of bone morphogenetic protein. It has recently been found that TGF-β applied to the implant via an HA/TCP carrier very effectively enhanced bone ingrowth; it was more effective than autogenous bone graft in the same model.

There is very little information in the literature on enhancing bone ingrowth in the presence of interface motion. In a canine model with 150 μm of initial interface motion and an interface gap of 0.75 mm, HA-treated implants had bone ingrowth at 16 weeks, whereas implants not treated by HA were encapsulated by a fibrous membrane.

The revision environment presents a severe challenge because the normal medullary contents have been replaced by granulation tissue, and loss of bone stock may adversely affect the ability to obtain initial rigid fixation of the prosthesis. It was recently reported that autogenous bone graft can be used to enhance bone ingrowth in this situation (Fig. 4).

Inhibition of Bone Ingrowth

In general, any treatment known to inhibit fracture healing has a dampening effect on bone ingrowth. Certain adjuvant treatments, which might be administered to patients receiving cementless joint replacements, can adversely affect bone ingrowth. Concern with formation of heterotopic bone following THR has led to the use of the bisphosphonate etidronic acid (EHDP), indomethacin, and low-dose radiation for prophylaxis. These therapies tend to delay or inhibit bone ingrowth. Thus, it has been suggested that low-dose radiation may be preferable in patients receiving cementless implants because it is possible to protect the interface by appropriate shielding.

Long-Term Maintenance of the Cementless Interface

Once bone ingrowth has occurred, the bone within and adjacent to the porous coating remodels. The long-term distribution of bone ingrowth within the prosthesis appears to be a reflection of the mechanical environment, which specifically reflects how the load is passed from the prosthesis to the surrounding skeleton. In a canine model of the femoral stem from THR, an even distribution of

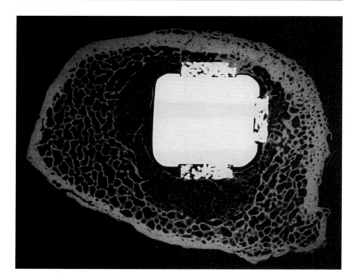

Fig. 4 Radiograph of a cross section of the proximal femur in a dog that had a cementless revision femoral stem placed with autogenous bone graft following aseptic loosening of a cemented component. Note the presence throughout the region, which had previously been cemented, of thin trabeculae, and the presence of some areas of bone ingrowth. Note also that the uncoated regions of the stem lack intimate bone-implant contact (original magnification × 4.3). (Reproduced with permission from Turner TM, Urban RM, Sumner DR, et al: Revision, without cement, of aseptically loose, cemented total hip prostheses: Quantitative comparison of the effects of four types of medullary treatment on bone ingrowth in a canine model. *J Bone Joint Surg* 1993;75A:845–862.)

bone ingrowth along the length of the device was observed at 1 month. However, at 6 and 24 months, there was more bone ingrowth in regions in which the interface stresses would be expected to be the highest—proximally and distally.

In most situations, the long-term distribution of bone ingrowth actually depends on a number of factors, including the degree of initial contact, component stability, and the inherent mode of stress transfer from the implant to the host. The canine study noted above showed such a clear-cut long-term influence of the stress transfer mechanism on the distribution of bone ingrowth because the initial contact and interface micromotion permitted bone ingrowth throughout the prosthesis. As this bone remodeled, the distribution of ingrowth reflected the stress-transfer mechanisms inherent in a well-bonded stem. Studies of components retrieved from patients also indicate that bone ingrowth can be patterned. For instance, in the femoral stem, bone ingrowth is greater medially than posteriorly and anteriorly in one proximally porous-coated design. This may be as much a reflection of the initial fit of the implant as the stress-transfer mechanism.

Roentgen stereophotogrammetric analysis (RSA) has been used to examine migration of cementless and ce-

mented total joint replacement components in vivo and is the most sensitive means of clinically assessing the long-term mechanical stability of the interface. Whereas migrations less than 2 mm are difficult to detect with conventional radiographic techniques, this technique can detect migrations as small as 200 μm. In several studies, prostheses that eventually developed late loosening were found to actually show early migration on RSA, indicating that aseptic loosening is called late only because it is not recognizable by conventional radiography (until the components have migrated 2 mm or more). These studies have also shown that implant design can have a profound impact on component migration. In addition, HA treatment of the proximal porous-coated region of one stem design was found to reduce migration significantly in the first postoperative year.

Two studies of implants retrieved at autopsy have indicated that motion at the bone-implant interface can be very small. In these studies of cementless femoral stems and cementless tibial components, inducible micromotions considerably smaller than 200 μm in magnitude (ie, below the sensitivity of RSA) were found.

Although cementless porous-coated devices are used because the "living" interface is expected to be less susceptible to fatigue failure than a cemented interface, data from two studies of femoral stems with limited areas of proximal porous coating have suggested that failure of a bone ingrown interface can occur because of fatigue failure of the connecting trabecular bone. An implication of this finding is that the area of coverage by the porous coating (and hence the area available for mechanical fixation) should not be severely restricted.

Long-Term Bone Loss

The severity of periprosthetic bone loss appears to be greater following cementless as opposed to cemented THR. Bone loss can lead to loosening or fracture of the host bone or implant and it makes further reconstruction difficult. Bone loss following total joint replacement is usually ascribed to one of two processes: adaptive bone remodeling or osteolysis.

Osteolytic bone loss occurs in loose and well-fixed cemented and cementless total joint replacement, and polyethylene wear debris is commonly hypothesized to be a major factor. Thus, a key current concern is whether polyethylene migration to the periprosthetic host bone occurs more commonly in cemented or cementless interfaces. It has become clear that uncoated regions of porous-coated femoral stems promote the development of periprosthetic cavities, which can serve as conduits for the migration of wear debris. Increased use of modularity with cementless devices may be partially responsible for the generation of particulates and, ultimately, reduction of the particulate burden should reduce the incidence of osteolysis. Many would agree that the porous coating should be applied cir-

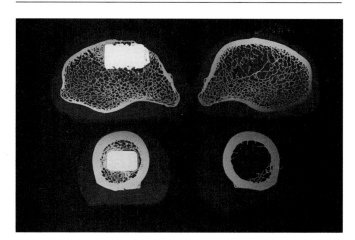

Fig. 5 Radiographs of cross sections from the operated and contralateral control femurs of a dog implanted with a porous-coated Ti6Al4V stem for 2 years. Note the extensive thinning of the proximal anteromedial cortex as a consequence of stress shielding and the hypertrophy of the distal medullary bone. Note also the lack of periprosthetic cavities in this circumferentially porous-coated stem. (Reproduced with permission from Sumner DR, Turner TM, Urban RM, et al: Remodeling and ingrowth of bone at two years in a canine cementless total hip-arthroplasty model. *J Bone Joint Surg* 1992;74A:239–250.)

cumferentially in the hope that circumferential bone ingrowth would prevent the ingress of wear debris to the interface. Some data indicate that dense fibrous tissue ingrowth into a porous surface can also act as a barrier. Osteolysis can often progress asymptomatically, necessitating careful radiographic follow-up of patients.

Adaptive bone remodeling in the femur following cementless THR has been extensively studied using animal models (Fig. 5), computer-based simulations, and, more recently, dual energy x-ray absorptiometry (DEXA) in patients. Proximal bone loss has been difficult to reduce, except with the use of more flexible stems. Because these stems are often based on composite technology, establishing and maintaining a cementless interface through bone ingrowth into a porous surface presents a significant design challenge.

Long-Term Biocompatibility

Use of foreign materials may have important local and systemic consequences for patients who have cemented or cementless total joint replacements. The rate of release of metal ions from an implant with a porous coating is probably as much as an order of magnitude higher than from a conventional cemented implant. Four basic areas concerning metal ion release need to be addressed: (1) amount, (2) destination, (3) chemical form, and (4) physiologic consequences.

Twofold elevations in serum titanium have been observed in patients with loose titanium-base alloy femoral stems compared to age-matched individuals without prostheses. No increases in serum titanium were reported for patients with well-functioning cementless porous-coated titanium-base alloy femoral components. None of the patients with prostheses had elevations of the constituent metals (titanium, aluminum, or vanadium) in their urine nor were there elevations of aluminum or vanadium in the serum of these patients. Loosening is also known to lead to increased levels of serum and urine cobalt in patients with cobalt-chromium (CoCr) alloy components.

Little is known about the destination, chemical form, and physiologic consequences of released metal ions. These are important issues because many constituents of both CoCr-base alloy and titanium-base alloy joint prostheses have known specific toxic effects. However, these effects are known mainly for the soluble forms of these elements and not necessarily for the species released in vivo. Malignant tumors have been reported to be associated with total joint replacement components, and two epidemiologic studies suggest a link between leukemia-lymphoma and patients with cobalt-base alloy total hip replacement.

Materials used in total joint replacement have functioned well for many years. It is not known if the use of porous coatings per se increases the risk of implant-site tumors or systemic effects. Certainly, this is an area requiring additional investigation given that porous-coated implants are often used in younger patients.

Summary

The papers reviewed herein suggest that cementless porous-coated interfaces can fail aseptically by one or a combination of four modes: (1) early mechanical loosening that is recognized only in intermediate to long-term follow-up; (2) fatigue of the trabeculae connecting an ingrown prosthesis to the host skeleton; (3) wear debris-related osteolysis; and (4) adaptive bone remodeling. No case of implant failure due to excessive adaptive bone remodeling has been reported, and failure due to fatigue may be limited to implant designs with highly restricted areas of porous coating. The relative importance of (unrecognized) early mechanical loosening and late osteolysis remains to be determined. Osteolysis may be more of a problem in components that are not mechanically well-integrated with the host skeleton.

Annotated Bibliography

Introduction

Callaghan JJ: The clinical results and basic science of total hip arthroplasty with porous-coated prostheses. *J Bone Joint Surg* 1993;75A:299–310.

Together, these three articles provide a detailed history through 1992 of bone ingrowth.

LeGeros RZ, Craig RG: Strategies to affect bone remodeling: Osteointegration. *J Bone Miner Res* 1993; 8(suppl):S583–S596.

This article provides an up-to-date summary of the concept of osseointegration—direct attachment of bone to an implant without an intervening layer of soft tissue at the level of light microscopy.

Sumner DR, Galante JO: Advances in osseointegration of cementless total hip replacements. *Curr Opin Orthop* 1992;3:427–435.

Sumner DR Jr, Galante JO: Bone ingrowth, in Evarts CM (ed): *Surgery of the Musculoskeletal System,* ed 2. New York, NY, Churchill Livingstone, 1990, pp 151–176.

Analysis of Retrieved Components

Bloebaum RD, Rubman MH, Hofmann AA: Bone ingrowth into porous-coated tibial components implanted with autograft bone chips: Analysis of ten consecutively retrieved implants. *J Arthroplasty* 1992;7:483–493.

This study of 10 primary porous-coated TKR tibial components (Natural-Knee) retrieved from 1 week to 48 months postoperatively showed that the volume fraction of bone ingrowth varied from 8% in the early cases to a plateau of ~20% in the five implants in place for more than 18 months. The authors suggested that the use of autogenous bone chips enhanced bone ingrowth, but it should also be noted that the initial stability of this implant was probably enhanced because of the inclusion of four pegs and two cancellous bone screws.

Engh CA, Zettl-Schaffer KF, Kukita Y, et al: Histological and radiographic assessment of well functioning porous-coated acetabular components: A human postmortem retrieval study. *J Bone Joint Surg* 1993;75A:814–824.

Nine porous-coated acetabular components (3 Arthropor, 2 Trilock, 4 AML) retrieved at autopsy from 17 to 87 months postoperatively had an average volume fraction of bone ingrowth of 13%. Six of the 9 components had 10% or more volume fraction of bone ingrowth. The authors observed no granulomatous formation in areas occupied by soft tissue and suggested that both fibrous tissue and bone ingrowth interfaces may be effective impediments to the migration of particulate debris.

Jacobs JJ, Sumner DR, Urban RM, et al: Retrieval: Successful uncemented implants, in Morrey BF (ed): *Biological, Material and Mechanical Considerations of Joint Replacement.* New York, NY, Raven Press, 1993, pp 185–196.

The burgeoning literature on analysis of tissue ingrowth into porous-coated orthopaedic implants is summarized in this book chapter. The incidence and amount of bone ingrowth found in implants retrieved for cause vary widely. Fewer studies of well-functioning implants retrieved at autopsy have been reported, but seem to indicate that bone ingrowth may occur more frequently at some anatomic sites than indicated by the initial studies.

Pidhorz LE, Urban RM, Jacobs JJ, et al: A quantitative study of bone and soft tissues in cementless porous-coated acetabular components retrieved at autopsy. *J Arthroplasty* 1993;8:213–225.

This study, besides describing the amount and distribution of bone ingrowth in 11 primary hemispheric porous-coated acetabular components (HG I) retrieved at autopsy at an average 41 months postoperatively, showed that wear debris can accumulate in screw holes. Although no osteolytic reactions were observed in the vicinity of the wear debris, its presence is worrisome because it is generally accepted that wear debris in sufficient quantity plays a key role in the formation of osteolytic lesions. The volume fraction of bone ingrowth within the porous coating was 12% (±8%). Bone ingrowth was greater adjacent to screw holes through which screws had been placed compared to empty screw holes.

Sumner DR, Kienapfel H, Jacobs JJ, et al: Bone ingrowth and wear debris in well-fixed cementless porous-coated tibial components removed from patients. *J Arthroplasty* 1995;10:1–11.

This study of 13 primary porous-coated TKR components (MG I) retrieved from 3 to 30 months postoperatively showed that the volume fraction of bone ingrowth was 10% (±8%), with five of the six implants in place for more than 18 months having 10% or more bone ingrowth. The authors suggested that the routine use of initial screw fixation led to sufficient initial stability of the device to permit bone ingrowth. The tibial bearing surfaces in these components contained carbon fiber, which facilitated histologic identification of wear debris migration. The carbon fiber debris was found in the vicinity of the hollow fixation pegs and at the periphery of the interface.

Vigorita VJ, Minkowitz B, Dichiara JF, et al: A histomorphometric and histologic analysis of the implant interface in five successful, autopsy-retrieved, noncemented porous-coated knee arthroplasties. *Clin Orthop* 1993;293:211–218.

This study of porous-coated TKR components (PCA) retrieved at autopsy from 5 patients at 13 to 56 months postoperatively showed that the volume fraction of bone ingrowth was 23% in the patellar component and 6% in both the femoral and tibial components.

Basic Biology of Bone Ingrowth

Caplan AI: Mesenchymal stem cells. *J Orthop Res* 1991;9: 641–650.

This useful review discusses the role of mesenchymal stem cells in bone and cartilage formation during development, repair, and remodeling.

Ibaraki K, Termine JD, Whitson SW, et al: Bone matrix mRNA expression in differentiating fetal bovine osteoblasts. *J Bone Miner Res* 1992;7:743–754.

The authors used an in vitro system to study gene expression during bone development and found that levels of expression vary over time, supporting the concept that differentiation involves precise regulation of genes and their products.

Liang CT, Barnes J, Seedor JG, et al: Impaired bone activity in aged rats: Alterations at the cellular and molecular levels. *Bone* 1992;13:435–441.

With the rat tibial marrow ablation model the authors determined that increased age led to decreased expression of bone-related genes and reduced bone formation.

Stein GS, Lain JB, Owen TA: Relationship of cell growth to the regulation of tissue-specific gene expression during osteoblast differentiation. *FASEB J* 1990;4:3111–3123.

Bone cell differentiation can be characterized by three periods: proliferation, extracellular matrix maturation, and mineralization. An in vitro model was used to determine that gene expression varies during these three periods. The authors suggest that transition from one period to the next represents points at which cell differentiation and, therefore, tissue development, can be halted.

Suva LJ, Seedor JG, Endo N, et al: Pattern of gene expression following rat tibial marrow ablation. *J Bone Miner Res* 1993;8:379–388.

The rat was used to determine the pattern of gene expression following ablation of the marrow, an experimental procedure which causes intramembranous bone formation analogous to the process of bone ingrowth. Insulin-like growth factor I was highly expressed, but transforming growth factor-β was only weakly expressed between days 5 and 12, leading the authors to suggest that the former growth factor but not the latter may play a significant role in initiating bone formation following marrow ablation.

Initial Interface Gaps

MacKenzie JR, Callaghan JJ, Pedersen DR, et al: Areas of contact and extent of gaps with implantation of oversized acetabular components in total hip arthroplasty. *Clin Orthop* 1994;298:127–136.

This study in cadaver acetabula showed that gaps wider than 3 mm can form at the polar region of the bone-implant interface with hemispherical porous-coated acetabular components press-fit into underreamed cavities.

Otani T, Whiteside LA, White SE: Cutting errors in preparation of femoral components in total knee arthroplasty. *J Arthroplasty* 1993;8:503–510.

This study using cadaver femurs showed that both saw blade toggle and motion between the cutting guide and skeleton lead to cutting errors and the creation of interface gaps of at least 0.5 mm in width in cementless TKR.

Toksvig-Larsen S, Ryd L: Surface characteristics following tibial preparation during total knee arthroplasty. *J Arthroplasty* 1994;9:63–66.

Flatness of the tibial cut in 26 clinical cases of cementless TKR was investigated and showed that the maximum roughness (distance between the highest and lowest points) was 1.71 mm,

indicating that significant bone-implant interface gaps exist in the initial postoperative period.

Initial Interface Micromotion

Berzins A, Sumner DR, Andriacchi TP, et al: Stem curvature and load angle influence the initial relative bone-implant motion of cementless femoral stems. *J Orthop Res* 1993;11:758–769.

Off-axis loading was an important contributor to the initial bone-implant motion and the curved stem had slightly greater proximal (though not distal) stability than the straight stem.

Curtis MJ, Jinnah RH, Wilson VD, et al: The initial stability of uncemented acetabular components. *J Bone Joint Surg* 1992;74B:372–376.

This study of press-fitting a cementless porous-coated CoCr hemispherical acetabular component showed that underreaming by 2 or 3 mm led to acceptable initial stability of the implant. Underreaming by 1 mm was not adequate and underreaming by 4 mm had a risk of fracture in addition to making it difficult to obtain good contact with host bone in the polar region of the prosthesis.

Jasty M, Krushell R, Zalenski E, et al: The contribution of the nonporous distal stem to the stability of proximally porous-coated canine femoral components. *J Arthroplasty* 1993;8:33–41.

In a canine model of THR, the nonporous-coated distal part of the femoral stem was an important contributor to the initial stability of the implant, but its role became negligible after bone ingrowth occurred.

Lee RW, Volz RG, Sheridan DC: The role of fixation and bone quality on the mechanical stability of tibial knee components. *Clin Orthop* 1991;273:177–183.

In a model system using "foam bone," the most important factor for achieving initial stability of the tibial component in TKR was the use of four peripheral cancellous bone screws. The addition of a central stem was important only in the presence of poor bone quality.

Soballe K, Hansen ES, Brockstedt-Rasmussen H, et al: Hydroxyapatite coating converts fibrous tissue to bone around loaded implants. *J Bone Joint Surg* 1993;75B:270–278.

Bone ingrowth was inhibited in the presence of 150 μm of initial motion, however, immobilization of the implants after the development of the fibrous tissue membrane at 4 weeks led to bone formation and increased fixation strength at 16 weeks. This study implies that immobilization of an initially unstable implant could permit development of adequate fixation by bone.

Soballe K, Hansen ES, Brockstedt-Rasmussen H, et al: Tissue ingrowth into titanium and hydroxyapatite-coated implants during stable and unstable mechanical conditions. *J Orthop Res* 1992;10:285–299.

This study introduced a model in which bone ingrowth was inhibited in the presence of 500 μm of initial motion.

Sumner DR, Berzins A, Turner TM, et al: Initial in vitro stability of the tibial component in a canine model of cementless total knee replacement. *J Biomech* 1994;27:929–939.

In a canine model of the tibial component in TKR, in the presence of four cancellous screws that usually gained purchase in cortical bone, the addition of four short porous-coated pegs provided no added initial stability.

Vanderby R Jr, Manley PA, Kohles SS, et al: Fixation stability of femoral components in a canine hip replacement model. *J Orthop Res* 1992;10:300–309.

Initial relative displacements between the femoral component of a canine THR model and the cortex with a 100-N axial load were on the order of 200 to 300 μm, but these motions were reduced by threefold after a 4 month period of in vivo use. By 4 months, cementless components were as stable as cemented controls, and there was a positive correlation between the amount of bone apposition to the implant and the stability of the device.

Wyatt RWB, Alpert JP, Daniels AU, et al: The effect of screw fixation on initial rigidity of tibial knee components. *J Appl Biomater* 1991;2:109–113.

Better initial stability of the tibial component of TKR was achieved with four peripherally placed screws than with three or two screws, and long cancellous screws and screws with cortical purchase provided more initial stability than short cancellous screws.

Yoshii I, Whiteside LA, Milliano MT, et al: The effect of central stem and stem length on micromovement of the tibial tray. *J Arthroplasty* 1992;7(suppl):S433–S438.

The initial stability of the tibial component of TKR fixed with four cancellous screws that gain purchase in the cortex can be improved with the use of a long central stem. Use of a short stem was not effective.

Enhancement of Bone Ingrowth

Kienapfel H, Sumner DR, Turner TM, et al: Efficacy of autograft and freeze-dried allograft to enhance fixation of porous coated implants in the presence of interface gaps. *J Orthop Res* 1992;10:423–433.

Grafting of a 3-mm gap at the bone-implant interface with autogenous bone led to a sevenfold increase in the strength of fixation and a threefold increase in the amount of bone ingrowth at 4 weeks in a canine model. Use of freeze-dried allograft was not efficacious.

Rubin CT, McLeod KJ: Promotion of bony ingrowth by frequency-specific, low-amplitude mechanical strain. *Clin Orthop* 1994;298:165–174.

Loads applied to the ulna in an avian model were controlled experimentally. Transcortical placement of a porous-coated implant was tested under various conditions. Bone ingrowth was enhanced in the presence of extremely low-amplitude mechanical strains (150 με), particularly when a 20-Hz frequency was used, whereas bone ingrowth was inhibited in the absence of applied loads.

Shen W, Chung KC, Wang GJ, et al: Demineralized bone matrix in the stabilization of porous-coated implants in bone defects in rabbits. *Clin Orthop* 1993;293:346–352.

Demineralized bone graft was as effective as autogenous iliac crest bone for enhancing bone ingrowth and fixation strength of porous-coated implants at 8 weeks in a rabbit model in which there was a 2-mm bone-implant interface gap.

Soballe K, Hansen ES, Brockstedt-Rasmussen H, et al: Gap healing enhanced by hydroxyapatite coating in dogs. *Clin Orthop* 1991;272:300–307.

HA-treatment of a porous-coated implant led to a twofold increase in the strength of fixation in normal bone and a threefold increase in osteopenic bone in a canine model at 4 weeks in the presence of a 1-mm gap at the bone-implant interface.

Soballe K, Hansen ES, Brockstedt-Rasmussen H, et al: Hydroxyapatite coating converts fibrous tissue to bone around loaded implants. *J Bone Joint Surg* 1993;75B: 270–278.

In a canine model with a 750-μm interface gap and 150 μm of initial motion, HA-treated porous-coated implants had bone ingrowth at 16 weeks, but porous-coated implants not treated with HA were surrounded by a fibrous membrane.

Sumner DR, Kienapfel H, Galante JO: Metallic implants, in Habal MB, Reddi AH (eds): *Bone Grafts & Bone Substitutes.* Philadelphia, PA, WB Saunders, 1992, pp 252–262.

This review chapter provides a useful summary of attempts to enhance bone ingrowth until approximately 1990.

Sumner DR, Turner TM, Purchio AF, et al: Enhancement of bone ingrowth by transforming growth factor beta. *J Bone Joint Surg,* in press.

TGFβ1 at a dose of 120 μg/implant applied to a HA/TCP carrier plasma flame sprayed to the porous surface, was found to enhance the volume fraction of bone ingrowth by threefold compared to implants treated only with the HA/TCP in the presence of a 3-mm gap at the bone-implant interface in a canine model.

Tisdel CL, Goldberg VM, Parr JA, et al: The influence of hydroxyapatite and tricalcium-phosphate coating on bone growth into titanium fiber-metal implants. *J Bone Joint Surg* 1994;76A:159–171.

These authors found a threefold increase in bone ingrowth in HA/TCP-treated porous-coated rods placed in rabbit femora compared to untreated control rods.

Turner TM, Urban RM, Sumner DR, et al: Revision, without cement, of aseptically loose, cemented total hip prostheses: Quantitative comparison of the effects of four types of medullary treatment on bone ingrowth in a canine model. *J Bone Joint Surg* 1993;75A:845–862.

A model replicating the radiographic and histologic features of aseptic loosening of the cemented femoral component in THR was created in canines to test the efficacy of graft materials for enhancing bone ingrowth in cementless revision. Autogenous bone graft was found to be an efficacious means of enhancing bone ingrowth, but a bone graft substitute consisting of HA/TCP particles was not effective.

Inhibition of Bone Ingrowth

Sumner DR, Turner TM, Pierson RH, et al: Effects of radiation on fixation of non-cemented porous-coated implants in a canine model. *J Bone Joint Surg* 1990; 72A:1527–1533.

Exposure of a porous-coated implant to 1000 rads inhibited bone ingrowth, whereas exposure to 500 rads had no significant effect in a canine model. The authors recommended that the implant should be shielded if radiation is used as a prophylactic for heterotopic ossification following THR.

Long-Term Maintenance of the Cementless Interface

Engh CA, O'Connor D, Jasty M, et al: Quantification of implant micromotion, strain shielding, and bone resorption with porous-coated anatomic medullary locking femoral prostheses. *Clin Orthop* 1992;285:13–29.

Relative displacement between the femoral stem and cortex was studied in 13 AML prostheses retrieved at autopsy 12 to 93 months after surgery.

Grewal R, Rimmer MG, Freeman MA: Early migration of prostheses related to long-term survivorship: Comparison of tibial components in knee replacement. *J Bone Joint Surg* 1992;74B:239–242.

This study indicates that migration of the tibial component of TKR as measured by RSA within the first postoperative year is an accurate predictor of late aseptic loosening as determined in conventional radiographic analyses or of the need for revision surgery.

Jasty M, Bragdon CR, Maloney WJ, et al: Ingrowth of bone in failed fixation of porous-coated femoral components. *J Bone Joint Surg* 1991;73A:1331–1337.

These authors describe bone ingrowth in 5 femoral stems (HG) removed because of loosening. They suggest that fatigue of the connecting trabeculae may have occurred.

Nilsson KG, Karrholm J: Increased varus-valgus tilting of screw-fixated knee prostheses: Stereoradiographic study of uncemented tibial components. *J Arthroplasty* 1993;8:529–540.

In general, migration with screw-fixed cementless tibial total knee replacement components occurred within the first 6 weeks to 3 months and then reached a plateau, whereas migration of the cemented components did not plateau at 3 months. Migration during this early period was less with the cemented components, but by 24 months most of the migrations were equivalent except for greater rotation about the sagittal axis in the cementless group.

Önssten I, Carlsson AS, Ohlin A, et al: Migration of acetabular components, inserted with and without cement, in one-stage bilateral hip arthroplasty: A controlled, randomized study using roentgen stereophotogrammetric analysis. *J Bone Joint Surg* 1994;76A:185.

This study indicates that in the intermediate term equivalent fixation can be obtained with cemented and cementless acetabular components.

Ryd L, Carlsson L, Herberts P: Micromotion of a noncemented tibial component with screw fixation: An in vivo roentgen stereophotogrammetric study of the Miller-Galante prosthesis. *Clin Orthop* 1993;295:218–225.

Data from an RSA study of migration of the MG I tibial component in 7 patients indicated that the mean total point migration during the first postoperative year was 0.6 mm. The amount of inducible displacement was usually less than 300 μm after 1 year.

Ryd L, Toksvig-Larsen S: Early postoperative fixation of tibial components: An in vivo roentgen stereophotogrammetric analysis. *J Orthop Res* 1993;11:142–148.

The amount of inducible motion did not differ between cemented and cementless tibial components of TKR of one design (PCA). However, displacements were large enough to have inhibited bone ingrowth, and they may play a role in the development of a fibrous membrane at the cement-bone interface.

Soballe K, Toksvig-Larsen S, Gelineck J, et al: Migration of hydroxyapatite coated femoral prostheses: A roentgen stereophotogrammetic study. *J Bone Joint Surg* 1993;75B:681–687.

These authors studied the migration of one type of femoral stem in cementless THR in which the proximal aspect of the stem had a porous surface of plasma flame spray. In one-half of the patients the porous surface was further treated with HA. The "maximum total point motion" was twofold higher in the group lacking the HA treatment after 12 months. Both groups had equivalent Harris hip scores preoperatively, but at follow-up these scores and visual analogue pain scores were improved in the group with HA treatment.

Sumner DR, Turner TM, Urban RM, et al: Remodeling and ingrowth of bone at two years in a canine cementless total hip-arthroplasty model. *J Bone Joint Surg* 1992;74A:239–250.

This study showed that the amount of bone ingrowth in the femoral stem of a canine model of THR was patterned as would be predicted by consideration of the distribution of interface stresses.

Long-Term Bone Loss

Bloebaum RD, Dupont JA: Osteolysis from a press-fit hydroxyapatite-coated implant: A case study. *J Arthroplasty* 1993;8:195–202.

The HA coating had separated from the femoral component of a cementless THR and migrated to the articulation, leading to the generation of considerable wear debris, which was associated with the development of osteolysis adjacent to both the femoral and acetabular components.

Bobyn JD, Mortimer ES, Glassman AH, et al: Producing and avoiding stress shielding: Laboratory and clinical observations of noncemented total hip arthroplasty. *Clin Orthop* 1992;274:79–96.

Use of a low stiffness stem in a canine model of cementless THR led to more retention of cortical bone than use of a stiffer stem. An analysis of human stems suggests that to reduce stress-shielding-related bone loss, the device should be 33% to 50% as stiff in bending as the femur.

Engh CA, McGovern TF, Bobyn JD, et al: A quantitative evaluation of periprosthetic bone-remodeling after cementless total hip arthroplasty. *J Bone Joint Surg* 1992;74A:1009–1020.

Dual energy x-ray absorptiometry was used in an autopsy study to compare the bone mineral content of five proximal femurs that had had an AML prosthesis in place from 17 to 84 months to that of the paired intact contralateral bones.

Engh CA, O'Connor D, Jasty M, et al: Quantification of implant micromotion, strain shielding, and bone resorption with porous-coated anatomic medullary locking femoral prostheses. *Clin Orthop* 1992;285:13–29.

Nine autopsy-retrieved femora with AML stems which had been in service in vivo were compared to their contralateral pairs in which similar stems were implanted acutely to simulate the immediate postoperative mechanical environment.

Jacobs JJ, Sumner DR, Galante JO: Mechanisms of bone loss associated with total hip replacement. *Orthop Clin North Am* 1993;24:583–590.

This recent review article discusses bone loss following THR due to adaptive bone remodeling (stress-shielding) and pathologic bone remodeling (osteolysis).

Kim KJ, Chiba J, Rubash HE: In vivo and in vitro analysis of membranes from hip prostheses inserted without cement. *J Bone Joint Surg* 1994;76A:172–180.

These authors investigated membranes from 64 femoral components in 63 patients with cementless THR, 57 from hips with polyethylene articulations, and seven from unipolar devices with no polyethylene articulation. Biochemical analyses supported the generally accepted view that polyethylene debris is critical in the development of osteolysis.

Peters PC Jr, Engh GA, Dwyer KA, et al: Osteolysis after total knee arthroplasty without cement. *J Bone Joint Surg* 1992;74A:864–876.

A 16% incidence of osteolysis was found following cementless TKR. The onset was typically at 35 months after surgery and was often progressive. The design investigated had extensive polyethylene wear and corrosion between titanium fixation screws and the cobalt chrome base plate.

Sumner DR, Galante JO: Determinants of stress shielding: Design vs. materials vs. interface. *Clin Orthop* 1992;274:202–212.

Sumner DR, Turner TM, Urban RM, et al: Experimental studies of bone remodeling in total hip replacement. *Clin Orthop* 1992;276:83–90.

These reviews of bone remodeling in cementless THR models indicate that the most reliable way to reduce periprosthetic bone loss in the femur is to reduce the stiffness of the femoral component.

Van Rietbergen B, Huiskes R, Weinans H, et al: The mechanism of bone remodeling and resorption around press-fitted THA stems. *J Biomech* 1993;26:369–382.

Ward WG, Johnston KS, Dorey FJ, et al: Extramedullary porous coating to prevent diaphyseal osteolysis and radiolucent lines around proximal tibial replacements: A preliminary report. *J Bone Joint Surg* 1993;75A:976–987.

These authors suggest that fibrous tissue ingrowth into a circumferential porous coating can impede migration of wear debris from the joint and the development of osteolysis.

Weinans H, Huiskes R, van Rietbergen B, et al: Adaptive bone remodeling around bonded noncemented total hip arthroplasty: A comparison between animal experiments and computer simulation. *J Orthop Res* 1993;11:500–513.

These studies show that the results of finite element-based predictions of bone remodeling around the femoral stem following cementless THR can accurately reflect experimental results.

Long-Term Biocompatibility

Jacobs JJ, Galante JO, Sumner DR: Cementless primary total hip arthroplasty, in Chapman MW (ed): *Operative Orthopedics.* Philadelphia, PA, JB Lippincott, 1993, vol 3, pp 1889–1909.

This is an extensive review of cementless primary total hip arthroplasty, including issues related to long-term biocompatibility.

9

Medical Treatment of Arthritis

Introduction

Advances in knowledge and evolving data on a variety of arthritic disorders are presented in this section. Common rheumatic disease issues, emphasis on differential diagnosis, advantages of conservative therapy, and drug toxicities are discussed.

Articular Tissues

Connective tissue is an important part of the large mass of tissues of the musculoskeletal system. Connective tissue cells are embedded in an abundant extracellular matrix composed of collagens, proteoglycans, and other extracellular proteins. This tissue has been characterized as a relatively inert structural tissue that is not very active metabolically and that has a sparse cell population. However, this characterization is misleading, because, even under normal conditions, turnover of connective tissues is relatively active. The individual macromolecular components of these tissues undergo continuous degradation and resynthesis.

The principal elements of connective tissue are the cells, including fibroblasts, chondrocytes, and endothelial cells; the macromolecules synthesized by the cells; and the interstitial fluid surrounding them. The macromolecules are either proteins or complex polysaccharides. The major proteins are the collagens, a family of proteins with common structural features, which provide an extracellular framework; fibronectin, an adhesive glycoprotein, which plays a role in the attachment of various macromolecular components to cell surfaces; and elastin, a polymer that gives some distensible tissues their elastic properties. The complex polysaccharides are mainly represented by proteoglycans, fundamental structural components of articular cartilage that permit compressibility.

Biochemistry

Proteoglycan monomers are complex macromolecules that contain a protein backbone to which are attached long chains of repeating disaccharide units, which are called glycosaminoglycans. Proteoglycan aggregates are formed when several monomers bind to a single linear backbone consisting of hyaluronic acid (Fig. 1). Arrayed at intervals along this backbone, like bristles on a bottle brush, are individual glycosaminoglycan molecules, each of which consists of a core protein to which is attached varying amounts of the glycosaminoglycans chondroitin sulfate or keratan sulfate. This proteoglycan is joined to the hyaluronic acid backbone by special link proteins. Turnover of proteoglycan molecules in the extracellular matrix is gen-

erally very slow; it is measured in terms of months or years. This slow turnover may allow changes resulting from injury or disease to persist long after the insult has passed.

The overall composition of cartilage glycosaminoglycans changes with age. The proportion of chondroitin sulfate falls with increasing age, whereas that of keratan sulfate and hyaluronate rises. It is possible, but not firmly established, that the changes in the properties of cartilage that occur with age, disuse, and injury may be related to the changes in its composition.

The collagens are the most abundant body protein. At least 15 different collagens have been identified. The various collagens are highly specialized; by means of subtle control of the polypeptide structures, diverse support structures for tendons, skin, transparent lenses, bone scaffold for mineralization, and compressible shock-absorbing articular cartilage can be formed. The major cartilage collagen is type II, which is a specific product of chondrocytes and vitreous cells of the eye. Type II collagen molecules contain a higher number of hydroxylysine amino acid residues than other collagens.

The definitive structure of all collagen molecules is the triple helix, which is composed of three polypeptide chains, known as alpha-chains. Multiple genes encode for the various collagen chains. In the triple helix, three chains are twisted around each other to form a rigid structure similar to a thin segment of rope. A complex set of steps is required from the synthesis of procollagen molecules by cells, association of chains in proper ratio, formation of a triple helix structure, and processing of collagen molecules to the formation of fibrils and ultimately of structural support members for tissues (Fig. 2).

Joint Structure

Differing designs of human joints have been classified according to histologic features of the union and the degree of motion the union permits. Synarthrodial joints consist primarily of the suture lines of the skull. The adjoining cranial plates are separated by only a thin fibrous tissue that permits no detectable motion, but provides for orderly intramembranous growth. When cranial growth ceases, the synarthrodial joints have no further use and regularly close. In cartilaginous joints, the bony elements are joined by intervening cartilage, which permits slight degrees of motion. The intervertebral disk and pubic symphysis are examples of this type of union, which is firm but allows some motion. The third class of joints include the most mobile joints, which possess a synovial membrane and

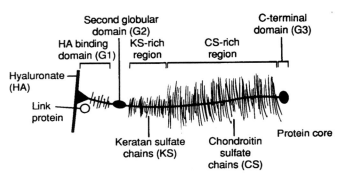

Fig. 1 A schematic diagram of the aggrecan molecule and its binding to hyaluronate. The protein core has several globular domains (G1, G2, and G3), with other regions containing the keratan sulfate and chondroitin sulfate glycosaminoglycan chains. The N-terminal G1 domain is able to bind specifically to hyaluronate. This binding is stabilized by link protein. (Reproduced with permission from Mankin HJ, Mow VC, Buckwalter JA, et al: Form and function of articular cartilage, in Simon SR (ed): *Orthopaedic Basic Science.* Rosemont, IL, American Academy of Orthopaedic Surgeons, 1994, pp 1–44.)

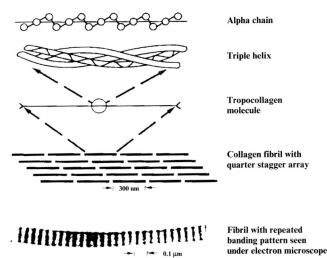

Fig. 2 A scheme for the formation of collagen fibrils. The triple helix is made from three α chains, forming a procollagen molecule. Outside the cell the N- and C-terminal globular domains of the α chains are cleaved off to allow fibril formation, which occurs in a specific quarter-staggered array that ultimately results in the typical banded fibrils seen under electron microscopy. (Reproduced with permission from Mow VC, Zhu W, Ratcliffe A: Structure and function of articular cartilage and meniscus, in Mow VC, Hayes WC (eds): *Basic Orthopaedic Biomechanics.* New York, NY, Raven Press, 1991, pp 143–198.)

contain synovial fluid. They are thus referred to as synovial joints.

Synovial joints are normally surrounded by a capsule that defines the boundary between articular and periarticular tissues. The capsule varies in thickness from a thin membrane to a strong ligamentous band. A reinforced synovial capsule may actually serve as an effective rein to prevent hyperextension of some joints, such as the interphalangeal joints. Reinforcing the capsule are additional ligaments that are sometimes extracapsular, and further support is provided by the tendons of those muscles that act across the joint.

The synovium is the principal intracapsular tissue. It is generally made up of one to three layers of cells that line all intracapsular structures other than the contact areas of cartilage. This lining is normally collapsed upon itself and the articular cartilage to minimize the volume of the joint space it encloses. The principal cells of normal synovium are type A (phagocytic) and type B (secretory) cells. Type A synoviocytes are derived from monocytes and have a high content of cytoplasmic organelles, including lysosomes, vacuoles, and micropinocytotic vesicles. In contrast, type B cells have fewer organelles and a more extensive endoplasmic reticulum; these features are consistent with the cells' presumed role in the synthesis of hyaluronate. Various other white blood cell types are sometimes seen in normal synovium. In synovitis, all the cells of the synovium proliferate and interact with the vasculature to produce the syndromes of acute and chronic arthritis.

Articular cartilage makes up the low friction facing that lines the opposing members of the synovial joint (Fig. 3). Of greatest importance is the framework of type II collagen fibrils, which are densely packed and arranged parallel

to the axis of motion at the surface. Deeper down, at the beginning of the calcified region of bone, the collagen fibrils become perpendicular to the osteochondral junction, firmly anchoring cartilage to bone. This framework of collagen contains the proteoglycan aggregates previously described. The substantial concentration of electronegative charge in the proteoglycan aggregates creates a powerful osmotic force, which attracts water molecules, as well as an electrostatic force, which results in a strong expansile force against the restraining force of the collagen fibrils. The net result is a resilient but turgid tissue that is normally 70% or more water and grossly appears firm with a smooth, glistening surface. Chondrocytes are distributed sparsely throughout the matrix of cartilage. These specialized fibroblasts synthesize the collagen and proteoglycans and provide for regular turnover and remodeling. No other cells are present.

In normal synovial joints, a thin film of synovial fluid covers the surfaces of synovium and cartilage within the joint space. Only in disease does the volume of fluid increase to provide a clinically apparent effusion. In the synovium, essential nutrients and other solutes are delivered via the bloodstream. Free diffusion through the narrow passage between synovial lining cells provides full equilibration between plasma and synovial fluid of nutrients, metabolic waste products, and small solutes. In addition, a special transport system enhances transport of glucose.

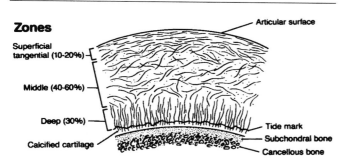

Zones

Superficial tangential (10-20%)

Middle (40-60%)

Deep (30%)

Calcified cartilage

Articular surface

Tide mark

Subchondral bone

Cancellous bone

Fig. 3 Diagram of collagen fiber architecture in a sagittal cross section showing the three salient zones of articular cartilage. (Reproduced with permission from Mow VC, Proctor CS, Kelly MA: Biomechanics of articular cartilage, in Nordin M, Frankel VH (eds): *Basic Biomechanics of the Musculoskeletal System*, ed 2. Philadelphia, PA, Lea & Febiger, 1989, pp 31–57.)

This process is clinically relevant in evaluating the delivery of therapeutic agents into joints. Levels of therapeutic agents in the plasma initially exceed, but eventually equilibrate with levels in synovial fluid. There is no evidence that any agent is specifically transported or selectively retained in joint fluid. Imbalance between synovial fluid and circulation occurs rarely. This imbalance, which occurs when synovial metabolic demand cannot be met by microvascular supply, results in oxygen deficit, high lactate and carbon dioxide levels, and low pH in synovial fluid. Because articular cartilage has no blood supply and the overlying synovial fluid normally meets its metabolic needs, this tissue is particularly at risk during imbalance. Imbalance of fluids is found regularly in septic arthritis, sometimes in rheumatoid disease, and occasionally in other kinds of synovitis.

Clinical Laboratory Tests

Erythrocyte Sedimentation Rate and C-Reactive Protein

The factors responsible for the erythrocyte sedimentation rate (ESR) are complex and only partially understood. In this test, anticoagulated blood is placed in a vertical tube, and the rate of sedimentation of the erythrocytes is measured, reflecting the production of proteins known as "acute phase reactants." Although abnormal results do not have diagnostic specificity and may accompany many abnormal states, this test can be used to screen a patient with vague musculoskeletal complaints because a high ESR increases the likelihood of important rheumatic or systemic illness. High ESR values are also usually seen in bacterial infections. The ESR is usually normal in mild viral infections, whereas in severe viral infections, such as poliomyelitis or mumps, the ESR is usually high. Conditions associated with significant tissue damage, such as trauma or surgery, will elevate the ESR in proportion to the amount of tissue injury. An ESR in excess of 100 mm/h is almost never associated with a benign process, and a

thorough investigation for an underlying cause is warranted. In a number of protracted and chronic illnesses, the course of the disease process is reflected by the rise and fall of the ESR.

Although measurement of C-reactive protein (CRP) has been suggested to differentiate fever due to infection from fever due to other illness, this procedure has not proven useful. Generally speaking, elevation of CRP occurs in the same variety of infectious, traumatic, and inflammatory states that elevate the ESR. However, the CRP level will fluctuate more rapidly than the ESR, and changes in it can occur from day to day or even hour to hour.

Antinuclear Antibodies

As diagnostic markers, antinuclear antibodies (ANAs) continue to be an important set of tests. In general, ANAs are associated with various collagen diseases and variants of systemic lupus erythematosus (SLE). Because arthritis is a component of many of these diseases, the presence of ANAs in an individual with arthritis increases the likelihood that a collagen disease or SLE is present. Many of these conditions are accompanied by other, potentially serious illnesses and, thus, require a thorough medical examination and evaluation. Many variants of SLE and collagen diseases are associated with a wide variety of antibodies, the more common of which are listed in Table 1. Moreover, because exposure to drugs, chronic infections, and many other unknown stimuli can be associated with the development of ANAs, in many cases, a thorough medical evaluation may reveal no specific cause or disease.

Rheumatoid Factors

Rheumatoid factors are antibodies directed against a specific portion of a particular antibody class, such as immunoglobulin G (IgG). Although rheumatoid factors of many types have been demonstrated, the usual clinical tests measure only one particular type. This type, IgM rheumatoid factor, is present in 80% of patients with rheumatoid arthritis (RA) but can also be observed in patients with other connective tissue diseases, chronic infections, and other chronic inflammatory diseases. Children with

Table 1. Autoantibodies in rheumatic diseases

Antibody to:	Disease association (% Prevalence)*
Antinuclear antibody	SLE (95%)
Native, double stranded DNA (dsDNA)	SLE (>50%)
Sm (Smith)	SLE (30%)
RNP (ribonuclear protein)	SLE (30%)
	Mixed connective tissue disease (95%)
Centromere	Limited scleroderma (70% to 90%)
Antineutrophil cytoplasmic antibody (ANCA)	Wegener granulomatosis, vasculitis (> 90%)

*SLE = systemic lupus erythematosus

juvenile onset RA rarely make this detected type of rheumatoid factor and, consequently, usually have a negative response to this conventional test. Highly elevated levels of rheumatoid factor are associated with a worse prognosis, in terms of both joint damage severity and the likelihood of systemic manifestations.

Synovial Fluid Analysis

There are a few disorders for which synovial fluid analysis is diagnostic, providing information that is not otherwise available. The only proper way to diagnose infectious arthritis and crystal-induced arthritis is through synovial fluid analysis. Results of synovial fluid analysis are important in differentiating inflammatory from noninflammatory arthritis, in attempting to identify the cause of inflammation, and in diagnosing infectious arthritis when the white blood cell (WBC) count is high. This analysis is used most frequently to differentiate between inflammatory and noninflammatory arthritis. For example, a diagnosis of simple osteoarthritis is ruled out by synovial fluid with a WBC count greater than 2,000/mm^3, and RA is unlikely in a joint with a WBC count less than 2,000/mm^3.

All synovial fluids should be sent for total WBC counts. Fluids with a WBC count less than 2,000/mm^3 are considered noninflammatory. Fluids with a cell count more than 100,000/mm^3 should be considered septic. Making diagnoses based on fluids that have cell counts between 50,000 and 100,000/mm^3 is more difficult, because some septic fluids will be in this range in the compromised or partially-treated patient. Very turbid fluids should be sent for culture. Although it is not necessary to send fluids routinely for fungal or tuberculosis cultures, refractory monoarthritis is an important indication for such cultures. All fluids should be examined under coverslip for crystalline material. Proper polarized microscopy requires a high quality, maintained microscope and a well-trained observer; these are lacking in many hospital laboratories. Glucose, viscosity, mucin clot, protein, and immunologic tests are of little or uncertain value.

Drug Therapies

Nonsteroidal Anti-inflammatory Drugs

Nonsteroidal anti-inflammatory drugs (NSAIDs) are among the most widely used classes of therapeutic agents. In the United States, the number of prescriptions written for NSAIDs increased from 27.5 million in 1973 to 66.5 million in 1988. NSAIDs block the synthesis of prostaglandins by inhibiting cyclooxygenase, the enzyme that catalyzes the conversion of arachidonic acid to prostaglandin precursors. This block is clinically important because prostaglandins mediate several inflammatory reactions. These agents may also have several other effects, including impairment of neutrophil migration and altered lymphocyte responsiveness, and they are also potent analgesic and antipyretic agents.

Table 2. Dosage of nonsteroidal anti-inflammatory drugs

Drug Category	Dosage Range (mg/day)	Half-life (hours)	Doses/Day
Carboxylic Acids			
Aspirin	1000–6000	4–15	2–4
Nonacetylated salicylates			
Choline magnesium	1500–4000	4–15	2–4
Salsalate	1500–5000	4–15	2–4
Diflunisal	500–1500	7–15	2
Acetic Acids			
Indomethacin	50–200	3–11	2–4
Sulindac	300–400	16	2
Tolmetin	600–2000	1–2	3–4
Diclofenac	100–200	22–24	
Etodolac	600–1200	2–4	3–4
Proprionic Acids			
Ibuprofen	1200–3200	23–24	
Naproxen	500–1500	13	2
Fenoprofen	1200–3200	23–24	
Ketoprofen	100–400	23–24	
Flurbiprofen	200–300	23–24	
Oxyprozin	600–1800	24	1–2
Enolic Acids			
Phenylbutazone	200–800	40–80	1–4
Piroxicam	20	30–86	1
Naphthylkanones			
Nambumetone	500–1500	19–30	1–2

NSAIDs are classified on the basis of their chemical composition (Table 2). They are rapidly absorbed from the gastrointestinal tract, and the majority are metabolized in the liver to inactive metabolites that are then excreted by the kidney. The only NSAID approved for nonoral administration for the treatment of arthritis is indomethacin, which is available as a rectal suppository. Parenteral NSAIDs have been approved for acute pain. In Europe, several NSAIDs have been approved for use in topical solutions for bursitis and tendinitis.

NSAIDs have many potential drug interactions. Phenylbutazone inhibits the metabolism of warfarin, potentially enhancing the anticoagulation effect. All NSAIDS, except for the nonacetylated salicylates, inhibit cyclooxygenase and platelet function, prolonging bleeding time. Because aspirin does this in an irreversible fashion, it should be discontinued at least 7 to 10 days before surgical procedures. The remaining agents can be discontinued 1 to 2 days before surgery. NSAIDs attenuate the effects of antihypertensive agents and can, therefore, raise blood pressure in hypertensive patients taking those agents.

Gastrointestinal side effects are reported in over 21% of patients taking NSAIDs, and 10% of patients discontinue these drugs because of side effects. Symptoms include nausea, dyspepsia, abdominal pain, gastric or duodenal ulcers, esophagitis, and rarely, life-threatening bleeding or perforation. Toxicity is dose related and occurs most commonly with aspirin. Enteric coated salicylates, nonacetylated salicylates, or nonsalicylate NSAIDs may give lower incidence of gastrointestinal symptoms. Pharmacologic interventions have been advocated to reduce gastric toxicity, including co-administration of H-2 blockers, sucralfate, or misoprostal. Misoprostal is the only agent with an FDA-approved indication for prevention of NSAID gastrointestinal side effects, but the economic impact of long-term use in all asymptomatic patients must be considered.

NSAIDs produce little change in renal function in normal persons, but a substantial decline can occur in patients who are volume depleted, or have congestive heart failure, renal disease, or cirrhosis. NSAIDs can also promote fluid retention and impair diuretic function, leading to edema. Elevation of liver function tests can occur with all NSAIDs. Bone marrow toxicity is rare, but has been more frequent with phenylbutazone; therefore, phenylbutazone should not be used as a first-line NSAID. Headaches, dizziness, blurred vision, and confusion have been reported most frequently with indomethacin, but may occur with any NSAID. Skin rashes have been seen in varying frequencies with NSAIDs.

NSAIDs should be used with caution in patients with known hypersensitivity to aspirin or other NSAIDs. Combinations of NSAIDs may increase toxicity and should not be used. If a therapeutic effect has not been achieved within 2 to 4 weeks at its maximum dose, the drug should be stopped and another NSAID substituted. The drugs should be given with food, and prophylactic anti-ulcer therapy should be considered for any patient with a prior history of ulcer disease. Hematologic, renal, and liver functions should be periodically monitored in patients using these drugs.

Disease-modifying antirheumatic drugs, also referred to as second-line, remittive, or slow-acting drugs, are indicated in RA when there is incomplete control of signs and symptoms with NSAIDs, when deformities develop, and when there is radiographic evidence of bone erosion. Because the majority of these more serious events occur within the first 2 years of disease onset, careful and close clinical observation of patients with RA is necessary if these complications are to be avoided. The disease-modifying agents have had some use in other conditions, such as SLE and the seronegative spondyloarthropathies, predominantly for control of joint symptoms in these multisystem diseases. These agents include the antimalarials, including chloroquine and hydroxychloroquine; oral and parenteral gold salts; D-penicillamine; and sulfasalazine. Each of these agents may require 3 to 6 months of administration before onset of action. In addition, they each have unique and more serious potential toxicities than NSAIDs, so that careful assessment of risk/benefit ratios and clinical monitoring for response and toxicity are required. Subspecialty consultation is usually required for this difficult assessment. These agents, when properly used, do not usually interfere with coagulation or bleeding, nor do they increase infection risk, so that they can be used routinely in the perioperative period.

The antimetabolites, including azathioprine, methotrexate, and cyclophosphamide, are reserved for patients with the most active and refractory disease, although earlier use of methotrexate is under study. These drugs are potent agents that act on rapidly dividing cells by slowing pathways of DNA synthesis. They inhibit the division of immune cells active in inflammatory pathways, thereby reducing inflammation. However, these drugs also have the potential for slowing division of rapidly dividing cells, such as bone marrow, gastrointestinal, and liver cells, accounting for these major sites of potential toxicity. Regular monitoring of blood count, renal function, and liver blood tests are thus required. Increased risk of infection is a potential consequence of antimetabolite use, but has in fact occurred very rarely in clinical practice. Studies of methotrexate have reported somewhat greater efficacy and similar toxicity when compared to other second-line agents, and this drug is gaining widespread popularity. A significant reduction in maintenance prednisone dose has also been noted with long-term methotrexate therapy. The drug is teratogenic and must be discontinued for a minimum of 30 days in women and 90 days in men prior to attempting conception. Liver toxicity rarely has been reported, but may be related to host factors, such as alcohol consumption, therapy with other hepatotoxins, and other concomitant diseases. Routine liver biopsies are no longer advocated.

Because of the potential for the antimetabolites to increase infection, their effect on perioperative infection rates has been questioned. A 10-year retrospective study has shown that treatment in the perioperative period with weekly low-dose methotrexate does not increase the risk of postoperative infections or affect wound healing in RA patients who undergo total joint replacement.

Specific Rheumatologic Illnesses

Rheumatoid Arthritis

RA is a complex disease that damages diarthrodial (synovial) joints. It can follow a monocyclic, polycyclic, or progressive pattern, with the prevailing pattern influencing both therapy and outcome. Extra-articular disease is common, may involve organ systems, may result in diagnostic confusion, and is associated with a poor prognosis. Although an infectious cause has been suspected for decades, attempts to identify a specific initiating organism have been unrewarding. There are convincing data that link susceptibility to seropositive RA with a genetic basis, in particular the human leukocyte antigen HLA-DR4. American Caucasians with this antigen have a several-fold increased risk of developing the disease.

The onset of rheumatoid disease is usually insidious but may be acute, sometimes with prominent systemic symptoms such as fever or fatigue. The illness often progresses inexorably, but about 10% to 15% of cases remit, and a larger percentage follow a relatively indolent course. The most frequently involved joints are the wrists and metacarpophalangeal, metatarsophalangeal, and proximal interphalangeal joints. Palpable swelling of deep-seated joints, such as the shoulder and hip, is rare. In far advanced cases, multiple deformities in upper and lower extremities can occur. Approximately one half of rheumatoid patients have cervical spine involvement, which may manifest as neck pain, loss of neck mobility, headache, and even dizziness. Atlantoaxial subluxation (best detected by lateral flexion/extension radiography or computed tomography) can result in cord compression and myelopathy. Thus, presurgical evaluation of cervical spine stability is important in rheumatoid patients because of potential cervical cord injury during extubation and/or movement of the anesthetized patient.

Diagnosis of RA may be difficult early in the course of the disease, especially if the individual patient is rheumatoid factor negative. Other potential diagnoses include viral and other infectious arthritides, other collagen diseases, seronegative spondyloarthropathies, Lyme disease, and human immunodeficiency virus (HIV) infection. The combined presence of morning stiffness, involvement of three or more joints with inflammatory synovitis, simultaneous involvement of the same joints on both sides of the body, and involvement of hand joints, when present for more than 6 weeks has a sensitivity and specificity of greater than 89%. Patients tend to develop radiographic evidence of irreversible joint damage (erosions and joint space narrowing) within 2 years of disease onset; therefore, effective early intervention is important.

The management of patients with RA involves skill in assessing the degree of synovitis, changes in function, and nonarticular status, and, in many cases, skill in the use of so-called second-line antirheumatic drugs. Suppression of inflammation and of immunologic pathways is the underlying goal of medical therapy. A general principle is to control inflammation first with a single NSAID, given for 2 to 4 weeks, while adjusting the dose to clinical response. Patients receiving NSAIDs should be monitored for occult gastrointestinal bleeding, liver and renal function, edema, and hypertension; elderly patients are at increased risk. If the response to the first NSAID is inadequate or the agent is poorly tolerated, the next step is to change to another NSAID. It is unwise to use two or more NSAIDs simultaneously because toxicity is additive while efficacy is not. In patients who have a prior history of ulcer disease and are taking NSAIDs, concomitant use of a gastroprotective agent such as misoprostal is indicated.

Second-line agents may be added after 3 to 12 months if NSAID treatment is insufficient. In most patients, this decision can be made within 3 to 6 months after initiation of treatment. Choices available include oral or injectable gold, an antimalarial drug, or methotrexate. Six months of uninterrupted treatment with most second-line agents is needed to assess efficacy. Close monitoring is necessary for all second-line agents, because of increased risk of organ toxicity.

The use of systemic corticosteroids in the therapy of RA remains controversial. Many authorities recommend low-dose corticosteroids only for severe, disabling disease, or while awaiting the onset of action of second-line agents. Intra-articular injection of corticosteroid may be used as an adjunct to systemic drug therapy throughout the disease course. It is unrealistic to expect or attempt to achieve complete symptomatic relief in every patient.

Juvenile Chronic Polyarthritis (Juvenile RA)

Juvenile chronic polyarthritis is arbitrarily defined as being present when the onset of inflammatory polyarthritis occurs before the age of 16 years. Three major subtypes can be identified: systemic, with fever, rash, and organomegaly; polyarticular, with or without rheumatoid factor detected; and pauciarticular, which usually affects large lower extremity joints. Wrist and cervical spine involvement is common in the polyarticular form. Because of the diverse constellation of findings and absence of laboratory tests specific for this illness, as well as lack of physician familiarity, this condition is often misdiagnosed as systemic infection. Evaluating children can be further compromised because the patients are too young to describe their problems accurately. Growth abnormalities are common in children with juvenile polyarthritis, either in individual bones or the entire skeleton. The management of these conditions is best done by an experienced team that is able to provide care for diverse conditions including growth abnormalities, psychological and developmental problems, and social issues.

Seronegative Spondyloarthropathies

The seronegative spondyloarthropathies are diseases affecting the spine and peripheral joints and are not associated with the presence of rheumatoid factor or ANAs. These diseases classically include ankylosing spondylitis, Reiter's syndrome or reactive arthritis, and psoriatic arthritis. Inflammatory bowel disease and Behçet's disease are two additional rare conditions sometimes included in this group. Ankylosing spondylitis and Reiter's syndrome occur with increased frequency in persons with the HLA-B27 genetic marker, but the B27 genotype is neither necessary nor sufficient by itself for the development of one of these conditions. Enthesopathy, the involvement of the insertion of ligaments and tendons into bone, is common to the spondyloarthropathies, and this feature distinguishes them from RA.

Of particular interest is the recent discovery that a six amino acid sequence of the B27 antigen is identical to a sequence of protein on a bacteria considered a possible trigger for the development of ankylosing spondylitis. This finding strongly supports the molecular mimicry hypothesis of pathogenesis, wherein a triggering organism induces misrecognition of B27 as a foreign antigen, or the organism modifies B27, rendering it foreign in appearance. Either situation results in perpetual autoimmune reaction and inflammatory arthritis.

Sacroiliitis is an obligatory finding of ankylosing spondylitis, and is an early lesion. Hip involvement occurs in those with a young age of onset. Back pain is insidious in onset, improved with exercise and activity, and worse with bed rest. Peripheral joint involvement is frequently asymmetric, and more common in large lower extremity joints.

Ten percent to 20% of patients with ankylosing spondylitis develop anterior uveitis (iritis).

Reactive arthritis and Reiter's syndrome are terms often used interchangeably. Both refer to a syndrome of asymmetric inflammatory arthritis of the lower extremity, along with urethritis, conjunctivitis, skin rash, or mucous membrane ulceration. Enthesopathy and unilateral sacroiliitis are frequently present. HLA-B27 is present in 85% of those affected, but is not necessary for the condition's development. The condition may follow a genitourinary infection with *Chlamydia;* or a gastrointestinal infection with *Yersinia, Shigella, or Salmonella;* or may occur spontaneously.

NSAIDs remain the treatment of choice for the spondyloarthropathies. Some patients are unable to tolerate or do not respond to NSAIDs. Trials of sulfasalazine suggest benefit, but the drug is not yet approved for this indication by the FDA.

Other Rheumatologic Illnesses

Osteoporosis is not a normal consequence of aging. Caucasian race, female sex, early menopause, positive family history, small build, high alcohol intake, and sedentary lifestyle all increase fracture risk. Black persons suffer less osteoporosis than do Caucasian and Asian persons matched for age and sex. From young adulthood until middle age, the rate of bone loss is constant. In women, bone loss accelerates after menopause. Thus, those who have a large peak bone mass in early adulthood will reach a fracture threshold later than those who have a small peak bone mass. In the average patient, the rate of bone loss cannot be measured by routine blood biochemical tests. Bone-scanning techniques are static measurements and also are insensitive to early disease. Serial scans may allow some estimation of bone loss over time. In adults, calcium supplementation alone is insufficient to prevent or treat osteoporosis, but it may be useful in children and young adults to ensure high peak bone mass. Sodium fluoride is falling into disfavor as a treatment because it has paradoxically increased fracture risk. Estrogen is currently accepted as the most important therapy for osteoporosis in women, with calcitonin or bisphosphonates as alternatives or for therapy in men.

Fibrositis is a common clinical syndrome. There are some estimates that it affects 5% of Americans. The syndrome occurs predominantly in women and is characterized by marked fatigue, diffuse aching pain, stiffness, and a sense of weakness. Physical examination is usually normal as are laboratory tests and radiographs. The pain is widespread, poorly localized, and referred to muscles or bony prominences. Upon questioning, most patients admit to sleeping poorly and feeling tired in the morning. The symptoms are chronic and tend to persist for months or years. Simple analgesics and NSAIDs provide minimal benefit; however, heat, massage, and an exercise program may result in improvement. Tricyclic antidepressants such as amitriptyline may improve symptoms and restore sleep, but it is not known if the sleep disturbance is causative or secondary. This disorder is associated with high rates of psychiatric symptoms and abnormalities on psychological tests.

Several rheumatic diseases may occur in persons with all stages of human immunodeficiency virus (HIV). Reiter's syndrome may be severe and unrelenting, with arthritis following an additive or migratory pattern. The arthritis usually affects a small number of joints and has a predilection for the lower extremities. Skin rashes may be severe. Response to first-line nonsteroidal agents is poor. Phenylbutazone and sulfasalazine have been effective in some patients. Psoriasis also appears with increased frequency in patients with HIV infection, and psoriatic arthritis occurs in this group. Involvement of interphalangeal joints and tendon/ligament insertions dominates the clinical picture. Low titer auto-antibodies such as rheumatoid factor and ANA occur in HIV infection and can lead to confusion in diagnosis.

Osteoarthritis

Although osteoarthritis (OA) commonly occurs in the elderly, it is clearly not due to aging alone. Forms of OA that are not associated with aging include posttraumatic OA and the inherited form of the illness, including a rapidly progressive OA with an associated chondrodystrophy that has been linked to a mutation in the gene for type II collagen. Other forms of OA not related to aging include inflammatory OA, chondrocalcinosis, hydroxyapatite degenerative disease, epiphyseal dysplasia, and hemochromatosis arthritis.

The pathogenesis of OA is not yet understood, but many contributory factors are known. Patients with OA are thought to have stiffer subchondral bone then persons without OA. The first sign of OA on a histopathologic level is loss of cartilage proteoglycan. In normal aging, proteoglycan aggregate decreases in size, allowing more rapid degradation by cartilage and synovial fluid enzymes. Biochemical markers of disease activity in synovial fluid or serum are an area of active investigation, but at the current time there are no tests that are useful in monitoring the progression of the condition.

Reassurance and education are important and often overlooked tools for management. A recent study confirmed the value of these by demonstrating that regular telephone contact of OA patients by medical personnel measurably improved their ability to function. Physical therapy should be available to all patients. They should be taught and encouraged to do gentle exercises each day to maintain muscle strength and maximum range of motion of affected joints. Quadriceps exercises in patients with knee OA are of special value in relieving symptoms and maintaining function. Reduction of stress on joints can relieve pain and affect outcome favorably. Obese patients with lower limb disease should be helped to lose weight.

Use of a cane can reduce loading on the contralateral hip or knee by 30% to 60%. The use of shock-absorbing insoles may be of benefit, and orthotic devices to correct leg length inequality or angulation deformities can be valuable. Activities that involve impact loading or result in prolonged postexercise pain should be avoided.

Drugs are of benefit, but there has been a tendency to rely on them alone. Simple analgesics such as acetaminophen are of value, either through regular or on demand use. NSAIDs relieve pain and stiffness to a significant degree in some patients. Long-term use can be associated with toxicity, and medical monitoring is important in these cases. Some NSAIDs depress proteoglycan synthesis; thus, their analgesic and anti-inflammatory benefits may be offset by inhibition of cartilage repair. The clinical importance of this finding is unclear, but it does raise questions about the use of nonsteroidal agents over the long term. As yet, no drug has been proved to have "chondroprotective" value in human OA. Intra-articular steroid injections are commonly used. Surprisingly, there are few data on their true value in management.

Crystal-Associated Arthritis

The prevalence of gout and calcium pyrophosphate dehydrate arthritis (pseudogout) increases as the population ages and as medicines that raise uric acid levels are more widely used. Gout is the more likely diagnosis in younger persons. The pathogenesis and causes of gout are better understood, but there is presently no known biochemical pathway to explain calcium pyrophosphate dehydrate arthritis. The most common cause of gout is primary renal deficiency in excretion, and this problem is often genetic. Excessive dietary purine intake, consumption of alcohol, and blood disorders account for many of the remaining cases. Gout can have myriad clinical presentations in virtually any synovial joint. In elderly persons, it may occur in osteoarthritic interphalangeal joints, leading to diagnostic confusion. Unrecognized gout can become polyarticular and chronic, again leading to diagnostic confusion if joints are not aspirated. The diagnosis rests on demonstration of uric acid crystals in synovial fluid, not upon serum level of uric acid, because there are many individuals with prolonged asymptomatic hyperuricemia in whom other causes for joint pain exist.

In addition to acute, gout-like attacks, calcium pyrophosphate dehydrate associated arthritis causes chondrocalcinosis and radiographic changes that resemble osteoarthritis but differ by occurring in unusual locations such as wrist, shoulder, elbow, and patellofemoral compartment of the knee. Occasionally, crystals other than monosodium urate or calcium pyrophosphate have been identified as causing acute arthritis; these crystals include calcium phosphates, calcium oxalate, and liquid lipid crystals. At the current time their detection is beyond the capabilities of most laboratories.

The treatment of acute crystal-induced arthritis is most effective when started as early in the attack as possible. Useful drugs include NSAIDs, colchicine, corticotropin (ACTH), and corticosteroids. Although it is clearly effective, colchicine has become controversial, and it should never be used in persons with reduced leukocyte count or in the presence of liver or kidney disease. In the absence of significant renal impairment or active peptic ulcer disease, indomethacin or naproxen in short courses of 50 mg four times daily or 500 mg three times daily, respectively, are effective. Prednisone, 40 mg daily, or 40 units of intramuscular corticotropin are appropriate for patients intolerant of NSAIDs or colchicine. Recurrent attacks of gout usually require subsequent prevention with one of the hypouricemic drugs, which should be used only after the acute attack and in doses sufficient to maintain the serum uric acid level at or below normal levels. Younger patients with good renal function may be managed on 3 g of probenecid daily, otherwise allopurinol is preferred in an average daily dose of 300 mg.

Infectious Arthritis

There are three major types of osteomyelitis in adults: hematogenous osteomyelitis, osteomyelitis from a contiguous focus of infection, and infection consequent to vascular insufficiency. Hematogenous osteomyelitis is common in children but rare in adults, and when present it most often involves the vertebrae. The symptoms may be subtle, with only malaise and back pain, and the most common infecting organism is *Staphylococcus aureus*. Aspiration of bone for culture is necessary for accurate treatment. Adequate surgical drainage is important when prompt clinical response does not take place. Antibiotic therapy should be continued for at least 4 weeks.

Septic arthritis is usually sudden in onset and is typically monoarticular. Suppurative arthritis usually occurs in large weightbearing joints, although gonococcal arthritis can also involve wrist and interphalangeal joints. Most adults with nongonococcal arthritis have a predisposing factor such as steroid use, preexisting arthritis, diabetes mellitus, trauma, malignancy, or intravenous drug use. The most common infecting organism is *Staphylococcus aureus*, followed by streptococcus. Gonococcus remains the most prevalent in sexually active young adults. In immunosuppressed persons, other organisms must be considered. Synovial fluid leukocyte counts are often greater than 100,000/mm³, with 90% or more polymorphonuclear leukocytes, but lower cell counts are common in gonococcal infection or in immunosuppressed hosts. In gonococcal arthritis, organisms are rarely recovered from the fluid; in nongonococcal disease, synovial fluid culture will usually show the infecting organism. A gram stain should always be done and may direct initial therapy. Radiographs show only nonspecific soft-tissue swelling and joint capsule distension early, but destructive changes can be seen if therapy is not begun rapidly. Treatment requires systemic antibiotics and drainage by frequent aspiration, which has been shown to be comparably effective to surgical drainage. When effective needle drainage cannot be obtained, arthroscopic debridement is useful; open drainage is reserved for the hip and for patients with thick exudative fluid, loculation, or lack of clinical response.

Lyme arthritis is a worldwide chronic progressive infectious disease caused by the spirochete *Borrelia burgdorferi*. Lyme disease primarily affects the skin, nervous system, heart, and musculoskeletal system. The earliest common manifestation is a characteristic spreading rash, called erythema migrans. About one-half of patients with Lyme disease will experience this rash. Disseminated infection will follow with symptoms of skin, nervous system, or musculoskeletal involvement consisting of migratory pain in the joints, bursae, tendons, muscle, and bones. Patients often appear systemically ill and may have profound malaise and fatigue. Within weeks, 50% will develop arthritis. The arthritis affects few, mostly large joints; it most commonly affects the knee. Arthrocentesis reveals leukocyte counts of 500 to 100,000/mm^3 with predominantly polymorpho-

nuclear leukocytes. Histologically, the synovium in Lyme arthritis resembles that in RA. The organism can be seen by Dieterle silver stain in 25% of biopsies. Rarely, the organism can be cultured from synovial fluid.

The difficulty in visualizing or culturing *B. burgdorferi* in serum can make diagnosis difficult. Antibody to the organism can be measured by several techniques. The results must be interpreted with caution, because false-positive results can occur in persons with autoimmune disease, and false-negative results can also occur within the first several weeks of disease and in later stages following incompletely effective therapy.

For early Lyme disease, oral tetracycline, 250 mg four times daily, or doxycycline, 100 mg twice daily, for 14 to 21 days is effective. Amoxicillin is an acceptable alternative and is the best choice for children. Optimal treatment of late Lyme disease, including joint synovitis, warrants the use of high doses of intravenous penicillin or ceftriaxone. Treatment with appropriate antibiotics is usually curative; early treatment is essential to prevent late complications.

Annotated Bibliography

Arnett FC, Edworthy SM, Bloch DA, et al: The American Rheumatism Association 1987 revised criteria for the classification of rheumatoid arthritis. *Arthritis Rheum* 1989;31:315–324.

This collaborative study of more than 500 subjects led to the development of a new, simplified set of noninvasive criteria for classifying rheumatoid arthritis, with a 91% sensitivity and 89% specificity.

Centers for Disease Control: Lyme disease: United States 1991–1992. *MMWR* 1993;42:345–350.

Current distribution and recommendations for treatment of Lyme disease in the United States are given.

Felson DT: Osteoarthritis. *Rheum Dis Clin North Am* 1990;16:499–512.

This is an authoritative overview of the epidemiology of osteoarthritis.

Fuchs HA, Kaye JJ, Callahan LF, et al: Evidence of significant radiographic damage in rheumatoid arthritis within the first two years of disease. *J Rheumatol* 1989; 16:585–591.

In 200 patients with rheumatoid arthritis there was a positive correlation between disease duration and radiographic joint space narrowing and hand and wrist malalignment. Joint damage was seen with less than 2 years of illness, supporting the need for early treatment with second-line drugs.

Furst DE: Clinically important interactions of nonsteroidal antiinflammatory drugs with other medications. *J Rheumatol* 1988;17(suppl):58–62.

The interactions of NSAIDs with commonly prescribed medications and the clinical implications are reviewed. Warfarin, oral hypoglycemics, antihypertensive agents, lithium, and methotrexate are reviewed.

Goldenberg DL, Brandt KD, Cohen AS, et al: Treatment of septic arthritis: Comparison of needle aspiration and surgery as initial modes of joint drainage. *Arthritis Rheum* 1975;18:83–90.

This article demonstrates that needle drainage of septic arthritis is associated with at least as good an outcome as surgical drainage.

Hurd ER: Extraarticular manifestations of rheumatoid arthritis. *Semin Arthritis Rheum* 1979;8:151–176.

This is a classic review with an extensive bibliography.

Katz LM, Love PY: NSAIDs and the liver, in Famey PJ, Paulus HE (eds): *Clinical Applications of NSAIDs, Subpopulation Therapy and New Formulations*. New York, NY, Marcel Dekker, 1992, pp 247–263.

This is a thorough analysis of NSAIDs and their clinical use in particular patient types, with emphasis on potential for toxicity in given patient populations.

Khan MA, van der Linden SM: A wider spectrum of spondyloarthropathies. *Semin Arthritis Rheum* 1990;20: 107–113.

This knowledgeable review describes the possible clinical manifestations associated with HLA-B27. The authors distinguish diagnostic criteria for individual patients from criteria to classify groups.

Knowlton RG, Katzenstein PL, Moskowitz RW, et al: Genetic linkage of a polymorphism in the type II procollagen gene (COL2A1) to primary osteoarthritis associated with mild chondrodysplasia. *N Engl J Med* 1990;322:526–530.

This is the original description of families in whom multiple cases of premature osteoarthritis are linked to abnormalities of collagen genes.

Mayne R: Cartilage collagens: What is their function, and are they involved in articular disease? *Arthritis Rheum* 1989;32:241–246.

Cartilage collagens and their contribution to cartilage structure are reviewed. The article includes hypotheses about the development of both osteoarthritis and rheumatoid arthritis.

Perhala RS, Wilke WS, Clough JD, et al: Local infectious complications following large joint replacement in rheumatoid arthritis patients treated with methotrexate versus those not treated with methotrexate. *Arthritis Rheum* 1991;34:146–152.

This is a 10-year retrospective review of local postoperative infectious complications in a total of 92 joint arthroplasties in patients treated with methotrexate. They were compared to a group of patients with 110 joint arthroplasties who were not treated with methotrexate. There were no significant differences between the groups in local infections or poor wound healing. Treatment in the perioperative period with methotrexate does not appear to increase risk of complications.

Rizkalla G, Reiner A, Bogoch E, et al: Studies of the articular cartilage proteoglycan in health and osteoarthritis. *J Clin Invest* 1992;90:2268–2277.

Evidence is provided for molecular heterogenity and extensive molecular changes in disease.

Weinberger M, Tierney WM, Cowper PA, et al: Cost-effectiveness of increased telephone contact for patients with osteoarthritis: A randomized, controlled trial. *Arthritis Rheum* 1993;36:243–246.

This randomized controlled trial demonstrates that, compared with usual care, a sustained program of telephone contacts with trained nonmedical interviewers was associated with improved physical health and decreased joint pain 1 year later in patients with osteoarthritis. It provides remarkable proof of the value of reassurance and education in patient management.

10

Total Joint Replacement in Special Medical Conditions

Hematologic Disorders

Hemophilic Arthropathy

Severe hemophilic arthropathy requiring total joint arthroplasty occurs much more frequently in the knee than in the hip joint. With excellent surgical technique and hematologic supervision, total joint arthroplasty with modern implants can provide both excellent relief of pain and improvement in motion and function in severely disabled patients. The preoperative evaluation should include determination of the level of factor VIII or IX, the presence of inhibitor, and a survival study of infused factor concentrate. Serologic testing for the HIV-I virus, skin testing, and determination of the absolute CD4 lymphocyte count is also recommended. In one study of elective orthopaedic surgical procedures in patients with hemophilia, the risk of infection was very low with a CD4 lymphocyte count greater than 400 x 10^9 per liter. Surgery should be avoided if the CD4 lymphocyte count is less than 200 x 10^9 per liter.

A three-plane deformity of the knee (flexion contracture, valgus, and external rotation of the tibia) is most commonly seen in patients with hemophilic arthropathy. However, in one series, 25% of knees had a preoperative varus deformity. Because of the usual presence of severe flexion contractures, a posterior stabilized total condylar prosthesis is recommended, with routine resurfacing of the patella with a polyethylene component. Less constrained models have had results inferior to the posterior stabilized prosthesis. Cement fixation of all three components is recommended for the most reliable pain relief and component stability.

In one study of 24 total knee arthroplasties, 21 knees had an excellent or good result at a median follow-up time of 3.6 years with use of the total condylar or posterior stabilized prostheses. There were two late infections requiring implant removal. In another series of 19 knees, there were six failures at a mean follow-up time of 9.5 years. Two knees required additional surgery for patella resurfacing, two required revision of a loose tibial component, and one knee with a deep infection had removal and arthrodesis. In a retrospective multicenter study of 93 knees in 76 patients, with a 1- to 14-year follow-up time, the major finding was the late development in ten knees of deep infection, usually from a distant source of infection. During the study period, there were nine deaths, seven from the complications of AIDS.

The ratio of total knee arthroplasties to total hip arthroplasties at any one hemophilia center is four-to-five

knees to one hip. Valgus deformity and protrusio acetabuli are frequently seen in the hemophilic hip (Fig. 1). There is a high rate of failure of cemented arthroplasties in these patients (Fig. 2). In one study of 22 Charnley total hip arthroplasties with a median follow-up time of 7.6 years, five hips had been revised and three additional hips had definite radiographic loosening (total failure 36%). Ten of the 21 patients were seropositive for the HIV-I virus, and 40% of that group were deceased. In a retrospective multicenter study of 34 hip arthroplasties, there was a 62% failure rate of cemented acetabular components and a 36% failure rate of cemented femoral components at a mean follow-up of 8.5 years. There were no failures of six hips with uncemented components, but the mean follow-up

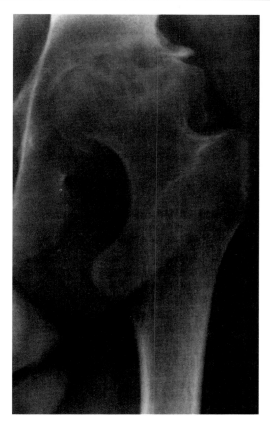

Fig. 1 Preoperative AP radiograph of an arthritic hip in a 35-year-old man with classic hemophilia, with valgus deformity of the proximal femur.

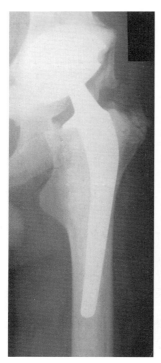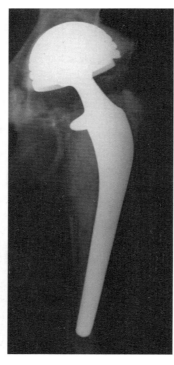

Fig. 2 **Left,** Postoperative radiograph of HD-2 components placed with modern cement techniques. **Right,** Ten-year radiograph showing loosening of both components and femoral osteolysis.

was only 2.7 years. Nine of the 27 patients were deceased at the time of review, and in six, death was related to an infectious complication of AIDS.

Gaucher's Disease

Gaucher's disease is an autosomal, recessively inherited systemic disorder, characterized by the accumulation of glucocerebroside in reticuloendothelial cells. There is a specific deficiency of the lysosomal acid hydrolase, beta-glucocerebrosidase. Gaucher cell infiltration eventually causes avascular necrosis of the femoral head, which usually has been treated by cemented total hip arthroplasty. In two small series of patients with Gaucher's disease who had total hip arthroplasties, increased intraoperative and postoperative bleeding was often encountered. There was a high rate of loosening (46%) of the cemented components, but no infections in these series. In another study of 15 hips in eight patients followed for a mean of 7.3 years, 27% of the hips had been revised for loosening. There are no reports of the results of cementless components in this patient population.

Sickle-Cell Disease

Osteonecrosis of the femoral head occurs frequently in patients with sickle-cell disease (SS), sickle-cell thalassemia (S-thal), and sickle-cell hemoglobin C (S-C) disease, and occasionally in patients with sickle-cell trait. A thorough preoperative medical and hematologic evaluation is required prior to total hip arthroplasty. Preoperative transfusion to a hemoglobin level of 10 g/dl, with or without exchange transfusions to decrease the level of hemoglobin S, is generally recommended. Epidural or spinal anesthesia, good oxygenation, hydration, prophylactic antibiotics, and thromboembolism prophylaxis (thigh-high pneumatic boots) are mandatory. In one series of 14 hips, there was a complication rate of 100%, with increased blood loss and transfusion requirements and prolonged hospitalization. Intraoperative blood loss was high in one series of 17 hips, averaging 1,390 ml in primary cases, and 2,850 ml in revision cases. The report of one study described difficulty in reaming the femur, which had hard sclerotic bone and obliteration of the medullary canal, and three perforations and four femoral fractures occurred. The rate of infection is very high, 16% to 20% was reported for several series, probably due to the high incidence of bacteremia in these patients.

There is a very high rate of failure of all types of hip arthroplasties in this patient population. In one series of 20 total hip arthroplasties, the revision rate was 50% at a mean follow-up of 10 years, and the infection rate was 10%. In another series, 38% of cemented primary hips failed, usually due to aseptic acetabular loosening. In a revision arthroplasty group, 43% of the hips had failed at 5.3 years. Although the follow-up is short, uncemented, porous-coated prostheses are currently recommended for primary and revision arthroplasties in this patient population.

Metabolic Disorders

Ochronosis

Ochronosis or alkaptonuria is a rare, autosomal recessive metabolic disorder, which is characterized by urinary excretion of homogentisic acid. There is absence of homogentisic acid oxidase in the liver and kidneys. Homogentisic acid binds to cartilage, which then becomes brittle and degenerates. In about one third of patients with ochronosis, a secondary degenerative arthritis develops, which affects the large joints and spine. The articular cartilage and femoral head contain black pigment on examination. There is one report of successful staged bilateral total hip arthroplasties in a patient with ochronosis and severe hip pain and disability.

Acromegaly

The clinical syndrome of acromegaly is the result of increased circulating growth hormone in a skeletally mature individual; it is usually caused by an acidophilic pituitary adenoma. In acromegalic arthropathy, which commonly affects the hips, cartilage hypertrophy and hyperplasia lead to a disruption of joint geometry and chondrocyte metabolism and, ultimately, to degenerative arthritis. An unusual proboscis-like medial osteophyte on the femoral heads, moderate synovial inflammation, subchondral bone pitting, and osteopenia suggested that this is a peculiar arthropathy distinct from osteoarthritis. In one report, six acromegalic patients underwent 11 cemented total hip arthroplasties. At follow-up of 1 to 9 years, only one hip arthroplasty failed.

Diabetes Mellitus

Diabetes mellitus is a common disorder that affects virtually every organ system. Many medical problems of diabetic patients are attributed to involvement of the vascular system. Large vessel involvement causes cerebral, coronary, and peripheral vascular disease. Microvascular involvement causes neuropathy, retinopathy, and renal disease. Preoperative cardiac and peripheral vascular evaluations are recommended for all diabetic patients undergoing total joint arthroplasty. The adverse effects of hyperglycemia on bone strength and fracture healing have been demonstrated in experimental models. Diabetic patients have an increased susceptibility to infections, which probably is due to a defect in the mechanism of phagocytosis.

In one study of 64 Charnley total hip arthroplasties in diabetic patients, four hips (6.5%) developed a deep infection. These procedures were performed in a clean-air enclosure, but without prophylactic antibiotics. This rate of infection was significantly higher than in non-diabetic osteoarthritic patients. However, in another study there was no superficial or deep infection in diabetic patients who had 93 total hip arthroplasties performed in a clean-air enclosure with laminar air flow, body-exhaust suits, and a second-generation cephalosporin prophylaxis. However, the overall complication rate was high (24.3%) in this patient group, and the most frequent complication (14.2%) was urinary tract infection. There was no increased loosening of cemented prostheses in diabetic patients.

In a study of 59 cemented total knee arthroplasties in 40 diabetic patients, there was an overall infection rate of 7% and there were 12% wound complications despite prophylactic antibiotics. The rate of deep joint infections in diabetic patients was statistically higher than in nondiabetic patients. There were two deaths due to myocardial infarction. The overall revision rate was 10% at a mean follow-up time of 4.3 years. Antibiotic-impregnated bone cement was recommended for use in these patients.

Renal Failure and Transplantation

Patients with chronic renal failure treated with either hemodialysis or chronic peritoneal dialysis usually have severe renal osteodystrophy from hyperparathyroidism and osteomalacia. In seven patients receiving chronic hemodialysis or peritoneal dialysis, femoral neck fractures were treated with bipolar endoprosthesis or hemiarthroplasty; there was a high complication rate and one postoperative death. Four patients developed prolonged narcotic-induced confusion. Six hip prostheses functioned well, with mean follow-up of 26 months.

In reports of total hip arthroplasties placed with modern cement techniques and prostheses, there has been early loosening of components in patients who continue to receive chronic dialysis. This loosening probably is due to osteomalacia and bone resorption at the bone–cement interface. Uncemented components may be a better choice, but there are no published reports of the results. More recent reports have noted a high infection rate in this population.

The early results of cemented total hip arthroplasty for osteonecrosis after renal transplantation were encouraging. However, with longer follow-up, the results in this patient population were less satisfactory due to loosening at the bone–cement interface. In one study of 24 cemented total hip arthroplasties followed for a mean of 86 months, six (25%) failed due to aseptic loosening. There was a high prevalence of dislocation. Iliac crest biopsies of these patients showed high-turnover osteoporosis and hyperosteoidosis, which probably contributed to the high failure rate. Uncemented porous-coated total hip arthroplasties may be preferable in this patient population. In one study of 27 cementless hips, all patients had good or excellent hip ratings at a mean of 48 months after surgery.

Neurologic Disorders

Neuropathic Arthropathy (Charcot Joint)

Neuropathic joints are associated with central or peripheral nerve lesions. The specific radiographic patterns seen in the knee, foot, and hip are usually associated with neurosyphilis (tabes dorsalis) or diabetes mellitus, but occasionally there is no known etiology. Many consider neuropathic arthropathy to be an absolute contraindication to total knee arthroplasty. However, the procedure is feasible provided that a surface replacement can be used, the joint is debrided, and correct alignment and stability are achieved (Fig. 3). A posterior stabilized or constrained condylar implant is usually required. In one series of nine Charcot knees followed for an average of 3 years, the results were excellent in eight, and there was no loosening or instability. Seven knees required custom prostheses with medial or lateral tibial wedges because of severe bone deficiencies. In 24 knees of various designs implanted at another center, with a mean follow-up time of only 2 years, there was a 50% rate of failure, which usually was due to loosening or instability. However, seven of eight condylar knees had a satisfactory result. Another study followed five condylar-type knees for 8 to 10 years. There were two knees with tibial component failure, one of which was successfully revised and followed for 8 years.

It is generally believed that total hip arthroplasty is contraindicated in a Charcot joint. Hip joint involvement requiring total hip arthroplasty is rare and there are only case reports: one cemented hip functioned well for 7 years in a patient without ataxia, one loosened within 1 year, and one had recurrent instability. An additional case re-

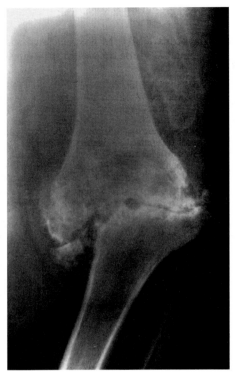 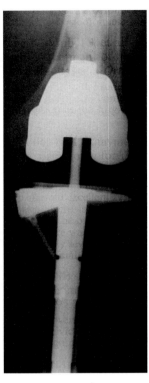

Fig. 3 **Left,** Radiographs of the left knee in a 73-year-old woman with neuropathic arthropathy (due to tabes dorsalis). **Right,** Knee reconstructed with constrained condylar implants with medial tibial wedge and long stem.

port described a Charnley prosthesis with recurrent dislocations, despite proper component alignment, which required removal of components at 1 year.

Neuromuscular Disease: Cerebral Palsy

Hip dislocation in cerebral palsy results from persistent coxa valga and excessive femoral anteversion associated with muscle imbalance. The painful dislocated or subluxed hip in the patient with cerebral palsy occurs in late adolescence or young adulthood. Girdlestone resection arthroplasty has failed to provide reliable relief of pain. Hip arthrodesis has been recommended for unilateral disease in patients who are unable to walk and in young, active patients. Cemented total hip arthroplasty is preferred for bilateral hip disease or in patients who are able to walk. In one series, six of eight hip arthrodeses were successful, and two had symptomatic pseudarthroses. Thirteen of 15 total hip arthroplasties in patients with cerebral palsy were clinically successful at a mean follow-up of over 6 years. There were two femoral component loosenings and two recurrent dislocations, both of which required revision. In another series of 12 total hip replacements in patients with mental retardation, Down syndrome, or cerebral palsy, there were no major complications, infections, or dislocations, but one cemented hip was revised at 4.5 years for loosening. In a long-term follow-up study (mean 10 years)

of 19 cemented total hip arthroplasties, 94% of patients had relief of pain and improved function. Hip spica casts were used postoperatively in almost all patients to minimize the incidence of dislocation and trochanteric nonunion. With revision surgery for any reason as the defined end point, survival at 10 years was 86%.

Poliomyelitis

Patients with anterior poliomyelitis often develop severe knee deformities and chronic instability. Due to altered knee kinematics, these patients eventually develop osteoarthritis. The knee deformities associated with poliomyelitis are external rotation of the tibia, unstable valgus deformity, and genu recurvatum. In the early stage, bracing with a knee-ankle-foot orthosis will sometimes provide symptomatic relief. Cemented condylar design total knee arthroplasty has been used in an attempt to relieve pain and improve stability. In one study, nine knees in nine patients (mean age 68 years) with poliomyelitis and knee arthritis had cemented total knee arthroplasty. At a mean follow-up of 6.8 years, three of the nine knees required revision knee arthroplasty, one for late infection and two for recurrent instability (one posterior subluxation and one recurvatum). Three knees developed recurrent recurvatum deformity, and bracing was unsuccessful in all cases. When performing a total knee arthroplasty in pa-

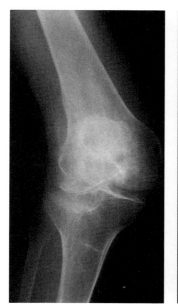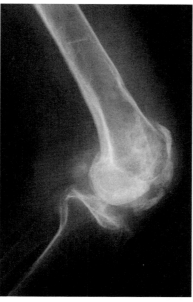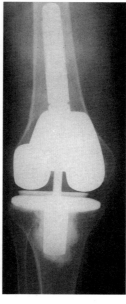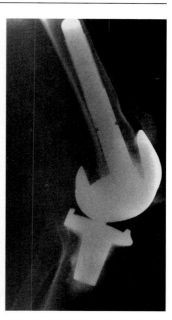

Fig. 4 Anteroposterior (**left**) and lateral (**center left**) radiographs of the knee in a wheelchair-bound 74-year-old woman with Parkinson's disease. There is a severe valgus deformity, notching of the anterior cortex of the femur, and severe destruction of the patella. **Center right and right,** Postoperative radiographs showing a constrained condylar knee with an uncemented femoral stem. The patella could not be resurfaced. Although she had complete relief of pain, the patient remained a nonambulator.

tients with multiaxial instability, a relatively constrained implant with intramedullary stems (posterior stabilized or constrained condylar) should be strongly considered. In addition, a recurvatum deformity may be addressed by resecting a less than usual segment of the distal femur, so that the extension gap is 2 to 3 mm less than the flexion gap. This method generates a flexion contracture of 5° to 10°, which is necessary to eliminate the recurvatum deformity. Patients with quadriceps weakness should be informed that bracing after surgery may be required. The functional status of many of the patients with poliomyelitis continued to decline despite a painless, stable total knee arthroplasty.

Parkinson's Disease

Parkinson's disease is a common geriatric neurologic disorder, which is characterized by tremor, muscular rigidity, and abnormalities of gait, posture, and facial expression. Patients with this disorder may develop severe osteoporosis with concomitant femoral neck fracture and, occasionally, severe osteoarthritis of the knees. In one report, it was suggested that Parkinson's disease is a contraindication to total knee arthroplasty. Three patients had total knee arthroplasties that were considered failures because of severe hamstring muscle rigidity, recurrent flexion contracture, and inability to ambulate despite medical treatment. However, in another report of 12 knees in nine patients with a mean age of 70 years, the results were rated as excellent in nine and good in three knees at a mean follow-up of 4.3 years. Four knees developed recurrent

flexion contractures. Total knee arthroplasty was successful for both the relief of pain and an increase in range of flexion (Fig. 4).

Controversy exists as to the optimal treatment for a fracture of the femoral neck in patients with Parkinson's disease. Some reports suggest that hemiarthroplasty should be avoided because of the increased frequency of dislocation (as high as 37%). Other reports describe a high rate of morbidity and mortality after internal fixation of these fractures. In one retrospective report of 50 hips (49 patients) treated with unipolar or bipolar hemiarthroplasty, there was a high rate of postoperative complications, including urinary tract infection (20%) and pneumonia (10%). However, there was only one dislocation, and 80% of the surviving patients could ambulate at a mean follow-up of 7.3 years. The early functional results of 56 elective total hip arthroplasties in 52 patients with Parkinson's disease were generally good. There were six dislocations (10.7%). The long-term functional results deteriorated due to the progression of the neurologic disability in 42% of patients.

Miscellaneous Disorders

Paget's Disease

Paget's disease of bone is a disorder in which there is a great increase in the rate of bone turnover. The primary abnormality is intense focal resorption of normal bone by abnormal osteoclasts followed by an attempt by osteoblasts to remodel and lay down new bone. There is some evidence to support a viral etiology, probably a paramyxovirus. The incidence of Paget's disease of bone is between 2% and 4% of the general population who are more than 40 years old. Symptomatic osteoarthritis will develop in the hip in 30% to 50% of patients and in the knee in 10% to 12%. Medical management with nonsteroidal anti-inflammatory drugs and/or calcitonin, diphosphonates, or both is usually successful, but total joint arthroplasty is occasionally indicated.

Coxa vara deformity is commonly seen with Paget's disease of the proximal femur and can lead to varus positioning of the femoral component. Severe coxa vara or femoral bowing may require an osteotomy. Mild protrusio acetabuli is frequently seen, but this condition does not usually require bone grafting. Reaming of the acetabulum and femur may be quite difficult due to hard, sclerotic bone. Preoperative treatment of patients with calcitonin and/or diphosphonates has been effective in decreasing intraoperative blood loss and is highly recommended. In one report of cemented total hip arthroplasty in 21 patients, there was a 9.5% incidence of revision and 52% incidence of heterotopic ossification at a mean follow-up of 5 years. In another study of 91 hips with a mean follow-up of 7.2 years, 13% had undergone revision of one or both components. Actuarial analysis of 52 hips with 10-year follow-up showed a statistically significant increase in the rate of revision (15%) compared to a group of cemented hips in patients who did not have Paget's disease. The incidence of heterotopic ossification was also high (37%). Uncemented, porous-coated arthroplasty is not recommended because of the high rate of bone turnover.

In one study of 16 cemented total knee arthroplasties in patients who had Paget's disease of bone at the knee, there was no loosening of ten total condylar knees followed for a mean of 5.4 years. There was no difference in blood loss between the patients who had preoperative treatment with calcitonin, diphosphonates, or fluoride and the patients who did not have such treatment. There were multiple technical intraoperative difficulties, and malalignment frequently occurred; extramedullary alignment devices were recommended.

Systemic Lupus Erythematosus

Systemic lupus erythematosus is a chronic, multisystemic inflammatory disorder, which predominantly affects women in the second and third decades. Osteonecrosis of the femoral head, usually associated with steroid treatment for this underlying immunologic disorder, frequently requires prosthetic arthroplasty. In one study of 43 hip arthroplasties (29 conventional total hip arthroplasties and 19 bipolar prostheses) in 31 patients followed for a mean of 57 months, there was a high rate of postoperative complications: delayed wound healing in 15%, superficial wound infection in 10%, and deep infection in 4.6%, which was unrelated to the use of steroids. Eight patients died

from complications (usually renal) of their disease at a mean of 54 months after surgery. No patient with a total hip replacement required revision, but five bipolar prostheses were revised for pain or loosening. Another study of 33 total hip arthroplasties was more optimistic, with 94.6% survival at 5 years and 81.8% survival at 9 years. There were no wound healing complications, no infections, and only one late death due to pneumonia. One cemented hip was revised for loosening and two acetabular components were radiographically loose. Uncemented or hybrid total hip arthroplasties are recommended for this patient population.

Psoriatic Arthritis

Psoriasis is a chronic skin disorder that affects 1% to 2% of the population. Approximately 7% of patients with psoriasis have an inflammatory arthritis that is similar to rheumatoid arthritis. Patients with psoriasis have characteristic plaques on the extensor surfaces and in body creases, which are known to harbor bacterial pathogens. In a study of 55 Charnley total hip arthroplasties in patients with psoriasis, there was a superficial infection rate of 9.1% and a deep infection rate of 5.5%. All operations were performed in a clean-air enclosure but without a prophylactic antibiotic. In a study of 24 cemented total knee arthroplasties in patients with psoriasis, performed with perioperative antibiotic prophylaxis, the rate of deep infection was 17% and the overall rate of revision was 21% at a mean follow-up time of 4 years. It is likely that patients with psoriasis have an increased rate of infection after total joint arthroplasty. Preoperative dermatologic consultation and skin treatment is strongly recommended.

Ankylosing Spondylitis

Arthritis of the hip joint occurs in approximately 30% of patients with ankylosing spondylitis and, when present, it is usually bilateral. Spinal involvement results in fixed thoracolumbar kyphosis and, in combination with severe hip flexion contractures, the patient's ability to ambulate is severely restricted. Cemented total hip arthroplasty has been shown to provide excellent relief of pain and improved ambulatory capacity. However, the improvement in the total range of motion of the hip was limited in several series due to the high incidence of heterotopic ossification. In one series of 29 hips, severe heterotopic ossification (Brooker Class III and IV) occurred in 23% of the hips.

Prophylaxis against heterotopic ossification by means of either low-dose radiation or indomethacin therapy is generally recommended. However, in a report of 53 total hip arthroplasties with a mean follow-up of 6.3 years, cemented total hip prostheses were very durable in this population. In this series, clinically important heterotopic bone formation (Brooker Class III and IV) developed in only 11% of patients, all of whom had a previous hip operation, postoperative infection, or complete ankylosis preoperatively.

Annotated Bibliography

Acurio MT, Friedman RJ: Hip arthroplasty in patients with sickle-cell haemoglobinopathy. *J Bone Joint Surg* 1992;74B:367–371.

The rate of revision was 50% at a mean follow-up of 10 years.

Alpert B, Waddell JP, Morton J, et al: Cementless total hip arthroplasty in renal transplant patients. *Clin Orthop* 1992;284:164–169.

All 27 uncemented total hip arthroplasties were successful at a mean follow-up of 48 months.

Buly RL, Huo M, Root L, et al: Total hip arthroplasty in cerebral palsy long-term follow-up results. *Clin Orthop* 1993;296:148–153.

Survival was 86% for 19 hips at 10 years.

Clarke HJ, Jinnah RH, Brooker AF, et al: Total replacement of the hip for avascular necrosis in sickle cell disease. *J Bone Joint Surg* 1989;71B:465–470.

There was a 59% rate of loosening in this series of 27 cemented and uncemented prostheses.

Devlin VJ, Einhorn TA, Gordon SL, et al: Total hip arthroplasty after renal transplantation: Long-term follow-up study and assessment of metabolic bone status. *J Arthroplasty* 1988;3:205–213.

There was a 25% incidence of aseptic loosening of cemented total hip arthroplasties at a mean follow-up of 86 months.

England SP, Stem SH, Insall JN, et al: Total knee arthroplasty in diabetes mellitus. *Clin Orthop* 1990; 260:130–134.

This study of 59 cemented total knees in diabetic patients showed an infection rate of 7% and overall revision rate of 10% at a mean follow-up of 4.3 years.

Figgie MP, Goldberg VM, Figgie HE III, et al: Total knee arthroplasty for the treatment of chronic hemophilic arthropathy. *Clin Orthop* 1989;248:98–107.

Six of 19 knees were failures at a mean follow-up of 9.5 years.

Gabel GT, Rand JA, Sim FH: Total knee arthroplasty for osteoarthritis in patients who have Paget disease of bone at the knee. *J Bone Joint Surg* 1991;73A:739–744.

Suboptimal alignment occurred in ten of 13 limbs.

Goldblatt J, Sacks S, Dall D, et al: Total hip arthroplasty in Gaucher's disease: Long-term prognosis. *Clin Orthop* 1988;228:94–98.

Only 73% of cemented arthroplasties were intact at a mean follow-up of 7.3 years.

Hansen AD, Cabanela ME, Michet CJ Jr: Hip arthroplasty in patients with systemic lupus erythematosus. *J Bone Joint Surg* 1987;69A:807–814.

There was an increased incidence of wound complications and of superficial and deep infections.

Huo MH, Salvati EA, Browne MG, et al: Primary total hip arthroplasty in systemic lupus erythematosus. *J Arthroplasty* 1992;7:51–56.

Perioperative morbidity was minimal and the 5-year survival was 94.6%.

Kilgus DJ, Namba RS, Gorek JE, et al: Total hip replacement for patients who have ankylosing spondylitis: The importance of the formation of heterotopic bone and of the durability of fixation of cemented components. *J Bone Joint Surg* 1990;72A:834–839.

Conventional cemented total hip arthroplasties were very durable at a mean follow-up of 6.3 years.

McDonald DJ, Sim FH: Total hip arthroplasty in Paget's disease: A follow-up note. *J Bone Joint Surg* 1987;69A: 766–772.

There was a 15% incidence of revision in hips followed for 10 years.

Menon TJ, Wroblewski BM: Charnley low-friction arthroplasty in patients with psoriasis. *Clin Orthop* 1983;176:127–128.

The rate of deep infection was 5.5% in this study of 55 Charnley total hips in patients with psoriasis.

Merkow RL, Pellicci PM, Hely DP, et al: Total hip replacement for Paget's disease of the hip. *J Bone Joint Surg* 1984;66A:752–758.

Revision surgery was necessary in 9.5% of hips.

Moeckel B, Huo MH, Salvati EA, et al: Total hip arthroplasty in patients with diabetes mellitus. *J Arthroplasty* 1993;8:279–284.

There was a high rate of complications in this series of 93 total hip arthroplasties in diabetic patients, but the rate of loosening was low.

Moran MC, Huo MH, Garvin KL, et al: Total hip arthroplasty in sickle cell hemoglobinopathy. *Clin Orthop* 1993;294:140–148.

Thirty-eight percent of cemented primary hips failed; failure usually was due to aseptic acetabular loosening.

Nelson IW, Sivamurugan S, Latham PD, et al: Total hip arthroplasty for hemophilic arthroplasty. *Clin Orthop* 1992;276:210–213.

The total rate of failure of 22 cemented Charnley total hip arthroplasties was 36% at a median follow-up of 7.6 years.

Oni OO, MacKenney RP: Total knee replacement in patients with Parkinson's disease. *J Bone Joint Surg* 1985;67:424–425.

All three knees were failures due to severe hamstring rigidity.

Patterson BM, Insall JN: Surgical management of gonarthrosis in patients with poliomyelitis. *J Arthroplasty* 1992;7(suppl):419–426.

Three of nine cemented condylar knees required revision knee arthroplasty.

Robb JE, Rymaszewski LA, Reeves BF, et al: Total hip replacement in a Charcot joint: Brief report. *J Bone Joint Surg* 1988;70B:489.

A Charnley prosthesis required removal because of recurrent dislocations.

Root L, Goss JR, Mendes J: The treatment of the painful hip in cerebral palsy by total hip replacement or hip arthrodesis. *J Bone Joint Surg* 1986;68A:590–598.

Six of eight arthrodeses and 13 of 15 total hip arthroplasties were clinically successful.

Skoff HD, Keggi K: Total hip replacement in the neuromuscularly impaired. *Orthop Rev* 1986;15:154–159.

There was one femoral component loosening in 12 hips.

Soudry M, Binazzi R, Johanson NA, et al: Total knee arthroplasty in Charcot and Charcot-like joints. *Clin Orthop* 1986;208:199–204.

Results were excellent in eight knees at a mean follow-up of 3 years.

Staeheli JW, Frassica FJ, Sim FH: Prosthetic replacement of the femoral head for fracture of the femoral neck in patients who have Parkinson's disease. *J Bone Joint Surg* 1988;70A:565–568.

There was a low dislocation rate (2%) and a high postoperative complication rate.

Stern SH, Insall JN, Windsor RE, et al: Total knee arthroplasty in patients with psoriasis. *Clin Orthop* 1989; 248:108–110.

The rate of deep infection was 17%.

Vince K, Insall J, Bannerman C: Total knee arthroplasty in the patient with Parkinson's disease. *J Bone Joint Surg* 1989;71B:51–54.

Nine of 12 knees were rated as excellent and three as good.

Walker LG, Sledge CB: Total hip arthroplasty in ankylosing spondylitis. *Clin Orthop* 1991;262:198–204.

There was complete relief of pain in 97% of patients, but there was a 23% incidence of grade III and IV myositis ossificans.

Yoshino S, Fujimori J, Kajino A, et al: Total knee arthroplasty in Charcot's Joint. *J Arthroplasty* 1993;8: 335–340.

In this report of an 8- to 10-year follow-up of five knees, two had tibial component loosening and one was revised successfully, with an 8-year follow-up.

11

Osteonecrosis

Introduction

Any discussion of management of osteonecrosis of the femoral head must include a discussion of the concepts on which its diagnosis and management are based. These concepts have evolved rapidly over the past decade as new technologies have allowed early recognition and identification of the disease and have raised questions concerning some of the basic tenets on which appropriate treatment is based. This chapter represents a summary of present knowledge regarding the epidemiology, etiology, pathogenesis, diagnosis, staging, and management of osteonecrosis of the femoral head.

ARCO, the Association Research Circulation Osseous, through its committee on Staging and Nomenclature has suggested the following definition: "Bone" is an organ that consists of mineralized and nonmineralized tissues. Bone necrosis is a disease that causes death of bone and is called "osteonecrosis." This consensus definition implies that because no one etiology explains all findings presently known about the disease, its definition should be all encompassing. Although avascular necrosis, aseptic necrosis, ischemic necrosis of the femoral head, and other names are applied to this disease state, investigators and clinicians are encouraged to use the term osteonecrosis.

Epidemiology

In studying the epidemiology of osteonecrosis, investigators are trying to address several questions: (1) Who is at risk for developing this disease; (2) how prevalent is this disease; and (3) what is its pattern of presentation (which joints are most likely to be affected, what age group, sex distribution, etc.). Over the years, a number of disease states have been identified that have a high association with necrosis of the femoral head. Initially these were the less common diseases, such as Caisson's disease, sickle disease, and Gaucher's disease. As understanding of the disease and the ability to find it in its early stages have grown, it has been found to occur more frequently in conditions such as systemic lupus erythematosus (SLE), corticosteroid usage, and alcohol abuse. Outline 1 lists disease states, medications, or afflictions felt to be strongly associated with the development of osteonecrosis, as well as those that may have some association with its development.

There have been few studies of populations large enough to provide meaningful epidemiologic information. Useful studies require a time frame and population size capable of providing information that can withstand rigid statistical evaluation. Prospective studies have been difficult to establish because they require agreement as to the data to be collected as well as appropriate diagnostic and staging criteria for the disease. Several recently reported studies meet these criteria and will be of interest.

An increase in the incidence of femoral head necrosis in Japan between 1984 and 1987 has been reported. The incidence of new patients with the disease was 1,131 in 1984 and rose to 2,364 by 1987. These figures included patients with posttraumatic osteonecrosis and were based on surveys carried out in 1,721 hospitals throughout Japan. There was no obvious gender preponderance (males: female, 1.41:1), although osteonecrosis seen in the collagen vascular diseases or autoimmune diseases associated with corticosteroid usage was more common in females while that associated with alcohol ingestion or idiopathic causes was more common in males. The origin of osteonecrosis was idiopathic in 39.5% of the studied patient population, whereas steroid and alcohol associated osteonecrosis accounted for 37% and 23% of the population, respectively.

Similar data on large populations are just beginning to become available from North American and European studies in which agreement on parameters of assessment have been more difficult to reach. In a recent North American study, 630 hips with osteonecrosis treated either by protected weightbearing (PWB), core decompression (CD), or pulsed electromagnetic fields (PEMFs) were identified. The same clinical and radiographic success criteria were applied to each of the groups, and an extensive statis-

Outline 1. Common clinical entities associated with osteonecrosis

Alcoholism
Dysbaric phenomena-decompression sickness
Hypercortisonism
Hyperlipemia
Pancreatitis
Hemoglobinopathies
Diabetes mellitus
Endotoxin reactions
Systemic lupus erythematosus
Serum sickness
Toxic shock
Inflammatory bowel disease
Chemotherapy
Brain/spinal surgery
Anticoagulant deficiencies
Storage diseases-Gaucher's disease
Sickle-cell crisis
Vascular disorders-arteriosclerosis
Nephrotic syndrome

tical evaluation of the entire population was performed. Although the entry criteria for each of the populations were slightly different (the PEMF study patients were all prospectively studied as part of an Investigational Device Exemption), the data for each of the groups were collected by the same individuals and evaluated in the same fashion. Thus, the analyses were consistent for the entire population.

The following findings were reported. The time of progression of each hip to failure, which was defined as either hip replacement or progression to advanced collapse and arthritis (Ficat stage IV), correlated with both radiographic and clinical indicators at the start of treatment. For all three treatment approaches, progression to failure was associated with the Ficat stage at entry. For Ficat stage II hips, progression was associated with the initial pain score, but not with the area of the lesion as described on the plain radiographs. For stage III hips, progression correlated with the degree of collapse, the area of the lesion, and the pain scores. No correlations with the etiology of the necrosis could be demonstrated. This information confirms that early identification increases the chance of success of limited surgical or nonsurgical interventions and raises questions as to the importance of the various etiologic factors in the ultimate outcome of these treatment approaches.

Of the risk factors most commonly associated with osteonecrosis in contemporary patient populations, several continue to remain major impediments for successful limited intervention. In the Japanese study, two subpopulation studies were performed to assess the risk associated with their two largest disease states: SLE (studied over 5 years in 212 patients), and regular alcohol intake (1988 to 1990). Data from the first study indicated that dosages of 30 mg/day of prednisolone, particularly if started rapidly without preloading, are harmful. In addition, certain clinical features were identified that place some SLE patients at greater risk for developing osteonecrosis.

The risk of alcohol intake and cigarette smoking combined was assessed in a population of 118 patients and 236 controls. A dose and duration relationship of alcohol to osteonecrosis development was identified. Using appropriate statistical techniques to identify relative risk rates, it was possible to determine that those individuals who regularly consume greater than 400 ml/week were at 13 times greater risk of developing osteonecrosis than those who never consume alcohol. Coupling this intake with cigarette smoking or underlying liver dysfunction did not increase this risk.

Etiology

Basic and applied scientific effort has been directed to the study of the etiology of osteonecrosis and has enhanced the orthopaedist's ability to apply treatment modalities. However, no one model of osteonecrosis has emerged as predictable and universal in reproducing the human entity in the laboratory. A number of observations (some conflicting) can explain observed phenomena, but these observations do not always translate to predictable treatment approaches. Several hypotheses of etiology do deserve to be highlighted, because they influence current approaches to diagnosis and management.

The major theories now advanced to explain the earliest changes inciting osteonecrosis are: (1) fat embolism with subsequent intravascular thrombosis; (2) intraosseous hypertension with a subsequent "compartment" syndrome of bone; (3) fatty overload and fat cell changes with subsequent vascular compression and compromise; and (4) abnormal extraosseous blood flow with absence of transcortical blood supply from the superior retinacular arteries.

Fat Embolism

In the first hypothesis, fatty osteocytic necrosis is felt to progress to ischemic degeneration of necrotic osteocytes and adipocytes when the volume of subchondral fat overload results in vascular stasis, local hypercoagulability, endothelial damage, and subsequent intravascular coagulation. In this situation, local mechanisms of repair are prevented in a vulnerable microcirculatory environment. Histologically observed phenomena include intraosseous thromboses and peripheral hemorrhages. These phenomena were observed in animals with induced intravascular coagulopathy and in children with disseminated intravascular coagulopathy and histologic evidence of interosseous thrombosis and osteonecrosis.

Intraosseous Hypertension and the Compartment Syndrome of Bone   Many investigators have been able to demonstrate intraosseous hypertension of bone in patients with both osteonecrosis and osteoarthritis of the femoral head. The entire role of intraosseous hypertension in the development of localized osteonecrotic lesions and the subsequent development of osteonecrosis have been clearly articulated. A role was suggested for microcirculatory compromise in the observed progressive histologic changes noted at biopsy. A functional exploration of bone was described that allows for the documentation of intraosseous venous hypertension in the femoral head and trochanteric region.

Fat Cell Abnormalities

Fat cell hypertrophy and fatty marrow overload have been demonstrated in animals as a consistent consequence of high-dose corticosteroid exposure. Histologic changes consistent with necrosis were frequently identified and femoral head blood flow was consistently diminished. The use of lipid clearing agents was shown to consistently improve this alteration in blood flow.

Abnormal Extraosseous Blood Flow

Superselective angiography of the medial circumflex artery has been used for extensive study of the extraosseous femoral head blood flow in patients with osteonecrosis of the femoral head. Consistent loss of transcortical blood flow from the superior retinacular arteries and alterations in the revascularization process in hips with radiographically and preradiographically defined osteonecrosis have been demonstrated. A mechanism of alteration of the process of revascularization has been considered to be a contributory feature of nonreversible osteonecrosis.

Pathogenesis

Over the past 5 years, it has become clear that separating the concept of pathogenesis of disease from its etiology is beneficial. Although the cause of the disease for a particular patient or associated disease state may not be explainable, the stages or common pathways that can lead to ultimate destruction of the femoral head can be identified. The concept of a compartment syndrome of bone and the application of Starling's hypothesis to bone blood flow and the compromise thereof incorporate a number of laboratory and clinically based observations, and these ideas can be applied clinically.

Attempts to diminish intraosseous hypertension through core decompression can be used to treat osteonecrosis if improving blood flow to the femoral head is sufficient to allow normal processes of healing to occur. Intraosseous hypertension can be demonstrated by intraoperative exploration of bone in a large percentage of patients who have symptoms of osteonecrosis. Venous hypertension is observed via intraosseous manometry, outflow obstruction is demonstrated by intraosseous venography in which delayed venous outflow and diaphyseal reflux of dye can be visualized and documented, and these phenomena are decreased by core biopsy with decompression (Fig. 1). The clinical results using this approach as a treatment modality are discussed below.

Diagnosis

Important advances in the recognition and diagnosis of osteonecrosis in its earliest state have been made in the past 5 years. Although plain radiography, technetium bone scans, and either whole bone or computed tomography have proven important tools for diagnosis of osteonecrosis in the past decade, it is the rapid developments in magnetic resonance imaging (MRI) and single photon emission computed tomographic (SPECT) imaging technology that have had the greatest impact on the ability to detect this disease at its earliest stages.

It is now documented that a number of abnormalities in the proximal femur can be identified using MRI. Only the single bandlike area of low signal intensity on the T1-weighted image (Fig. 2, *left*), or the double line sign seen on the T2-weighted image (Fig. 2, *right*) in which an isointense central area is surrounded by a band of low signal intensity can be accepted as diagnostic for osteonecrosis.

A problem over the past several years has been that all femoral head abnormalities have tended to be considered

osteonecrosis by either orthopaedists or radiologists. Controversy remains as to the significance of many of the other abnormalities that can be identified on MRI. However, substantial evidence is being advanced that the bone marrow edema syndrome is a reversible entity (Fig. 3) that is representative of a transient condition with marrow histologic changes comparable to those seen with osteonecrosis.

SPECT imaging is a three-dimensional scanning technique initially developed for analysis of cardiac blood flow abnormalities. It has been shown to be useful in the analysis of bone graft healing and in the identification of early osteonecrosis. Because of its ability to three dimensionally visualize bone reactivity, it is particularly helpful in identifying an area of decreased activity (a cold spot) within an

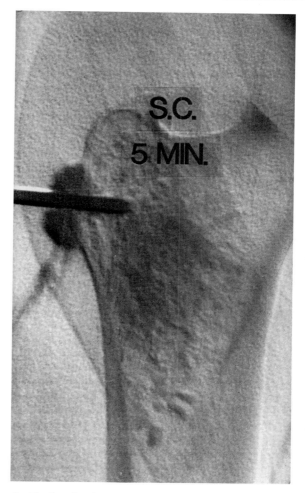

Fig. 1 The functional exploration of bone includes the injection of up to 10 cc of radiopaque dye. The femoral head with venous hypertension demonstrates outflow obstruction. Dye present within the trabecular spaces more than 5 minutes following injection and the presence of diaphyseal reflux of dye are indicative of venous hypertension and are consistent with the diagnosis of osteonecrosis.

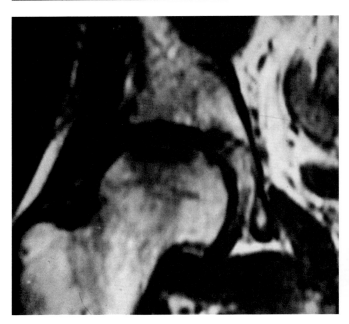
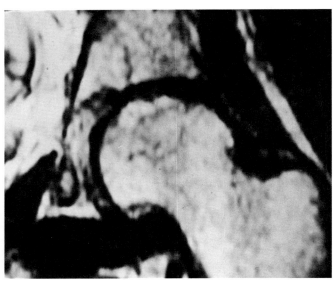

Fig. 2 Magnetic resonance imaging findings in early stages of osteonecrosis. **Left,** The decreased signal intensity on a T1-weighted image, in a band-like pattern, is diagnostic of osteonecrosis. **Right,** An isointense area of uptake surrounded by a dark band, seen on the T2-weighted image, is diagnostic of osteonecrosis.

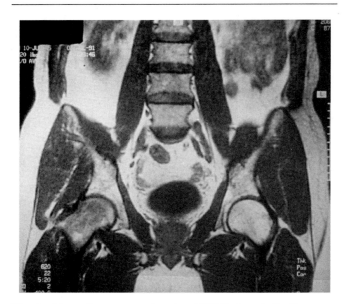

Fig. 3 Magnetic resonance imaging (MRI) findings in the Bone Marrow Edema Syndrome show decreased marrow signal uptake that is more widespread. While the MRI signal is clearly abnormal, the absence of the specific findings of Figure 2 make this a nondiagnostic MRI study for osteonecrosis.

area of increased reactivity. This clinical picture can be seen in a very early stage of osteonecrosis (Fig. 4).

Diagnostic Algorithms

The identification of appropriate diagnostic algorithms is important to the development of therapeutic intervention for the patient with osteonecrosis. It is in the patient's best interest to use diagnostic modalities efficiently and effectively. One diagnostic algorithm (Fig. 5) calls for use of MRI and SPECT for the early disease states, when the radiographic evaluation is normal or equivocal, or for the contralateral hip of an obviously involved hip in a high-risk patient. For the radiographically apparent disease, either computed or whole bone tomography would be used to identify the volume of head involvement and the integrity of the subchondral plate.

Staging

Probably most important to the development of a true understanding of the disease, and to its ultimate control and prevention, is the development of a universally accepted staging system that can allow the assembly of consistently collected information from a large number of investigators with sufficiently large populations of patients. The usefulness of the large body of literature on osteonecrosis has been hampered by small patient populations, lack of rigid prospective protocols, and the absence of standardized as-

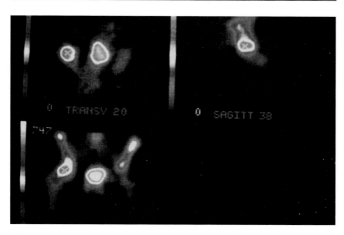

Fig. 4 Single Photon Emission Computerized Tomography (SPECT) imaging findings in osteonecrosis are the area of decreased uptake surrounded by an area of increased activity. (Reproduced with permission from Stulberg BN, Levine M, Bauer TW, et al: Multimodality approach to osteonecrosis of the femoral head. *Clin Orthop* 1989;240:181–193.)

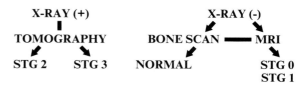

Fig. 5 The diagnostic algorithm pictured here uses magnetic resonance imaging and single photon emission computed tomography imaging when the plain radiographic images fail to reveal signs of disease in the femoral head. When the radiographic findings are apparent, this algorithm calls for the use of tomographic studies to identify the extent of disease within the femoral head. (Reproduced with permission from Stulberg BN, Bauer TW, Belhobek GH, et al: A diagnostic algorithm for osteonecrosis of the femoral head. *Clin Orthop* 1989;249:176–182.)

Table 1. The five-stage system proposed by ARCO

Stage	Finding
0	Histology only
1	(+) Diagnostic test
2	(+) X-ray: no collapse
3	(+) X-ray: collapse
4	(+) X-ray: osteoarthritis

sessments of outcome. ARCO has suggested a uniform staging system that is acceptable to investigators from around the world. This staging system draws on the positive attributes of established systems. Its goals are to standardize the criteria for diagnosis of the disease, to outline steps required to standardize the method of reaching the diagnosis, and to suggest minimum requirements for the reporting of results. Such a system must be clear and usable, employ standard terminology, and be based on quantifiable parameters.

The ARCO five-stage system (Table 1) suggests a stage 0, perhaps not yet seen but likely in the future, in which early histologic changes can be identified but all available noninvasive diagnostic studies are normal. In stage 1, the plain radiograph is normal, but one of the newer diagnostic methods is positive. Stage 2 is radiographically apparent disease without subchondral collapse. Stage 3 is radiographic disease with subchondral collapse but without arthritis. Stage 4 involves disease with arthritis.

A schema involving subclassification and quantitation is shown in Figure 6 and Table 2. It is based on plain radiographic appearance and requires a measure of mild, moderate, or severe head involvement. Radiographic types of involvement of the femoral head are based on quantitative relationships to the dome of the acetabulum on the anteroposterior (AP) radiograph. This latter approach to quantitation apparently is also applicable to the MRI findings identified in preradiographic disease states. Progressive radiographic collapse and failure was seen in greater than 90% of hips with involvement extending to the entire dome of the acetabulum, slight subchondral irregularity, or cystic involvement of the femoral head under the lateral third of the dome.

Investigators also must adopt a minimum standard of information for reporting results relating to the treatment of osteonecrosis. ARCO requires clinical quantitation of performance based on an accepted hip scoring system (eg, the Harris Hip Rating), information as to radiographic progression (using quantitation), and information regarding hip survival. In this fashion the literature will begin to allow comparison of differing therapeutic interventions in a reliable manner.

Treatment Modalities

Although many modalities are currently being suggested for the treatment of osteonecrosis in both its early and advanced stages, most studies evaluating these methods have serious flaws either in design, diagnosis of true disease, consistency of therapeutic intervention, or in the manner in which the results are reported. Only one study in the treatment literature is based on randomization of therapeutic options. In that study, limitation of weight-bearing was shown both clinically and radiographically to be statistically less successful than core decompression in stabilizing Ficat stage I and stage II hips. These findings have been replicated in several concurrently studied populations.

Early Stages

The most commonly applied interventions for early stages of osteonecrosis of the femoral head include limited

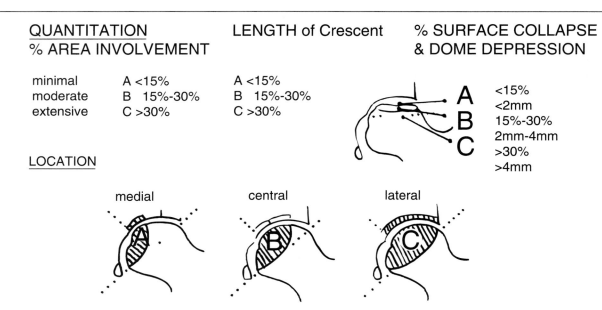

Fig. 6 The ARCO staging system encompasses a radiographic subclassification system that requires quantitation of the amount of femoral head involvement. This subclassification is to accompany the stages outlined in Table 1.

Table 2. Subclassification system for ARCO staging

Subclassification	Quantitation (% area)	Surface Collapse
A Minimal	< 15	< 15 or < 2 mm
B Moderate	15 to 30	15% to 30% or 2 to 4 mm
C Extensive	> 30	> 30% or > 4 mm

weightbearing, core decompression, fibular grafting, electrical stimulation (noninvasive or semi-invasive), proximal femoral osteotomy (varus or rotational), and vascularized fibular grafting.

Protective Weightbearing This intervention has been shown to be a relatively poor choice for most patients. However, under some circumstances protective weightbearing may be an appropriate initial treatment choice. It may be the correct choice for the elderly patient who develops osteonecrosis and for whom total hip arthroplasty may represent the best ultimate treatment intervention. It may also be the correct choice for the hip with limited disease as characterized by the newer classification schemas, or for those patients with other areas of compromised health in whom other alternatives are not realistic alternatives. An appropriate protective weightbearing approach would start with nonweightbearing, and follow the patient closely. Progression in weightbearing would be allowed as clinical symptoms and signs demonstrate that the hip is less irritable. Radiographic and clinical follow-up are used at 6-week intervals until pain has subsided and motion has returned to an optimum level. It is likely that such a course

of protective weightbearing would take a minimum of 3 to 6 months to return a patient to full weightbearing status without walking aids. Success for stage I and stage II hips has been reported to range from less than 5% to 20% at 3- to 5-year follow-up.

Core Decompression This procedure often is used in concert with the functional exploration of bone. The goal of this procedure is to demonstrate intraosseous venous hypertension and remove a central core of bone from the lesional area to effectively lower intraosseous pressure. The biopsy obtained can confirm the disease histologically. The procedure is performed under fluoroscopy, and when properly done involves minimal morbidity. Patients remain nonweightbearing for a 6-week period following the procedure to protect the lateral cortical window. There is a real but small risk of fracture if either patients or surgeons deviate from the details of surgery and postoperative care. There has been substantial controversy as to the effectiveness of this procedure. The success rates reported vary from 45% to 95% for stage 1 hips, 30% to 85% for stage 2 hips, and 15% to 60% for stage 3 hips. This procedure appears to be best suited for the stage 1 and early stage 2 hips in which pain relief and preservation of the femoral head are predictable (>70%).

Electrical Stimulation This procedure has been used in several different ways. The use of adaptive coupling in conjunction with core decompression and grafting was not found to be beneficial. The use of PEMFs with external coils in a large multicenter study was successful for stage

1, 2, and 3 hips, irrespective of the etiology of the condition. This approach appears as effective as core decompression for stages 1 and 2, but is more effective for stage 3 hips. This relatively uncomplicated treatment offers great promise, but is awaiting final FDA approval before it can become widely available for use.

Proximal Femoral Osteotomy This procedure directly addresses the mechanical aspects of osteonecrosis of the femoral head, an aspect of the disease that is important but poorly understood. The goal of this type of intervention is preservation of the femoral head by altering the pattern of stress transfer in the diseased head. Varus osteotomy attempts to shift the most involved portion of the head medially, and is likely to work best for those lesions that are less extensive laterally. Success has been reported in 74% of stage 3 hips in one series. The rotational osteotomy is designed to shift the diseased portion of the head medially, inferiorly, and posteriorly. Although it is a structurally more appropriate treatment for this disease, it is technically difficult. Its reported success rates are 100% if the intact area was greater than 60% of the weightbearing surface after transposition, 93% if the transposed area was greater than 36%, 65% if the transposed area was between 21% and 35%, and 29% if the transposed area was less than 20% of the weightbearing surface. This approach can be associated with substantially greater morbidity, and may be best reserved for those hips in which subchondral collapse has occurred.

Fibular Grafting This procedure, either of the Bonfiglio nonvascularized type or using a vascularized grafting technique, may also be used in the treatment of radiographically apparent disease and in the early collapse stage. The former technique has been applied for several decades and

seems to be effective if the graft is placed carefully in the subchondral region. The limitations of this technique may be in its inability to effectively alter the stress-transfer patterns in the upper femoral regions. The addition of a vascularized approach to fibular grafting appears to be evolving. Some investigators advocate an aggressive debridement of the necrotic and reparative zone and augment the vascularized graft with cancellous bone graft; others use a less aggressive debridement and rely on the revascularization aspect of this approach. Although early reports are encouraging, studies to date are not sufficient to support widespread application.

Advanced Stages

In hips in which collapse is severe or there is evidence for advancing arthritic involvement, arthroplasty remains the treatment of choice. Although arthrodesis and hemiarthroplasty are options for treatment in these advanced stages, the former is probably best reserved for the young, posttraumatic necrosis in which the appropriate indications for fusion exist. The high percentage of bilateral involvement favors treatment that relieves pain and provides for a mobile hip. The areas of concern are obviously those related to the fate of devices placed in otherwise healthy individuals with high activity levels or to the use of arthroplasty for patients in whom an underlying disease state may complicate the success of the arthroplasty. Both uncemented and cemented total hip arthroplasty have been used in this population, and the reported success rates are below what appear to be expected from series in other patient populations. To date, these studies are of insufficient size to be able to delineate the important underlying patient issues that may make one choice more appropriate than another.

Annotated Bibliography

General Review

Schoutens A, Arlet J, Gardeniers JW, et al: *Bone Circulation and Vascularization in Normal and Pathological Conditions.* New York, NY, Plenum Press, 1993.

This volume represents a collection of manuscripts summarizing a two-day symposium held in Brussels, Belgium, in late fall of 1992. It provides an understanding of the depth and breadth of current research in bone circulation, whether related to osteonecrosis, fracture healing, or other abnormalities of bone blood flow. It will be of interest to the orthopaedist who has research interests in these areas.

Steinberg ME: Osteonecrosis of the hip. *Semin Arthroplasty* 1991;2:159–249.

This series of invited review articles covers the range of current thought related to osteonecrosis. Taken as a whole, it provides a

suitable background for current research efforts in osteonecrosis and provides a background (well-referenced) for the controversial areas that remain.

Epidemiology

Aaron RK, Galante JO, Rosenberg AG, et al: Osteonecrosis of the femoral head, Part I: Risk factors for progression with treatment by protected weight bearing, core decompression or pulsed electromagnetic fields. *J Bone Joint Surg,* in press.

Patients evaluated by three different therapeutic approaches were studied by analysis of similar clinical, radiographic, and success criteria. While core decompression and pulsed electromagnetic field therapy were found to be statistically more beneficial than protected weightbearing, the authors identified risk factors common to all groups, as well as to each specific treatment. The degree of radiographic involvement at presentation, and the accompaniment of symptoms, were most predictive of the ultimate outcome.

Ono K, Sugioka Y: Epidemiology and risk factors in avascular osteonecrosis of the femoral head, in Schoutens A, Arlet J, Gardeniers JW, et al (eds): *Bone Circulation and Vascularization in Normal and Pathological Conditions.* New York, NY, Plenum Press, 1993, pp 243–248.

This article presents ongoing epidemiologic information from the Investigation Committee for ONFH (osteonecrosis of the femoral head). The large population studies allow the authors to perform extensive statistical analysis to identify key risk factors. Radiographic evidence of bilateral involvement was seen in 31.4% with a greater preponderance in those treated with corticosteroids. Dosage levels above 30 mg/day of prednisolone for at least 30 days were associated with an increased rate of ONFH in the population of those with systemic lupus erythematosus, especially in cases involving the sudden introduction of corticosteroids at dosages above this level. Alcohol-related osteonecrosis was greater if intake was greater than 400 ml/day, and was not influenced by cigarette smoking.

Etiology

Atsumi T, Kuroki Y: Role of impairment of blood supply of the femoral head in the pathogenesis of idiopathic osteonecrosis. *Clin Orthop* 1992;277:22–30.

The authors have applied the technique of superselective microangiography to 16 hips with bone-scan documented osteonecrosis, to 22 normal contralateral hips of patients with unilateral osteonecrosis, and to 22 normal hips in patients on corticosteroids. Radiographic follow-up was used to determine progression to osteonecrosis. Abnormal patterns of revascularization from the superior lateral retinacular arteries were identified, and disruption of revascularization appears to be related to progression of necrotic changes. The authors suggest a possible mechanism by which these altered changes may influence the course of development of osteonecrosis.

Ficat RP: Idiopathic bone necrosis of the femoral head: Early diagnosis and treatment. *J Bone Joint Surg* 1985; 67B:3–9.

In this classic article, the author articulates the rationale for decompression as a treatment modality for early stages of osteonecrosis. He outlines the clinical, radiographic, and histological correlations that demonstrate the marrow effects of ischemia and progressive elevations of extravascular intraosseous hypertension.

Hungerford DS: Core decompression for the treatment of avascular necrosis of the femoral head. *Semin Arthroplasty* 1991;2:182–188.

In discussing the current controversy over the use of decompression in the treatment of osteonecrosis, the author articulates the concepts behind the theory of intracompartmental pressure and its role in the disease process.

Jones JP Jr: Etiology and pathogenesis of osteonecrosis. *Semin Arthroplasty* 1991;2:160–168.

Jones JP Jr: Intravascular coagulation and osteonecrosis. *Clin Orthop* 1992;277:41–53.

In these two articles the author articulates his concept of the development of osteonecrosis. While it is clearly influenced by

the author's longstanding belief in the embolism of fat, his extensive understanding of cellular changes occurring in the femoral head, and his broad grasp of this condition in clinical, basic, and applied research, and even nonorthopaedic arenas, make this a useful and important article for all orthopaedists and researchers. An excellent bibliography should allow the reader to trace the evolution of the understanding of osteonecrosis.

Wang GJ: Improvement of femoral head blood flow in steroid-treated rabbits using lipid-clearing agent, in Brand RA (ed): *The Hip: Proceedings of the Fourteenth Open Scientific Meeting of the Hip Society.* St. Louis, MO, CV Mosby, 1987, pp 87–93.

This series of articles describes use of a rabbit model of osteonecrosis to demonstrate consistent changes of fat cell size (hypertrophy), with resultant pressure elevation within the femoral head and sinusoidal compromise related to engorgement with fat. In the latter article, the author demonstrates reversal of diminished blood flow by blocking these fat cell changes.

Wang GJ, Sweet DE, Reger SI, et al: Fat-cell changes as a mechanism of avascular necrosis of the femoral head in cortisone-treated rabbits. *J Bone Joint Surg* 1977;59A: 729–735.

Pathogenesis

Baker KJ, Brown TD, Brand RA: A finite-element analysis of the effects of intertrochanteric osteotomy on stresses in femoral head osteonecrosis. *Clin Orthop* 1989;249:183–198.

Finite element analysis is used to assess loads experienced in the subchondral bone and femoral neck in the diseased femoral head with osteonecrotic lesions. The effect of surgical intervention has been analyzed using this approach. The varus osteotomy of greater than 30° resulted in diminished stresses, whereas valgus osteotomies and anteversion/retroversion osteotomies were less effective. This approach represents an important additional source of information regarding the structural aspects of osteonecrosis.

Diagnosis
Assessment

Hofmann S, Engel A, Neuhold A, et al: Bone-marrow oedema syndrome and transient osteoporosis of the hip: An MRI-controlled study of treatment by core decompression. *J Bone Joint Surg* 1993;75B:210–216.

A characteristic magnetic resonance imaging (MRI) pattern, in conjunction with nonspecific radiologic density decreases and positive bone scanning, was used to follow nine patients (10 hips). All had core decompression. Histologic evaluation of undecalcified sections confirmed bone marrow edema, with marrow and bone necrosis and repair processes seen. Serial MRI was continued for 24 months. All patients remained symptom free at 33 months. The authors suggest that this condition may be a self-limiting form of early osteonecrosis.

Ohzono K, Saito M, Sugano N, et al: The fate of nontraumatic avascular necrosis of the femoral head: A radiologic classification to formulate prognosis. *Clin Orthop* 1992;277:73–78.

A quantitative schema relating the radiographic involvement of the femoral head to the acetabular dome on the anteroposterior view was used to assess the progress of 115 hips in 87 patients. Six distinct types of radiographic findings were noted.

Owen RS, Dalinka MK: Imaging modalities for early diagnosis of osteonecrosis of the hip. *Semin Arthroplasty* 1991;2:169–174.

This is a review of recent advances in radiologic assessment and their ability to identify early changes in the femoral head consistent with osteonecrosis. It serves as a review of current controversies from the radiologists' perspective.

Robinson HJ Jr, Hartleben PD, Lund G, et al: Evaluation of magnetic resonance imaging in the diagnosis of osteonecrosis of the femoral head: Accuracy compared with radiographs, core biopsy, and intraosseous pressure measurements. *J Bone Joint Surg* 1989;71A:650–663.

Using magnetic resonance imaging (MRI) in conjunction with other available means of diagnosis, the authors determined the accuracy of MRI in the assessment of early osteonecrosis in the pre-radiographic stages.

Stulberg BN, Levine M, Bauer TW, et al: Multimodality approach to osteonecrosis of the femoral head. *Clin Orthop* 1989;240:181–193.

Eighty patients underwent radiographic assessment using multiple modalities, including plain radiographs, tomography, magnetic resonance imaging (MRI) (T1-weighted images only), bone scanning with single photon emission computed tomography (SPECT), the functional exploration of bone, and core biopsy. Results indicated that no single study was 100% sensitive and specific for osteonecrosis. Results suggested MRI was most appropriate for the uninvolved side of a symptomatic hip, and SPECT imaging increased the sensitivity and specificity of technetium bone scanning.

Takatori Y, Kokubo T, Ninomiya S, et al : Avascular necrosis of the femoral head: Natural history and magnetic resonance imaging. *J Bone Joint Surg* 1993;75B: 217–221.

Twenty-five patients (32 hips) considered at high risk for osteonecrosis from corticosteroid or alcohol usage were studied using magnetic resonance imaging (MRI). All had radiographically normal hips at the time of MRI. Patients were not treated. Four patterns of involvement were noted, from minimal to greater than half of the femoral head. Results showed differing behavior between minimal involvement and greater involvement. Incidence of collapse was 0/15 and 14/17, respectively. Time interval to collapse averaged 15 months (range 2 to 43).

Staging Systems

Gardeniers JMW: The ARCO perspective for reaching one uniform staging system of osteonecrosis, in Schoutens A, Arlet J, Gardeniers JW, et al (eds): *Bone Circulation and Vascularization in Normal and Pathological Conditions.* New York, NY, Plenum Press, 1993, pp 375–380.

The five-stage system that is being proposed as an international system for staging and reporting osteonecrosis of the femoral head is proposed in this chapter. It is presently being used by many investigators and is enumerated in the text.

Steinberg ME, Steinberg DR : Evaluation and staging of avascular necrosis. *Semin Arthroplasty* 1991;2:175–181.

The authors' six-stage system for osteonecrosis is articulated in this article. It includes careful quantitative measures that have become a part of the ARCO staging system.

Treatment Modalities: Early Stages

Aaron RK, Steinberg ME: Electrical stimulation of osteonecrosis of the femoral head. *Semin Arthroplasty* 1991;2:214–221.

The authors discuss the rationale of the use of inductive coupling and pulsed electromagnetic fields (PEMFs) as either a primary or adjunctive treatment for osteonecrosis. Results suggest that PEMF treatment does stabilize the hip with stage 1, stage 2, and early stage 3 osteonecrosis and is as good as, if not better than, other minimally invasive approaches. They correctly note the limitations of understanding as to why it works and the most appropriate signals for use.

Nelson LM, Clark CR: Efficacy of Phemister bone grafting in nontraumatic aseptic necrosis of the femoral head. *J Arthroplasty* 1993;8:253–258.

Fifty-two Phemister bone grafting procedures in 40 patients were followed a minimum of 2 years. Twenty-three percent had undergone total hip arthroplasty or femoral head replacement at the time of follow-up. Progression radiographically was seen in 76% of (Marcus/Enneking) stage 2 and 64% of stage 3 hips. Progression was 88% for stage 2, 82% for stage 3, and 95% of stage 4 hips. The authors confirm that this procedure is of limited usefulness once collapse has occurred.

Scher MA, Jakim I: Intertrochanteric osteotomy and autogenous bone-grafting for avascular necrosis of the femoral head. *J Bone Joint Surg* 1993;75A:1119–1133.

Forty-five hips with Ficat stage 3 osteonecrosis were followed an average 65 months following flexion-valgus osteotomy. Survivorship was 87% based on Harris hip score less than 70 or subsequent need for total hip arthroplasty. Significant exclusions included patients over 45 years of age, those receiving corticosteroids, those with large lesions, and those with continuing systemic illness.

Stulberg BN, Bauer TW, Belhobek GH: Making core decompression work. *Clin Orthop* 1990;261:186–195.

The diagnostic, technical, and clinical aspects of applying this modality are outlined. The authors stress the importance of accurate diagnosis as to the location and extent of the lesion, discuss important aspects of the technique, and suggest that the literature supports the use of this procedure in early disease if these steps are followed.

Stulberg BN, Davis AW, Bauer TW, et al: Osteonecrosis of the femoral head: A prospective randomized treatment protocol. *Clin Orthop* 1991;268:140–151.

Fifty-five hips in 36 patients were randomized to either a program of protected weightbearing or core decompression. Criteria for entry, staging, and results reporting were standardized. Statistically better results were obtained with decompression for stage 2 hips, significance was approached for stage 1 hips, and results were better for stage 3 hips. Average success for decompression was near 70% for all three stages randomized. While small, the early significant differences led the authors to discontinue the study.

Sugioka Y, Hotokebuchi T, Tsutsui H: Transtrochanteric anterior rotational osteotomy for idiopathic and steroid-induced necrosis of the femoral head: Indications and long-term results. *Clin Orthop* 1992;277:111–120.

Between 1972 and 1988, 474 hips in 378 patients were treated. Results of anterior rotational osteotomy were excellent in 295 hips (78%) with a follow-up period of at least 3 years. The outcome was directly related to the amount of transposed articular surface under the acetabular dome.

Yoo MC, Chung DW, Hahn CS: Free vascularized fibula grafting for the treatment of osteonecrosis of the femoral head. *Clin Orthop* 1992;277:128–138.

Eighty-one hips followed an average 62 months underwent vascularized fibular grafting. There were 91% good/excellent results with 71% showing radiographic improvement and 11% showing radiographic progression. Fifty-nine hips were stage 2 (Ficat) and 22 were stage 3 disease prior to intervention.

Treatment Modalities: Advanced Stages

Alpert B, Waddell JP, Morton J, et al: Cementless total hip arthroplasty in renal transplant patients. *Clin Orthop* 1992;284:164–169.

Twenty-seven total hip arthroplasties (THAs) in 17 corticosteroid-dependent transplant patients were followed-up an average of 4 years. All patients had good and excellent results at this follow-up interval despite chronic steroid administration. Uncemented THA is suggested to be a reasonable option for this patient population.

Cornell CN, Salvati EA, Pellicci PM: Long-term follow-up of total hip replacement in patients with osteonecrosis. *Orthop Clin North Am* 1985;16:757–769.

Twenty-eight cemented total hip arthroplasties in 24 patients were followed an average of 8 years. A 39% failure rate included five due to acetabular loosening, one femoral loosening, three femoral stem fractures, and two deep infections. This represented first generation cementing techniques. Factors associated with a greater rate of failure included male sex, young age, increased weight, and alcoholic and corticosteroid causes of osteonecrosis.

Piston RW, Engh CA, De Carvalho PI, et al: Osteonecrosis of the femoral head treated with total hip arthroplasty without cement. *J Bone Joint Surg* 1994;76A:202–214.

Thirty-five hips in 30 patients underwent uncemented total hip arthroplasty using the AML (DePuy, Warsaw, IN) prosthesis for stages 3 and 4 osteonecrosis. Average follow-up was 7.5 years with the average age being 32 years (range 21 to 40). Osseointegration was seen in 94% of the femoral stems. Revision rate was 3% on the femoral side and 6% on the acetabular side. Stress shielding was prominent (17% of patients) as was osteolysis (17%). Because of concern about osteolytic reaction (presumably related to acetabular wear), the authors recommend this procedure with caution.

12

Trauma: Hip

Introduction

Hip fractures represent a common problem encountered by the vast majority of orthopaedic surgeons. Epidemiological data indicate that the number of hip fractures that occur annually is increasing and is expected to double (to 500,000 per year) by the year 2040. Most occur in elderly patients with preexisting medical comorbidities and functional limitations. Fracture treatment should take into consideration the medical, surgical, and psychological problems frequently encountered in these patients. Successful fracture outcomes (union, alignment) do not necessarily result in successful functional outcomes (ambulation, return to the community, independence in activities in daily living).

General Considerations: Hip Fractures

Risk Factors

Hip fracture becomes more common as people get older; its incidence doubles for each decade beyond 50 years of age. One third of women and one sixth of men 90 years and older will have sustained a hip fracture. Females are more commonly affected by a ratio of two or three to one. The incidence in white females is two to three times higher than that reported for black and Hispanic women. Additional risk factors include urban dwelling, excessive alcohol and caffeine intake, physical inactivity, previous hip fracture, use of psychotropic medication (hypnotics-anxiolytics, tricyclic antidepressants, and antipsychotics), and senile dementia.

Coxarthrosis of the ipsilateral hip is rarely associated with an intracapsular femoral neck fracture, whereas intertrochanteric fractures do occur in the presence of degenerative changes.

Approximately 90% of hip fractures occur as the result of a simple fall. The exceptions are hip fractures in young adults which usually result from the high energy trauma of motor vehicle accidents. The contribution of osteoporosis and osteomalacia to the incidence of hip fracture has been studied extensively. In general, osteoporosis should not be considered the cause of hip fractures in the elderly, but rather a potential contributing factor along with the other risk factors described. The relationship between osteoporosis and hip fracture remains unclear; in two large series, bone density between hip fracture patients and age-matched controls displayed no significant difference. Osteomalacia has not been shown to be a risk factor for hip fractures.

Age-related changes in neuromuscular function may increase the likelihood that a fall will result in a hip fracture. These changes include decreased speed of ambulation (which makes it more likely that the point of impact from a fall will be near the hip) and decreased reaction time (which limits the potential for a protective response).

Mortality

Because the vast majority of hip fractures occur in elderly patients who often have significant medical comorbidities, mortality following hip fracture is significant. The current overall mortality rate in elderly patients 1 year following hip fracture ranges from 14% to 36%. There is general agreement that the increased mortality is seen primarily in the first year after injury. After 1 year, mortality rate returns to that for age- and sex-matched controls. Factors associated with increased mortality include advanced age, significant medical comorbidities, male sex, institutionalized living, and dementia. Disagreement exists as to whether fracture type, delay in surgical treatment, or type of surgical procedure are consistent risk factors for increased mortality.

The influence of nutrition on the mortality and morbidity of hip fracture patients is well documented. Serum albumin level has been found to closely correlate with mortality. In a recent study, the value of lymphocyte counts was reported to be a prognostic indicator of survival following femoral neck fracture.

Treatment Principles

The primary goal of treatment of hip fractures in the elderly is to return the patients to their prefracture level of function. There is general agreement that this can be accomplished best by surgical management followed by early mobilization. Historically, nonsurgical management resulted in an excessive rate of medical morbidity and mortality, as well as malunion and nonunion. Today, nonsurgical management may be appropriate in selected elderly demented patients who were nonambulators prior to the fracture, and who experience minimal discomfort from the injury. In these patients "return to prefracture level of function" can be accomplished without surgery. However, they should be mobilized as quickly as possible to avoid the complications of prolonged recumbency. Overall, nonsurgical management should be utilized cautiously in carefully selected patients.

Elderly hip fracture patients should be stabilized medically prior to surgery. The vast majority of patients can undergo surgery within 24 hours of injury. Longer delays that are necessary for stabilization of medical problems have not been shown to increase morbidity or mortality. Rather, surgical treatment of medically unstable patients significantly increases the risk of mortality. The choice of anesthesia (spinal versus general) has not been shown to significantly affect the incidence of postoperative confusion or mortality in elderly hip fracture patients. The use of broad-spectrum antibiotics has been shown to significantly decrease the incidence of postoperative infection. However, prolonged use (greater than 24 hours) has not been demonstrated to be advantageous.

Postoperative management is directed at early mobilization to avoid the complications of recumbency. The ability to ambulate within 2 weeks following surgery has been shown to correlate with living at home 1 year after surgery. Prevention of decubitus ulcers is extremely important. Decubitus ulcers occur in up to one third of patients, usually within the first week after admission. Patients with decubiti have a significantly longer length of stay and higher mortality rate. Prevention of decubiti by meticulous nursing care remains the best treatment approach.

Thromboembolic Disease

The significant incidence of thromboembolic disease (deep venous thrombosis, pulmonary emboli) in hip fracture patients has resulted in the development of different prophylactic regimens. The use of some of these regimens has been extrapolated from their use in patients undergoing total hip replacement. Aspirin is effective and has the advantages of low cost and easy administration. However, demonstration of its effectiveness has been primarily in men. Warfarin has been shown to be effective, but results in an increased incidence of bleeding problems (hematoma), particularly if the prothrombin time exceeds 1.5 times control. Dextran alone or in combination with dihydroergotamine has also been shown to be effective. However, use of Dextran requires a large fluid administration, which increases the risk of fluid overload in these elderly patients, especially in the presence of preexisting cardiopulmonary problems. Low-dose intravenous heparin or heparin in combination with dihydroergotamine has been effective specifically in hip fracture patients; low-dose subcutaneous heparin has not been shown to be effective.

Subcutaneous injection of low-molecular-weight heparin has recently been shown to be effective prophylaxis in patients undergoing total joint and hip fracture surgery. Intermittent external pneumatic compression may also be of value, but the cost of specialized equipment and the need for recumbency limit its usefulness.

Compression ultrasonography has been shown to be a very effective technique for diagnosing venous thrombosis in hip fracture patients. This technique has a reported accuracy of 97%, sensitivity of 100%, and specificity of 97% when compared to venography. It is safe, quickly performed, readily repeated, and carries no inherent risks.

Imaging Studies

The vast majority of hip fractures can be identified on standard radiographs. However, occult hip fractures require additional imaging studies. It may require 2 to 3 days for bone scintigraphy to become positive in the elderly patient with a hip fracture. Magnetic resonance imaging (MRI) has been shown to be as accurate as bone scanning in the assessment of occult fractures of the hip and can be performed within 24 hours of fracture (Fig. 1). However, MRI within 48 hours of injury does not appear to be useful for assessing femoral head viability/vascularity or predicting the development of osteonecrosis or healing complications.

Hip Fractures in Young Adults

This is a small but significant subgroup of hip fracture patients. In young adults, hip fractures are the result of high energy trauma (motor vehicle accidents, falls from heights), which results in multiple injuries in over 50% of cases. It is essential to carefully evaluate these patients for head, neck, chest, abdominal, and other long bone or pelvic injuries. Immediate stabilization of orthopaedic injuries in these frequently multiply injured patients is essential. Specific attention must be given to the treatment of the hip fracture to minimize the possibility of complications.

Functional Recovery

Successful treatment of elderly hip fracture patients is frequently measured by those patients who are able to regain their prefracture level of function. However, this goal of management may be quite difficult to achieve. Among patients who were functionally independent and living at

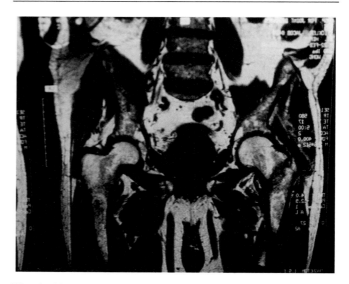

Fig. 1 Magnetic resonance imaging study of a minimally displaced left hip fracture. This fracture was not apparent on plain radiographs.

home before hip fracture, 15% to 40% will require institutionalized care for more than a year after fracture. Only 50% to 60% of patients will regain their prefracture ambulatory status within a year after fracture. Approximately 50% to 83% of patients will regain independent ambulation using assistive devices. The factors associated with regaining prefracture ambulatory status following hip fracture include younger age, male sex, and the absence of preexisting dementia.

To achieve functional independence, the patient must be able to perform certain activities of daily living (ADLs). The functions necessary for community dwelling have been identified and divided into two categories: basic activities of daily living (BADLs) and instrumental activities of daily living (IADLs). BADLs include feeding, bathing, dressing, and toileting, whereas IADLs include food shopping, food preparation, banking, laundry, housework, and use of public transportation. The vast majority of patients will require assistance in performing ADLs. Of those that were independent in ADLs before fracture, only 20% to 35% will regain their prefracture ADL independence. The factors reported to be predictive of recovery of ADLs are younger age, absence of dementia or delirium in nondemented patients, and greater contact with one's social network.

Stress Fractures

Stress fractures of the femoral neck are relatively uncommon injuries that usually occur in military recruits and athletes. These fractures are classified as either tension or compression fractures. Tension fractures are found on the superior aspect of the femoral neck, are potentially unstable, and require surgical stabilization. Compression fractures occur on the inferior aspect of the femoral neck, are more stable than tension fractures, and can be treated nonsurgically; treatment should consist of a short period of rest followed by protected weightbearing. Nonsurgical treatment must include frequent serial radiographs to detect any changes in fracture pattern or displacement. Radiographic evidence of fracture widening or disruption of both cortices is an indication for internal fixation.

Pathologic Fractures

The proximal femur is a common site for metastatic lesions, which result in pathologic fractures or impending fractures. The indications for stabilization of impending fractures include a lesion more than 2.5 cm in diameter or with destruction of 50% or more of the cortex of a long bone. Patients treated prophylactically for impending fractures have less surgical mortality, fewer complications, less stabilization failures, and more successful rehabilitation than those undergoing surgery with pathologic fractures. In addition, stabilization of an impending fracture is easier and spares the patient the pain and disability associated with fracture. Life expectancy has been used as an indication for surgical treatment. Some have recommended at

least a 90-day life expectancy, and others have used 30 days. Although there is no universal agreement, surgical treatment of impending and pathologic fractures is indicated in patients whose quality of life will be enhanced, regardless of the anticipated life expectancy. Surgical management provides for pain relief and allows mobilization of the patient.

Preoperative evaluation and preparation of the patient must be meticulous because these patients are often quite debilitated. Particular attention should be given to serum calcium levels, because hypercalcemia is commonly encountered. Metastatic lesions that are radiosensitive should undergo radiotherapy preoperatively or immediately after stabilization of the fracture. Radiotherapy has not been shown to decrease soft-tissue healing, but does interfere with incorporation of bone graft. Polymethylmethacrylate (PMMA) is an important adjunct for stabilization of these fractures. It is used to fill defects that remain after tumor removal and for fixation of prostheses. Surgical management usually consists of internal fixation using adjunctive PMMA or prosthetic replacement. The choice depends on location and size of the lesion and sensitivity to radiotherapy.

Femoral Neck Fractures

The Garden classification of femoral neck fractures is the one most commonly used in the literature. However, there is difficulty in differentiating the four types of fractures as shown by studies of interobserver reliability. Therefore, it may be more accurate to classify femoral neck fractures as nondisplaced (Garden types I and II) or displaced (Garden types III and IV).

There is general agreement that treatment of nondisplaced femoral neck fractures (Garden types I and II) should consist of internal fixation using multiple lag screws or pins placed in parallel. There has been no consensus as to the optimal number of pins, although most authors report successful treatment using three or four pins or screws for both nondisplaced and displaced fractures. Nonunion and osteonecrosis are uncommon complications following nondisplaced fractures, with nonunion occurring in less than 5% of cases and osteonecrosis in less than 10%.

Treatment of displaced femoral neck fractures remains controversial. Most authors advocate closed/open reduction and internal fixation in younger active patients and primary prosthetic replacement in older, less active patients. There is general agreement that when internal fixation is used, achieving anatomic reduction is probably the most important factor in avoiding healing complications. An acceptable reduction may have up to 15° of valgus angulation and less than 10° of anterior or posterior angulation. Prompt reduction of displaced fractures has been advocated, but has not consistently been shown to decrease the incidence of nonunion or osteonecrosis. Following

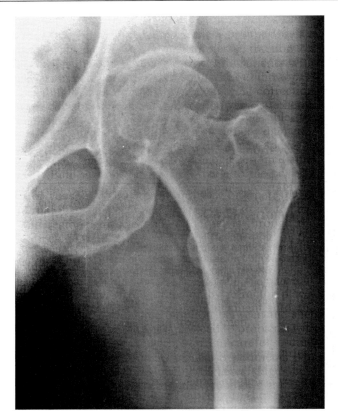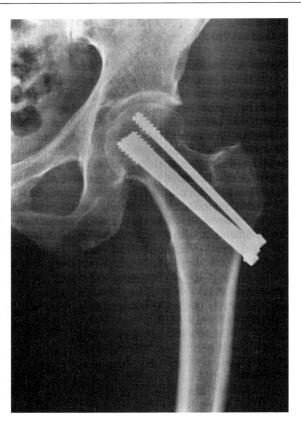

Fig. 2   Displaced femoral neck fracture (**left**) treated with an open reduction and internal fixation using three cannulated cancellous screws (**right**).

closed reduction, good quality anteroposterior (AP) and lateral radiographs are necessary to determine the adequacy of reduction. If a closed reduction is not acceptable, open reduction may be required. Multiple lag screws or pins placed in parallel are most commonly used for internal fixation of displaced fractures (Fig. 2). Previously, sliding screw devices have been utilized, but results were found to be inferior. Nonunion and osteonecrosis continue to be a problem following displaced femoral neck fractures. The incidence of nonunion has ranged from 10% to 30% and for osteonecrosis, 15% to 33%. Adequacy of reduction has consistently been reported as the most important prognostic factor for the development of these complications. Capsular distension and increased intracapsular pressure have been implicated as a possible cause of posttraumatic avascular necrosis. However, the clinical usefulness of immediate joint aspiration following femoral neck fracture is unclear. The need for additional surgery following internal fixation of displaced fractures has been variable. Approximately one third of patients with osteonecrosis will require additional surgery; approximately 75% of patients with nonunion or early fixation failure will require additional surgery.

Hemiarthroplasty is a treatment alternative that has been advocated for older and less active patients who have displaced femoral neck fractures. Progressive acetabular erosion has been found to be a problem in some series of cemented unipolar hemiarthroplasties; the factors that have best correlated with the severity of acetabular erosion were patient activity level and duration of follow-up. The bipolar prosthesis was designed to decrease the incidence of acetabular erosion (Fig. 3). However, controversy remains regarding the indications for its use as well as the amount of motion that occurs at the outer and inner surfaces of the bipolar prosthesis.

The role for prosthesis cementation was evaluated in a prospective randomized study of cemented versus noncemented bipolar hemiarthroplasties in previously ambulatory individuals. The incidence of postoperative complications, the early mortality rate, and the operating time and blood loss were not significantly different. However, there was a significant difference in the incidence of pain at 18 months follow-up: 32% in the cemented group and 80% in the noncemented group.

The results of primary cemented total replacement after femoral neck fracture have been disappointing. At an average follow-up of 56 months, 18 of 37 patients (49%) less than 70 years old who had a primary total hip replacement

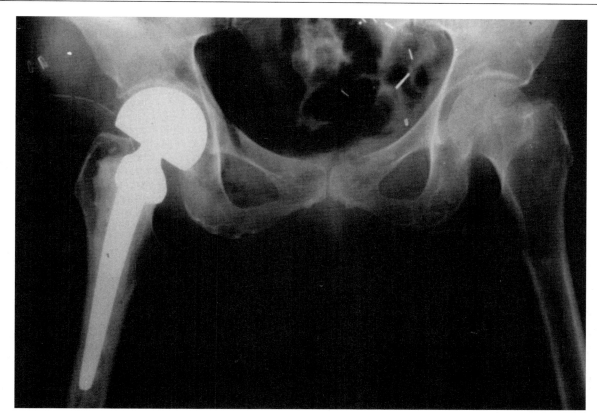

Fig. 3 A cemented bipolar prosthesis.

after fracture had undergone or were waiting revision surgery. A further four (11%) had definitive radiologic signs of loosening. Activity level correlated with early failure. A prospective study comparing range of hip motion following total hip replacement for arthritis and fracture reported significantly greater motion in the fracture group, a possible predisposing factor for early loosening and dislocation. The results of secondary total hip replacement performed after failed internal fixation of a femoral neck fracture are reported to be comparable to those obtained after primary arthroplasty for femoral neck fracture.

Young Adults

In most cases, femoral neck fractures in young adults occur as a result of high energy trauma (motor vehicle accidents, falls from heights). However, in those that occur from a simple fall, a predisposing factor is often present (alcoholism, medication use). When these fractures result from high energy trauma, careful evaluation for other injuries should be performed. Specific consideration should be given to the possibility of ipsilateral femoral neck and shaft fractures.

There is general agreement that femoral neck fractures in young patients represent an orthopaedic emergency that requires prompt evaluation and definitive management.

Nondisplaced fractures should be treated by multiple lag screw or pin fixation. Care should be taken to avoid any loss of reduction during the surgical procedure. Nonunion and osteonecrosis are very uncommon following nondisplaced fractures, except in cases where the fracture was not identified initially. Successful treatment of displaced fractures is related to achieving anatomic reduction and stable internal fixation as soon as possible after the injury. A gentle, closed reduction should be attempted. If the reduction is unacceptable, an open reduction should be performed followed by multiple lag screw or pin fixation. When the principles of prompt anatomic reduction and internal fixation are followed, the incidence of nonunion should be less than 10% and of osteonecrosis 20% to 33%.

Special Problems

Neurologically impaired patients include those with Parkinson's disease, previous stroke, and severe dementia. For patients with Parkinson's disease who sustain a femoral neck fracture, both internal fixation and prosthetic replacement have been recommended. The treatment chosen in these patients should be based on patient age, fracture type, and severity of disease. All of these patients require meticulous medical and nursing care to avoid complications. If prosthetic replacement is chosen, correction of a hip adduction contracture by tenotomy and an anterior surgical approach should be considered. Both measures may decrease the risk of dislocation. Patients with previous strokes are at increased risk for hip fractures, primarily because of residual balance and gait problems and osteoporosis of the paretic limb. Treatment approach depends on fracture type and functional status. When the fracture occurs within 1 week of the stroke, poor functional recovery can be anticipated. If prosthetic replacement is chosen, hip contractures may require tenotomy and an anterior approach may be preferred. Institutionalized patients with severe dementia present a particular challenge. In-hospital mortality has been reported as high as 50%. Nondisplaced fractures should be treated by internal fixation. Displaced fractures that require prosthetic replacement should be performed through an anterior approach to decrease the risk of dislocation and infection from wound contamination in incontinent patients. In nonambulatory patients with severe dementia who do not experience significant discomfort from the injury, nonoperative management with early bed to chair mobilization should be considered.

Femoral neck fractures in patients with rheumatoid arthritis are associated with an increased incidence of complications. In general, nondisplaced fractures can be successfully treated by internal fixation. However, internal fixation of displaced fractures results in a high complication rate. Therefore, prosthetic replacement is recommended. If significant acetabular degeneration is present, total hip arthroplasty is indicated. Femoral neck fractures are very uncommon in patients with underlying osteoarthritis of the hip. When they do occur, total hip arthroplasty is preferred.

Femoral neck fractures (nondisplaced and displaced) in patients with chronic renal disease or hyperparathyroidism are at increased risk for complications of internal fixation because of associated metabolic bone disease. In these patients, cemented primary prosthetic replacement is recommended.

Femoral neck fractures in patients with Paget disease should be evaluated carefully because of the potential for preexisting acetabular degeneration and deformity of the proximal femur. Nondisplaced fractures can be treated by internal fixation. For displaced fractures, prosthetic replacement is preferred. If there were prefracture symptoms of hip pain in the presence of acetabular degeneration, total hip arthroplasty is preferred; if acetabular degeneration is not present, cemented hemiarthroplasty should be performed. Deformity of the proximal femur and the tendency for excessive bleeding are technical difficulties often encountered.

Femoral neck fractures that occur as a result of metastatic disease require prosthetic replacement. With involvement of the entire proximal femur, a calcar or proximal femoral replacement may be necessary. For patients with acetabular involvement, a cemented acetabular component should be used. If acetabular involvement is extensive, portions of the ilium may have to be reconstructed using PMMA, wire mesh, and specialized acetabular com-

ponents. Before performing prosthetic replacement for pathologic fractures of the proximal femur, it is important to identify any metastatic lesions that may be present in the femoral shaft. This will decrease the risk of intraoperative fracture or shaft perforation.

Intertrochanteric Fractures

Intertrochanteric fractures occur with approximately the same frequency as femoral neck fractures in patients with similar demographic characteristics. The most important aspect of fracture classification is determination of stability. Evans, in 1949, introduced a classification system based on fracture pattern and stability of the fracture after reduction. He recognized that stability is provided by the presence of an intact posteromedial cortical buttress (Fig. 4). Comminution of this area or inability to restore a medial buttress allows the fracture to collapse into varus. Unstable fracture patterns also include intertrochanteric fractures with subtrochanteric extension and reverse obliquity fractures.

Surgical treatment of intertrochanteric fractures has undergone an important evolution over the past 40 years. Operative management using rigid nail-plate devices resulted in complication rates of up to 40% for unstable frac-

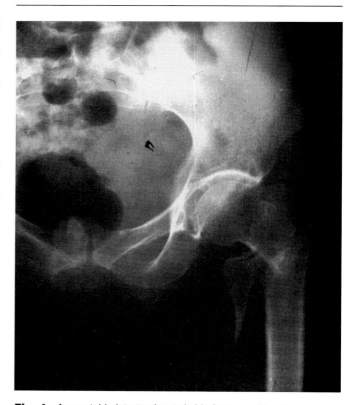

Fig. 4 An unstable intertrochanteric hip fracture with a large posteromedial fragment.

tures. These devices did not allow impaction at the fracture site. Mechanical complications, including nail penetration, nail breakage, and superior "cut-out," resulted as unstable fractures impacted into a more stable position. In the 1960s, in an effort to overcome these mechanical problems, displacement osteotomies were developed to convert unstable fractures to more stable patterns. The Dimon and Hughston medial displacement osteotomy and the Sarmiento valgus osteotomy successfully decreased the rate of mechanical complications when rigid nail-plate devices were used. However, because additional impaction occurred after osteotomy and fixation, mechanical problems persisted with use of rigid nail-plate devices.

In the 1970s, sliding nail and screw devices were developed. These devices provided secure fixation of the proximal (head and neck) fragment to the distal (shaft) fragment, but more importantly, they allowed controlled impaction at the fracture site. Sliding screw devices were preferred over sliding nail devices because the screw provided better fixation in the proximal fragment. These sliding devices are "load-sharing" devices, compared to rigid nail-plates, which are "load-bearing" devices. They permit early mobilization and weightbearing without the high risk of fixation failure associated with rigid nail-plate devices. Also in the 1970s, intramedullary fixation of intertrochanteric fractures became popular. These flexible condylocephalic nails were inserted in a retrograde manner, through an insertion point in the distal aspect of the femur. It was hoped that postoperative morbidity would be decreased by utilizing a less extensive surgical procedure that avoided exposure of the fracture site. In the 1980s, calcar replacement endoprostheses were used to treat selected, comminuted, intertrochanteric fractures.

Sliding Hip Screws

Sliding hip screws are the devices most commonly used for the treatment of both stable and unstable intertrochanteric fractures. They are available in plate angles from 130° to 150° in 5° increments. Theoretically, the 150° plate angle is closer to the resultant forces acting across the hip, thereby facilitating sliding and fracture impaction. In addition, a smaller varus moment arm acts on this implant, theoretically reducing the risk of implant failure. However, clinically, it is difficult to consistently insert a 150° device into the center of the femoral head and neck. In addition, newer implant designs have almost eliminated the problem of implant breakage regardless of the plate angle chosen. The 135° devices are used most commonly; these devices are easier to insert in the desired central position of the femoral head and neck. In addition, the insertion point is in metaphyseal bone, which produces less of a stress riser effect than the diaphyseal insertion point required for 150° devices. Clinical studies have not shown a significant difference in the amount of sliding and impaction for these two plate angles.

Based on available information, the most important aspect of device insertion is secure placement of the screw within the proximal fragment. This requires insertion of the screw to within 1 cm of the subchondral bone. A central position within the femoral head and neck is most commonly recommended (Fig. 5). If a central position is not possible, a posteroinferior position is preferred. Anterosuperior positions should be avoided because the bone is weakest in this area, thereby increasing the likelihood of superior cut-out of the screw.

The necessity of a medial displacement osteotomy with use of the sliding hip screw remains controversial. Because the sliding hip screw allows controlled collapse at the fracture site, unstable fractures anatomically reduced can be expected to impact to a stable pattern, which is often medially displaced. This usually results in less shortening of the extremity than a formal medial displacement osteotomy. No advantage of medial displacement over anatomic reduction was found in recent clinical studies comparing their use for unstable fractures.

Sliding hip screw fixation of intertrochanteric fractures has resulted in a 4% to 12% incidence of loss of fixation. This most commonly occurs with unstable fractures. Most fixation failures can be attributed to technical problems of screw placement and fracture reduction. Although the sliding hip screw allows postoperative impaction at the fracture site, it is essential to obtain an impacted reduction at the time of surgery. This reduction avoids excessive collapse postoperatively that may exceed the sliding capacity of the device. If screw sliding brings the screw threads in contact with the plate barrel, additional impaction will not be possible, and the device becomes the biomechanical equivalent of a rigid nail-plate.

PMMA has been advocated as adjunctive fixation in extremely osteoporotic, unstable fractures treated by a sliding hip screw. However, currently, its routine use with sliding hip screw fixation for nonpathologic fractures is not recommended.

Intramedullary Devices

Intramedullary devices have been used extensively for the treatment of intertrochanteric fractures. The largest experience has been with Ender nails (Smith & Nephews, Richards, Memphis, TN). The results have been variable and, in general, disappointing. The stated advantages of these devices were decreased surgical time and decreased blood loss due to the distal insertion site and lack of necessity to expose the fracture site. The procedure is technically demanding and requires use of the image intensifier. Complication rates have ranged from 16% to 71%, with the most common being varus deformity, knee pain caused by distal migration of the nails, and external rotation deformity. An early subsequent procedure has been required in up to 19% of cases. The highest complication rates were reported when these devices were used for unstable fractures. At present, the indications for Ender nailing of intertrochanteric fractures remain undefined. This technically demanding procedure may be most useful in elderly, debilitated patients with stable fractures who can tolerate only

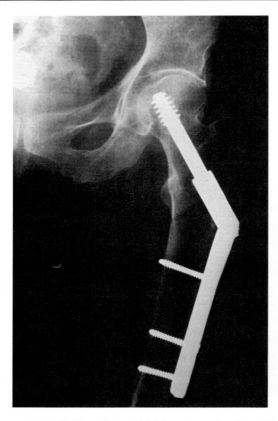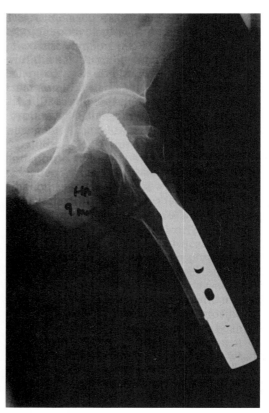

Fig. 5 Anteroposterior (**left**) and lateral (**right**) radiographs of a stable intertrochanteric fracture stabilized with a sliding hip screw. The screw is positioned in the center of the femoral head and neck, within 1 cm of the joint.

minimal surgical intervention or those with skin compromise over the hip that precludes surgery in that area. An adequate number of nails must be used, and they should be driven deeply into the femoral head with prebending into anteversion to prevent postoperative external rotation deformity. They should not be used for unstable intertrochanteric fractures.

The Gamma nail (Howmedica Inc, Rutherford, NJ) is an intramedullary nail/sliding hip screw device that has been used for the treatment of intertrochanteric hip fractures (Fig. 6). Its theoretical advantages are both technical (limited exposure, "closed insertion," reduced operating room time, decreased blood loss) and mechanical (shorter lever arm and bending moment on the device due to its intramedullary design) compared to the sliding hip screw. However, recent studies comparing the Gamma nail and a sliding hip screw found no differences with respect to operating time, blood loss, duration of hospital stay, infection rate or wound complications, implant failure, screw cut-out, or screw sliding. However, the patients treated with the Gamma nail were at risk for femoral shaft fractures at the nail tip or the insertion sites of the distal locking bolts. The Gamma nail may be best used in the treat-

ment of comminuted intertrochanteric fractures with subtrochanteric extension, reverse obliquity fractures, or high subtrochanteric fractures.

A biomechanical evaluation of the Gamma nail in an experimentally created stable and unstable intertrochanteric fracture model was recently reported. The Gamma nail was shown to transmit decreasing load to the calcar with decreasing fracture stability. Virtually no strain on the bone was seen in four-part fractures with the posteromedial fragment removed. Insertion of the distal locking screws did not change the pattern of proximal femoral strain.

Prosthetic Replacement

Prosthetic replacement for intertrochanteric fractures has been used successfully to treat postoperative loss of fixation when repeat open reduction and internal fixation is not possible or desirable. A calcar replacement prosthesis is necessary because of the level of the fracture. Primary prosthetic replacement for comminuted, unstable fractures has also been used successfully in a limited number of patients. The disadvantages include a larger and more extensive surgical procedure and the potential for dislocation.

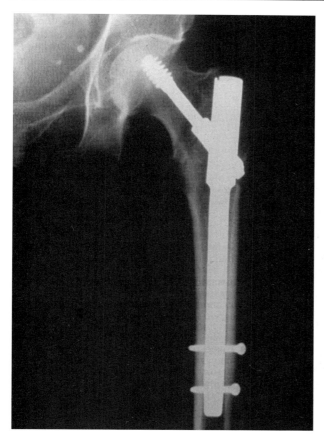

Fig. 6 Stabilization of an intertrochanteric fracture with an intramedullary hip screw.

The indications for its use in the treatment of acute intertrochanteric fractures have not been defined. It does not appear to offer any advantages over a properly inserted sliding hip screw.

Subtrochanteric Fractures

Subtrochanteric fractures account for approximately 15% of all proximal femur fractures. These fractures start at or below the lesser trochanter and involve the proximal femoral shaft. They are generally seen in three groups of patients: (1) young patients with normal bones who are involved in high energy trauma; (2) older patients with weakened bone whose fracture occurs as a result of a minor fall; and (3) older patients with pathologic or impending pathologic fractures from metastatic lesions. The subtrochanteric area experiences some of the highest biomechanical stresses in the body. The medial and posteromedial cortex is a site of high compressive forces, whereas the lateral cortex experiences high tensile stresses. This

stress distribution has important implications in fracture fixation and healing.

Various classification systems have been proposed, but as yet, one has not been universally accepted. The determination of fracture stability is essential in planning treatment. As in intertrochanteric fractures, fracture stability is based on the presence or absence of a posteromedial buttress. In stable fractures, medial and posteromedial cortical support is intact or can be re-established. In unstable fractures, comminution results in loss of medial cortical continuity. These fractures are at highest risk for healing complications and implant failure.

Surgical management of subtrochanteric fractures has involved the use of various implants, including intramedullary devices, sliding hip screws, and screw/plate assemblies (Fig. 7). The use of intramedullary devices has been a significant improvement over previously used rigid nail-plates. Available devices include Ender nails, the Zickel nail (Howmedica Inc, Rutherford, NJ), and interlocking rods. The results of Ender nailing of subtrochanteric fractures continue to be variable. Early repeated surgery rate has ranged from 10% to 32%. The Zickel nail has been used extensively for subtrochanteric fractures. Insertion was initially described as an open procedure with exposure of the fracture site. For unstable fractures, supplemental fixation (cerclage wires) is necessary to restore stability and prevent shortening. When significant medial comminution is present, bone grafting should be performed. Zickel nailing can also be performed using a closed technique, which avoids exposure of the fracture site. Closed Zickel nailing may result in shorter operating time, decreased blood loss, and decreased postoperative morbidity. However, closed insertion is most applicable in impending pathologic fractures and fractures with minimal displacement.

Problems resulting from removal of the Zickel nail have been described. A small but significant number of patients develop a subtrochanteric fracture at the time of nail removal. In each case, refracture occurs at a level different than the original fracture. This complication may require re-evaluation of the use of the Zickel nail in younger patients, in whom eventual nail removal can be expected.

Interlocking nails have become the standard of care for subtrochanteric femur fractures. Essentially all nonpathologic subtrochanteric fractures can be stabilized by interlocking nailing, regardless of the fracture pattern or degree of comminution. Favorable mechanical characteristics of interlocking nails have eliminated the requirement of surgically reconstituting the medial femoral cortex. High rates of union have been reported in large series of subtrochanteric femur fractures with both first and second generation interlocking nails.

Sliding hip screws have also been used, particularly in low energy subtrochanteric fractures in the elderly. A 95% rate of union was reported for one series. For this device to function optimally, the sliding component of the device must cross the fracture site. Therefore, subtrochanteric/in-

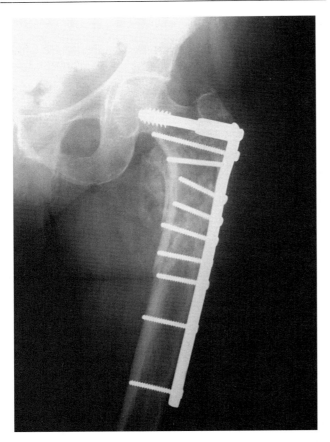

Fig. 7 Subtrochanteric femur fracture stabilized with a 95° screw/plate device and bone graft.

tertrochanteric fractures are most suitable for this device. More distal fractures can be treated by use of a 95° fixed angle device: the condylar blade plate or condylar screw. These devices provide improved fixation of the proximal fragment and act as a lateral tension band if the medial cortex is intact. The condylar screw is technically easier to insert than the blade plate; similar results have been reported for recent series with use of either device for the treatment of subtrochanteric fractures. These 95° devices appear to be most useful when an anatomic reduction is feasible. Complication rates up to 20% have been reported after their use, complications usually are related to the inability to restore the medial femoral cortex. It may be possible to minimize these complication rates by using indirect reduction techniques to minimize soft-tissue stripping. If significant medial cortical comminution or soft-tissue stripping is present, bone grafting should be performed.

Postoperative management depends on the fracture pattern and the method of fixation. For subtrochanteric/intertrochanteric fractures treated with a sliding hip screw that allows impaction at the fracture site, early weightbearing can be started. Stable fractures treated with intramedullary devices can also be treated with early weightbearing. Fractures with medial comminution or segmental comminution must be protected, regardless of the device used, for at least 6 to 8 weeks until early healing is evident.

Pathologic fractures and impending pathologic fractures in the subtrochanteric region have been treated successfully with both Zickel or interlocking nails, both with and without adjunctive PMMA. Insertion by closed technique has been particularly beneficial for the treatment of impending fractures in this patient population. These devices provide the benefits of proximal fixation with an intramedullary rod that can bridge more distal lesions.

Annotated Bibliography

Thromboembolic Disease

Froehlich JA, Dorfman GS, Cronan JJ, et al: Compression ultrasonography for the detection of deep vein thrombosis in patients who have a fracture of the hip: A prospective study. *J Bone Joint Surg* 1989;71A:249–256.

The effectiveness of compression ultrasonography for the detection of femoral and popliteal venous thrombosis was prospectively evaluated. Venography was the standard with which all ultrasonic studies were compared. The incidence of venous thrombosis in 112 hip fractures (detected by venography) was 12.5%. The compression ultrasonic technique had an accuracy of 97%, a sensitivity of 100%, and a specificity of 97%.

Gerhart TN, Yett HS, Robertson LK, et al: Low-molecular-weight heparinoid compared with warfarin for prophylaxis of deep-vein thrombosis in patients who are operated on for fracture of the hip: A prospective, randomized trial. *J Bone Joint Surg* 1991;73A:494–502.

In a randomized, prospective trial, a low-molecular-weight heparinoid was compared with warfarin for efficacy and safety in preventing deep vein thrombosis in 263 surgically treated hip fracture patients. The incidence of deep vein thrombosis was 7% in those patients receiving the low-molecular-weight heparinoid, compared to 21% in those receiving warfarin. Adverse reactions were not significantly different between the two groups. The authors conclude that low-molecular-weight heparinoid is a safe, effective, antithrombotic agent for the prevention of venous thrombosis after hip fracture surgery.

Imaging Studies

Rizzo PF, Gould ES, Lyden JP, et al: Diagnosis of occult fractures about the hip: Magnetic resonance imaging compared with bone-scanning. *J Bone Joint Surg* 1993; 75A:395–401.

Magnetic resonance imaging (MRI) and bone scanning were performed in 62 patients in whom a fracture about the hip was clinically suspected, but not radiographically evident. MRI was performed within 24 hours of hospital admission; bone scanning was performed within 72 hours of hospital admission. MRI was as accurate as bone scanning in the detection of occult hip fractures, took less than 15 minutes to perform, and was well tolerated by the patient.

Functional Recovery

Magaziner J, Simonsick EM, Kashner TM, et al: Predictors of functional recovery one year following hospital discharge for hip fracture: A prospective study. *J Gerontol* 1990;45:M101–M107.

The authors followed 536 geriatric hip fracture patients in order to evaluate the predictors of recovery in walking ability, physical activities of daily living (eating, grooming, dressing, transferring, bathing, and toileting), and instrumental activities of daily living (taking medication, using the telephone, getting to places out of walking distance, shopping, preparing meals, doing housework, and handling money) 1 year following hospital discharge. Most recovery occurred by 6 months; however, a large proportion of patients did not regain prefracture activities of daily living level. Patients who were older, had acute or chronic cognitive deficits or depressive symptomatology, or required a longer hospital stay or readmission exhibited poorer recovery. Greater contact with one's social network after discharge was associated with greater recovery.

Femoral Neck Fractures

Frandsen PA, Andersen E, Madsen F, et al: Garden's classification of femoral neck fractures: An assessment of inter-observer variation. *J Bone Joint Surg* 1988;70B: 588–590.

Radiographs of 100 femoral neck fractures were assessed by eight observers using Garden's classification. The radiographs were classified identically by all eight in only 22 cases. Between the different observers, the number of displaced fractures varied from 63 to 89. The authors conclude that there is a high interobserver variability with use of the Garden's classification for femoral neck fracture.

Franzen H, Nilsson LT, Stromqvist B, et al: Secondary total hip replacement after fractures of the femoral neck. *J Bone Joint Surg* 1990;72B:784–787.

The rate of revision in 84 consecutive total hip replacements performed for failed osteosynthesis of femoral neck fractures was compared to that of primary arthroplasty for osteoarthritis. The age and sex adjusted risk of prosthetic failure was 2.5 times higher after failure of fixation; however, the results of secondary replacement were no worse than those obtained after primary arthroplasty for femoral neck fracture.

Greenough CG, Jones JR: Primary total hip replacement for displaced subcapital fracture of the femur. *J Bone Joint Surg* 1988;70B:639–643.

The authors report a series of 37 patients less than 70 years old with displaced subcapital fractures without preexisting degenerative changes of the acetabulum. At an average follow-up of 56 months, 49% had undergone or were waiting revision surgery. An additional 11% had radiographic signs of loosening.

Phillips TW: Thompson hemiarthroplasty and acetabular erosion. *J Bone Joint Surg* 1989;71A:913–917.

Acetabular erosion was measured in 72 hips treated with a Thompson hemiarthroplasty. Follow-up averaged 7.7 years. Level of activity and duration of follow-up correlated most with erosion, occurring in 34 of 38 hips in active patients and 0 of 34 hips in inactive patients. Severity of erosion increased with time, but only in active patients. The Thompson hemiarthroplasty had consistently good results in inactive patients.

Intertrochanteric Fractures

Bridle SH, Patel AD, Bircher M, et al: Fixation of intertrochanteric fractures of the femur: A randomised prospective comparison of the Gamma nail and the Dynamic Hip Screw. *J Bone Joint Surg* 1991;73B:330–334.

The results of fixation of 100 intertrochanteric hip fractures using the DHS and Gamma nail were compared. Proposed advantages of the Gamma nail—decreased operative time and blood loss, lower infection rate, and lower implant failure rate—were not confirmed. The major finding was a tendency toward femur fracture at the nail tip or distal locking bolts with Gamma nail use.

Desjardins AL, Roy A, Paiement G, et al: Unstable intertrochanteric fracture of the femur: A prospective randomised study comparing anatomical reduction and medial displacement osteotomy. *J Bone Joint Surg* 1993; 75B:445–447.

A prospective randomized study was performed on 127 consecutive patients with unstable intertrochanteric hip fractures, to compare the results of anatomic reduction to medial displacement osteotomy. At an average follow-up of 11 months, no difference was found in walking ability or fixation failure. No significant differences were found in the early mortality or postoperative complication rates; however, operating time and blood loss were significantly higher in the osteotomy group. The authors conclude that with use of the sliding hip screw, medial displacement osteotomy is rarely indicated.

Gehrchen PM, Nielsen JO, Olesen B: Poor reproducibility of Evans' classification of the trochanteric fracture: Assessment of 4 observers in 52 cases. *Acta Orthop Scand* 1993;64:71–72.

The radiographs of 52 consecutive intertrochanteric hip fractures were assessed by four observers, using the Evans' classification. Only 23 of 52 radiographs were classified identically by all four observers. When only assessing stability, the four observers agreed in only 34 of 52 cases.

Meislin RJ, Zuckerman JD, Kummer FJ, et al: A biomechanical analysis of the sliding hip screw: The question of plate angle. *J Orthop Trauma* 1990;4:130–136.

A cadaver-based biomechanical analysis was performed in order to determine the effects of plate angle on plate strain and proximal femoral strain distribution in stable and unstable intertrochanteric fractures. There was no statistical difference in either strain location among plates with 130° to 150° angles. However, there were mechanical complications with the 130° and 150° plates. The 130° plate had a tendency to jam during testing of unstable fractures while the 150° plate had a propensity for cut-out, probably related to superior screw placement. The authors conclude that the 135° or 140° plate is preferable for the fixation of intertrochanteric fractures.

Rosenblum SF, Zuckerman JD, Kummer FJ, et al: A biomechanical evaluation of the Gamma nail. *J Bone Joint Surg* 1992;74B:352–357.

A biomechanical evaluation of the Gamma nail was performed in an experimentally created stable and unstable intertrochanteric fracture model. The Gamma nail was shown to transmit decreasing load to the calcar with decreasing fracture stability. Virtually no strain on the bone was seen in four-part fractures with the posteromedial fragment removed. Insertion of the distal locking screws did not change the pattern of proximal femoral strain.

Subtrochanteric Fractures

Mullaji AB, Thomas TL: Low-energy subtrochanteric fractures in elderly patients: Results of fixation with the sliding screw plate. *J Trauma* 1993;34:56–61.

Thirty-one patients above 70 years old with low energy subtrochanteric hip fractures were internally stabilized using a sliding hip screw. Interfragmentary lag screws were placed whenever possible. Of those patients alive at 6 month follow-up, 91% had successful union. The authors conclude that the sliding hip screw is a reliable implant for low energy subtrochanteric hip fractures in elderly patients.

Wiss DA, Brien WW: Subtrochanteric fractures of the femur: Results of treatment by interlocking nailing. *Clin Orthop* 1992;283:231–236.

The authors report a series of 95 subtrochanteric fractures treated with an interlocking nail. Closed nailing was performed in 94% of cases. The union rate was 95%. The average time to healing was 25 weeks. The authors conclude that closed interlocking nailing is the treatment of choice for subtrochanteric fractures.

13
Hip Reconstruction: Nonarthroplasty

Introduction

Reconstructive hip surgery encompasses several procedures that do not involve prosthetic implantation. This chapter will focus on the current role of arthrodesis, osteotomy, and cup arthroplasty in the spectrum of available options. Despite the many advances in total hip surgery, including the use of superalloys for strength, fibermetal and bead-technology for cementless fixation, vacuum mixing of the cement, and pressurization techniques, the reliability and longevity of total hip replacement in young patients is not significantly greater than it was two decades ago. Osteolysis, chronic dislocation, and subsidence are ever-present concerns. In the final decade of his life, Charnley emphasized the need to avoid total hip replacements in the young. This admonition is just as valid today. Moreover, there is a growing recognition of the role of antecedent factors in premature adult arthritis of the hip. These factors include developmental dysplasia, osteonecrosis, Perthes, slipped capital femoral epiphysis, and trauma. Carefully chosen intervention in well-selected patients has been validated by numerous long-term follow-up studies. Clearly, the vast majority of patients with established arthrosis of the hip are best managed by complete total hip replacement arthroplasty. The purpose of this chapter is not to argue for inappropriate application of osteotomy in such cases, but rather to more carefully define the indications for, and best choice of, alternative procedures, given unique clinical circumstances.

Radiographic Assessment

Most decisions regarding reconstructive surgery of the hip can be made on the basis of high-quality plain radiographs. All patients should have an anteroposterior (AP) view of the pelvis, including both hip joints and upper femoral shafts, as well as AP and lateral radiographs centered over the involved hip. A magnification marker in the plane of the bone on the AP radiograph will allow its future use for computer-based surgical planning, using either surface perimeter digitization or direct optical scanning. In dysplastic hips, the false profile radiograph is extremely useful. This radiograph is taken in the standing position and represents an oblique of the pelvis and true lateral of the upper femur. It allows better visualization of the anterior coverage parameters of the femoral head than any other plain radiographic view. An AP radiograph of the extremity, which has been placed in abduction internal rotation, as well as an AP radiograph in adduction, permit

full characterization of potential coverage enhancements. Where indicated, the AP radiographs can be combined with flexion at the hip joint to replicate the effects of combined coronal plane angulation correction with sagittal plane extension osteotomy.

Three-dimensional (3-D) reconstruction of the hip based on computed tomography (CT) taped data can be used, both for enhanced characterization of qualitative and quantitative coverage deficiencies and as a source of data for generation of actual 3-D plastic models in exceptional cases. These radiographs are not mandatory, however, for satisfactory decision-making in selection of surgical candidates. In fact, there is no way yet to correlate intraoperative correction in three planes with 3-D CT images.

In osteonecrosis, spatial localization of the necrotic sector is important. This localization is enhanced by obtaining two specialized AP radiographs. One radiograph is centered over the hip, with the thigh flexed approximately 40°. This permits visualization of anteriorly-localized necrotic sectors. In the second view, the thigh is in full extension, and the beam of the machine is tilted 30° and angled from superior proximal to inferior distal. This radiograph captures the posterior portion of the femoral head. Magnetic resonance imaging (MRI) of the hips is indicated in osteonecrosis, both for evaluation of the extent of head involvement and for assessment of the contralateral hip, because bilateral involvement in nontraumatic cases is approximately 60%. Because spatial localization is superior with CT, a CT scan is also indicated occasionally to verify subchondral collapse when it is suspected but not convincingly demonstrated on plain radiographs.

Arthrodesis

In unilateral, posttraumatic arthritis of the hip in young patients, arthrodesis is indicated. Prerequisites include normal back and ipsilateral knee status. Placing a prospective candidate in touch with a successful arthrodesis patient is useful in overcoming understandable reluctance to accept the concept of permanent loss of all hip motion. Contrary to commonly-held beliefs, the operation is equally valuable for male and female patients. Patients of both genders report satisfactory sexual function in several long-term follow-up studies of North American patients. Preservation of the abductors for use in later total hip reconstruction conversion surgery is important and can be incorporated into most techniques. The Cobra plate has emerged as the most reliable and widely-used fixation device. It can be used in combination with trochanteric osteotomy to protect and preserve the abductors for later total hip replacement.

Position of the limb is important. Sufficient flexion in the sagittal plane of approximately 20° is necessary to balance the need for adequate flexion to permit modified sitting and the need to stand and walk without a limp. Neutral or slight adduction and neutral or slight external rotation are the other positions of choice.

Other acceptable techniques use compression screw and plate devices, Barr bolts, and multiple lag screws. These devices usually require adjunctive use of a postoperative spica or partial spica cast until consolidation has been achieved.

Several studies have proven the long-term success of arthrodesis. Patients can anticipate doing well for more than 20 years. Occupations that involve manual labor and farming can be undertaken by patients with fused hips. Failure modes over time include degenerative arthrosis of the low back and ipsilateral knee. Disabling low back pain is the best indication for take-down of the arthrodesis and conversion to total hip replacement. Low back pain is often effectively managed by the hip replacement surgery. Degenerative arthritis of the knee does not respond as well to conversion arthroplasty of the hip, and total knee surgery is often necessary as well.

Malposition of an arthrodesis that is functioning well is best treated by corrective osteotomy, rather than by take-down arthroplasty. Arthroplasty after arthrodesis has a significantly higher incidence of complications, including dislocation, limp due to muscle insufficiency, stiffness, and heterotopic ossification. In a young patient with posttraumatic unilateral arthritis of the hip, a good 20-year result is much more likely to emerge after arthrodesis than arthroplasty.

Osteonecrosis

Osteonecrosis (avascular necrosis, ischemic necrosis) is a condition, not a disease of bone, in which impairment of blood supply from various etiologies commonly results in irreversible loss of bone structure and function. As recently as 1962, only 22 cases were reported in the English literature. It is now frequently diagnosed, and is one of the principal diagnostic subgroups in any series of total hip replacement patients. Although there remains no scientifically proven direct causal linkage between steroids and osteonecrosis, the association between patients who have been treated with corticosteroids and the onset of osteonecrosis is compelling. The widespread use of corticosteroids is probably the principal reason for the high number of nontraumatic cases of osteonecrosis seen over the last three decades. Even brief, low-dose exposure is sufficient. The vast majority of patients who receive steroids never develop the condition. A combination of host susceptibility and exposure to the medication needs to exist, it would seem, which is similar to the low statistical risk of

developing aplastic anemia from exposure to chloramphenicol. Other etiologies in adult patients include trauma, specifically femoral neck fractures and hip dislocations; alcohol ingestion; coagulopathy (eg, sickle cell anemia, etc.); ionizing radiation; and dysbarism. The condition frequently affects patients in the prime of life and is bilateral in greater than 60% of cases. It may involve other major joints, such as the shoulder and knee, although much less frequently. Both the pathogenesis and natural history are not fully understood. Not all cases result in irreversible arthrosis. Spontaneous reversal does occur in a small number of cases. Very little is known about carefully studied prospective groups of untreated patients. In general, however, conservative treatment is not effective in approximately 85% to 90% of cases and progression to disabling arthritis over time is to be expected.

Staging

Historically, the four-stage classification of Ficat and Arlet has been the most widely used. The Steinberg classification in six stages incorporates MRI results and the size of involvement, and it is emerging as the most comprehensive classification system for the 1990s.

Treatment

There is no truly effective treatment of osteonecrosis, whether medical or surgical. Even total hip replacement has a higher failure rate among osteonecrotic patients. Various heroic surgical procedures have been attempted and continue to be attempted, with mixed results at best. A careful review of the world's literature does reveal one common and compelling theme. The size of the necrotic sector appears to be the single most important variable in predicting efficacy of nonarthroplastic treatment. When the size of the lesion is less than 50% of the femoral head, reasonable success with various alternative procedures has been documented. These include core decompression, osteotomy, osteocartilaginous allograft, and pulsed electromagnetic stimulation, among others. Alternatively, when the size of the lesion is greater than 50%, virtually all the above have a dismal success rate. It is not worth pursuing aggressive, expensive surgery, such as osteotomy or microvascular bone grafting, unless reasonable probability for success exists. In general, total hip replacement is indicated once disability factors warrant surgery in cases in which the size of involvement represents greater than 50% of the femoral head.

Unfortunately, very few studies cross-reference outcomes with size of lesion. This makes review of the literature frustrating and difficult. Recently, microvascular fibular autograft transplantation has been pursued in several European and North American centers. There has been no report to date stratifying the results versus the size of the lesion. Until such data exist, it will be impossible to justly compare this extremely aggressive approach, which involves donor site morbidity and considerable expense, with much less costly alternatives, such as core decompression, external pulsed electrostimulation, or biplane intertrochanteric osteotomy.

MRI has added greatly to the ability to make an early diagnosis, and it is particularly useful in screening the opposite hip. Because of the greater than 60% incidence of bilaterality, the opposite hip should be screened routinely in all cases. The size of the lesion can be quantified by plain radiographs for established lesions and MRI for earlier lesions. The 50% Rule outlined above refers to measurements on plain radiographs and correlates with published data on outcomes. Size parameters using MRI techniques are not yet available to guide decisions concerning nonarthroplastic versus arthroplastic treatments.

Core decompression is effective in relief of pain in early stages of osteonecrosis. This welcome side effect of a biopsy procedure was first recognized by Ficat during the course of his histologic research on osteonecrosis. He subsequently adapted it as a therapeutic method. Forage, or drilling of bone to relieve pain, was practiced for years before the advent of arthroplasty surgery for the relief of pain in degenerative arthrosis of the hip. The efficacy of core decompression in reversing the pathogenesis of osteonecrosis is more controversial. In general, good results correlate with smaller lesions in earlier stages. Good results are uncommon in stage III and beyond. There have been no convincing data to demonstrate added benefit of adjunctive, autogenous, or allograft bone grafting at the time of core drilling.

Osteotomy is useful in a small subset of patients, in whom involvement is focal and small (less then 50% of the femoral head). This size criterion is equally applicable to rotational and angulation osteotomies. Many types of intertrochanteric osteotomies have been espoused without the emergence of any clearly superior approach. In general, for superolateral lesions with collapse of the femoral head at the lateral aspect of the femoral head, valgus or flexion valgus is indicated. Alternatively, when the superolateral segment of the femoral head is involved and the lesion is more central, varus or flexion varus is preferable. When considering osteotomy, the surgeon should anticipate the need for eventual total hip stem insertion and avoid excessive lengthening or shortening of the limb.

Dysplasia

Whenever possible, rotational osteotomy of the acetabulum should be performed. As a general rule, these major procedures should be reserved for cases in which the CE-angle is less than 10°. When concomitant valgus of the femoral neck shaft angle is greater than 145°, adjunctive varus or varus extension should also be considered. There are no data that compare prospectively controlled adult patients with and without surgical treatment for dysplasia. The decision to recommend major osteotomy surgery for an adult who is just beginning to have symptoms is a difficult one. It is now known that a vast majority of patients who have surgically significant arthritis of the hip in the sixth decade of life also have radiographic evidence of

an antecedent developmental hip condition. It is not known, as a matter of scientific fact, whether aggressive surgery earlier in life would have eliminated the need for the total hip replacement. There are good long-term data, however, for the surgically treated patients without control groups.

For rotational pelvic osteotomies, a congruent mobile hip with minimal or no degenerative changes is preferable. Decisions can be made with plain radiographs, as noted above. The most important x-rays are the false profile and the AP in abduction and internal rotation. In cases of mild subluxation in addition to the dysplasia, centering of the femoral head into the socket on the abducted and internal rotation view is an important selection criteria. Until the advent of the false profile view, the magnitude of coverage deficiency anteriorly was not appreciated, except at the time of surgery.

Among the pelvic osteotomies, the periacetabular osteotomy developed by Swiss and American surgeons in the early 1980s offers the most advantages. This operation preserves the integrity of the posterior column by using a series of precise and interrelated geometric cuts, which isolate the acetabulum and its surrounding bone from the ilium, ischium, and pubis. Rotational correction in three dimensions and medial displacement are both possible; this advantage sets this operation apart from dome and other rotational osteotomies previously described in the literature. The operation requires careful study and preparation. Serious vascular and nerve injuries can occur and must be avoided. Because of the free mobility of the fragment, overcorrection is as frequent a problem as undercorrection. Furthermore, retroversion or anteversion of the acetabulum can occur and must be carefully avoided by use of intraoperative AP pelvis check radiographs. This operation is technically challenging even in the hands of very experienced hip and osteotomy surgeons.

Recent data indicate that approximately 20% of patients require some form of major subsequent reconstructive procedure within 5 years of the index osteotomy. The results closely parallel the status of the joint at the time of surgery. Those patients with moderate to severe arthrosis at the time of rotational pelvic osteotomy have a much higher failure rate during the follow-up period, as might be expected. Patients with minimal evidence of joint space loss or arthrosis do much better during the first 5-year follow-up interval. The complication rate, the repeated surgery rate, and the technical difficulty need to be weighed against the advantages to the patient of this surgery.

The Chiari osteotomy still has a role in subluxing painful hips that do not satisfy criteria for rotational reconstructive osteotomy. When the femoral head apex is beaked on the AP radiograph, adjunctive valgus intertrochanteric osteotomy is indicated to present a flatter, smoother surface to the bony shelf. Conceptually, the Chiari is a type of shelf arthroplasty. Displacement of the upper fragment anteriorly, as well as laterally, is desirable. Because the true width of the ilium narrows dramatically proximal to the immediate subchondral region of the acetabulum, the bone cut should be as close to the joint capsule as possible. When the femoral head is subluxated proximally, very little bone is actually available for coverage. Degenerative arthritis is common after Chiari osteotomy. Many of the long-term follow-up reports in the literature are based on the use of Chiari in skeletally immature patients for whom rotation reconstructive osteotomies would now be performed instead. Prior Chiari makes the acetabular portion of total hip replacement much more difficult, contrary to common assumption. This is not true of rotational pelvic osteotomies, which actually facilitate conversion to total hip replacement. A common consequence of Chiari osteotomy is abductor weakness and resultant limping. Factors responsible for the limp include the operative stripping of the rectus and gluteal muscles from the lateral iliac wall, lateral translation of the abductor origin, verticalization of the abductor lever arm vector, and shortening of the muscle mass. Minimal surgical dissection and careful repair are important at the time of the original surgery. In an otherwise satisfactory result, trochanteric lateral and distal transfer as a secondary procedure is indicated.

The status of the labrum may influence outcomes of osteotomy surgery more than commonly recognized. In the late 1980s data from a Japanese study demonstrated close correspondence between a detachment of the acetabular labrum and failure of Chiari osteotomy. A preoperative diagnosis of torn or detached labrum can be difficult. MRI has proven disappointing. Arthrogram CT is the best option. Arthroscopy has been used in some centers with good results. When a tear is confirmed or suspected, arthrotomy at the time of osteotomy can be performed for its inspection and resection. There are no data on outcomes after combined osteotomy and labral resection.

Nonunion

Single-plane valgus-producing intertrochanteric osteotomy is indicated for nonunion of a femoral neck fracture. Biomechanical consequences of valgus include reduction of the sheer forces at the nonunion site and enhancement of compressive forces. Exposure and grafting of the nonunion can be accomplished at the same time. This is not necessary, however, and risks embarrassment to femoral head circulation. Is it worth performing an osteotomy if the head is necrotic? If the patient is physiologically young, the answer is yes. Approximately 60% of patients will do well for the initial 5 years, even in the face of proven avascular status of the femoral head prior to osteotomy. In the elderly, prosthetic replacement is indicated. If the ipsilateral leg is short, the inherent lengthening effect of valgus osteotomies can be exploited to make up the difference. When the leg lengths are equal, full wedge resection is advisable to avoid unintended lengthening. Patients dislike lengthening of legs after osteotomies as much as they do after total hip replacement. Careful preoperative planning is required to select the angle and length of the fixation device, the level of cut, the base of wedge, and position of fragments for osteosynthesis. Single-plane valgus osteotomy for biomechanical and biologic enhancement of healing of nonunions of the femoral neck was one of the original indications for which osteotomy surgery was developed in the early portion of the Twentieth century. It remains a valid and useful technique in contemporary hip surgery. This osteotomy, like all femoral osteotomies, should be done in such a way as to not unduly complicate the possible subsequent need for insertion of a total hip stem. Simple attention to preoperation planning details should minimize these difficulties.

Slipped Capital Femoral Epiphysis

There have been major advances over the last decade in the understanding of the pathogenesis of slipped capital femoral epiphysis. The major deformity is in the sagittal plane and is posterior in nature. The posterior displacement of the upper femoral capital epiphysis creates a secondary appearance of varus on the AP projection. Consequently, the surgical approach suited for biomechanical correction is primarily a flexion osteotomy and secondarily a valgus osteotomy. Concomitant with the biplane correction in the coronal and sagittal planes, rotational abnormalities can be easily rectified by positioning the foot and ankle in an anterior orientation at the time of osteotomy. The so-called triplane intertrochanteric osteotomy for slipped capital femoral epiphysis involving flexion, valgus, and derotation is a useful procedure in grade II slips with symptoms of a rotational or painful limp. Once again, it is important to acknowledge that there is no series of prospective randomly controlled matched subgroups treated with and without intertrochanteric osteotomy. It is known, however, that a history of a prior slip is found in a significant number of patients with premature secondary arthritis who require total hip replacement surgery, and that patients who have had a slip in adolescence have a much higher incidence of ultimate degenerative arthrosis than the general population.

Comments Regarding Upper Femoral Osteotomy

The ability to reverse a hip flexion contracture, to correct a rotational imbalance, to lengthen or shorten an extremity, are particular assets of the osteotomy on the femoral side, which cannot be duplicated as well or as easily during pelvic osteotomy. In general, the recovery time from surgery is 4 to 6 months before walking without support is regained. A period of at least this much time is necessary before return to work in moderately demanding occupations. For light duty, return to work is possible within 5 to 6 weeks after surgery with the use of two crutches. Before subjecting a patient to such a significant period of disability, the indication for the operation must be secure, and the patient's understanding of the realistic goals and consequences of the surgery must be clear.

Valgus and Varus Intertrochanteric Osteotomy

Valgus Osteotomy

Valgus osteotomy refers to an osteotomy that repositions the proximal fragment as if the leg were placed in adduction. It depicts the positioning of the distal fragment as if it were abducted at the osteotomy site. Valgus in the frontal plane is frequently combined with extension in the sagittal plane, which is equivalent to extension of the distal fragment on the proximal fragment at the osteotomy site. Indications include dysplasia with mushroom-capped deformity of the femoral head that is associated with at least 15° of passive adduction, comfort in adduction, and improved radiographic appearance in adduction. Other indications include nonunion of the femoral neck, acquired varus deformity, certain cases of osteonecrosis, and hinged abduction impingement as a sequelae of Perthes' disease. Valgus osteotomies inherently lengthen the femur. This can be offset by appropriate wedge resection. It is important to understand that even full wedge resection is often insufficient to prevent unintended lengthening, and additional block resection may be necessary. Planning is essential to avoid this unwanted side effect.

Varus Osteotomy

Varus is equivalent to abduction of the leg at the hip level, or adduction of the distal fragment at the osteotomy level. Indications include coxa valga subluxans or high valgus neck shaft angle in a patient with dysplasia that is associated with round congruent femoral head, at least 15° of passive abduction, comfort in abduction, and improved radiographic appearance in abduction. Other indications include certain cases of osteonecrosis and idiopathic osteoarthritis. Varus inherently shortens. Open-hinged techniques can reduce shortening to an absolute minimum when necessary. Beware of the capacity of severe shortening when full wedges are resected. Varus of greater than 20° is rarely indicated.

Cup Arthroplasty

Few indications remain for interpositional arthroplasty without fixation. Historically, only approximately 10% of the patients were rated as excellent, even in the period of maximum enthusiasm for the procedure. The use of ceramic as an alternative to cobalt chrome has had no impact on the reliability of the surgical result. Cup arthroplasty is a rational alternative to fusion in the unilateral posttraumatic arthritis patient who is willing to trade preservation of motion for incomplete pain relief, permanent mild to moderate limp, and possible lifelong use of a cane. It is contraindicated for osteonecrosis, one condition for which it has theoretical appeal, ie, young, active patients known for high-failure rate after total hip replacement surgery.

Annotated Bibliography

Alternatives to Total Hip Arthroplasty

General

Duncan CP (ed): Symposium on surgical management of hip disease in young adults. *Can J Surg* 1995;38(supp 1): S4–S68.

Contributions from multiple authors cover radiologic evaluation, clinical assessment, and surgical procedures for the management of arthritic conditions in young patients. Subjects include hip arthroscopy, core decompression, pelvic osteotomy, femoral osteotomy, hip arthrodesis, and primary cemented and cementless arthroplasty.

Harris WH: Etiology of osteoarthritis of the hip. *Clin Orthop* 1986;213:20–33.

An excellent review of the relationship between antecedent pediatric hip conditions and ultimate development of adult osteoarthritis. This paper amplifies work previously presented by Harris and Stulberg in 1974 in the Proceedings of the Hip Society.

Arthrodesis

Callaghan JJ, Brand RA, Pedersen DR: Hip arthrodesis: A long-term follow-up. *J Bone Joint Surg* 1985:67A: 1328–1335.

This is a retrospective review of 28 patients with average 35-year follow-up after arthrodesis. Only one patient at the time of final follow-up had disabling back or knee pain. Six patients had undergone conversion to THA for either low back pain or ipsilateral knee pain. All patients with low back pain were successfully managed by total hip conversion, and 50% of patients with knee pain experienced relief. Abduction of the hip at the time of arthrodesis was found to correlate with a greater incidence of ipsilateral knee and back pain.

Liechti R (ed): *Hip Arthrodesis and Associated Problems.* Berlin, Germany, Springer-Verlag, 1978.

This is an excellent review of the technique for use of the Cobra plate and follow-up of an extensive number of patients with good clinical examples. Over 40% of the patients were female. No problems were encountered with hip arthrodesis opposite a total hip. Successful conversion to total hip was associated with protection of abductors during the index arthrodesis.

Sponseller PD, McBeath AA, Perpich M: Hip arthrodesis in young patients: A long-term follow-up study. *J Bone Joint Surg* 1984;66A:853–859.

This reports average 38-year follow-up in 53 patients, 80% of whom were working and satisfied with the result. When asked to do so, 34% of patients could not think of any significant functional limitation. No patient had disabling back pain or radicular symptoms, and none required lumbar surgery. Of the seven conversions to THA, three were done for ipsilateral knee complaints and three for low back pain. These conversions were successful for relief of back pain, but two of the three knee problems required subsequent TKA.

Osteonecrosis

Katz RL, Bourne RB, Rorabeck CH, et al: Total hip arthroplasty in patients with avascular necrosis of the hip: Follow-up observations on cementless and cemented operations. *Clin Orthop* 1992;281:145–151.

This review of 42 total hips, including cemented and cementless techniques, demonstrated a high success rate using modern cement technique and cementless technology in a group of patients with osteonecrosis. The overall postoperative Harris scores at minimum 2-year and average 46-month follow-up were 88 in the cemented group and 84 in the noncemented group. Thigh pain was a problem in 29% of the patients in the cementless group.

Osteotomy

Aronson J: Osteoarthritis of the young adult hip: Etiology and treatment, in Anderson LD (ed): *American Academy of Orthopaedic Surgeons Instructional Course Lectures XXXV.* St. Louis, MO, CV Mosby, 1986, pp 119–128.

A solid review of the relationship between childhood afflictions and later secondary arthritis. Of adult hip arthritis, 65% is attributable to either developmental dysplasia, slipped capital femoral epiphysis, or Legg-Calve-Perthes disease. Angulation osteotomy was shown to be more effective than medial displacement osteotomy at long-term follow-up. Bibliography is excellent.

Aronson J, Schatzker J (eds): *The Intertrochanteric Osteotomy.* Berlin, Springer-Verlag, 1984.

This book contains contributions from many leading osteotomy surgeons. It is an excellent review of natural history, classical planning, biomechanics, case examples, and results.

Benson MK, Evans DC: The pelvic osteotomy of Chiari: An anatomical study of the hazards and misleading radiographic appearances. *J Bone Joint Surg* 1976;58B: 164–168.

The authors provide an anatomic demonstration of 1.5-cm true lateral coverage with proper displacement of the pelvis. The vulnerability of the sciatic nerve and gluteal vessels is demonstrated, as well as the technical error of hinging on the sciatic notch.

Bombelli R (ed): *Structure and Function in Normal and Abnormal Hips: How to Rescue Mechanically Jeopardized Hips,* ed 3. Berlin, Germany, Springer-Verlag, 1993.

This book reviews theoretical mechanics of the hip and

numerous examples of osteotomy technique in dysplastic hips, including varus and valgus osteotomies and combined intertrochanteric Chiari osteotomies.

Ganz R, Klaue K, Vinh TS, et al: A new periacetabular osteotomy for the treatment of hip dysplasias, technique and preliminary results. *Clin Orthop* 1988;232:26–36.

This paper reviews the initial series of 75 periacetabular osteotomies with relatively low complication rate. Included are an extensive description of the surgical technique and clinical examples.

Marti RK, Schuller HM, Raaymakers EL: Intertrochanteric osteotomy for non-union of the femoral neck. *J Bone Joint Surg* 1989;71B:782–787.

This review of 50 patients under the age of 70, with minimum 7-year follow-up showed excellent results with osteotomy, both in patients with known necrosis of the femoral head and with viable femoral heads prior to the osteotomy. Successful results were achieved as long as there was no collapse of the femoral head prior to osteotomy. Only seven patients had required conversion to THA at the time of final follow-up.

Millis MB, Murphy SB, Poss R: Osteotomies about the hip for the prevention and treatment of osteoarthrosis. *J Bone Joint Surg* 1995;77A:626–647.

This is an excellent overall review of the clinical evaluation in patient selection for pelvic and intertrochanteric osteotomies. It has an excellent bibliography.

Morscher E, Feinstein R: Results of intertrochanteric osteotomy in the treatment of osteoarthritis of the hip, in Aronson J, Schatzker J (eds): *The Intertrochanteric Osteotomy.* Berlin, Springer-Verlag, 1984, pp 169–177.

This is a review of the Swiss multicenter study of 2,251 intertrochanteric osteotomies. One third had enduring good results, one third were acceptable, and one third fared poorly. Of the patients, 84% were satisfied with the relief of pain; 71% returned to their previous occupations.

Ninomiya S, Tagawa H: Rotational acetabular osteotomy for the dysplastic hip. *J Bone Joint Surg* 1984;66A:430–436.

A minimum 3-year follow-up of 45 hips in 41 patients demonstrated 35 with no pain and six with mild pain at follow-up. One case of necrosis of the acetabulum with subsequent healing was reported, as were two cases of penetration of the joint by osteotome.

Santore R, Bombelli R: Long-term follow-up of the Bombelli experience with osteotomy for osteoarthritis: Results at 11 years, in Hungerford DS (ed): *The Hip Proceedings of the Eleventh Open Scientific Meeting of the Hip Society.* St. Louis, MO, CV Mosby, 1983, pp 106–128.

Thirty-four of 45 patients (75%) followed for a minimum of 11 years after intertrochanteric osteotomy were rated excellent or good. No patient had required conversion to THA. Operations included 40 valgus osteotomies for advanced arthritis secondary to residual supplication and 10 varus intertrochanteric osteotomies for less advanced arthritic changes in a dysplastic population.

Schreiber A: Long-term results of Chiari pelvic osteotomies, in Weil UH (ed): *Joint Preserving Procedures of the Lower Extremity.* Berlin, Springer-Verlag, 1980, pp 31–37.

Ten- to 19-year follow-up of 51 adult patients showed radiographic evidence of arrest or regression of arthritis in 80%. Valgus intertrochanteric osteotomy was done in nearly 50% of cases and was felt to contribute significantly to the result.

Steel HH: Triple osteotomy of the innominate bone. *J Bone Joint Surg* 1973;55A:343–350.

This is a historically significant initial report of the triple innominate osteotomy. Results were successful in dysplasia and disappointing in myelodysplasia and cerebral palsy. Forty of 52 reported cases were satisfactory, with minimum 2- to 10-year follow-up.

Trousdale RT, Ekkernkamp A, Ganz R, et al: Periacetabular and intertrochanteric osteotomy for the treatment of osteoarthrosis in dysplastic hips. *J Bone Joint Surg* 1995;77A:73–85.

Minimum 5-year results of 42 patients with osteoarthritis at the time of rotational pelvic osteotomy are reported. Osteoarthritis was graded into three levels according to Tönnis.

Thirty-two of 33 patients with grade I (minimal) or grade II (moderate) osteoarthritis had good or excellent results. Eight of the nine patients with grade III osteoarthritis preoperatively fared poorly. Pelvic osteotomy is contradictory in patients with significant osteoarthritis. The complication rate was 33% for heterotopic ossification, 5% for pubic nonunion, 21% for hardware bursitis. Nine of the 42 patients required a subsequent operation within 5 years, either for a THA or adjunctive intertrochanteric osteotomy.

Slipped Capital Femoral Epiphysis

Aronson J, Bombelli R, Benedini A, et al: Slipped capital femoral epiphysis: A functional comparison of in situ pinning and primary osteotomy. *Techniques in Orthopedics* 1989;4:64–73.

This is a review of 39 consecutive triplane intertrochanteric osteotomies performed between 1972 and 1983. There were 24 triplane osteotomies for grade II slips. Complication rate was low, with no cases of chondrolysis, osteonecrosis, pain, or limited abduction.

14

Biomechanics of the Hip

Kinesiology of the Hip Joint

The hip is a enarthrosis or ball and socket joint. By virtue of its shape and surrounding soft-tissue elements, it is structured to permit mobility during function. The maximum total range of motion of the hip joint is approximately 140° of flexion–extension, 75° of abduction–adduction, and 90° of rotation. The maximum ranges may change based on the starting position. In walking, the functional range motion of the hip is markedly less than these potential maximums. In level walking, the flexion and extension range is up to 50° or 60° of motion with minimal abduction–adduction and rotation. In the activities of daily living, the maximal total motion required is the activity of putting on one's socks or shoes, and this activity requires approximately 160° to 170° of total motion, which includes flexion, abduction, and external rotation.

Hip Joint Contact Areas

During the stance phase of gait the entire articular surface of the acetabulum is involved in weightbearing and approximately 70% to 80% of the femoral head is in contact with the acetabulum. The areas of articular cartilage on the inferior and parafoveal regions always remain non-weightbearing. This corresponds to the area of the femoral head covered by the ligamentum teres and the soft tissue of the acetabular fossa. In the swing phase of gait, the dome of the acetabulum is no longer loaded, and only the anterior and posterior aspects of the femoral head maintain contact. Using an instrumented endoprosthesis, contact pressures were found to be as high as 18 MPa in the posterosuperior region of the acetabulum when the patient was rising from a chair. This transition from partial contact during swing phase to maximum contact during load bearing is responsible for the change in femoral head contact areas during gait. The presence of incongruity during weightbearing could create high contact areas; however, this does not occur because of the compliance made possible through deformation of the two layers of articular cartilage and of the underlying subchondral bone, all of which accommodate the transition from incongruence during swing phase to congruence during load bearing. This transition allows the joint to distribute large forces efficiently. However, this change from incongruence to congruence has been shown to create high pressures in the hip, up to 300 lb/in² during gait. These pressure environments appear to be well tolerated in the normal hip joint, but there is some question as to whether these high joint pressures are responsible for transporting debris from the bearing surface to the acetabular and femoral prosthetic interfaces in total hip arthroplasty.

Hip Joint Forces

A general understanding of hip joint forces can be obtained by simplified frontal plane static analysis of forces on the hip for one-legged stance. Two other methods of predicting hip joint forces are to make direct measurements with instrumented implants and to make mathematical predictions using various modeling techniques and gait analysis. These types of studies are important to better understand the function of normal and diseased joints; to design better treatments in terms of implant design, osteotomy considerations, and rehabilitation protocols; to evaluate the effects of treatment; to optimize performance; and to obtain clues to the pathogenesis of hip disease processes.

Using simplified frontal plane static analysis, joint contact forces can be approximated using a simple lever system. Such analyses have been used to predict joint contact forces in single limb stance (Fig. 1) and with the use of a cane in the contralateral hand (Fig. 2). The relative length of the lever arms of muscle and body weight is generally considered to be in the range of two to three to one. Assuming a ratio of 3.0, there is a mechanical advantage of three for the body weight force versus a muscle force. Therefore, the abductor muscle force must operate at a negative mechanical advantage using the lever system approach. To provide a crude estimate of muscle and joint forces, the problem is reduced to a simple lever system and equilibrium on which all forces acting parallel in the anatomic angles are ignored. Thus, the muscle force is simply five-sixths body weight (taking away the weight of the lower extremity below the hip joint) times three. For a person weighing 660 N, five-sixths body weight would be 550 N, and the abductor muscle force would be three times 550 or 1,650 N. This figure represents the vertical component of the muscle force, which is actually about 90% of the total resultant muscle force, because a 30°, 60°, 90° triangle is formed when the direction of the abductor muscle to the trochanter is included. To compute the joint reactive force, it must be realized that a fulcrum force must act upward and be equal to the sum of the two forces acting downward if the system is to remain static and the forces to be balanced. Accordingly, the total load on the fulcrum, ie, the hip joint, would be approximated by 550 plus 1,650

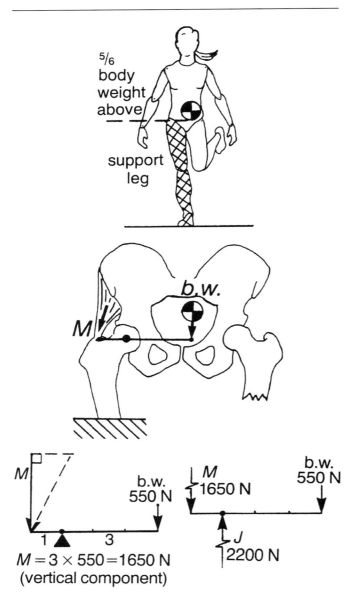

Fig. 1 Determination of joint contact forces during single limb stance using simplified frontal plane static analysis and a simple lever system. (Reproduced with permission from Cochran G: *A Primer of Orthopaedic Biomechanics.* New York, NY, Churchill Livingstone, 1982, p 241.) **Top,** Subject in single limb stance with center of gravity noted. **Center,** Contribution of body weight and abductor muscles on hip joint contact force. **Bottom left,** Simple lever system calculation of abductor muscle force. **Bottom right,** Calculation of hip joint contact force (J) from static analysis.

to the hip in stance phase. If the body weight lever arm with the arm held laterally is 15 cm and the abductor moment arm is 5 cm, the mechanical advantage of the body weight over the abductors would be three because the ratio of the two lever arms is three to one. However, the ratio between the cane lever arm and the abductor lever arm is ten to one. Compared to the abductor muscle force, a given amount of cane force would be ten times as effective in counteracting body weight. The abductors have a negative mechanical advantage of three compared to the body weight, but the cane has a positive mechanical advantage of 3.3, that is, 50/15 over the body weight. In a gait analysis study, use of a cane decreased the joint contact forces by approximately 20% when compared to not using a cane in level walking.

Gait analysis has also been used to predict hip joint contact forces. By tracking exterior landmarks, which are used later to identify the centers of the hip, knee, and ankle, joint contact forces can be calculated by the summation of resultant forces that contribute to the foot floor forces. The resultant intersegmental forces and moments are calculated using Newtonian formulation of the equations of motion with both kinematics (ie, displacement history or motion of the body segments) and kinetics (ie, external reaction or foot floor forces) and body segment inertial property data as input. A diagram of these resultant forces is demonstrated in Figure 3. By adding muscle force optimization techniques in these calculations more realistic predictions can be obtained. Using these methods of predicting forces, hip contact forces of three to six times body weight have been demonstrated in level walking, up to six or eight times body weight in stair climbing, 1.5 to 2.5 times body weight using canes, and three to four times body weight when rising from a chair. Although these predictions generally have been higher than those obtained with instrumented prostheses, the peak loads demonstrated with these techniques simulate those of instrumented prostheses. These gait analysis and modeling techniques have demonstrated the benefit of inferior medial placement of acetabular components to decrease joint contact forces, with medial placement more important than inferior placement. This information can help the surgeon decide whether to use high versus low hip center component positioning. The benefit of lateral trochanteric placement predicted by these models has aided in the development of offset considerations in femoral component design. These models have also provided a better understanding of the effect of osteotomies on joint contact forces.

Important data have been obtained from instrumented prostheses. The most recent device was a triaxial telemeterized total hip replacement prosthesis. The measured joint contact force during double limb stance was one body weight. Ipsilateral single limb stance demonstrated joint contact forces of 2.1 times body weight and the stance phase of gait demonstrated peak forces of 2.6 to 2.8 times body weight. Stair climbing demonstrated forces of 2.6 times body weight. In addition to demonstrating the

or 2,200 N, which is just over three times body weight assuming the three to one lever arm ratio.

The same fulcrum analysis can be used to explain why using a cane in the opposite hand can decrease the joint-contact force to the contralateral hip. To determine the relative lever arms, consider the cane to be 50 cm lateral

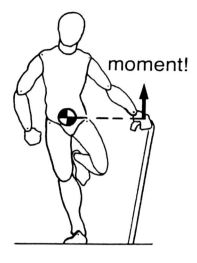

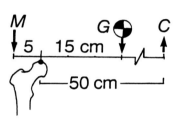

Fig. 2 Determination of the mechanical advantage obtained in reducing hip contact forces by the use of a cane in the contralateral hand. (Reproduced with permission from Cochran G: *A Primer of Orthopaedic Biomechanics*. New York, NY, Churchill Livingstone, 1982, p 247.) **Top,** Subject in single limb stance and cane in contralateral hand. Center of gravity is noted. **Bottom,** Lever arms and forces contributing to hip joint contact force when subject uses a cane in the contralateral hand.

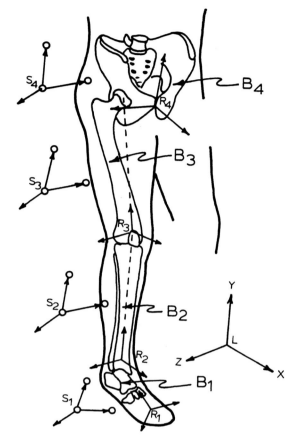

Fig. 3 Forces at B_1 through B_4 can be calculated using Newtonian equations when the force at foot floor contact is known and when external reference coordinate systems (S_1 through S_4) are used to reference internal anatomic landmarks. (Reproduced with permission from Johnston RC, Brand RA, Crowninshield RD: Reconstruction of the hip. *J Bone Joint Surg* 1979;61A:639–652.)

magnitude of force, the telemetric force measurements have demonstrated large out-of-plane forces, which produce torque around the femoral head or femoral prosthesis, with measurements as high as 22 N·m recorded.

Findings from the gait analysis and telemeterized implant studies have aided in the experimental testing of prosthetic devices, allowing researchers to apply more physiologic loads to the implants during testing. The need to obtain initial torsional stability at the time of the prosthesis insertion, and the need to design torsionally stable prostheses, especially with uncemented devices, have come from these observations. In addition, this loading information has provided more realistic boundary conditions for finite element models.

Annotated Bibliography

Blount W: Don't throw away the cane. *J Bone Joint Surg* 1956;38A:695–708.

This classic article using static lever arm analysis demonstrates the benefit of using a cane in the contralateral hand to markedly reduce the joint contact forces to the ipsilateral hip.

Brand RA, Pedersen DR, Davy DT, et al: Comparison of hip force calculations and measurements in the same patient. *J Arthroplasty* 1994;9:45–51.

This study compared the hip contact forces calculated using gait analysis versus those of an instrumented prosthesis. Force predictions from gait analysis were reasonably similar to the output of the instrumented implant.

Burke DW, O'Connor DO, Zalenski EB, et al: Micromotion of cemented and uncemented femoral components. *J Bone Joint Surg* 1991;73B:33–37.

This study demonstrated minimal differences in bone-prosthesis micromotion between cemented and cementless prostheses in quasi physiologic axial loading. However, there was a marked increase in bone prosthesis micromotion for the uncemented device but not for the cemented device in stair climbing where torsional loads were applied.

Davy DT, Kotzar GM, Brown RH, et al: Telemetric force measurements across the hip after total arthroplasty. *J Bone Joint Surg* 1988;70A:45–50.

In this study a triaxial telemetrized total hip replacement prosthesis was inserted in a patient and studied at 30 days after the insertion. Ipsilateral single-limb stance joint contact forces were 2.1 body weight, stance phase gait peak forces were 2.6 to 2.8 body weight, and stair climbing forces were 2.6 times body weight. In addition, in stair climbing high out-of-plane forces were noted with up to 22 Newton meter moments being generated around the femoral prosthesis.

Hodge WA, Carlson KL, Fijan RS, et al: Contact pressures from an instrumented hip endoprosthesis. *J Bone Joint Surg* 1989;71A:1378–1386.

Measurements were obtained from a pressure-measuring Moore type endoprosthesis. Contact pressures as high as 18 MPa were recorded 1 year postoperatively while a patient was rising from a chair. High pressures occurred in the superior and posterior aspects of the acetabulum.

Johnston RC, Brand RA, Crowninshield RD: Reconstruction of the hip, a mathematical approach to determine optimum geometric relationships. *J Bone Joint Surg* 1979;61A:639–652.

This gait analysis study demonstrated that locating the hip center inferior and medially and lateralization of the greater trochanter decreased the joint contact forces in the hip.

15

Hip Assessment and Outcomes

Since World War II, medicine has undergone an era of unprecedented expansion. The volume, intensity, and cost of patient services have increased dramatically. Most countries are now faced with a crisis in terms of controlling medical expenditures. Competition for funding exists among various health-care providers. This competition has prompted the emergence of new methodologies to assess the cost effectiveness of competing medical services. The last 50 years have witnessed the eras of expansion, cost containment (1980s), and assessment and accountability (1990s). Although hip replacement patients and orthopaedic surgeons are well aware of the benefits of total hip arthroplasty, few data exist with regard to the cost effectiveness of total hip replacement, particularly in comparison to other forms of medical intervention. The various forms of assessment will be outlined and these data combined with accurate costing information to provide a method for comparing the cost effectiveness of total hip arthroplasty to other medical and surgical interventions.

Various Forms of Outcome Measures

Disease-Specific Outcome Measures

Orthopaedic surgeons have long recognized the need for outcome measures to assess the results of total hip arthroplasty and other surgical interventions. By and large, most traditional hip outcome measures (eg, Harris, D'Aubigne, Mayo, and Iowa Hip Scores) are disease specific. Assessment of hip pain, function, and range of motion form the bases of these assessment tools. Statistically significant improvement in preoperative to postoperative scores emerge after total hip arthroplasty. Unfortunately, these tests have not proved sensitive enough to distinguish whether one total hip implant is superior to another (ie, cemented versus cementless total hip arthroplasty). Dissatisfied cementless total hip arthroplasty patients with significant thigh pain often had satisfactory hip scores. In addition, some studies have indicated that these scales often do not address some of the most important reasons why a patient has gone to a physician for total hip arthroplasty.

Epidemiologists have pointed out that most disease specific outcome measures have not been validated. The WOMAC (Western Ontario McMaster) hip assessment is an example of one of the newer, validated disease-specific outcome measures. This assessment uses visual analog or Linkert scales to document pain, function, and stiffness

before and after total hip arthroplasty. The use of a visual analog scale enables patients to indicate where they fall in a range from no symptoms to very severe symptoms. At each visit, the patient is shown where he or she marked the scale on the previous visit, allowing an indication as to improvement, deterioration, or no change in the patient's progress with regards to the function being assessed. This form of assessment is much less prone to observer bias than trying to pigeonhole the patient into mild, moderate, or severe disabilities.

Patient-Specific Outcome Measures

Patient-specific outcome measures prioritize the reasons why a patient sought medical intervention. After treatment, the patient is re-assessed and the efficacy of treatment determined for each of the parameters listed. An example of a patient-specific outcome measure would be the MACTAR (McMaster Toronto Arthritis) scale in which the patient is asked to list the primary reasons why he or she is undergoing total hip arthroplasty. The process is aided by a list of prompts indicating some of the commonest reasons that other patients have listed before undergoing total hip arthroplasty. The patient then compiles a prioritized list of the main reasons why he or she is undergoing total hip replacement. Postoperatively, the patient is assessed on a 10-point visual analog scale as to the completeness of each complaint's relief and the quality of outcome. This form of patient-specific outcome measure is individual for each patient and is a valuable assessment tool.

Functional Capacity Outcome Measures

Functional capacity measures assess exercise capacity before and after a medical treatment. The six-minute walk utilizing the same course and prompts has proven useful in assessing hip-replacement patients.

Global Outcome Measures

Health-care providers are interested not only in disease-specific and patient-specific outcome measures, but also in the overall health of a patient following a medical or surgical intervention. In other words, the providers want to know which patients are most disabled and which form of medical treatment is the most efficacious in restoring normal health. Therefore, a number of global outcome measures have emerged (eg, Sickness Impact Profile, Nottingham Scale, SF–36). These global tests provide a measure of the severity of patient morbidity before treatment and the degree of restoration of normal health following medical intervention. These measures also allow a comparison of different disease states and the quality of result following treatment of each of these.

Cost to Quality Adjusted Life Year Outcome Measures

Recently, there has been considerable interest in providing health care in the most cost effective manner. Cost to quality adjusted life years is an example of this form of assessment. To perform this type of study, the patient is first assessed clinically using an assessment tool such as the time trade-off in which the patient is assessed on a scale from 0 to 1, with 0 being virtual death and 1 being normal health. In this way, the patient's clinical status is given a particular number at any point in time. Coupled with this approach is accurate costing data, generated by an independent observer for each medical intervention. The clinical status using time trade-off and the costing data are then combined to give cost to quality adjusted life year data. These data can then be used to compare one form of medical intervention with another.

Effectiveness Versus Efficacy Research

Effectiveness Research

Health-care providers have noted significant variations in operation rates, hospital beds per capita, and the cost for a given medical intervention, to mention a few, without any apparent effect on outcomes (eg, life expectancy, perinatal mortality). Indeed, the issue of quality assurance has been raised, particularly when operation rates seem out of line. Cost also is a major issue. Various Health Management Organizations (HMOs) are very interested in controlling costs while at the same time providing effective health care. Issues such as doctor to patient ratios, the number of hospital beds per capita, and the expenditure for a given medical intervention are extremely important in this type of research.

Medicare in the United States and the various provincial health ministries in Canada act as large HMOs. These organizations have large databases that were developed largely for billing purposes. Recently, these large databases have been used for effectiveness research. The strengths of these studies rest in the large number of patients assessed and the generalizability of the patient groups studied. The weakness of such an approach rests on the fact that these systems were developed for billing rather than research. In addition, the accuracy of data input, particularly in terms of diagnostic codes, is often in question, and because the databases were developed for billing, important disease categories often are missing. For instance, the Medicare database does not differentiate between unicompartmental knee replacement, total knee replacement, or revision total knee replacement. In addition, a right knee replacement is not differentiated from a left knee replacement;

therefore, a patient with two knee replacements in 1 year may have had the right and left sides replaced or may have had to have one operation redone. These shortcomings lead to considerable contamination of data. Nevertheless, the value of large database studies in terms of effectiveness research is well recognized, and large databases will be improved to get around many of these shortcomings.

The Patient Outcome Research Team (PORT) studies funded by the U.S. Health Care Finance Agency represent contemporary effectiveness studies. These studies usually incorporate meta-analysis (evaluation of published evidence), physician preferences, medical-care guidelines, and dissemination of information components. The first six PORT studies incorporated more than 50% of inpatient surgery and included hip fractures, total hip arthroplasty, and low back pain treatments. Total knee replacement was added when seven more common treatment domains were added.

Efficacy Research

To determine the efficacy of one medical intervention as compared to another, a precise, scientific research plan must be used. Randomized clinical trials have emerged as the gold standard for this type of research. The risks of using traditional clinical research methods have been demonstrated. Chalmers and associates assessed 145 publications on the medical treatment of acute myocardial infarcts with death as the end point. In those publications where the newer form of medical treatment was compared to historic controls, it appeared that there was a 58% improvement in patient survival. When nonrandomized clinical trials were used, the physician chose what treatment a specific patient might get. For instance, if the new medical treatment was more expensive, the physician might tend to give this treatment to younger, healthier patients, whereas the old, less expensive treatment was given to elderly, frail individuals. Despite this shortcoming, nonrandomized clinical trials demonstrated that the new medical treatment improved the survival of acute myocardial infarct by only 24%. When randomized clinical trials in which the physician had no control as to which patient group got the new or old treatment therapy were reviewed, it was found that only 9% of patients benefited from the new medical management of acute myocardial infarct. The power of a randomized clinical trial is obvious.

Recently, meta-analysis has become a popular means of reviewing medical literature. In this process, the leading medical publications are reviewed and graded. Randomized clinical trials get the highest grading. Publications are also examined as to whether there is a control group, whether various patient groups are mixed (eg, whether open and closed tibial fractures are mixed), or whether follow-up is appropriate. Meta-analysis is virtually impossible in current surgical literature, owing to serious flaws in research methodology.

WOMAC Pain Score

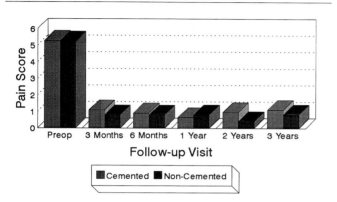

Fig. 1 Comparison of cemented to cementless total hip replacements using the disease-specific Western Ontario McMaster scale for pain. Note the severity of the preoperative pain and the virtual obliteration of this symptom after surgery.

RCT: MACTAR PATIENT SPECIFIC MEASURES

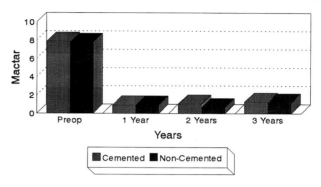

Fig. 2 Comparison of cemented to cementless total hip replacements (THR) using the patient-specific McMaster Toronto Arthritis scale. Before surgery, patients list why they had their THR. After surgery, these patients are questioned to determine whether their complaints were remedied. Note the marked improvement with both cemented and cementless implants.

Example: A Randomized Clinical Trial Comparing Cemented to Cementless Total Hip Replacements in Terms of Health Related Quality of Life and Cost Effectiveness

In the mid 1980s, orthopaedic surgeons were still reeling from the failure of many popular surgical interventions (eg, surface replacement total hip arthroplasty and metal-backed patellar components). When cementless total hip replacements appeared, some seemed to perform better than others. The advantages of cementless fixation were attractive to many orthopaedic surgeons. To truly investigate cementless versus cemented total hip replacement, a peer-reviewed, externally funded, multidisciplinary clinical trial comparing second-generation cementless and cemented total hip arthroplasties was attempted.

This clinical trial required the expertise of an epidemiologist, an assessment tool expert, a statistician, a medical economist, a data entry expert, two clinical investigators, and two orthopaedic surgeons. The protocol was to study 250 osteoarthritic patients between the ages of 18 and 75 years of age. Definite inclusion and exclusion criteria were developed, leaving only Charnley Type A patients in the study. The patient groups were stratified according to surgeon, whether they were over or under 60 years of age, and whether they received a cemented or cementless device. Randomization from a computer-generated list of random numbers was performed within each stratum.

Seventy-nine percent of eligible patients agreed to participate in this study. The patient and clinical investigators remained blinded as to whether a cementless or a ce-

mented total hip replacement was inserted. Each patient was assessed preoperatively and at 3 months, 6 months, 12 months, and yearly thereafter by the same, blinded clinical investigators. Disease-specific (Harris, D'Aubigne, and WOMAC scales), patient-specific (MACTAR), global (Sickness Impact Profile), functional capacity (6-minute walk), utility (Time Trade-off), and economic analyses were performed. Accurate inpatient costing was performed on 100 consecutive patients. Outpatient costing was performed using patient diaries and frequent follow-up. At each follow-up, clinical data were assessed by the clinical investigators. Radiographic data were gathered by the surgeons, without the patient being able to look at his or her radiographs. All data were then entered into a computer database with 10% perpetual repeat entry to minimize any data-entry errors.

This study is ongoing and it is recognized that the most important data will be available at 10 or more years follow-up. The first patient was entered in October 1987 and the last patient in October 1991. To date, no difference has been found in the disease-specific, patient-specific, global, or functional capacity data between the cemented and cementless devices (Figs. 1–4).

Special note was made of the marked disability that preoperative osteoarthritic hip patients have as determined by both the Sickness Impact Profile (global) and Time Trade-off (utility) scales. The levels of disability were similar to those of patients with intractable angina, chronic renal failure, or even malignancy. What is even more striking is the dramatic improvement in both indices. Following total

SIP: GLOBAL PHYSICAL

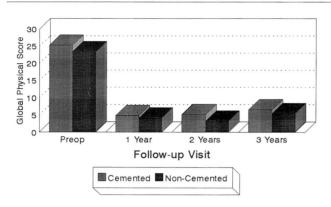

Fig. 3 Comparison of cemented to cementless total hip replacements using the global Sickness Impact Profile. Note the severity of disability before surgery (similar to intractable angina or renal failure requiring hemodialysis) and almost complete restoration of normal health.

COMPARATIVE COST-UTILITY RATIOS

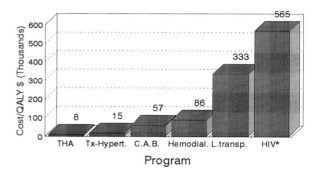

*cost/additional life saved

Fig. 5 Cost to quality adjusted life years (QALY) ratios comparing various surgical and medical interventions. THA = total hip arthroplasty; Tx-Hypert = treatment of moderate hypertension; C.A.B. = coronary artery bypass; Hemodial. = renal hemodialysis; L. Transp = liver transplantation; HIV = universal human immunodeficiency virus precautions.

SIX MINUTE WALK

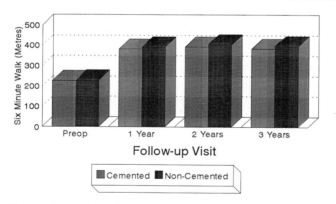

Fig. 4 Comparison of cemented to cementless total hip replacements (THR) using the functional capacity measure, the six-minute walk. Exercise capacity was dramatically enhanced with both forms of THR.

hip replacement, osteoarthritic hip patients are virtually reverted to normal health. This is in contradistinction to the much less dramatic improvement that follows coronary artery bypass or renal dialysis.

Accurate costing data (in contradistinction to hospital charges) has revealed that a cemented or cementless total hip replacement could be performed for approximately

$10,000 in inpatient costs (1988 Canadian dollars). After surgery, first year costs were approximately $1,100 and second and third year costs were $500 each. Unfortunately, outpatient costs borne by the patient, the patient's family, and the health-care system prior to total hip replacement were not collected.

Combining the Time Trade-off utility score and the accurate costing data allowed determination of the cost to quality adjusted life year data. These data can then be compared to data for other medical interventions. Figure 5 demonstrates that total hip replacement is at least as efficacious as most other medical and surgical interventions, if not much more so. A cost to quality adjusted life years ratio of less than $20,000 is considered very cost effective, whereas those between $20,000 and $100,000 are moderately so. Items with a cost to quality adjusted life years ratio of greater than $100,000 are considered not to be cost efficient. Obviously, ratios such as cost to quality adjusted life years raise many ethical and methodologic issues. Some have questioned the accuracy of both the utility and costing data. These figures can obviously be manipulated to one's advantage. In addition, withholding treatment (eg, transplantation) to patients who would otherwise succumb is a real moral issue.

The value of the randomized clinical trial in assessing a surgical intervention is obvious. This study has demonstrated that patients will participate in a randomized clinical trial involving a surgical operation. In addition, there does not appear to be any difference in the clinical results between cemented and cementless total hip replacements, with up to 5 years of follow-up. Finally, it is possible to argue that total hip replacement is as efficacious as any medical or surgical intervention performed today. When such analyses are more broadly applied, health care pro-

viders might be given more concrete information on which to make funding decisions for various health-care interventions available.

Annotated Bibliography

Bellamy N, Buchanan WW, Goldsmith CH, et al: Validation study of WOMAC: A health status instrument for measuring clinically important patient relevant outcomes to antirheumatic drug therapy in patients with osteoarthritis of the hip or knee. *J Rheumatol* 1988;15: 1833–1840.

This study describes a validated, disease-specific scale to assess the results of treatment of osteoarthritic hip and knee patients. Pain, function, and stiffness are analyzed using 10 cm visual analog scales in which the patient can indicate improvement or deterioration in health status by marking higher or lower points on the scale in comparison to previous visits.

Chalmers TC, Celano P, Sacks HS, et al: Bias in treatment assignment in controlled clinical trials. *N Engl J Med* 1983;309:1358–1361.

This important paper demonstrates the power of randomized clinical trials. A group of 145 papers on the treatment of acute myocardial infarction was divided into those in which the randomization process was blinded (57 papers), unblinded (45 papers), or selected by a non-random process (eg, historic controls, 43 papers). Differences in the fatality rates between treatment and control groups ($p < 0.05$) were found in 8.8% of the blinded-randomization studies, 24.4% of the unblinded randomization studies, and 58.1% of the unrandomized studies!

Gartland JJ: Orthopaedic clinical research: Deficiencies in experimental design and determinations of outcome. *J Bone Joint Surg* 1988;70A:1357–1364.

A review of ten published articles on the long-term follow-up of total hip arthroplasty patients. All ten studies were found to be deficient in study design, to be flawed by confusing data, and to contain data of doubtful validity. The emphasis was on the prosthetic device rather than the health of the patients in whom the prosthetic device had been used.

Guyatt G, Sullivan MJ, Thompson PJ, et al: The 6-minute walk: A new measure of exercise capacity in patients with chronic heart failure. *Can Med Assoc J* 1985;132:919–923.

A new functional capacity measure is described that can be used to assess exercise capacity before and after medical treatment.

Keller RB: Outcomes research in orthopaedics. *J Am Acad Orthop Surg* 1993;1:122–129.

This is an excellent review of the outcomes movement. Rapidly increasing health-care costs, marked variations in utilization, and deficiencies of the literature are cited as the stimulus. Outcomes

research includes analyses of large databases, structured literature reviews (meta-analysis), prospective clinical trials, decision analysis, and guideline development.

Laupacis A, Bourne RB, Rorabeck CH, et al: The effect of elective total hip replacement on health-related quality of life. *J Bone Joint Surg* 1993;75A:1619–1626.

The effect of total hip replacement (THR) on health-related quality of life of patients who have osteoarthrosis was examined as part of a randomized clinical trial comparing cemented to cementless implants. Disease-specific, patient-specific, global, functional capacity, and utility measures were assessed. Both forms of THR had a profound effect on patient outcome.

Laupacis A, Feeny D, Detsky AS, et al: Tentative guidelines for using clinical and economic evaluations revised. *Can Med Assoc J* 1993;148:921–924.

This is an excellent review of quality-adjusted life-years (QALY) as a measure of outcomes in economic evaluations of medical care. The shortcomings of utility measures and costing are outlined. Despite these drawbacks, QALYs are supported in medical evaluations.

Laupacis A, Rorabeck CH, Bourne RB, et al: Randomized trials in orthopaedics: Why, how, and when? *J Bone Joint Surg* 1989;71A:535–543.

This manuscript suggests that new procedures or technologies should be rigorously evaluated before being applied to general clinical use. Randomized clinical trials provide the most unbiased assessment of the risks and benefits of these therapies. The key points in conducting a randomized clinical trial are discussed.

Naylor CD, Williams JI, Basinski A, et al: Technology assessment and cost-effectiveness analysis: Misguided guidelines? *Can Med Assoc J* 1993;148:921–924.

In this critique of cost-effectiveness evaluations of medical treatment, the need for refinement of utility and costing methods is urged. Ethical concerns are raised, and the risk of cost-effectiveness data abuse stressed.

Relman AS: Assessment and accountability: The third revolution in medical care. *N Engl J Med* 1988;319: 1220–1222.

The eras of expansion, cost containment, and assessment and accountability since World War II and the reasons for each of these eras are described.

Rorabeck CH, Bourne RB, Laupacis A, et al: A double-blind study of 250 cases comparing cemented with cementless total hip arthroplasty: Cost-effectiveness and its impact on health-related quality of life. *Clin Orthop* 1994;298:156–164.

This randomized clinical trial compared cemented to cementless total hip arthroplasty demonstrating comparable disease-specific, global functional capacity, and cost outcome measures. Total hip arthroplasty was extremely cost effective, comparing favorably to other medical and surgical interventions.

Tugwell P, Bombardier C, Buchanan WW, et al: The MACTAR patient preference disability questionnaire: An individualized functional priority approach for assessing improvement in physical disability in clinical trials in rheumatoid arthritis. *J Rheumatol* 1987;14:446–451.

Patients are asked to list the reasons they sought medical treatment, aided by a number of suggestions before treatment is initiated. Following treatment, the investigator seeks to determine the degree to which each reason for seeking treatment has been resolved.

Wennberg JE: Outcomes research, cost containment and the fear of health care rationing. *N Engl J Med* 1990;323:1202–1204.

This editorial outlines the rationale for research on medical outcomes and the need to develop guidelines for practice. Variations in hospital beds and expenditures per capita without discernible differences in outcome parameters and cost containment issues are used to support this approach.

16

The Design of Cementless Femoral Prostheses

Introduction

Over the past 50 years, efforts to restore normal, pain-free function to the diseased hip joint have resulted in the development of a wide assortment of designs of femoral prostheses. Initially, attempts to anchor prostheses within the femoral canal without the use of acrylic cement failed to provide consistent pain relief because of excessive motion of the femoral stem within the femur. It was this observation that led Charnley and others to experiment with acrylic cement as a means of stabilizing the implant, thereby reducing interface motion and the associated symptomatology. Despite the successes of cemented hip replacement, cementless fixation has reemerged because of aseptic loosening of cemented hips in young, active, and heavy patients.

Mechanical and biologic challenges confront designers of cementless hip prostheses. First and foremost is stabilization of the implant within the femur. This is essential for asymptomatic performance of the joint replacement. While there has been great interest in the potential benefits of bony attachment to the surfaces of cementless prostheses as a means of providing rigid, long-term fixation, formation of stable interfaces is possible only if rigid implant fixation is achieved at surgery. Consequently, the primary focus of the surgeon is to stabilize the implant–bone interface intraoperatively so that normal joint function may be regained rapidly. Once this is achieved, biologic stabilization of the prosthesis will occur through tissue attachment, leading to durable fixation in the long term.

A second requirement of all femoral stem designs is the ability to allow reconstruction of a stable hip joint with a functional range of motion. Because dislocation is one of the principal short-term complications of total hip replacement, attention to the impact of implant design on the biomechanics of the joint can give the surgeon maximum flexibility in providing a stable hip without compromising leg length.

Cementless hip prostheses can also have dramatic biologic effects upon the femur. The key determinant of the longevity of total hip replacement is prevention of osteolysis. The incidence and location of this potentially devastating complication vary dramatically with the design of the implant and the duration of implantation. Nonetheless, the underlying cause in most cases appears to be a biologic response to particulate debris generated by wear of the acetabular liner. While one solution to this problem is the elimination of ultra-high molecular weight polyethylene from the acetabulum, the design of current prostheses can be changed to significantly reduce the exposure of the stem–bone interface to wear particles. The presence of an intramedullary stem within the femur also causes profound changes in the distribution of mechanical stresses within the femur, leading to loss of cortical and cancellous bone. Because the severity of bone loss is determined by the design of the implant and its mode of fixation, measures may be adopted to minimize adverse remodeling.

This chapter will discuss the interrelation of each of these considerations with the design of cementless hip replacement and how, through a critical approach to the design, selection, and implantation of prosthetic implants, the performance and longevity of these prostheses may be optimized.

Factors Affecting the Stability of Cementless Fixation

For a cementless hip replacement to function without pain or limp, almost all relative motion between the implant and the supporting bone must be eliminated; however, every femoral prosthesis undergoes some displacement within the femur when subjected to physiologic loads (Fig. 1). Some of this motion represents settling and is not recovered with unloading the femur; this component of displacement is commonly termed migration or subsidence. Typically, the subsidence of the prosthesis is greatest during the immediate postoperative period and decreases progressively with increasing weightbearing. Once the patient returns to normal function, most of the motion at the interface occurs through elastic deformation between loading and unloading and is referred to as micromotion.

The micromotion and migration of a femoral prosthesis may be described in terms of three components of translation (medial-lateral, anterior-posterior, and superior-inferior) and three components of rotation (varus-valgus, anteroposterior [AP] toggling, and rotation about the femoral axis) (Fig. 2). The magnitude of interfacial micromotion is determined primarily by the geometric distribution of points of contact between the implant and bone, the stiffness of the bone at each contact point, and the coefficient of friction of the stem–bone interface. Rotational micromotion of the prosthesis about the femoral axis appears to be the source of much of the symptomatology of inadequately fixed components. Migration of the prosthesis within the femur is also important and can potentially lead to shortening of the extremity and instability of the joint. In practice, cementless stems undergo relatively little (1 to 3 mm) subsidence within the medullary canal. How-

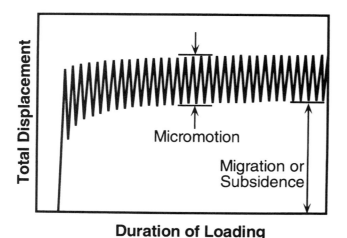

Duration of Loading

Fig. 1 Schematic representation of the relative displacement of the stem–bone interface during repetitive loading. (Reproduced with permission from Noble PC: Biomechanical advances in total hip replacement, in Niwa S, Perren SM, Hattori T (eds): *Biomechanics in Orthopaedics*. Tokyo, Japan, Springer-Verlag, 1992, pp 46–75.)

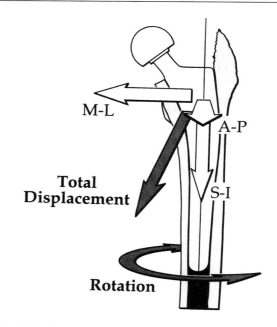

Fig. 2 Typical components of translation and rotation of a cementless prosthesis within the femur. (Reproduced with permission from Noble PC: Biomechanical advances in total hip replacement, in Niwa S, Perren SM, Hattori T (eds): *Biomechanics in Orthopaedics*. Tokyo, Japan, Springer-Verlag, 1992, pp 46–75.)

ever, loosening occurs through progressive rotation about the femoral axis, leading to significant retroversion of the prosthesis.

The presence of motion at the implant–bone interface also determines the biologic response of the host to the prosthesis. At low levels of micromotion (0 to 50 μm), bone will form in contact with the surface of an implant; however, once the displacement of the interface exceeds 50 to 100 μm, fibrous tissue forms in continuity with the prosthesis. Consequently, a critical factor in the development of successful cementless femoral prostheses has been the development of methods of mechanical fixation to minimize micromotion of the bone–stem interface.

In the United States, two different design philosophies have been adopted to maximize the stability of cementless femoral stems. The first has held that the most reliable method of stabilizing the prosthesis is through fixation of the distal stem with the hard cortical bone of the femoral diaphysis. This may be achieved by driving a prosthesis with a porous-coated, cylindrical distal stem into a slightly undersized medullary canal. During this process, the porous coating cuts into the cortical walls, thereby providing resistance to rotational forces developed during weight-bearing. This mode of fixation may be referred to as diaphyseal-locking and can be provided by an assortment of surface features in addition to beaded coatings, including sharp longitudinal flutes and plasma-sprayed coatings of titanium and cobalt-chromium.

The second design philosophy proposes that the prosthesis should be stabilized primarily within the metaphysis. Implants of this design may be termed metaphyseal-locking. In this case, initial fixation is provided by the fit of

the prosthesis to the endosteal cavity. Unlike diaphyseal-locking prostheses, implant stability depends on the geometry of the prosthesis with respect to the proximal femur, rather than on the presence of surface features (eg, a porous coating) that cut into the endosteal surface. Over the past 10 years, numerous prostheses have been developed in keeping with the metaphyseal loading concept. Some designs are asymmetric in the sagittal plane in order to allow contact with the anterior and posterior cortices of the proximal femur. Others are symmetric in the lateral view to increase the ease of implantation and to avoid the need for separate prostheses to fit right and left femora. Metaphyseal locking prostheses are relatively bulky in order to maximize contact with the medial, anterior, and posterior cortices of the proximal femur, thereby increasing resistance to rotational and anterior-posterior micromotion.

The Fit of Cementless Implants to the Femur

One of the most important factors controlling stem–bone micromotion is the fit of the implant to the femur. Though simple in concept, the term fit is used in several ways to describe the geometric relationship between a prosthesis and the femur. Primarily, a prosthesis that fits the femur is one that achieves contact with points on opposite cortices within the femoral canal, as projected on the AP and lateral radiographs. Thus, in the AP view, a correctly-fitting implant would have at least one point of cortical contact medially and another laterally; in the lateral view, contact would be present at some point anteriorly and posteriorly. The quality of fit may be expressed by the total area of contact between the prosthesis and the endosteal surface. Within the metaphysis, no prosthesis fills the femur in the sense that there is line-to-line contact with cortical bone. In cross section, discrete areas of cortical contact are present, but most of the implant is separated from the cortex by a layer of cancellous bone of at least same thickness. In many cases, gaps are present between the implant and the cancellous surface as a result of errors in machining and implantation. The presence of these gaps prevents transfer of forces between the prosthesis and the bone and can dramatically affect the rigidity of fixation. Thus, two different measures of the fit of the implant have functional significance: (1) the presence of cortical contact, especially with the medial cortex proximally, and (2) the area of contact of the prosthesis with the cancellous bone lining the implantation cavity.

Data from laboratory studies have shown that contemporary prostheses do not attain a line-to-line, "hand-in-glove" fit with the femur. In fact, approximately 70% of the surface of the implant is separated from bone by gaps larger than 1 mm (Fig. 3). In diaphyseal-locking implants, direct cortical contact occurs over 10 to 30 mm of the medial and lateral surfaces of the distal stem, depending on the degree to which the canal is enlarged by intramedullary reaming. Contact between the distal stem and the anterior and posterior cortices is more variable due to the elliptical shape of the isthmus; the medullary canal of the average femur is 4 mm wider in the sagittal plane than the coronal plane. Proximally, the patterns of contact of diaphyseal-locking implants are less predictable because the alignment of the implant is dictated by the distal femur. Generally, the implant will come into contact with the femur medially, often around the level of the lesser trochanter. Medially and laterally the proximal stem is more often in contact with cancellous than cortical bone, although gaps are present between much of the stem and the implantation site, especially anteriorly and posteriorly, and may extend distally all the way to the tip of the prosthesis.

Metaphyseal-locking prostheses present a somewhat similar picture. However, cortical contact is normally observed at three key areas: proximally, along the medial aspect of the stem extending both anteriorly and posteriorly; laterally, in the mid-stem region, close to the level of the metaphyseal-diaphyseal junction; and distally, in isolated areas, most frequently over the medial aspect of the tip of the prosthesis. Due to the anterior-posterior taper of the implant, cancellous contact often occurs over a larger area of the proximal stem of metaphyseal- than diaphyseal-loading designs, although gaps are still common, especially at the level of the femoral neck osteotomy. Given that much of the surface of most cementless prostheses is not in contact with bone, it is not surprising that many prostheses retrieved at autopsy show relatively few areas of direct bony attachment.

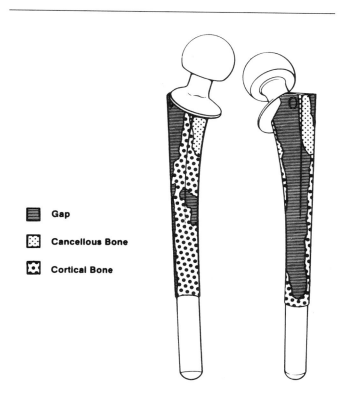

Gap

Cancellous Bone

Cortical Bone

Fig. 3 Schematic representation of the distribution of bony contact between a symmetric prosthesis and the femur. (Reproduced with permission from Noble PC: Biomechanical advances in total hip replacement, in Niwa S, Perren SM, Hattori T (eds): *Biomechanics in Orthopaedics.* Tokyo, Japan, Springer-Verlag, 1992, pp 46–75.)

Several key variables determine the fit of a cementless prosthesis within the femur. These variables include the design of the implant and the extent to which it reproduces femoral anatomy, the shape of the implantation site formed at surgery, and the relationship between the shape of the prosthesis and the corresponding bone-shaping instrument. For stable fixation, it is essential that the prosthesis implanted at surgery match the basic endosteal dimensions of the femur, either proximally or distally. Undersized implants generally do not gain adequate cortical contact and must therefore be supported by cancellous bone, which cannot sustain the loads of weightbearing without excessive micromotion of the implant–bone interface. In the past, this led to the conclusion that an essential feature of metaphyseal-loading implants is their ability to fill the endosteal contours of the proximal femur; thus, it was assumed that the bulkier the implant, the greater its mechanical stability. Biomechanical studies have shown that this conclusion is not necessarily true, because stabilization of prostheses depends on contact with rigid bone that is suitably situated to resist the multiaxial forces applied to the femoral head. Thus the fit and not the fill of

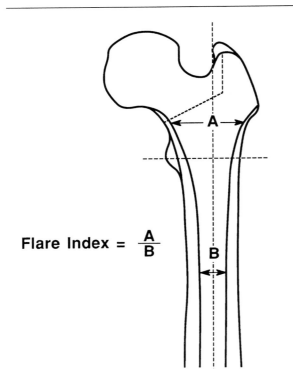

Flare Index = $\dfrac{A}{B}$

Fig. 4 The canal flare index, defined as the ratio of the proximal and distal widths of the medullary canal in the anteroposterior view. (Reproduced with permission from Noble PC: Biomechanical advances in total hip replacement, in Niwa S, Perren SM, Hattori T (eds): *Biomechanics in Orthopaedics.* Tokyo, Japan, Springer-Verlag, 1992, pp 46–75.)

a cementless prosthesis within the metaphysis determines its stability.

The Shape of the Femoral Canal

Because the primary method of stabilizing cementless implants is contact with the endosteal surface, the three-dimensional shape of the implant must precisely match key dimensions of the intramedullary canal, despite the geometric variations between femora. Several studies have shown that the quantitative anatomy of the femur is highly variable, both in terms of intramedullary and extramedullary dimensions. This morphologic diversity may be measured in many ways. Statistical correlation between individual dimensions of the femur may be determined to describe the shape of each femur, independent of its overall size. These correlations can be expressed as dimensionless ratios. One example of such a parameter is the canal flare index, which is the ratio of the widths of the femoral canal at two levels—20 mm proximal to the center of the lesser trochanter and at the canal isthmus (Fig. 4).

The canal flare index expresses the overall shape of the medullary canal in the coronal plane and can be used to identify three distinctly different shapes of medullary canals. Very straight or stove-pipe femora have a canal flare index less than 3.0 and are present in about 10% of the population. At the other extreme, highly flared or champagne-fluted bones have canal flare indices greater than 4.7 and, again, are present in approximately 10% of cases. Between these two extremes lies the range of femora of normal radiographic appearance, which have canal flare indices of 3.0 to 4.7. In patients who undergo cementless hip replacement, the overall shape of the medullary canal varies continuously between the stove-pipe and the champagne-fluted extremes. Although some shapes are encountered more frequently than others, it is not possible to designate any one shape as normal.

A confounding factor is the fact that the dimensions of the medullary canal do not vary proportionally with the size of the bone. Individuals of the same stature have femora of similar lengths, but widely varying endosteal geometries. This is contrary to the assumption that all femora have one basic endosteal shape that can be scaled proportionally to derive the canal geometries of larger and smaller bones, an assumption that has been fundamental to the design of many cementless prostheses in the past.

Computer-based anatomic studies have shown that at least nine separate shapes are needed to represent the contours of the human femur in the coronal plane. These shapes are not proportionally related and do not have a fixed medial curvature, unlike most cementless prostheses. The shape of the femur is also found to vary with overall canal size and is strongly influenced by the inclination of the neck with respect to the medullary axis.

An anatomic consideration that can lead to selection of an undersized implant is impingement of the prosthesis with the medullary canal. The curvature of the femur in the sagittal plane varies extensively, partly as a function of sex, race, and bone length. Straight-stemmed prostheses of excessive length can impinge against the anterior cortex of the femur during implantation, preventing seating of the prosthesis within the metaphysis or causing a distal fracture of the femur. This impingement may be prevented by selection of shorter femoral stems or by use of implants with curved or slit distal stems that can negate the effects of the anterior bow of the femur during implantation.

The Effect of Bone-Shaping Instruments

A second factor affecting the fit of a prosthesis within the femur is the effect of bone-shaping instruments on the implantation site. Although in theory the metaphyseal cavity formed by broaching or rasping is of exactly the same dimensions as the instrument itself, in practice, passage of an instrument enlarges the implantation site. This enlargement occurs because orthopaedic rasps and broaches must remove a considerable volume of cancellous bone. They consequently have coarse, widely spaced teeth that crush and drag bone during implantation and removal, thereby eroding the surface of the cavity. If a prosthesis of exactly the same shape as the broaching instrument is implanted, gaps will inevitably be present at the implant–bone interface. Gaps prevent the bone from supporting the implant, regardless of the design of either the broach or the prosthesis. Moreover, many of the gaps at the interface may not fill in with bone and can become permanent conduits for the transport of polymeric debris, thus expanding the effective volume of the joint space and the area of the interface at risk of osteolysis.

Several approaches have been proposed to minimize gap formation between the prosthesis and metaphyseal bone. The surgeon can use broaching instruments sparingly and can remove as much bone as possible using reamers. He or she can also select broaching instruments that remove bone slowly, causing less expansion of the cavity, and can avoid twisting and tilting the broach within the femur in order to minimize enlargement of the implantation site. Another method under clinical evaluation is robotic reaming of the medullary canal using CAD-CAM (computer-automated design and manufacturing) techniques. This method uses an initial computed tomography (CT) scan of the femur, prepared after metallic markers have been implanted in the greater trochanter and the femoral condyles. Using the CT scan, a suitable prosthesis is selected and its ideal orientation within the femur is determined. This information is used to direct a high speed reamer that machines the implantation site to precisely fit the shape of the prosthesis, eliminating almost all gaps at the implant–bone interface. Alternately, the prosthesis may be designed to be slightly larger than the corresponding broach so that the cancellous bone within the metaphysis is compressed during the implantation of the prosthesis, filling many of the gaps left by broaching. Biomechanical measurements have shown that this strategy leads to an almost threefold reduction in rotational micromotion.

Stem Design Factors Affecting Implant Stability

Numerous factors affect the relative motion of the prosthesis and the femur under physiologic loads. Factors related to the patient include the intracortical geometry of the femur; the quality of the cancellous and cortical bone stock; and the weight, height, and activity of the individual. Factors that come under the control of the surgeon include the accuracy with which a selected prosthesis matches the anatomy of the femur, the position of implantation of the prosthesis within the bone (including the level of the femoral neck osteotomy), the fit of the implant to the endosteal contours of the femur, and the presence of any gaps between the prosthesis and the implantation site.

The contributions of many of these interrelated variables have been systematically examined in few studies; however, laboratory studies have been performed in which prostheses of different designs have been implanted in cadaveric and synthetic femora and loaded in torsion and compression. Arrays of measuring devices have been used to monitor the motion occurring at the stem–bone interface during loading. Data from these studies have demonstrated that the proximal and distal micromotion of most

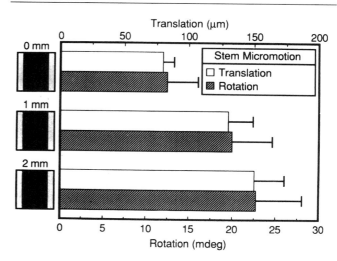

Fig. 5 The effect of distal canal fit on the rotational and translational micromotion of the proximal stem–bone interface. The values for distal fit refer to the difference in diameter between the stem and the canal. (Reproduced with permission from Noble PC: Biomechanical advances in total hip replacement, in Niwa S, Perren SM, Hattori T (eds): *Biomechanics in Orthopaedics*. Tokyo, Japan, Springer-Verlag, 1992, pp 46–75.)

designs of prostheses is relatively small under conditions simulating single-legged stance but increases dramatically with the application of torsional loading. This observation supports the conclusion that torsional stability is a good indicator of the clinical performance of femoral stems and can be used to differentiate between satisfactory and unsatisfactory designs. The following conclusions may be drawn about the contribution of specific factors to the stability of the stem–bone interface.

Stem–Bone Fit The rotational resistance of a cementless prosthesis within the femur is determined primarily by the distance between areas of stem–bone contact and the axis of rotation of the implant, which may be approximated by the longitudinal axis of the medullary canal. Thus, contact between the femur and the medial surface of the prosthesis at the level of the femoral neck osteotomy will produce the greatest reduction in rotational micromotion, especially if the area of contact includes part of the anterior and posterior surfaces of the prosthesis (Fig. 5). In a similar manner, a higher femoral neck osteotomy has the potential to reduce micromotion by shifting the position of areas of contact between the proximal stem and the femur medially. Raising the level of the osteotomy by 10 mm can lead to reduction in micromotion of 45%.

Proximal-Distal Fit Although cementless prostheses may be designed primarily to fit the metaphysis or the diaphysis of the femur, simultaneous proximal and distal stabilization is important to minimize the incidence of symptoms following cementless hip replacement. This fact is con-

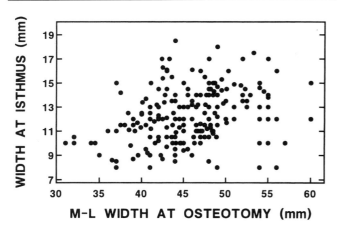

Fig. 6   The width of the medullary canal of 200 femora, as measured at the canal isthmus and the level of the femoral neck osteotomy (see Fig. 4). (Reproduced with permission from Noble PC: Biomechanical advances in total hip replacement, in Niwa S, Perren SM, Hattori T (eds): *Biomechanics in Orthopaedics*. Tokyo, Japan, Springer-Verlag, 1992, pp 46–75.)

firmed by the results of biomechanical experiments performed with metaphyseal-loading prostheses (Fig. 5). In these studies, the proximal fit of the prosthesis has been kept constant and the gap between the reamed femoral isthmus and the distal stem has been varied systematically. The presence of a gap between the bone and the implant dramatically increases the micromotion of the proximal stem; a gap of 0.5 mm increases micromotion by almost 100%.

Simultaneous proximal and distal fit is extremely difficult to achieve with stems of fixed dimensions because of the variability of the proximal and distal geometry of the medullary canal (Fig. 6). Even if optimum stem fit is achieved in the proximal femur, the variation present within the isthmus prevents distal stabilization of many components. Advocates of diaphyseal-loading prostheses approach this problem by extensively reaming the canal isthmus to allow distal fixation of a large enough prosthesis to fill the proximal femur. In a significant proportion of femora, distal fixation requires removal of more than 25% of the original cortical thickness with enlargement of the isthmus by up to 5 mm in diameter. This requirement has led to the development of modular prostheses that allow independent proximal and distal components to be assembled to form implants of different combinations of proximal and distal dimensions. Another approach has been the use of monolithic stems manufactured with a variety of distal sizes for each fixed proximal geometry.

Anterior-Posterior Width   Femoral stems may be designed with a fixed shape in the coronal plane but different widths in the sagittal plane. Although narrower prostheses are easier to implant within the femur, anterior-posterior

bulk significantly increases the stability of metaphyseal-loading prostheses, presumably because fixation is obtained in stronger bone with increased cortical contact.

Symmetric Versus Asymmetric Stems   The results of published studies are contradictory, because past experiments have been performed on commercial prostheses with several differences in design in addition to the presence of an asymmetric stem. Data from several studies have demonstrated that implants that are asymmetric in the sagittal plane can provide increased rotational stability. This increase may be due to the curvature of the distal stem, which allows the point of contact between the distal tip of the prosthesis and the femur to be displaced from the axis of the medullary canal. Another factor may be the increased area of contact between the implant and strong metaphyseal bone, which can be obtained using a prosthesis with a flared anterior surface.

Porous Coating   No systematic study has provided data that show whether differences in the frictional properties of porous coatings translate into variations in implant micromotion. In prostheses that load through the diaphysis, the presence of a porous coating is essential for cementless fixation because the uncoated component is not inherently stable within the femur. Moreover, the greater the area of contact between the distal stem and the diaphysis, the greater the resistance of the prosthesis to torsional moments. Metaphyseal-loading implants present the opposite picture. In this case, the presence of a beaded surface tends to increase micromotion, partly because bony contact is concentrated over the peaks of the beaded coating. The potential benefits of the biologic ingrowth into the surface of the prosthesis must be weighed against the possibility of instability of the interface in the immediate postoperative period.

Proximal Stem–Bone Interference   The presence of gaps between the cementless stem and metaphyseal bone profoundly affects the stability of cementless fixation, especially in rotation. In some designs of cementless prostheses, the impact of this factor is reduced by the presence of an interference fit between the cancellous bone of the metaphysis and the cementless prosthesis. This is achieved by designing a prosthesis that is oversized compared with the corresponding broaching instrument and, hence, the implantation site within the proximal femur. This strategy can lead to a reduction in rotational micromotion of 60% to 70%.

Restoration of the Joint Center

One of the most important factors influencing stability of a hip replacement is the accuracy with which the normal anatomic relationship between the femur and the pelvis is restored. At the extremes of joint motion, the mechanical stability of the artificial hip is critically affected by the tone

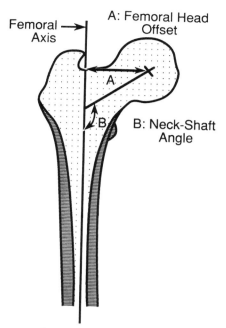

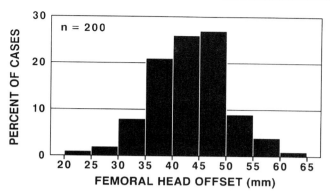

Fig. 8 Distribution of values of the medial offset of the femoral head. (Reproduced with permission from Noble PC: Biomechanical advances in total hip replacement, in Niwa S, Perren SM, Hattori T (eds): *Biomechanics in Orthopaedics.* Tokyo, Japan, Springer-Verlag, 1992, pp 46–75.)

Fig. 7 Diagrammatic representation of the position of the femoral head with respect to the axis of the medullary canal. (Reproduced with permission from Noble PC: Biomechanical advances in total hip replacement, in Niwa S, Perren SM, Hattori T (eds): *Biomechanics in Orthopaedics.* Tokyo, Japan, Springer-Verlag, 1992, pp 46–75.)

of the abductor muscles. The length of these muscles and the compressive force developed in the hip joint are determined by the inferior and lateral position of the greater trochanter with respect to the ilium. If the joint replacement displaces the femur medially, the mechanical efficiency of the abductor mechanism will be reduced so that a larger muscle force will be needed to balance the hip joint. This increased muscle force will increase the joint reaction force and the loading of the acetabular component.

Shortening of the medial offset of the prosthesis also reduces the range of motion and allows dislocation of the joint with less applied torque. In this situation, joint stability can be restored by lengthening the extremity or by changing the position of the trochanter on the femur. Because few patients will accept lengthening of the leg and most surgeons do not favor a trochanteric osteotomy, the prosthesis itself must allow sufficient variation in neck length to restore the original head position without lengthening the extremity. This restoration is achieved by matching the medial offset of the prosthesis to the original offset of the femur, with an additional allowance for the effects of any deformity and for medialization of the acetabulum.

In the coronal plane, the medial offset of the femoral head from the medullary axis varies from approximately 29 to 57 mm (95% confidence limits), a range of 28 mm (Figs. 7 and 8). This range is due to the combined effect of

differences in the neck inclination and the overall size of the femur. The range of head offset may be reduced to approximately 20 mm if the size and range of offset of the prosthesis are changed concurrently (Fig. 9). However, because the femoral neck is inclined with respect to the medial–lateral axis of the femur, this change necessitates a 28-mm range in prosthetic neck length in comparison with the 15- to 20-mm range provided by most standard hip systems with modular femoral heads.

A similar problem is presented by the variable anterior position of the femoral head in the sagittal plane. Although the anteversion of the femur varies by approximately 35° (95% confidence limits), cementless prostheses generally become stable within the femoral canal in only one rotational position. Fortunately, most prostheses rotate into anteversion during implantation, so that the femoral head generally ends up within 5 mm of its original anterior position. However, in some instances, the shape of the canal and/or the femoral head and neck cause the femoral head to be displaced posteriorly by up to 10 mm, leading to a potentially unstable joint.

Several approaches have been adopted to improve restoration of femoral head position. One is the use of custom prostheses that allow the relationship between the center of the femoral head and the body of the implant to be set prior to fabrication of the prosthesis to match the individual anatomy of each patient. Though effective in restoring extramedullary anatomy, this approach is presently too expensive for routine use and is not entirely accurate, because the implanted position of the acetabular cup cannot be precisely defined by preoperative planning. Some modular prostheses provide great versatility in allowing the anteversion of the femoral neck to be varied intraoperatively. In most cases, however, the superior and medial position of the femoral head cannot be varied to any greater degree than is possible using standard, monolithic femoral prostheses with modular femoral heads.

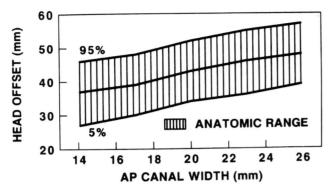

Fig. 9 The variation of medial head offset with the size of the femur, as defined by the width of the medullary canal, 20 mm distal to the center of the lesser trochanter. (Reproduced with permission from Noble PC: Biomechanical advances in total hip replacement, in Niwa S, Perren SM, Hattori T (eds): *Biomechanics in Orthopaedics.* Tokyo, Japan, Springer-Verlag, 1992, pp 46–75.)

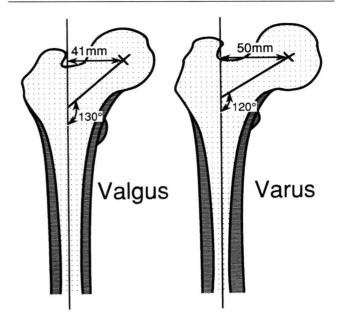

Fig. 10 The position of the femoral head varies with the neck–shaft angle and endosteal shape of each femur. (Reproduced with permission from Noble PC: Biomechanical advances in total hip replacement, in Niwa S, Perren SM, Hattori T (eds): *Biomechanics in Orthopaedics.* Tokyo, Japan, Springer-Verlag, 1992, pp 46–75.)

Another solution is for the implant manufacturer to supply each size of prosthesis in several different neck lengths. Although this solution expands the anatomic capabilities of the implant system, it also necessitates a large inventory of prosthetic components with additional inconvenience for the operating room. An alternate approach is a system of prostheses in which the fixed neck-shaft angle of each prosthesis is varied as a function of both its size and medial curvature. Because varus femora (neck-shaft angle < 120°) have larger medial head offsets than those with a valgus configuration (neck-shaft angle > 140°), this strategy enables much of the anatomic variation present within the normal bone population to be accommodated with a single implant system (Fig. 10).

The Response of the Femur to the Prosthesis

Osteolysis

A disturbing radiographic observation in a significant number of cementless femoral prostheses is the development of lytic lesions, typically within the exposed cancellous bone of the greater trochanter or the cortical wall near the tip of the implant. Osteolysis, or periprosthetic bone loss, has been identified in association with both cemented and cementless prostheses. Both focal (or localized) and linear (or diffuse) osteolytic lesions have been identified in radiographic studies. Focal lesions, especially those in conjunction with stable, asymptomatic prostheses, are the source of the greatest clinical concern and can lead to substantial bony destruction with attendant complications, including prosthetic loosening and periprosthetic femoral fractures.

Osteolytic destruction can be difficult to detect in its early stages; in cementless implants, it often involves areas of bone exposed by the proximal femoral osteotomy, in-

cluding any soft cancellous bone within the greater trochanter and the medial neck. In some implants, especially those without circumferential porous coating, lesions are observed distally as areas of endosteal scalloping or as a linear radiolucent halo surrounding the distal tip of the prosthesis. The pathogenesis of this process appears to involve proliferation of macrophages, which phagocytize wear debris consisting of micrometer- and submicrometer-sized particles of polyethylene. Generation of excessive quantities of these particles causes intercellular secretion of a variety of soluble mediators, principally interleukin-1 and prostaglandin E2. These mediators stimulate osteoclasts, which resorb bone adjacent to the implant–bone interface. Other particulates (metal, polymethylmethacrylate, hydroxyapatite) can also play a role in this process, either directly at the cellular level, or indirectly by scratching the polished surface of the femoral head leading to accelerated polyethylene wear.

The reported incidence of osteolysis following cementless hip replacement ranges extensively, from 16% to 56% at 5 to 7 years. Factors that influence the frequency of this observation include the methods used to identify lesions, the design of the prosthesis, and the number of implants within each study that achieve stable biologic fixation. Whereas only 5% to 10% of femoral stems with stable bony fixation show signs of osteolytic lesions at 5-year follow-up, rates of 30% to 40% are reported in association with undersized or unstable components. These data suggest that micromotion at the implant–bone interface or the formation of fibrous membrane assists the processes of particle transport and bone destruction. Consequently, mechanical stabilization of cementless prostheses leading to bony attachment at the stem–bone interface is the first defense against the invasion of particulate debris.

Interfaces are believed to play a critical role in the transport of particulate debris generated within the joint (Fig. 11). However, bony ingrowth appears to prevent or significantly impede the progress of osteolytic lesions. Osteolysis occurs more frequently when the femoral prosthesis has discrete pads of ingrowth coating that do not extend around the circumference of the implant. In these designs, the uncoated areas between the pads do not support attachment of bone or fibrous tissue and act as conduits for the transport of particulate debris. For this reason, implants with circumferential porous coatings or bioactive surfaces (eg, hydroxyapatite) are recommended to maximize the durability of cementless fixation. Although it is not known whether the presence of circumferential coating will reduce the total incidence of osteolysis within both the pelvis and the femur, lesions at or below the coated areas of these prostheses are relatively uncommon.

The principal method of preventing osteolysis is to minimize the rate of production of polyethylene particles. In practice, this necessitates selection of an acetabular cup with a liner of at least 5 mm in thickness, coupled with a femoral head having a diameter of 28 mm or smaller and the smoothest possible surface finish. Ceramic femoral heads also appear to significantly reduce the rate of wear of the prosthetic joint. Other measures may be adopted to reduce forces acting on the acetabular insert. These include placement of the acetabular cup in no more than 45° of abduction and restoration of the medial offset of the femoral head. All sources of hard foreign particles must also be excluded from the body to minimize third-body wear. These sources may include some porous coatings as metal particles can be generated through internal abrasion of flexible metal wires or repetitive motion of the stem in contact with bone. Particulate debris can also be generated at modular connections, including the modular head–taper junction and interfaces formed between bone screws and acetabular shells. By minimizing the use of modularity, the chances of particulate contamination of the prosthetic articulation may be further reduced.

Stress-induced Femoral Remodeling

The presence of a femoral stem within the femur radically changes the distribution of stress within cortical and cancellous bone. This change, in turn, leads to remodeling of the proximal femur through cortical thinning and increased intracortical and trabecular porosity. In the presence of bony ingrowth, the femur and the prosthesis act as a composite beam in bending and torsion. Because the mechanical stiffness of the prosthesis is comparable to that of the femur, a significant proportion of the joint reaction

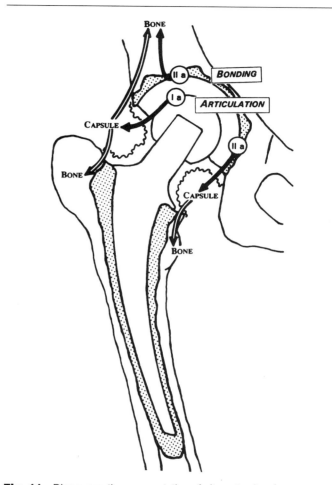

Fig. 11 Diagrammatic representation of alternate sites for generation and transport of particulate wear debris in cementless hip replacements. (Reproduced with permission from Willert HG, Buchhorn GH: Particle disease due to wear of ultrahigh molecular weight polyethylene: Findings from retrieval studies, in Morrey BF (ed): *Biological, Material, and Mechanical Considerations of Joint Replacement.* New York, NY, Raven Press, 1993, pp 87–102.)

force passes through the prosthesis and not through the proximal femur. This reduction in loading of the bone is called stress-shielding, and can amount to 50% to 80% of normal physiologic levels.

Once bone becomes attached to a cementless prosthesis, load transfer occurs through the areas of bony attachment, which often are localized to the distal edge of any ingrowth coating. This transfer leads to hypertrophy of the bone at the point of contact (spotwelding) and atrophy of adjacent bone, which is not attached to the prosthesis. Loss of bone is most pronounced in cases where circumferential bony ingrowth is present distally and is absent proximally. This situation may occur if gaps are present at the proximal implant–bone interface or if there is excessive micromotion between the implant and the proximal femur.

Extensive proximal bone loss is a common feature of

diaphyseal-locking prostheses and is the principal factor limiting the use of this mode of implant fixation, at least in primary hip arthroplasty. After implantation of a diaphyseal-locking prosthesis, most bone loss occurs in the first 2 years postoperatively, although some additional atrophy is observed between the second and fifth years. Moderate to severe femoral resorption has been reported in approximately 20% of extensively porous-coated devices, most frequently in stems of larger distal diameter (ie, greater than 13.5 mm) and in patients 50 years of age or older with osteoporotic bone.

The clinical significance of proximal bone loss has yet to be fully elucidated. Failure of well-fixed implants with femoral resorption is rare, but the lack of proximal bone can make reconstruction of the femur difficult and may lead to increased susceptibility of the proximal femur to osteolysis through increased penetration of polyethylene wear debris into the porous, osteoporotic cancellous bone. The incidence of proximal bone loss following cementless hip replacement may be minimized by restricting the use of extensively porous-coated implants to younger patients with thick cortices. In older patients, especially those with enlarged canals and osteoporotic bone, cemented prostheses cause less stress-shielding and provide proximal and distal fit to the medullary canal. This may lead to less resorption with time, although some studies suggest that adverse remodeling occurs in the osteoporotic femur regardless of the mode of implant fixation. Several measures have been proposed to reduce resorption of the femur, including reduction of the stiffness of the prosthesis through use of a hollow or slit distal stem or fabrication of the prosthesis from carbon fiber-reinforced composite materials. Clinical evidence of the success of these approaches is still awaited.

Annotated Bibliography

General

Engh CA, McGovern TF, Engh CA Jr, et al: Clinical experience with the anatomic medullary locking (AML) prosthesis for primary total hip replacement, in Morrey BF (ed): *Biological, Material, and Mechanical Considerations of Joint Replacement.* New York, NY, Raven Press, 1993, pp 167–184.

This is an excellent discussion of the development and results of the most popular diaphyseal-locking prosthesis. Interesting data are presented on the incidence and severity of bony remodeling following use of these devices. The results of radiologic studies and retrieval analysis are elegantly interwoven. This reference provides useful insight into the issues that remain controversial in implant design and selection.

Friedman RJ, Black J, Galante JO, et al: Current concepts in orthopaedic biomaterials and implant fixation. *J Bone Joint Surg* 1993;75A:1086–1109.

This is an excellent review of current knowledge of the properties, selection, and biological interactions of orthopaedic biomaterials. Special emphasis is given to current issues in the design of implants, especially those involving local and systemic responses, including bone lysis. A summary of advances and directions in implant fixation is also presented with an extensive bibliography.

Hungerford DS, Hedley A, Habermann E, et al: *Total Hip Arthroplasty: A New Approach.* Baltimore, MD, University Park Press, 1984.

This is an interesting, comprehensive review of the design philosophy of the first metaphyseal-loading prosthesis to gain widespread use in the United States.

Noble PC, Alexander JW, Lindahl LJ, et al: The anatomic basis of femoral component design. *Clin Orthop* 1988;235: 148–165.

This very informative review of the morphology of the femur in the context of femoral prosthesis design presents a great deal of anatomic data, based upon an analysis of 200 human femora. Interesting factors are presented concerning the variability of femoral anatomy and the difficulties inherent in standardizing canal geometry for implant design. Femoral dimensions are shown to be roughly proportional externally but nonproportional internally, due in part to the effects of aging of bony structure. Useful concepts are also developed, including the use of the canal flare index to describe the shape of the medullary canal and the classification of femora by characteristic shapes termed somatypes.

Bone Remodeling Following Cementless Hip Replacement

Bobyn JD, Glassman AH, Goto H, et al: The effect of stem stiffness on femoral bone resorption after canine porous-coated total hip arthroplasty. *Clin Orthop* 1990; 261:196–213.

In this ingenious experimental study, bilateral cementless hip replacements were performed in eight dogs using two prostheses of identical external shape but a difference in bending stiffness of approximately four-fold. The stiff prosthesis was fabricated from solid CoCr, whereas the flexible prosthesis was machined from titanium alloy and hollowed out to a distal wall thickness of only 1 mm. Both stems were extensively porous coated. At sacrifice, 1 year after surgery, femora implanted with flexible stems had 25% to 35% more cortical bone within the diaphysis than their contralateral pairs. Moreover, severe cortical resorption was observed in three quarters of the animals with stiff stems and none with flexible stems. This is the first study to provide unequivocal proof that implant flexibility and adverse osseous remodeling are related, as suggested by previous radiographic observations of patients with extensively coated prostheses.

Engh CA, Bobyn JD: The influence of stem size and extent of porous coating on femoral bone resorption after primary cementless hip arthroplasty. *Clin Orthop* 1988; 231:7–28.

This is a classic paper in which the incidence and severity of proximal bone loss are related to a variety of design variables following implantation of a diaphyseal-loading prosthesis. Pronounced resorption was observed in 18% of all 411 cases and increased once the stem diameter exceeded 13.5 mm (28%), in the presence of extensive porous coating (22%), and in patients older than 50 years of age (23%). The most severe bone loss occurred in fully porous-coated stems larger than 13.5 mm in diameter (54%). The incidence and severity of bone loss were found to correlate closely with theoretical calculations of the reduction of physiologic loading of the femoral shaft as a function of intramedullary diameter.

Sumner DR, Turner TM, Urban RM, et al: Remodeling and ingrowth of bone at two years in a canine cementless total hip-arthroplasty model. *J Bone Joint Surg* 1992;74A: 239–250.

This paper presents data from experiments in which bone remodeling was measured in terms of the change in the total area of cortical bone at cross sections taken along the length of the femur, 2 years after implantation of cementless prostheses in dogs. Unilateral cementless stems were implanted with fiber-metal, beaded, and plasma-sprayed titanium coatings. The extent of ingrowth varied between the different designs, but overall 10% to 20% of cortical bone was lost adjacent to the porous-coated sections of each prosthesis. There was a significant increase in medullary bone formed around the distal third of the prosthesis.

The Biomechanics of Cementless Femoral Stems

Callaghan JJ, Fulghum CS, Glisson RR, et al: The effect of femoral stem geometry on interface motion in uncemented porous-coated total hip prostheses: Comparison of straight-stem and curved-stem designs. *J Bone Joint Surg* 1992;74A:839–848.

This is the report of an elegant experimental study in which straight-stemmed and curved-stemmed prostheses were compared. Whereas no differences were observed under mechanical conditions simulating single leg stance or at low levels of torsional loading, large torsional moments (22 N·m) caused substantially less rotational motion in the curved prosthesis than in the straight-stemmed design, suggesting that the curvature of the stem leads to increased stability. This conclusion must be applied with caution to implants other than the two designs tested in this study. Because commercial devices were used, several factors may explain the differences observed. The design with reduced micromotion was not only curved but was bulkier proximally and was implanted with different instruments than the straight-stemmed design. The authors also showed that proximal bony ingrowth, simulated by proximal cementing, led to a reduction in proximal and distal implant bone motion.

Capello WN: Technical aspects of cementless total hip arthroplasty. *Clin Orthop* 1990;261:102–106.

This is a rare description of the interaction of prosthetic design, bone quality, and surgical technique on the stability of cementless hip prostheses. Through experimental data, the author demonstrates that the two factors leading to unstable rotating fixation are the retention of soft cancellous bone and line-to-line preparation of the implantation site. Curved stems and lateral pins led to no significant change in rotational micromotion. The author also emphasized the importance of prophylactic wiring of the femur to reduce the incidence of

fractures during impaction of the prosthesis and intraoperative testing of torsional stability.

Noble PC: Biomechanical advances in total hip replacement, in Niwa S, Perren SM, Hattori T (eds): *Biomechanics in Orthopedics*. Tokyo, Japan, Springer-Verlag, 1992, pp 46–75.

This is an interesting overview of the interaction between anatomy, bone morphometry, and the biomechanical function of implants. Original information is presented concerning the fit of cementless prostheses to the femur and the emergence of different philosophies of femoral stem design in order to accommodate variations in the shape of the medullary canal. This chapter also discusses the relationship between the extramedullary position of the femoral head and prosthetic design.

Noble PC, Kamaric E, Alexander JW: Abstract: Distal stem centralization critically affects the acute fixation of cementless femoral stems. *Orthop Trans* 1989;13:383.

This study was performed to explore the effect of distal stem fit on the stability of symmetric cementless prostheses. Standard prostheses were fitted with modular distal sleeves and then loaded in compression and torsion. The most stable fixation was produced with a line-to-line distal fit, which allowed axial sliding of the prosthesis without lateral motion. Use of a 1-mm undersized distal stem increased micromotion by almost 100%. This study supports the concept that simultaneous proximal and distal fit is a potent method for increasing the stability of cementless prostheses.

Poss R, Walker P, Spector M, et al: Strategies for improving fixation of femoral components in total hip arthroplasty. *Clin Orthop* 1988;235:181–194.

This is an interesting review of the considerations inherent in the design of cementless prostheses. The authors describe the rationale for the use of cementless implants and then present the dilemma of balancing maximum canal fill with increased interface stability against increased stress shielding and adverse remodeling of the proximal femur. The role of interface interactions is emphasized. The authors emphasize that the stiffness of the connection formed between the prosthesis and the femur strongly influences the degree of stress shielding of the host bone and, thus, the severity of remodeling observed postoperatively.

Schneider E, Kinast C, Eulenberger J, et al: A comparative study of the initial stability of cementless hip prosthesis. *Clin Orthop* 1989;248:200–209.

This elegant experimental study shows how implant–bone motion is measured in the biomechanics laboratory. The complexity of the motions generated and the dependence on the design of the prosthesis are well demonstrated. An intriguing finding was that substantial differences in the stability of different straight-stemmed prostheses were observed despite the apparent similarity of the stem designs. This study also demonstrated that the lowest and most consistent values of micromotion were observed with an asymmetric, curved prosthesis.

Whiteside LA, Easley JC: The effect of collar and distal stem fixation on micromotion of the femoral stem in uncemented total hip arthroplasty. *Clin Orthop* 1989;239:145–153.

In this experimental study, the role of distal canal fit in stabilizing cementless femoral stems is investigated for collared and collarless prostheses. While collar-calcar contact prevented distal migration, it had no effect on micromotion in the medial-lateral and anterior-posterior directions. The lowest values of micromotion were observed with a tight distal and proximal fit.

Osteolysis

Amstutz HC, Campbell P, Kossovsky N, et al: Mechanism and clinical significance of wear debris-induced osteolysis. *Clin Orthop* 1992;276:7–18.

This paper reviewed the issues related to wear particle-induced osteolysis. Macrophages, activated by the phagocytosis of particulate debris, are the key cells in this process, which can potentially occur in any implant system regardless of implant design or fixation mode.

Schmalzried TP, Jasty M, Harris KW: Periprosthetic bone loss in total hip arthroplasty: Polyethylene wear debris and the concept of the effective joint space. *J Bone Joint Surg* 1992;74A:849–863.

This is a landmark paper in the study of osteolysis and the penetration of wear debris into the implant-bone interface. The authors examine 34 cases of prosthetic revisions with diffuse or localized bone loss around the prosthesis. Intracellular particles of less than 1 μm in size were found in macrophages from every case, the predominant particle being polyethylene. The number of macrophages was also directly related to the number of polyethylene particles visible by light microscopy. These findings were true even in cases of well-fixed prostheses in which osteolytic lesions were observed at sites far from the articulating joint surfaces. These data led the authors to conclude that all of the periprosthetic interface is accessible to particulate debris and is thus susceptible to osteolysis, despite the findings of atrophy.

Willert HG, Buchhorn GH: Particle disease due to wear of ultrahigh molecular weight polyethylene: Findings from retrieval studies, in Morrey BF (ed): *Biological, Material, and Mechanical Considerations of Joint Replacement*. New York, NY, Raven Press, 1993, pp 87–102.

This is an outstanding summary of issues related to particle-induced osteolysis in cementless hip replacement. Many subjects relating to polyethylene particles are discussed, including mode of particle formation, transport methods for histologic identification, and the size and quantities of particles generated by implants within the body. The authors argue that macrophages are activated not in response to the toxicity of the polymeric particles themselves, but in response to ingestion of excessive amounts of particles. An interesting discussion is also presented regarding alternate methods of transport of wear particles.

Biologic Response to Implants

Galante JP, Lemons J, Spector M, et al: The biologic effects of implant materials. *J Orthop Res* 1991;9:760–775.

This review addresses issues related to the biodegradation of orthopaedic biomaterials, paradigms for prosthesis loosening, the local and systemic responses to materials (including carcinogenicity), and the remodeling of bone around femoral stems.

Robotic Surgery

Paul HA, Bargar WL, Mittlestadt B, et al: Development of a surgical robot for cementless total hip arthroplasty. *Clin Orthop* 1992;285:57–66.

This is a fascinating description of the development of computerized methods for templating the femur for cementless hip replacement combined with robotic machining of the implantation cavity under computer control. Data are presented showing the effects of manual preparation of the femur by broaching in comparison with robotic machining. After broaching, the average linear gap between the broach and the femur averaged 1.20 mm with only 20.8% of the surface of the implant in contact with bone. Robotic machining reduced the average gap width to 0.05 mm, with 95.8% bony contact. The implications of robotic machining for improved performance of cementless hip replacements are discussed.

Implant Retrieval Studies

Collier JP, Bauer TW, Bloebaum RD, et al: Results of implant retrieval from postmortem specimens in patients with well-functioning, long-term total hip replacement. *Clin Orthop* 1992;274:97–112.

This unusual report represents the key findings of eight institutions that cooperated with the Hip Society in the evaluation of a total of 85 hip prostheses retrieved at postmortem. The findings reported are important because much of the knowledge of the implant–bone interface has been skewed by observations from loose, poorly-functioning components. The studies performed at postmortem show that bony ingrowth into porous implants is slower than was originally reported, starts to occur at about 3 months, and may take 3 to 4 years to stabilize. The amount of the porous surface that becomes attached to bone is highly variable, averaging around 40%, although only 5% to 15% of the available pore volume for bony ingrowth is normally occupied by bone. This study suggests that bony attachment is a secondary, although highly effective, method of stabilizing the implant—host interface. Its unpredictability supports attempts to maximize or strategize the placement of coating on the prosthesis to enhance the probability of bony ingrowth.

17

Cemented Total Hip Replacement Design

Design Principles

A cemented joint replacement is a load bearing structure and must, therefore, follow engineering principles. The metal femoral stem placed within the proximal femoral shaft is held in place with polymethylmethacrylate (PMMA). The presence of the stiff metal stem alters the stress distribution within the femur, with the stem bearing most of the load. At the tip of the stem, a stress concentration or riser results from the difference in material properties (change in stiffness) that occurs. The stem is subjected to significant bending, axial, and torsional forces. These cause internal stresses on the component and place shear forces on the fixation interface. Fortunately, the more flexible cement acts as a cushion of sorts, absorbing stresses and allowing their distribution over a maximal surface area. Unlike the femoral component, the acetabular socket is captured within the bony acetabulum and is inherently stable because the forces that act across the joint are largely compressive rather than shear forces.

Manufacturing Variables

Metals can be machined more accurately than polymers. The surface metal may be peeled from the substrate with little deformation. Thus, an accurate cut is easier to achieve in metals. However, changes in temperature in the metal can result in variation in the outer dimensions, which must be checked for tolerances after the part has returned to room temperature.

Machining of polymers occurs by a combination of cutting and pushing the underlying material out of the way. Polymers thus deform during the cutting process and then return to their normal shape after the tool has passed, making precise cuts more difficult. Most polymers cannot be machined with shallow cuts, because the tool tends to push the material out of the way, resulting in a poor surface finish.

Articular surfaces of joint replacements intended for use with cement must be highly polished and matched with extremely close tolerances. The nonarticular segment can accept larger tolerances because the polymethylmethacrylate will act as a grout or filler between the component and the bone. In press-fit devices, tolerances are more important for the nonarticular segments. Extremely tight tolerances are necessary for mating parts so that the connections will be tight to avoid fretting and wear. This is a problem for components designed for assembly in the operating room that must have tolerances to allow assembly

with only hand held tools. Particularly important are the dimensional tolerances between polyethylene liners and their metal shells. There must be no deformation of the polyethylene allowed at the articular interface. Concern has been raised about the possibility of wear at the interface between the metal shell and the back of the polyethylene insert. If tolerances between the femoral head and the acetabular polyethylene allow overlap so that the femoral ball is unable to fully seat within the socket, then higher stresses will result and polyethylene wear will be increased. The amount of contact stress is directly affected by even small variations in the articular surface tolerances. A typical specification for the metal femoral ball would be 28.00 ± 0.08 mm diameter. For the mating ultra-high molecular weight polyethylene socket, the specification could be 28.19 ± 0.08 mm in diameter. Extremely tight tolerances could thus result in the acetabular component being 0.03 mm larger in diameter than the metal ball with exact dimensions of 28.08 and 28.11 mm, respectively. On the other hand, the ultra-high molecular weight polyethylene inner diameter could be 28.27 and the metal ball outer diameter 27.92, with a total difference of 0.35 mm. The peak stress for the closely matched system is 1.64 MPa under 500 pounds of joint load. For the extreme tolerance mismatch, contact stress is calculated as 9.95 MPa, which represents a sixfold increase in stress.

Stress Concentrations

Stress concentrations may occur in the femoral stem as a result of design, manufacturing, or surgical technique. Stress concentrations reduce the fatigue performance of femoral components, particularly if they occur on the tensile surfaces, for example, the lateral surface of femoral stems. Titanium and its alloys are inherently more sensitive to stress concentration than other available metal alloys. For this reason, titanium is referred to as being notch sensitive. Ideally, the femoral design should minimize the stress concentrations. Both internal and external corners should be rounded to minimize stress concentration effects on the cement.

Surface Treatments

Data from some studies have suggested that ridges and serrations on the cemented implant surface improve stress transfer to the surrounding bone cement; however, these ridges also represent stress concentrations and may provide not only a place for cracks to initiate but also a rough surface once debonding occurs. Although holes in the stem may provide a convenient place for attachment of a removal device or for placement of a rotational control device during implantation, the holes must be placed in an area of redundant material that is not essential for structural safety. Adequate manufacturing will require that the surface of the implant be free of cracks, machine tool marks, and scratches.

Porous Surfaces

The application of porous surfaces by either heat sintering or diffusion bonding may have the side effect of introducing stress concentrations at the individual sites where beads or wire fibers are attached to the substrate material. This reduction in fatigue strength may be compensated for by increased stem cross section; however, there have been cases of fatigue fracture of porous-coated stems. Porous-coated devices do not have fatigue strengths comparable to those of nonporous devices made with the superalloys. Due to their decreased strength and increased cost, porous-coated devices should not be used for cemented fixation.

Femoral Stem Components

Total hip arthroplasty can theoretically provide a painless, low-friction joint that restores reasonable function to the hip over a 20-year period. The most important goal of any cemented femoral design is the removal of pain with no adverse bone remodeling changes. In addition, if revision is required, the stem should be removable with little or no additional bone loss. Hip loads may reach five to six times body weight. These high loads can contribute to subsidence, varus bending of the neck, and posteriorly directed torsion of the component. Of the hip force, 80% is directed axially, contributing to subsidence; 60% contributes to varus bending at the neck; and 30% is directed in the out of plane or torsional direction, forcing the component into retroversion. The combination of bone and cement must provide sufficient support to counteract these forces. Design and technical considerations also affect force transmission to the bone and cement. These considerations include neck length, varus or valgus placement of the stem, extent of bone reaming, stem geometry, and material properties of the stem.

Offset

The further the center of rotation of the femoral ball from the neutral axis of the stem, the higher will be the femoral compressive and bending stresses. These forces then translate into compressive, tensile, and shear stresses within the supporting material. The magnitudes of these stresses depend highly on the interface conditions and material properties of the substrate materials. When the stresses exceed the strength of the host materials or interfaces, debonding will occur. However, increasing the femoral component offset lateralizes the insertion of the abductor mechanism and decreases the joint contact forces.

The geometry of the femoral stem contributes directly to the overall stability of the femoral component and to the distribution of forces to the supporting structures. Cemented femoral components should have wide medial surfaces with rounded corners to prevent excessive cement strains.

Cement Fixation

The goal of all cemented stem designs is to transfer loads from the femoral head to the proximal femoral bone without causing pain or bone loss. Cemented stem designs must be compatible with the surrounding cement mantle. Voids in the cement and thin cement mantles should be avoided to help prevent cracks in the cement. Reducing porosity in the cement by use of centrifugation or vacuum mixing can prevent voids in the cement. The stem should be able to function for millions of cycles without cracks or other defects developing in either the stem or its surrounding cement mantle. Deformation or creep of the surrounding cement mantle should be minimized. There are many factors affecting the ability of a femoral stem to withstand cyclic forces. These include stem design, preparation of the bone, skill of the surgeon, and quality of the patient's bone stock. Placing a stiff metal stem inside the proximal femur results in abnormal physiologic loading. This is true for all current cementless and cemented designs regardless of their material composition. Therefore, some stress shielding of bone must occur.

Bonding of the Stem to the Cement

In a finite element model comparing unbonded or loose condition to the bonded condition, there was a 300% increase in proximal cement stresses during simulated stair climbing and a six hundred fold stress increase at the cement plug distal to the stem tip when the stem was unbonded. Thus, attempts have been made to bond the stem to the cement for efficient strain transfer and to eliminate any possibility of micromotion between the stem and the cement. Laboratory studies of loose stems have demonstrated significant increases in the stresses in nonbonded femoral stems, with much higher cortical bone strains in the lateral medial direction. Thus, a fully bonded interface will behave as a stiffer construct that decreases the stresses on the proximal cement.

PMMA cement is not glue. Cement is a grouting material that adapts to and fills the endosteal spaces with no adhesion between the acrylic cement and the stem surface. A frequent finding at revision surgery is a soft-tissue or fibrous interface of up to 100 μm in diameter between the stem and the cement. In 17 retrieved femurs with primary stems, which were implanted for up to 17 years, the cement bone interfaces were noted to be free of interface membranes; however, all specimens showed some interface separation between the stem and the cement. Any implant that had been in place more than 3 years had cracks originating at the stem–cement interface. Although a perfect bond between the cement and the metal is possible within theoretical mathematical constructs (finite element analyses), it is much more difficult to achieve clinically. The coefficient of friction between cement and metal has been measured as 0.3 under dry conditions; however, clinically, with the presence of fluids that lubricate the interface surfaces, incomplete bonding of the cement to the stem occurs interfering with fixation.

Mechanical Interlocking of Cement With the Stem

The cement may be mechanically interlocked to the stem with ridges, grooves, scallops, textured surfaces, or porous coatings. Lateral stem flanges were added to the Charnley "Cobra" design, to increase surface area and facilitate stress transfer. Unfortunately, surface treatments potentially provide stress risers in the cement. Surface treatments may also make stem removal more difficult.

Although achieving an initial mechanical interlock between stem and cement is intuitively desirable, in clinical studies better results were achieved with smooth, highly polished stems than with identical stems that had undergone surface treatments such as sand blasting. The authors of one study concluded that the stem should be able to subside slightly within the cement mantle, thus compensating for creep of the cement. According to this argument, any mechanism that prevents stem subsidence distally within the cement mantle may interfere with engagement of a tapered stem. In general, no feature of the stem design should compartmentalize the cement mantle. Compartmentalization may produce a defect in the cement sheath that results in an egress point for particulate debris or may lead to stem cement micromotion that causes particulate debris. The worst combination would be a textured stem combined with cement debonding that resulted in a loose stem with a rough surface. Subsequent micromotion and abrasive wear of the rough metal surface on the cement surface could lead to massive debris lysis, bone loss, and, ultimately, stem failure.

The Tapered Wedge Stem Design

The tapered wedge stem design offers predictable stress transfer to the cement by wedging itself into the cement mantle. This design results in reactive hoop stresses in the cement that tend to counterbalance the total load applied to the stem. The wedging of the stem into the cement anchors the stem and prevents micromotion. The stability achieved by the fit of a tapered stem in the cement mantle is analogous to a Morse taper type fit. Thus, the more external force, the tighter the fit should become. The stem should remain securely in place even when the external force is removed. Tapered stem designs have functioned well clinically when used with cement. The Charnley stem (Thackray, Orlando, FL) is tapered only in the medial to lateral direction. The Exeter stem (Howmedica, Rutherford, NJ) is tapered in both the anterior–posterior and medial–lateral planes. Thus, a continuous taper along the full length of the stem may provide excellent fixation.

The Calcar Collar

The importance of a collar in cemented stem designs has been controversial since the 1970s. Designers who prefer a collar argue that there is improved loading. Physiologic stressing of the proximal medial bone occurs because the bone is loaded in an axial plane rather than by hoop stresses. A finite element analysis study predicted a 300% increase in proximal bone and cement stress with a collared design. Loading the calcar with a collar can theoretically increase the stresses in this region. Designers who prefer collarless devices argue that, despite the biomechanical tests in the laboratory, the clinical reality is lack of contact or calcar bone loss with cortical cancellization, osteopenia, and rounding off under the collar. They argue that even large collars such as found on the CAD (Computer Assisted Design by Howmedica, Rutherford, NJ) were ineffective in transferring stress because resorption occurred in many CAD hips where initial contact was achieved. Data from one prospective randomized study demonstrate better cement-bone interfaces at 5-year follow-up when calcar collar contact is maintained.

Stem Centralization

Most designers prefer to have the stem placed in either neutral or slight valgus relative to the femoral axis. Stems placed in varus may be subject to larger bending moments and bending stresses. A neutral position of the stem in the canal will also minimize the risk of mid and distal stem contact with the endosteal wall of the femur, thus maintaining the integrity of the cement mantle. Data from several studies have indicated an increased incidence of endosteal cysts and progressive loosening, which appeared to initiate at sites of cement defects or metal–bone contact. These defects may result in abrasion of the stem against the bone and fracture of the cement, with production of particulate debris and the initiation of osteolysis. Several designers have advocated the use of distal stem centralizers in order to keep the stem positioned centrally in the canal, thereby providing an intact cement mantle surrounding the tip of the stem. The use of proximal stem centralizers is more controversial. There are now several proximal centralizers available, and most consist of pre-formed PMMA attached to the anterior, posterior, and medial aspects of the proximal stem. Air bubbles have been noted around these centralizers.

Materials for Cemented Total Hip Arthroplasty

Materials

Placing a metallic stem into the proximal femur alters the physiologic stresses in every case. In extreme cases, stress shielding will result in significant bone resorption proximally. The choice of material for any given geometric cross section will affect the stiffness of the construct, and thus, affect the ultimate stresses on cement and bone surrounding the stem. Finite element analyses have demonstrated that lower modulus stems, such as those made of titanium alloys, increase the stresses in the cement and bone proximally. Cemented designs used in the 1980s generally had larger cross-sectional areas than those used in the 1960s and 1970s. These larger stems were often stiffer than the Charnley stem even when lower modulus materials such as titanium were used. With the stainless steel versions of the Charnley and Exeter stems, very few problems with stress shielding were noted. The material characteristics of chrome-cobalt alloys are similar to those of stainless steel; however, higher fatigue strengths can be achieved with these alloys.

Titanium alloys have been advocated in total hip arthroplasty because their lower modulus is closer to that of bone than those of stainless steel and chrome cobalt. In cemented stem designs, however, this more flexible alloy will increase the stress in the proximal medial cement, possibly leading to cement failure and ultimate debonding of the titanium stem from the cement mantle. Once this debonding occurs, pistoning of the stem within the cement mantle may create both PMMA debris and metal particulates from the abraded stem surface. Because titanium alloy is not as abrasion resistant as cobalt chromium alloy, there may be more metal debris around a loose titanium stem. If a titanium femoral head is present, problems may arise because of scratching of the femoral head and increased wear. Metal particulates may also be shed from porous-coated or cemented metal-backed or textured acetabular components.

Cementation Technique

Cementation technique is generally considered at least as important as stem design in the ultimate outcome of hip arthroplasty. Most authors currently recommend removal of poor quality cancellous bone with containment of the bleeding bone, bone lavage, drying techniques, distal canal plugs, cement centrifugation, retrograde filling of the canal, and cement spacers. Reaming of the femoral diaphysis should be avoided. The goal is penetration of cement in the supporting bone stock with complete canal filling and avoidance of particulates (air, blood, or bone chips) in the cement. Porosity reduction has been achieved with centrifugation and vacuum mixing of the cement. Both processes have been demonstrated to increase cement fatigue strength.

Acetabular Cemented Cup Design

Conventional all polyethylene acetabular cups are secured to the pelvis with PMMA, which acts as a grout between the bony bed and the outer surface of the polyethylene component. Because PMMA is not an adhesive or glue, fixation must be achieved through interdigitation of the PMMA to the bone and to the polyethylene. Thus, cancellous bone must be exposed or fixation holes must be placed on smooth cortical surfaces. The polyethylene component must have external grooves of sufficient depth and width to interlock with the cement. In general, these grooves should be rectangular or dovetailed and profiled to ensure strong mechanical interlock. Tapered grooves may predispose the polyethylene socket to dissociate from the cement. Beveling the component at its mouth may allow better stability of the femoral head while avoiding impingement.

The newer metal-backed polyethylene components introduced during the 1980s may provide a more uniform distribution of stresses to the cement and pelvic bone. This improvement of stress transfer has been demonstrated by finite element analysis. In the absence of metal backing, a minimum thickness of 8 mm of polyethylene is necessary for comparable stress transfer. Metal-backed components achieve fixation through interdigitation of the cement with a metal plasma spray coating fused to the exterior of the shell. Polyethylene is mechanically interlocked to the metal shell. Despite the early finite element analysis projections, clinical results have not demonstrated measurably improved fixation with these metal-backed devices. Three-dimensional finite element analysis suggests the possibility that metal backing may cause harmful tensile stresses when eccentric loading of the metal-backed components occurs. In one clinical study, results with a particular metal-backed design acetabular component were inferior to results with an all polyethylene design when both were cemented.

Discussion

Although there have been numerous cement designs presented in the past 30 years, few have had clinical results superior to those of the early smooth surfaced 316 stainless steel Charnley and Exeter designs. However, some data demonstrate comparable or better results when matte-finished stems are inserted using newer cementing techniques. Stems are now available with distal tip centralizers to better achieve adequate cement mantles. Newer cement techniques also allow the surgeon to more predictably obtain adequate cement mantles. The value of a collar on the prosthesis remains controversial, and collared stems have not demonstrated increased clinical success over the initial collarless designs. Similarly, textured, PMMA precoated, sand blasted, or macro interlocking surfaces on the stem may decrease cement stresses; however, no clinical studies have demonstrated superior results using these components. Chrome cobalt or stainless steel (higher modulus) cemented femoral components have outperformed titanium components (lower modulus). Reasons for this difference include the potentially deleterious increase in cement strains and the potential increase in particulate debris associated with the lower modulus material.

Annotated Bibliography

Barrack RL: Modularity of prosthetic implants. *J Am Acad Orthop Surg* 1994;2:16–25.

The advantages and disadvantages of modular prosthetic implants are reviewed. Disadvantages include increased fretting, wear debris, and dissociation, as well as mismatching of components. Advantages include decreasing inventory and allowing additional flexibility in revision surgery for dealing with bone loss or adding screws. Along with increasing modularity of the components there has been an increase in the incidence and extent of bone lysis, rate of polyethylene wear and generation of particulate debris. The extent to which modularity contributes to these problems remains unclear. Optimal design features of modular components include tightening of tolerances to minimize dimensional mismatch, minimizing fretting and corrosion, and hardening by nitriding or nitrogen implantation to improve strength and wear resistance of the Morse taper.

Collier JP, Mayor MB, Jensen RE, et al: Mechanisms of failure of modular prostheses. *Clin Orthop* 1992;285: 129–139.

One hundred eleven acetabular hip prostheses and 139 femoral prostheses, all of modular configuration, were analyzed. Component characteristics found to correlate with early failure included acetabular designs with thin polyethylene bearings, poor fixation of the polyethylene to the metal shell, and geometries that permitted a moment to be applied to the bearing insert, tending to cause it to rotate in the metal shell. Modular femoral components were susceptible to corrosion, and titanium alloy stems joined with cast cobalt alloy heads were at greatest risk for galvanic corrosion. All modular connections of femoral and acetabular components were at risk for dissociation and fretting. Precision machining was recommended to decrease the risks associated with modularity.

Crowninshield RD, Brand RA, Johnston RC, et al: An analysis of femoral component stem design in total hip arthroplasty. *J Bone Joint Surg* 1980;62A:68–78.

This finite element analysis demonstrated a decrease in femoral cement strains when a high modulus femoral component with large proximal stem cross-sectional area and a broad rounded medial surface was inserted.

Ebramzadeh E, Sarmiento A, McKellop HA, et al: The cement mantle in total hip arthroplasty, analysis of long-term radiographic results. *J Bone Joint Surg* 1994; 76A:77–87.

Eight hundred thirty-six cemented femoral stems were reviewed and assessed with survivor analysis. A 2- to 5-mm thick cement mantle in the proximal medial region resulted in better outcome than stems with thicker or thinner cement mantles. Proximal medial cancellous bone should be less than 2 mm. Stems should fill more than half of the medullary canal. More than 5° of varus predisposed to progressive loosening, fracture of the cement, and radiolucent lines at the stem-cement or bone-cement interfaces.

Harris WH: Is it advantageous to strengthen the cement-metal interface and use a collar for cemented femoral components in total hip replacements? *Clin Orthop* 1992;285:67–72.

The mechanism of initiation of loosening of cemented femoral components is debonding at the cement metal interface. Using contemporary instrumentation, collar calcar contact can be achieved regularly and once achieved is well maintained for years. Calcar collar contact in conjunction with pre-coating to improve the cement metal interface and newer cementing techniques contribute to extended longevity of the hip reconstruction.

Joshi AB, Porter ML, Trail IA, et al: Long-term results of charnley low-friction arthroplasty in young patients. *J Bone Surg* 1993;75B:616–623.

Two hundred and eighteen hips in patients aged 40 years or less were reviewed. The mean age at surgery was 32 years. The minimum follow-up was 10 years with a mean of 16 years. Complications occurred in 25 hips (11.5%). Fifteen were revised for a loose cup, eight for a loose femoral stem, four for loosening of both components, three for infection, one for dislocation, and two for removal of trochanteric wires. The probability of implant survival at 20 years was 75% for both components. The probability of survival of the femoral component was 86% at 20 years. Clinical assessment of the 103 patients who returned for review showed 94% with little or no pain. The femoral component had subsided 2 mm or less in 79.5% of 132 hips. In only 4% was subsidence more than 5 mm.

Kelley SS, Fitzgerald RH Jr, Rand JA, et al: A prospective randomized study of a collar vs. a collarless femoral prosthesis. *Clin Orthop* 1993;294:114–122.

Seventy hips were randomly assigned a collared or collarless Harris II prosthesis. The patients were examined at an average of 4.6 years after total hip arthroplasty. At final follow-up, 33 of 38 patients with collared prostheses had no or slight pain, four had moderate pain, and one had severe pain. Twenty-seven of the 32 patients with collarless prostheses had no or slight pain, four had moderate pain, and one had severe pain. The Harris hip score was 89.5 for patients with a collared prosthesis and 86.7 for patients with a collarless prosthesis. Two patients with collared and three with collarless prostheses needed revision for aseptic loosening. An increased frequency and width of radiolucent lines was seen in Gruen zone II of patients with collarless prostheses. There was no statistically significant difference in acetabular radiolucent lines in patients with collared or collarless prostheses. Cement fracture in zone 7 occurred more frequently in the collarless patients. There was also statistically less bone resorption of the medial femoral neck with a collar at average 4.6 years after surgery.

Ling RS: The use of a collar and precoating on cemented femoral stems is unnecessary and detrimental. *Clin Orthop* 1992;285: 73–83.

Evidence is presented from clinical sources that a large collar is not necessary for the transfer of load to the proximal femur in cemented total hip arthroplasty. The potential deleterious side effects of the use of a collar are presented as well as concern over possible problems with the use of pre-coated femoral stems. Problems associated with the collar included debris production and the "calcar pivot" phenomenon, as well as nonphysiologic loading of the cut surface of the femoral neck. Problems associated with pre-coating included a risk of separation from the stem in clinical practice. Concerns about adverse effects on the cement–bone interface were also raised.

Pedersen DR, Crowninshield RD, Brand RA, et al: An axisymmetric model of acetabular components in total hip arthroplasty. *J Biomech* 1982;15:305–315.

This finite element analysis demonstrated decreased acetabular bone and cement strains when a metal-backed component was placed into the acetabulum versus when a nonmetal-backed component was placed.

Rorabeck CH, Bourne RB, Laupacis A, et al: A double-blind study of two hundred fifty cases comparing cemented with cementless total hip arthroplasty: Cost-effectiveness and its impact on health-related quality of life. *Clin Orthop* 1994;298:156–164.

A randomized controlled clinical trial of 250 patients revealed that total hip arthroplasty was an extremely effective intervention with regards to its impact on patient's health-related quality of life, with no difference between cement versus cementless devices at 2 years follow-up examination.

Schulte KR, Callaghan JJ, Kelley SS, et al: The outcome of charnley total hip arthroplasty with cement after a minimum twenty-year follow-up: The results of one surgeon. *J Bone Joint Surg* 1993;75A:961–975.

Three hundred thirty total hip replacements performed by one physician are reviewed at a minimum of 20-year follow-up with the Charnley hip prosthesis and a polished stainless steel stem with a 22.25-mm head. (Average age at index surgery was 65 years.) Ninety-eight hips were followed for 20 years. Eleven hips were revised because of aseptic loosening, three because of loosening with infection, and one because of dislocation. The mean rate of acetabular wear was 0.074 mm per year. After 20 years, 80 of 83 patients were satisfied with their hips and 70 patients continued to live in their own home.

Wroblewski BM, Siney PD: Charnley low-friction arthroplasty in the young patient. *Clin Orthop* 1992;285:45–47.

At an average of 10 years, 4 months after surgery, 1,342 Charnley low friction arthroplasties were reviewed. The patient's average age was 41 years. The clinical results at follow-up remained excellent. Seventy-nine percent were pain free and 11% had no more than occasional discomfort. One hundred forty-one (10.5%) have been revised. Revision for stem loosening was below 1% and revision for socket loosening was also low. There were no stem fractures. A long-term problem was felt to be socket wear with subsequent socket migration.

Classic Bibliography

Agins HJ, Alcock NW, Bansal M, et al: Metallic wear in failed titanium-alloy total hip replacements: A histological and quantitative analysis. *J Bone Joint Surg* 1988;70A:347–356.

Carlsson AS, Gentz CF: Mechanical loosening of the femoral head prosthesis in the Charnley total hip arthroplasty. *Clin Orthop* 1980;147:262–270.

Charnley J (ed): *Low Friction Arthroplasty of the Hip: Theory and Practice.* Berlin, Germany, Springer-Verlag, 1979, 20–24.

Crowninshield RD, Johnston RC, Andrews JG, et al: A biomechanical investigation of the human hip. *J Biomech* 1978;11:75–85.

Crowninshield RD, Tolbert JR: Cement strain measurement surrounding loose and well-fixed femoral component stems. *J Biomed Mater Res* 1983;17:819–828.

Davy DT, Kotzar GM, Brown RH, et al: Telemetric force measurements across the hip after total arthroplasty. *J Bone Joint Surg* 1988;70A:45–50.

Fornasier VL, Cameron HU: The femoral stem/cement interface in total hip replacement. *Clin Orthop* 1976;116:248–252.

Fowler JL, Gie GA, Lee AJ, et al: Experience with the Exeter total hip replacement since 1970. *Orthop Clin North Am* 1988;19:477–489.

Harrigan TP, Kareh JA, Harris WH: Abstract: A failure criterion based on crack initiation at pores in cement applied to the loosening of femoral stems. Proceedings of the Society for Biomaterials 16th Annual Meeting, 1990, p 52.

Huddleston HD: Femoral lysis after cemented hip arthroplasty. *J Arthroplasty* 1988;3:285–297.

Jacobs J, Urban R, Kienapfel R, et al: Particulate associated endosteal osteolysis in titanium base alloy cementless total hip replacement. Presented at the ASTM Symposium on Particulate Biomaterials, San Antonio, 1990.

Maloney WJ, Jasty M, Bragdon CR, et al: Abstract: Long term histological evaluation of the bone cement interface: An autopsy study. Proceedings of the Society for Biomaterials 16th Annual Meeting, 1990, p 119.

Markolf KL, Amstutz HC: A comparative experimental study of stresses in femoral total hip replacement components: The effects of prosthesis orientation and acrylic fixation. *J Biomech* 1976;9:73–79.

McCoy TH, Salvati EA, Ranawat CS, et al: A fifteen-year follow-up study of one hundred Charnley low-friction arthroplasties. *Orthop Clin North Am* 1988;19:467–476.

McKellop H, Grogan W, Ebramzadeh E, at al: Abstract: Metal: Metal wear in metal-plastic prosthetic joints.

Proceedings of the Society for Biomaterials 16th Annual Meeting, 1990, p 114.

Paul JP, McGrouther DA: Forces transmitted at the hip and knee joint of normal and disabled persons during a range of activities. *Acta Orthop Belg* 1975;41(suppl 1): S78–S88.

Robinson RP, Lovell TP, Green TM, et al: Early femoral component loosening in DF-80 total hip arthroplasty. *J Arthroplasty* 1989;4:55–64.

Stauffer RN: Ten-year follow-up study of total hip replacement. *J Bone Joint Surg* 1982;64A:983–990.

Thomas BJ, Salvati EA, Small RD: The CAD hip arthroplasty: Five to ten-year follow-up. *J Bone Joint Surg* 1986;68A:640–646.

Willert HG, Bretram H, Buchhorn GH: Osteolysis in alloarthroplasty of the hip: The role of ultra-high molecular weight polythylene wear particles. *Clin Orthop* 1990;258:95–107.

18

Aseptic Loosening in Total Hip Arthroplasty

Introduction

Osteolysis and aseptic loosening have become the major problems limiting the longevity and clinical success of total hip arthroplasty (THA). As early as 1968, Sir John Charnley described a lytic lesion around a cemented femoral component and attributed this finding to possible infection. Subsequent assessment of cemented components noted periprosthetic radiolucencies and endosteal lytic lesions as a common finding, and it became apparent that a process of aseptic loosening was occurring. Early reviews found symptomatic loosening of the socket in up to 12% of patients and femoral loosening requiring revision arthroplasty in as many as 20%. Series that included radiographic assessment of loosening as well as reoperation had even higher rates. The early failure of cemented femoral components was followed by a disheartening exponential rate of late loosening of the acetabulum. The common denominator incorrectly seemed to be an adverse reaction to acrylic cement. Consequently, the fear of failure from "cement disease" prompted improvements in bone preparation, prosthetic design, and cementing technique. In addition, it prompted, in the last decade, the increasing use of uncemented femoral and acetabular components.

Time has proven, however, that aseptic loosening and osteolysis are not unique to the cemented hip. These findings have been reported in both stable and unstable cemented and uncemented implants and remain a major source of pain and failure in THA. This chapter will describe the current modes by which aseptic failure occurs in cemented and uncemented THA.

Radiographic Findings of Aseptic Loosening

Cemented Acetabular Component

Acetabular loosening is often a relatively late finding in patients with a cemented socket. Whereas femoral component loosening occurs at a linear rate, cemented cup loosening increases exponentially after the tenth postoperative year. Radiographic findings in loosened sockets include radiolucencies and demarcations at the cement–bone interface as well as migration and tilting of the component. Migration of the component or a crack in the surrounding cement mantle indicates definite loosening, whereas impending loosening is heralded by a continuous radiolucent line of 2 mm or more.

Radiolucencies of the cemented cup are described in three radiographic zones as seen on the anteroposterior

(AP) view. Zone 1 corresponds to the superior 45° arc, zone 2 to the middle 90°, and zone 3 to the inferomedial arc. In a study that correlated radiographic and intraoperative findings, a continuous radiolucent line, regardless of width, correlated with a loose socket 94% of the time, and a radiolucent line around two thirds of the component corresponded with loose sockets in 74%. If the line was in zones 1 and 3 only, the loosening rate was 7%.

It has been estimated that routine radiography could accurately predict the presence of socket loosening an average of 63% to 69% of the time. Special views improve the accuracy considerably. In a retrieval study, the commonly used AP view of the socket underrepresented the radiolucent zone. Oblique projections were necessary to visualize complete radiolucencies; the obturator oblique view showed the maximum extent and thickness of the radiolucent zone particularly well. In a 5-year follow-up series of 81 cemented cups, 42% were loose on the AP view alone, and the obturator oblique view increased the detection of radiolucency by 15%.

The use of intra-articular contrast improves the accuracy of predicting socket loosening to an average rate of 69% to 96%. Socket loosening is defined as contrast at the cement–bone interface in zones 1 and 2, zones 2 and 3, or all zones, or as a rim of contrast greater than 2 mm in any zone. These criteria are associated with intraoperative findings of loosening in at least 90% of cases. The contrast-enhanced radiographic study is improved by the digital subtraction technique, high-injection pressures, or inclusion of a postambulation view. Nonetheless, careful analysis of the plain radiograph and often the arthrogram are usually needed to make a definite diagnosis of a loose cup.

Uncemented Acetabular Component

Radiolucencies at the implant–bone interface, component migration, or implant mechanical failure are the major radiographic considerations in determining loosening of the uncemented socket. The significance of radiolucent lines around the uncemented socket is uncertain, but a static line may be less worrisome than a progressive demarcation, which traditionally signifies cup loosening. Migration of greater than 5 mm, on the other hand, is a definite sign of component loosening and can be quantified on serial films. Migration may be associated with broken transacetabular screws, shedding of the porous surface, or implant fracture. Vertical migration is measured by the distance between a perpendicular line from the center of the hip and a line through the bottom of the teardrop. Horizontal migration is gauged by the change in horizontal distance along this line, from the base of the teardrop to the perpendicular line from the hip center. Component position on follow-up films of pelvic rotation should be compared to increase accuracy of the evaluation.

In one study, a series of 83 porous-coated sockets was reviewed at a minimum of 5 years after primary THA fixed with screws. Although no migration was noted, 49 components (59%) had new radiolucent lines at 2 years, and in 27% of these, the lines progressed after an additional 2 years. No component was surrounded by a continuous radiolucency. One component developed an area of osteolysis around a fixation screw. The authors suggested that implantation technique (line-to-line reaming versus press fitting) may be an important factor in the longevity of uncemented acetabular prostheses, and that an initial peripheral gap may herald progressive radiolucency. The clinical significance of this gap has yet to be determined.

Acetabular and Pelvic Osteolysis

Acetabular osteolysis and pelvic osteolysis are noted in radiographically stable and loose cups, both cemented and uncemented. Several radiographic patterns have been described. Bone resorption around cemented cups commonly occurs as a progressive linear radiolucency at the cement–bone interface. Recently, central infiltrative, cystic lesions have been seen in porous-coated acetabular components inserted without cement. This study included both titanium and chrome-cobalt implants, with polyethylene liners 8 mm thick or less and most having 32-mm heads. The average time to diagnosis of osteolysis was 65 months, and despite significant destruction of bone, most patients were asymptomatic. The lesions were expansile, destructive, and ballooning into the trabecular bone of the supra-acetabular ilium. No component had a complete radiolucency at the implant–bone interface, and routine radiographs usually underestimated the actual bone loss found at revision surgery. Despite artifacts generated by the metal, the authors found computed tomography (CT) scanning to be helpful in preoperatively assessing the extent of bone loss in patients with pelvic osteolysis.

Cemented Femoral Components

Plain radiographs predict loosening with greater accuracy for femoral components (84% to 92%) than for acetabular components. Zones of loosening for cemented femoral components have been described. On the AP view of the hip, the seven zones progress from zone 1 at the greater trochanter through zone 4 at the tip of the prosthesis to zone 7 at the medial calcar. A lateral view provides seven additional zones for evaluation, with zone 8 anteriorly at the medial cortex and zone 11 at the tip of the stem progressing to zone 14 posterosuperiorly.

A classification of loosening has been proposed for cemented femoral components. Definite loosening is represented by migration or subsidence of the component, a radiolucency at the metal–cement interface, stem bending or fracture, or cement fracture. Probable loosening is defined as a complete radiolucent zone at the bone–cement interface on any view. A cemented femoral component is possibly loose if surrounded 50% to 100% by a radiolucency.

Four modes of loosening of the cemented stem have been described based on the pattern of loss of acrylic support as defined on radiographs. In the "piston mode," the entire stem is loose and has migrated. "Medial midstem pivot" is shown by complete loosening with motion of the stem in the proximal–medial and distal–lateral directions. In the "calcar-pivot mode," the stem has a fixed proximal center of rotation, allowing rocking of the loosened distal stem in a windshield-wiper fashion. In the "cantilever mode," the distal stem is well fixed, but proximal fixation is inadequate, allowing eventual component deformation or fracture. These radiographic patterns are useful in understanding the mechanical determinants of cemented stem failure.

The significance of radiolucent lines in cemented femoral components is questioned in several reports. In reports published in 1989 and 1992, retrieved cemented femoral components were stable despite the presence of radiolucency. Some radiolucent lines were interpreted as representing internal bone remodeling. The cement mantle had become surrounded by a dense shell of new bone apposed to the cement, apparently causing the endosteal cortex to become cancellous and thin. These osteoporotic changes appeared as a radiolucency. On retrieval, the remodeling-induced radiolucencies were not associated with intervening fibrous tissue at the cement–bone interface. In contrast, separations at the cement–metal interface were associated with cement-mantle deficiencies, fragmentation, fibrous membrane formation, and osteolytic lesions, with subsequent destruction of the cement–bone interface. Several hallmarks of radiolucencies that indicate a loosened prosthesis rather than natural bone remodeling are progression of the radiolucent zone on serial radiographs, a continuous radiolucent zone greater than or equal to 2 mm, and migration of the component within the cement mantle, shown by a distinct line at the prosthesis–cement interface.

Nuclear medicine studies are often used to evaluate the painful cemented THA. Following cemented THA, most technetium nuclear scans will return to baseline after 6 to 12 months. But even in the asymptomatic, stable cemented hip, the Tc^{99} may show definite, increased uptake in 10% of patients. Radioisotope studies have been found to be more accurate in the detection of femoral component loosening than acetabular loosening. In several series, sensitivity and specificity have ranged from 70% to 90% in evaluation of the femoral component, with an overall accuracy of 89% as opposed to 77% for acetabular loosening. Although the increased uptake seen in a positive study represents increased bone turnover, the result does not differentiate aseptic loosening from infection or other causes of increased osseous metabolism.

Uncemented Femoral Components

With the most commonly used uncemented femoral stems, fixation is achieved using either a proximally porous-coated stem with metaphyseal fit or an extensively porous-coated straight stem with diaphyseal fit. The radiographic finding that most reliably distinguishes an unstable uncemented femoral stem in any system is implant migration and subsidence. In addition, specific radiographic findings have been associated with aseptic loosening for various prosthetic designs. In the anatomically shaped stems with porous coating on the proximal one third, subsidence greater than 2 mm, cortical hypertrophy at the stem tip, and cancellous hypertrophy (platform sclerosis) at the tip have been associated with failure. Based on radiographic and retrieval experience, the extensively porous-coated, straight-stem, anatomic medullary locking (AML, Depuy, Warsaw, IN) type of prosthesis, which is intended for diaphyseal stability, is stabilized by bony ingrowth rather than fibrous ingrowth. Migration of the stem is a reliable indicator of instability. Additional signs of instability include widening circumferential radiolucencies adjacent to the porous surface, divergent lines of demarcation, shedding of particulate porous coating, absence of stress shielding, calcar hypertrophy, and an intramedullary pedestal at the tip of an unstable stem. With this prosthetic design, investigators have found that radiographic findings reliably predict the likelihood of stable bony or fibrous fixation.

In the evaluation of uncemented components, arthrography is associated with high rates of false-positive and false-negative results. However, arthroscintigraphy, wherein a radioisotope is injected into the joint to produce scintigraphic images, is reported to improve sensitivity.

The results of nuclear isotope scintigraphy in evaluation of the uncemented femoral component vary with stem design and the extent of porous coating. For patients with painful hips, a technetium scan may be helpful as an initial study. Although this technique is nonspecific in differentiating septic from aseptic loosening, infection is unlikely in patients with negative findings. Technetium scanning in conjunction with additional isotope studies, gallium or indium for example, can increase the value of radioisotope studies in the differential diagnosis.

Finally, the dynamic CT scan is being investigated as a means of quantifying loosening of the uncemented femoral component. With this modality, motion of the femoral component is measured after proximal and distal cuts have been obtained with maximal internal and external rotation of the limb.

Incidence of Aseptic Loosening

Acetabular Components

Loosening is reported as a late finding in the long-term (> 10 years) follow-up of cemented sockets, increasing exponentially after 10 years. In the report of a follow-up series of 680 cemented cups, radiographic parameters of early and late loosening were described. Early loosening evidenced by cup migration occurred within 10 years of surgery and was associated with a preoperative acetabular deficiency, congenital dysplasia, fracture, or protrusio. Late loosening was more commonly associated with radiolucent lines of more than 2 mm in all zones than with cup migration. A minimum 20-year follow-up of 330 cemented total hip arthroplasties in 262 patients was reported. In the group of 94 hips that survived at least 20 years, definitive radiographic signs of loosening, including migration and complete radiolucency, were present in 18%. Eight percent of surviving sockets were revised due to aseptic loosening. When the rates of radiographic loosening were combined with loosening confirmed at revision surgery, 22% of surviving acetabula had loosened.

At intermediate (5 to 10 years) follow-up, uncemented sockets generally have a low incidence of loosening and almost universally have negligible rates of revision. A 2-year follow-up of porous-coated anatomic (PCA, Howmedica, Rutherford, NJ) cups found an 18% incidence of bead loosening, with progressive radiolucencies in 8%. Later follow-up (5 to 7 years) showed radiographic evidence of loosening in 6%, with 3% requiring revision. Other investigators also have reported finding progressive radiolucent lines, but significantly lower rates of revision. For example, after a minimum of 5 years, progressive radiolucent lines in 22 of 83 porous-coated hemispherical Harris-Galante (HG, Zimmer, Warsaw, IN) cups reamed to size (line-to-line) with screw fixation were reported. No continuous radiolucencies were found, and no components required revision. The significance of the radiolucencies in these clinically well-functioning prostheses is unknown and will require further evaluation.

Outcome differs substantially with various designs of uncemented sockets. For example, although threaded cups provided excellent initial stability experimentally, approximately 30% have loosened. Unlike conical, cylindrical, or ellipsoidal cups, hemispheric cups transmit force physiologically, preserve the medial wall, and cause minimal iatrogenic bone loss. Because the hemispheric component placed in a bed reamed to size does not provide intrinsic stability, underreaming, screw fixation, or both, are required.

In summary, the cemented all-polyethylene cup, although continuing to function satisfactorily in most cases, has both a high rate of late revisions and a significantly higher incidence of radiographic loosening. Moreover, these rates have not been improved with either metal backing or improved cementing technique in the socket. In comparison, the uncemented socket has relatively better radiographic results at intermediate follow-up, with a significantly lower rate of revision for aseptic failure.

Femoral Components

Early radiographic studies of cemented femoral components identified significant rates of loosening, notably, 20% at 5 years and as high as 40% at 10 years. In young, active patients, the loosening rate approached 60%, with 20% requiring revision.

The use of improved second-generation cementing techniques, specifically canal plugging, careful curettage of the canal, lavage, drying, and retrograde delivery with a cement gun has reduced the reported incidence of femoral loosening from 30% to 40% to 3% or less. When these second-generation techniques were used, 97% of these components were rigidly fixed at 11 years. Moreover, the incidence of postoperative pain has fallen from 19.1% to 6.8%. With a follow-up of more than 20 years, one author found loosening in only 7% of surviving cemented Charnley femoral components. Some would consider the longevity provided by an excellent cement mantle, achieved with careful cementing technique, to be the standard for comparisons of other femoral fixation.

The introduction of additional modifications constitute third-generation cementing techniques. These include a roughened surface in some areas of the stem, precoating with a thin layer of polymethylmethacrylate (PMMA), porosity reduction of the cement through centrifugation or vacuum mixing, pressurization of the column after delivery, and centralization. The contribution of these modifications to the durability of cemented fixation has yet to be determined.

Femoral lysis and associated loosening have been reported for different designs of uncemented first-generation femoral components as well. The PCA used a curved, cast chromium-cobalt alloy (vitallium) stem with a proximal circumferentially beaded surface. After 5 to 7 years, 15% of patients with these implants had mild thigh pain, 3% had progressive femoral loosening, and 5% to 8% subsidence; overall, this design provided at least 90% good to excellent clinical results. The Harris-Galante system, using a forged, straight titanium alloy stem with mesh pads on the proximal anterior, posterior, and medial surfaces, resulted in a 28% rate of mild thigh pain, a 9% incidence of femoral loosening, and an ultimate revision rate of 4%. Straight diaphyseal fitted stems are reported to have a 10-year clinical survival of greater than 90% and a radiographic loosening rate of 9%. Intermediate follow-up of the AML femoral implants, a cast cobalt-chrome alloy stem with an extensive circumferential sintered porous surface designed for diaphyseal fit, has noted mild thigh pain in 14% of patients. The fully porous-coated design is reported to have a lower incidence of thigh pain. The overall failure rate in follow-up of 411 patients is 1.4%, including three revisions for symptomatic loosening and three stems with radiographic signs of instability. This success rate rivals those of second-generation cemented stems.

Mechanisms of Aseptic Loosening

Acetabular Components

Patient characteristics associated with reduced longevity of the acetabular components include young age, active life style, increased body weight, and female gender. Several other preoperative conditions also are associated with high rates of acetabular loosening, including developmental dysplasia, rheumatoid arthritis, acetabular fracture, and revision of a fused hip to THA. Less significant correlations also have been found with preoperative protrusio, avascular necrosis, and Paget disease. These risk factors may affect both the cemented and uncemented sockets.

The relevance of cup orientation and loosening is controversial. Certainly, orientation of the implanted socket determines the direction of force transmission to the pelvis and contributes to stability and range of motion of the joint. However, there was disparity in the results of several series in which a correlation was sought between orientation and loosening. The more important factor seems to be containment of the prosthetic component within the bony acetabulum. Well-seated cups with full containment were consistently associated with lower incidences of radiolucencies in several series.

In general, the use of improved cementing techniques for fixation of the socket has not reduced the rate of acetabular loosening. In the early 1980s, finite element analyses indicated that metal backing of cemented polyethylene sockets would reduce strain in trabecular bone, cement, and polyethylene. The expected outcome was better force transmission and decreased polyethylene cold flow, resulting in less loosening of the cup. This postulate has not been supported by radiographic or clinical data. That is, reducing strain distribution does not reduce failure rates in sockets. In short, various recent modifications in cementing technique and metal backing of the cemented socket have shown no benefit when compared to the results of the all-polyethylene cemented cup.

These observations led to the investigation of the biologic aspects of socket failure, namely, the progressive resorption of bone adjacent to the cup. In an autopsy retrieval study, acetabular specimens were examined radiologically and histologically and tested for stability. The authors of this study found progressive, three-dimensional resorption of bone, beginning peripherally at the socket margin and progressing toward the dome. Histologic analysis of the transition area in cemented cups, which corresponded to radiolucent areas, revealed thick membranes filled with macrophages, occasional giant cells, and particulate extracellular and intracellular polyethylene. The cutting wedge of active bone resorption represented an area in which small polyethylene particles migrate along the cement–bone interface, inciting macrophage proliferation and activation and, ultimately, osteoclastic bone resorption. This set of retrieved specimens helped to clarify the process of cemented socket loosening, from the initiating events of peripheral bone resorption to gross loosening and failure. In a study of membranes obtained at revision surgery from the cement–bone interface of aseptically loosened cemented polyethylene acetabular components, immunohistochemical techniques and in situ hybridization were used to demonstrate that potent cytokines are produced at the interface membrane. In this study, abundant particulate debris was present in all specimens. Macrophages were the predominant cell type, in association with fibroblasts. The in situ hybridization technique by showing messenger RNA specific for cytokines (interleukin-1β [IL-1β] and platelet-derived growth factor [PDGF]) demonstrated that these factors were produced at the membrane and that macrophages were responsible for their production. The above studies supported a biologic, rather than mechanical, mode of cemented acetabular loosening.

In contrast, the uncemented socket has provided excellent intermediate results. In an attempt to understand the mechanism of acetabular component loosening, several series have looked at the familiar signs of failure, namely migration and progressive radiolucencies, as well as extent of bony ingrowth.

A recent article reported autopsy findings of nine well-functioning porous-coated implants in which radiography significantly underestimated gap areas and overestimated bony apposition. Bone ingrowth occupied a mean 32% (range, 3% to 84%) of the component surface area. Histologically, the radiolucent areas consisted of dense, well-organized fibrous tissue with no evidence of granuloma formation or particulate debris.

An additional autopsy retrieval study of porous cups reamed to size and fixed with screws revealed bone ingrowth over an average surface area of 12%, with fibrous tissue in the remaining areas. The pattern of bone ingrowth was influenced by the presence of screws, with 50% more bone ingrowth at filled screw holes as compared to unfilled holes. The amount of metal debris was similar for filled or unfilled screw holes. Generally, the degree of radiolucency was inversely proportional to bone ingrowth.

In a series of 83 porous-coated HG acetabular components implanted with line-to-line reaming and fixed by screws, no migration was noted, but peripheral gaps present at implantation were associated with a greater chance of progressive radiolucency at 5 years. This is in comparison to a series of 122 press-fit acetabular components in which initial areas of noncontact at the dome were mostly resolved at 2 years. When data from both series were reviewed, zone 2 gaps tended to resolve, whereas peripheral gaps persisted. In addition, a press-fit insertion resulted in significantly higher percentages of pristine interfaces at final follow-up, which suggested a limitation to the ingress of particulate debris.

Although multiple factors may contribute to failure of the uncemented acetabular component, including inadequate preparation of the bony bed, poor initial fixation, or malposition, the findings of persistent and progressive radiolucencies at intermediate follow-up may represent early resorption of bone in reaction to particulate debris or motion. Particulate debris may also gain access to the interface membrane through peripheral implant–bone gaps or the retroacetabular space through screw holes in the metal backing. Maximizing peripheral contact through press fitting may be advantageous in limiting the ingress of particulate debris, while on the other hand, a

tight peripheral fit without concentric seating may allow debris through unfilled screw holes to initiate bone resorption in that area.

The volume of wear debris in the uncemented socket correlates with several factors, including the smoothness of the convex surface of the shell, the tolerance between the high density polyethylene insert and the shell, the stability of the insert within the shell, and polyethylene thickness. Metallic debris was noted mainly around loose implants; a possible source is fretting between the screws and shell. This report and others have led to the increased use of a solid metal-backed cup without screw holes.

In summary, early studies support the mechanism of failure of both cemented and uncemented acetabular components to be a host response to particulate debris at the implant–bone interface with subsequent bone resorption and osteolysis. Further studies will be needed to better understand the process.

Femoral Component

Aseptic loosening rates for cemented femoral components implanted for 10 years have improved from 30% to 40% in early studies to 1.3% to 3% in more recent follow-ups. The reductions in loosening have been attributed to improvements in stem design, as well as to improved cementing techniques. To elucidate the mechanisms that initiate loosening of cemented stems, femora from 16 asymptomatic patients were retrieved 2 weeks to 17 years after arthroplasty and were examined histologically, radiographically, and mechanically. All showed varying degrees of radiolucency at the cement–bone interface, which was generally intact with rare areas of fibrous tissue. Separations at the cement–prosthesis interface were common in areas of highest strain during activities, usually at the most proximal and distal ends of the prosthesis. Debonding at the cement–prosthesis interface was a frequent early finding, and later follow-up showed progression to fractures of the cement mantle. These fractures were both circumferential near the cement–metal interface and radial extending from the interface into the cement. In addition, fractures initiated at sharp corners of the prostheses or in deficient areas of the mantle.

A more recent study analyzed the quality of the cement mantle in relation to long-term outcome of 836 cemented femoral components over 21 years. Better outcomes correlated with the finding that less than 2 mm of cancellous bone remained in the proximal medial region in association with a 2- to 5-mm thick cement mantle. Better radiographic results were obtained when stems filled one half or more of the canal. Signs of failure, including radiolucent lines and cement fracture, occurred more often in stems oriented in 5° of varus, as compared to neutral or valgus alignment. This study indicates that appropriate stem size and implantation technique may prolong the longevity of cemented stems.

The value of using a precoated or a roughened stem surface to strengthen the cement-prosthesis interface and thus prevent debonding has been examined. Data from several studies indicate that precoating strengthens the weak bond between cement and metal precoating and that a roughened surface protects fatigue failure of this interface in shear. In an additional study, the torsional fatigue strength was tested using 15 specimens both with and without PMMA precoating. The precoating resulted in a statistically significant increase of the interfacial shear strength between the cement and metal. In contrast, a smooth-surfaced or polished component would allow slip at the cement–prosthesis interface and permit settling of the component while maintaining the cement in compression. The polished, tapered, collarless stem theoretically increases compression of the cement, and decreases shear at the metal–PMMA–bone interfaces, as well as within the cement. The ultimate resolution of the controversy between polished or augmented stem surfaces is not apparent, and the relevance of surface treatments to the improved longevity of the cemented stem has yet to be proven.

Multiple factors contribute to the potential for aseptic loosening of the uncemented femoral component. The process involves the interaction of mechanical and biologic factors, including implant material and design, quality of initial fixation, the tissue response to the implant and wear particles, and the bone's response to the postoperative change in applied stress. Theories of loosening include micromotion, variable contributions of material failure and wear debris, stress-shielding, and osteolysis.

Several studies have attempted to describe bone ingrowth relative to implant micromotion. In a study in which porous-coated cobalt-chromium stems were used, bone ingrowth occurred when relative displacements were less than 28 μm but was inhibited with motion greater than 150 μm, the latter resulting in fibrous fixation. A finite element model was developed to investigate the relationship between micromotion and the extent of porous coating. In this study, proximal porous coating of as little as one third of the femoral stem resulted in significantly less micromotion in all regions of the stem. Extending the coating did not improve stability in this model. Other authors, however, found the amount of micromotion to be directly related to the extent of porous coating in an autopsy retrieval study of 14 AML prostheses under simulated physiologic loading. When ingrown stems were compared, micromotion was greatest at the uncoated portion of the stem, with more interface motion at the tips of less-extensively coated stems. The greatest amount of micromotion was noted in the implant stabilized by fibrous versus bony ingrowth.

The contribution of the host response to particulate debris in loosening of the uncemented stem has recently received significant attention. Wear occurs partly because implant surfaces have irregularities and variable degrees of hardness. High stresses occur at contact areas of surface irregularities, and the consequent erosion, mostly from the softer material, produces wear particles. The mechanisms of wear-debris production are described as abrasion, adhesion, fatigue, and third-body wear. Abrasion depends on contact stress, surface hardness, and finish (roughness). Surface hardness may be increased, and abrasion wear reduced, by treatments such as nitriding or ion implantation, for example, in titanium components. Adhesive wear occurs when the interatomic forces between surfaces surpass the intrinsic molecular forces of the material, causing material to adhere to the opposing surface. This mechanism allows ultra-high molecular weight polyethylene (UHMWPE) to adhere to the harder bearing surface and, ultimately, to be shed into the effective joint space. High contact stresses can overcome the fatigue strength of a surface, causing subsurface stress that leads to crack formation and the production of wear debris. The third-body wear phenomenon occurs when particulate debris acts as a stress concentrator on another surface, abrading and generating additional debris.

Metal debris, PMMA, polyethylene, various contaminants, and materials used in the preparation of components provide the materials of biologically active wear debris, which incites a host macrophage response. One author noted that cellular response varied with particle quantity, size, and composition. In a retrieval study of membranes from 11 titanium-alloy stems retrieved an average of 62 months after arthroplasty, three major types of debris were documented. The major contribution to debris was from polyethylene, followed by calcium-phosphate rich particles and titanium fragments.

The predominant particle isolated from biologically active periprosthetic membranes is polyethylene. Various studies have estimated polyethylene wear by comparing the linear measurement of the polyethylene on serial radiographs. In early studies, an average of 1.2-mm wear at 10 years was reported. Another author measured wear in retrieved specimens at revision surgery and found the range of 0.017 to 0.52 mm/yr (mean, 0.19 mm/yr), which correlated well with measurements on radiographs. In a recent study, average wear was reported to be 0.13 mm/yr, with increased wear noted in men younger than 50 years old and subjects weighing more than 80 kg. All of these studies were of Charnley THAs with 22.25-mm femoral heads. Femoral head size has a well-documented correlation with polyethylene wear. The smaller (22 mm) heads show a higher rate of penetration into the cup, resulting in more linear wear, than the larger (32 mm) heads. However, the larger head generates greater volumetric wear owing to the larger articulating surface area, and it is a significant cause of wear-debris induced loosening and bone loss. Other authors examined 64 membranes retrieved from failed cementless porous-coated cobalt-chromium and titanium implants, as well as failed endoprostheses without UHMWPE. A significant finding was that the presence of polyethylene evoked a more intense histiocytic and giant-cell response as compared to the membranes retrieved from the nonpolyethylene-bearing endoprostheses.

Several investigations have addressed the issue of particle size in relation to host response. In one study, membranes retrieved from cemented and uncemented hip and knee prostheses were compared. Small polyethylene particles, generally less than 5 μm, were retrieved from hip membranes, particularly the uncemented group. These particles were contained within macrophages, as compared to larger (10 to 100 μm) particles retrieved from knee membranes, and were associated with a giant-cell response.

The significance of particle size has also been investigated in the cemented hip system. In a recent study, the significance of PMMA particle size was related to macrophage phagocytosis, cell toxicity, and release of inflammatory mediators that resulted in bone resorption and prosthetic loosening. In summary, retrieved tissue from the interface of loose cemented femoral components showed that particles small enough to be phagocytosed (1 to 12 μm) correlated with bone resorption. The investigators also prepared an in vitro model and thereby demonstrated that the phagocytosis of particles smaller than 12 μm resulted in cell toxicity and the production of tumor necrosis factor (TNF). Larger particles did not have this effect.

Metallic particles are also noted in periprosthetic tissues, most commonly from loose implants. These may result from fretting between the metallic implant and adjacent bone or cement surface or between acetabular fixation screws and metal cup backing. Another possible cause is burnishing at the cup and liner interface. The gradual degradation of metals through the chemical attack that occurs in corrosion is another source of metal debris.

The stresses normally experienced by the femur are reduced by transfer through the stiffer prosthesis, thereby causing the bone to adapt by reduction of its mass, via either subperiosteal resorption (external remodeling) or cancellization of the endosteal surface (internal remodeling). Important determinants include stem stiffness and the extent and location of porous coatings, with stem stiffness being the most significant factor. A predictable correlation has been noted between overall bone loss and bone-density reductions in the greater trochanter. Stress-shielding is noted with cemented stems but appears to be more prevalent around larger-diameter, extensively porous-coated stems with a high modulus of elasticity.

An additional manifestation of periprosthetic bone loss in patients with cemented and uncemented systems is localized or diffuse osteolysis. This osteolysis involves periacetabular as well as proximal femoral metaphyseal and diaphyseal cortical bone. Osteolysis was first noted early on in loose cemented stems. Later, focal osteolysis in cemented stems that showed no radiographic signs of loosening was described. In one study, the time to osteolysis ranged from 40 to 168 months, and in 60% of subjects, the area of osteolysis was related to deficiencies in the cement mantle. These and other investigators also described focal osteolytic lesions in radiographically stable uncemented femoral stems.

The histologic findings are similar in loose cemented and uncemented prostheses. A synovial-like membrane forms at the interface between implant and bone or bone and cement in reaction to particulate debris. Macrophage recruitment and proliferation are stimulated, resulting in phagocytosis and the release of cell mediators and cytokines. In general, cytokines result in tissue proliferation (eg, fibrous tissue) or in increased secretory capacity of cells. The relevant cell mediators include PDGF, IL-1, and TNF. IL-1 and TNF are produced primarily by macrophage membranes. PDGF may be produced by macrophages, fibroblasts, or osteoblasts. These probably act by both direct stimulation of osteoclasts and indirect inhibition of osteoblasts, thereby leading to bone resorption. Authors compared the cytokine activity of membranes retrieved from failed uncemented THA with and without focal osteolysis. The membranes of the group with osteolysis revealed more macrophages and small polyethylene particles, as well as increased activity of IL-1, IL-6, and TNF. The authors postulate that these cytokines contribute to osteolysis in failed uncemented hip arthroplasties.

Summary

Aseptic loosening is the prevailing cause of failure that necessitates revision of THA. Clinically significant loosening and osteolysis occur in both stable and radiographically unstable cemented and uncemented components. The mechanism of aseptic acetabular loosening may be the biologic response to particulate wear debris in both the cemented and uncemented constructs. Biologically active wear debris may be produced by each component of the prosthesis, including those parts made of metal, PMMA, or polyethylene. Particulate debris is distributed throughout the effective joint space and may migrate far from the synovial cavity even in well-fixed implants, leading to the release of cytokines and inflammatory mediators, a granulomatous response, and osteolysis.

Improvements in cement technique have had little effect on the acetabular side, but have significantly improved the radiographic appearance and performance of the cemented stem, thereby providing durable, long-term fixation. Failure of the cemented stem is related to component malposition and deficiencies of the cement mantle. One theory holds that cemented stem failure is initiated by debonding at the cement–metal interface. Whether precoating or other augmentation of the stem surface is beneficial has yet to be determined.

The femoral component inserted without cement is also subject to failure through an interaction of mechanical and biologic factors. Whether designed for metaphyseal or diaphyseal fixation, achieving rigid stability at the time of implantation to optimize bony ingrowth is of utmost importance.

A current emphasis of research concerning aseptic loosening is the contribution of the host biologic response. In vitro studies have investigated the role of PMMA, metallic debris, and other materials. Many authors hypothesize that this debris may stimulate membrane formation around prostheses, providing not only a biologically active membrane, but a potential conduit for other materials.

The production of and biologic response to particulate debris are believed to be significant components of aseptic loosening and failure of THA. Improved implant longevity will be the result of mechanical and material innovations achieved with better understanding of and the ability to affect the biologic host response.

Annotated Bibliography

Callaghan JJ: The clinical results and basic science of total hip arthroplasty with porous-coated prostheses. *J Bone Joint Surg* 1993;75A:299–310.

This is a comprehensive history of the development of porous-coated implants for biologic fixation in hip arthroplasty. This includes an extensive review of the science and clinical results of both femoral and acetabular porous-coated components.

Chiba J, Rubash HE, Kim KJ, et al: The characterization of cytokines in the interface tissue obtained from failed cementless total hip arthroplasty with and without femoral osteolysis. *Clin Orthop* 1994;300:304–312.

The histologic, biochemical, and immunohistologic characteristics of interface membranes retrieved from failed cementless total hip arthroplasty were studied. Membranes from hips that showed evidence of focal osteolysis also were associated with an increased number of macrophages, small particles of polyethylene debris, and increased activity level of interleukin-1 (IL-1), tumor necrosis factor (TNF), and IL-6. The authors suggest that these cytokines may play a role in focal femoral osteolysis in failed cementless hip prostheses.

Collier JP, Mayor MB, Jensen RE, et al: Mechanisms of failure of modular prostheses. *Clin Orthop* 1992;285:129–139.

Two hundred fifty modular hip prostheses were examined after retrieval. The authors correlate prostheses design and material factor that may lead to early radiologic and clinical failure.

Ebramzadeh E, Sarmiento A, McKellop HA, et al: The cement mantle in total hip arthroplasty: Analysis of long-term radiographic results. *J Bone Joint Surg* 1994;76A:77–87.

Eight hundred and thirty-six cemented femoral components were assessed by survival analysis over a 21-year period. Characteristics of canal preparation, cement mantle and stem size, shape, and position are identified that correlate with improved long-term results.

Engh CA, Massin P, Suthers KE: Roentgenographic assessment of the biologic fixation of porous-surfaced femoral components. *Clin Orthop* 1990:257;107–128.

Radiographic assessment of the anatomic medullary locking femoral prosthesis is a reliable indicator of the state of fixation of the prosthesis and stability. Radiographic findings and signs of instability are described.

Engh CA, O'Connor D, Jasty M, et al: Quantification of implant micromotion, strain shielding, and bone resorption with porous-coated anatomic medullary locking femoral prostheses. *Clin Orthop* 1992;285:13–29.

A retrieval study of 14 anatomic medullary locking prostheses addresses micromotion and relation to extent of porous coating and bony ingrowth and the resultant quantity and extent of stress shielding and resultant bone loss in the proximal femur.

Engh CA, Zettl-Schaffer KF, Kukita Y, et al: Histological and radiographic assessment of well functioning porous-coated acetabular components: A human postmortem retrieval study. *J Bone Joint Surg* 1993;75A:814–824.

The radiography and histology of nine well-functioning porous-coated acetabular components retrieved at autopsy are compared. Bony ingrowth was noted over an average area of 32% of the components and in most cases was overestimated by radiographs.

Evans BG, Cuckler JM: Evaluation of the painful total hip arthroplasty. *Orthop Clin North Am* 1992;23:303–311.

An algorithm including history, physical exam, laboratory, and radiographic studies is suggested for the systematic approach to the vexing clinical problem of the painful total hip arthroplasty.

Garcia-Cimbrelo E, Munuera L: Early and late loosening of the acetabular cup after low-friction arthroplasty. *J Bone Joint Surg* 1992;74A:1119–1129.

The radiographic findings of early and late patterns of loosening in 680 low-friction arthroplasties reviewed at 12 years are compared. Migration and extensive bony resorption exemplify early loosening, whereas late loosening correlates with depth of acetabular wear and radiolucencies.

Horowitz SM, Doty SB, Lane JM, et al: Studies of the mechanism by which the mechanical failure of polymethylmethacrylate leads to bone resorption. *J Bone Joint Surg* 1993;75A:802–813.

Membranes retrieved from 18 aseptically loosened femoral components in addition to an in vitro macrophage preparation showed phagocytosis of polyethylene particles less than 12 μm with resultant increased release of mediators of bone resorption.

Jacobs JJ, Sumner DR, Galante JO: Mechanisms of bone loss associated with total hip replacement. *Orthop Clin North Am* 1993;24:583–590.

Periprosthetic bone loss in total hip arthroplasty is described in terms of two separate mechanisms, adaptive bone remodeling and osteolysis. The pathogenesis of each is discussed and research to reduce the detrimental effects of these processes is summarized.

Jasty M, Maloney WJ, Brogden CR, et al: The initiation of failure in cemented femoral components of hip arthroplasties. *J Bone Joint Surg* 1991;73B:551–558.

Sixteen well-functioning post-mortem cemented femurs are

presented. These show intact bone–cement interfaces, but frequent cement–metal separations (debonding) with subsequent cement mantle failure. The authors suggest a mechanical mode of failure.

Jiranek WA, Machado M, Jasty M, et al: Production of cytokines around loosened cemented acetabular components: Analysis with immunohistochemical techniques and in situ hybridization. *J Bone Joint Surg* 1993;75A:863–879.

Immunohistochemical techniques and in situ hybridization were used to evaluate membranes retrieved from 10 aseptically loosened cemented polyethylene sockets. This study demonstrated potent cytokine production from macrophages at the membrane. The authors concluded that cytokines were produced at the membrane and not transported in, and were produced by macrophages.

Kim KJ, Chiba J, Rubash HE: In vivo and in vitro analysis of membranes from hip prostheses inserted without cement. *J Bone Joint Surg* 1994;76A:172–180.

Sixty-four membranes retrieved from failed cementless, porous-coated implants showed intense histiocytic and giant-cell response in the presence of polyethylene debris. This is compared to a nonpolyethylene bearing endoprosthesis membrane with significantly less activity.

Kwong LM, Jasty M, Mulroy RD, et al: The histology of the radiolucent line. *J Bone Joint Surg* 1992;74B:67–73.

A retrieval study of 15 cemented femurs demonstrates that radiolucent lines occur with well-fixed components. These lines may represent the remodeling and osteoporosis rather than a fibrous membrane at the cement-bone interface.

Maloney WJ, Jasty M, Harris WH, et al: Endosteal erosion in association with stable uncemented femoral components. *J Bone Joint Surg* 1990;72A:1025–1034.

Focal femoral osteolysis was identified in 14 uncemented radiographically stable implants. Lesions that were biopsied showed aggregates of macrophages with particulate polyethylene and metallic debris.

Maloney WJ, Peters P, Engh CA, et al: Severe osteolysis of the pelvis in association with acetabular replacement without cement. *J Bone Joint Surg* 1993;75A:1627–1635.

Fifteen uncemented acetabular components were noted on routine radiographic follow-up to have extensive osteolytic lesions. The patients were asymptomatic and functioning well clinically. Eleven of 15 components had screw holes, and 11 of 15 were articulating with a 32-mm head.

Maloney WJ, Smith RL, Castro F, et al: Fibroblast response to metallic debris in vitro: Enzyme induction, cell proliferation, and toxicity. *J Bone Joint Surg* 1993;75A:835–844.

Bovine synovial fibroblasts exposed in vitro to low concentrations of titanium, titanium-aluminum, and chromium particles responded with proliferation. The authors suggest that metallic debris may be an inciting factor in the formation of fibrous membranes around uncemented implants, and that those membranes may then provide a conduit for migration of polyethylene debris.

Morscher EW: Current status of acetabular fixation in primary total hip arthroplasty. *Clin Orthop* 1992;274:172–193.

This is a comprehensive review of acetabular reconstruction. The author provides a detailed history, a review of materials used, technique, and current recommendations in acetabular reconstruction.

Mulroy RD Jr, Harris WH: The effect of improved cementing techniques on component loosening in total hip replacement: An 11-year radiographic review. *J Bone Joint Surg* 1990;72B:757–760.

The results of improved cementing techniques in total hip replacement including use of a canal plug, cement gun, doughy cement, and a collared prosthesis are reported in 105 reconstructions at an average of 11.2 years. The authors show a marked reduction in the rate of aseptic loosening on the femoral side, with acetabular results remaining relatively unaffected.

Pidhorz LE, Urban RM, Jacobs JJ, et al: A quantitative study of bone and soft tissues in cementless porous-coated acetabular components retrieved at autopsy. *J Arthroplasty* 1993;8:213–225.

In an autopsy retrieval study, 11 cementless acetabular components were examined histologically at an average of 41 months postoperatively. The authors note an average volume of bone ingrowth of 12%. More bone was noted adjacent to screw holes. A correlation was drawn between radiolucency and decreased bone ingrowth.

Sarmiento A, Ebramzadeh E, Gogan WJ, et al: Cup containment and orientation in cemented total hip arthroplasties. *J Bone Joint Surg* 1990;72B:996–1002.

Radiographs of 864 Charnley and STH (Sarmiento Total Hip) cemented total hip arthroplasties with an average follow-up of 7 years were reviewed. Cups that were completely contained had significantly lower incidences of complete cement-bone radiolucencies and of wear. All vertically oriented cups were noted to be completely contained in comparison to horizontal cups. The authors stress the importance of complete bony containment and advise that it is better to accept vertical orientation and full bony coverage rather than horizontal orientation with partial containment.

Schmalzried TP, Harris WH: The Harris-Galante porous-coated acetabular component with screw fixation: Radiographic analysis of eighty-three primary hip replacements at a minimum of five years. *J Bone Joint Surg* 1992;74A:1130–1139.

Eighty-three consecutive porous-coated Harris-Galante acetabular components implanted with line-to-line reaming and screw fixation were reviewed at a minimum 5-year follow-up. No components in this study were revised for loosening. A progressive radiolucent line developed in 40% of cups that had a peripheral gap at the time of implantation. The authors suggest a prognostic significance for initial peripheral gaps in uncemented sockets.

Schmalzried TP, Jasty M, Harris WH: Periprosthetic bone loss in total hip arthroplasty: Polyethylene wear debris and the concept of the effective joint space. *J Bone Joint Surg* 1992;74A:849–863.

Membranes from 34 hips selected due to evidence of osteolysis showed bone resorption in association with polyethylene laden macrophages. The concept of the effective joint space is suggested to explain debris and biologic activity found far from the synovial cavity, even in well-fixed components.

Schmalzried TP, Kwong LM, Jasty M, et al: The mechanism of loosening of cemented acetabular components in total hip arthroplasty: Analysis of specimens retrieved at autopsy. *Clin Orthop* 1992;274:60–78.

An autopsy retrieval study of 14 cemented all-polyethylene acetabular components was undertaken. Bone resorption was initiated circumferentially and progressed towards the dome, fueled by small particles of polyethylene that incited an inflammatory response. This study supports a biologic rather than mechanical mode of late aseptic loosening of cemented acetabular components.

Schulte KR, Callaghan JJ, Kelley SS, et al: The outcome of Charnley total hip arthroplasty with cement after a minimum twenty-year follow-up: The results of one surgeon. *J Bone Joint Surg* 1993;75A:961–975.

Three hundred thirty Charnley cemented hip arthroplasties were followed for greater than 20 years. The authors showed 18% of surviving sockets with definitive radiographic loosening; 8% were revised. Only 7% of surviving femoral components had signs of definite radiographic loosening.

Shanbhag AS, Jacobs JJ, Glant TT, et al: Composition and morphology of wear debris in failed uncemented total hip replacement. *J Bone Joint Surg* 1994;76B:60–67.

Membranes retrieved from 11 failed uncemented femoral prostheses were examined by electron microscopy, microchemical spectroscopy, and particle size analysis. Most particles were submicron polyethylene which was noted by the authors to be similar to particles of base resin seen in the manufacture of acetabular implants. The authors note that this may be an important factor in the production of wear debris.

Sumner DR, Galante JO: Determinants of stress shielding: Design versus materials versus interface. *Clin Orthop* 1992;274:202–212.

A review of bone remodeling after total hip arthroplasty is presented with special attention to canine models, design variables, the implant–bone interface, and patterns of remodeling. The authors report that the dominant long-term design feature controlling bone remodeling appears to be stem stiffness.

19

Infection Following Total Hip Arthroplasty

Etiology and Incidence of Infection

The incidence of deep infection following total hip arthroplasty has fallen dramatically in the three decades since the introduction of the procedure. Unfortunately, even at the current rate of only 1% over the lifetime of the prosthesis, over 10,000 patients will be diagnosed as having deep sepsis involving total hip replacements in the United States over the next year.

Sepsis in the immediate postoperative period, Stage I sepsis, is most commonly associated with postoperative hematomas infected by *Staphylococcus aureus* or Group B streptococci. Such infections are usually easy to identify due to their fulminant course. Stage II sepsis poses more of a diagnostic challenge because it is more indolent, with usual onset of symptoms 6 to 24 or more months following surgery. The organisms involved, such as coagulase negative staphylococcus, are usually considered less virulent. Unfortunately, the pattern of antimicrobial resistance of these organisms has changed in recent years. At many institutions, methicillin-resistant *S. epidermidis* is now the most frequently identified pathogen in Stage II sepsis. There is evidence to suggest that these infections are related to intraoperative contamination that is suppressed by the prophylactic antibiotics.

An infection that causes symptoms more than 2 years after surgery in a previously asymptomatic patient is considered Stage III sepsis. These infections are thought to arise from sources elsewhere in the body, such as the urinary tract, and as such may be caused by a wide variety of gram-positive and negative pathogens. While the incidence of Stage I sepsis has fallen steadily to its current level of less than 0.05% (primarily as a result of the widespread use of antibiotic prophylaxis), Stage III sepsis has not been so affected and now accounts for more than half of all periprosthetic infections. As the long-term results of total hip arthroplasty are examined, it appears that the danger of Stage III sepsis remains significant over the lifetime of the prosthesis and may increase with wear of the prosthetic joint, perhaps as a result of local alterations of the immune response secondary to that wear. Thus, current Medicare statistics indicate the overall incidence of infection remains over 1% despite the decrease in the perioperative infection rate.

The rate of sepsis after revision surgery is at least double that following primary total hip arthroplasty. The reason for this markedly increased rate of sepsis is multifactorial. Longer operating times and larger surgical exposures result in an increased potential for contamination. The exposures required for revision surgery result in greater volumes of devascularized bone and soft tissue and larger dead space, all of which increase the likelihood of bacterial colonization. Patients who require major bone grafting have been found to have an even greater infection rate than other patients undergoing revision surgery.

Prevention

Antibiotic prophylaxis remains the single best method of preventing sepsis. Prophylaxis usually consists of administration of a first-generation cephalosporin (most commonly cephalothin or an equivalent) just prior to surgery and every 8 hours for 48 hours thereafter. A recent study indicates that a second-generation cephalosporin with a longer half-life (cefuroxime) administered less frequently for a shorter period is equally effective in preventing Stage I sepsis at a potentially lower overall expense. Although additional improvement may theoretically be offered by ultra-clean air systems, body exhausts, ultraviolet lighting, and other similar environmental measures, their efficacy in conjunction with antibiotic prophylaxis remains to be demonstrated. Further, each has additional drawbacks, not the least of which is the problem of added expenditure in an era of cost-containment.

Because Stage III sepsis has emerged as an ever-increasing problem, it would be advantageous if an effective method of prophylaxis could be devised to prevent these infections. Although anecdotal reports of sepsis following dental work and other bacteremia-producing procedures are common, well-documented accounts are rare. Furthermore, case reports by their nature often focus on the unusual infecting organism, such as *Citrobacter freundii* following endoscopy, rather than on more common pathogens. As a result, it is almost impossible to accurately determine whether antimicrobials should be given for a particular procedure and, if appropriate, which would be most effective. The cost-benefit ratio of late prophylaxis has, therefore, been questioned. Nevertheless, there are few surgeons who would willingly expose a patient to a potential infection without some effort at antibiotic prophylaxis, despite the lack of supportive evidence. Studies are currently being designed to evaluate the efficacy of antibiotic prophylaxis for dental procedures in a statistically valid manner.

Diagnosis

The onset in a previously asymptomatic hip of pain that cannot be related to other factors must be considered septic in origin until proven otherwise. Laboratory evaluation will usually show an elevation of the erythrocyte sedimentation rate (ESR) and of the C-reactive protein, but in general such studies are suggestive, not diagnostic. Plain-film anteroposterior and lateral radiographs are the most common form of imaging for the patient with a painful total hip arthroplasty. Rapid lysis of periprosthetic bone associated with pain and other constitutional signs is most frequently indicative of a high-grade septic process. Unfortunately, plain radiographs are rarely diagnostic in the differentiation between low-grade sepsis and aseptic loosening. In only a small percentage of patients will lacy periosteal new bone formation, indicative of infection, be identified (Fig. 1).

Because of the general inability of plain-film radiographs to distinguish sepsis, other forms of imaging may be necessary to evaluate the patient with a painful prosthetic hip. Arthrography may demonstrate pocketing of the radiopaque medium in the area of the pseudocapsule, suggesting infection (Fig. 2), but this finding is also uncommon. The true value of arthrography is that it provides an opportunity to aspirate the joint. Aerobic and anaerobic incubation of the hip aspirate permits recovery of the causal organism in over two thirds of patients with an infected total hip arthroplasty. Because the infecting organism may be a bacteria, such as *S. epidermidis,* that is often considered a contaminant, the laboratory must be informed that all organisms isolated from the aspirate are

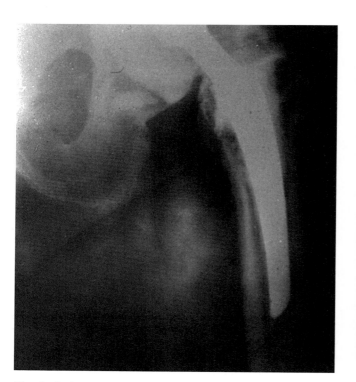
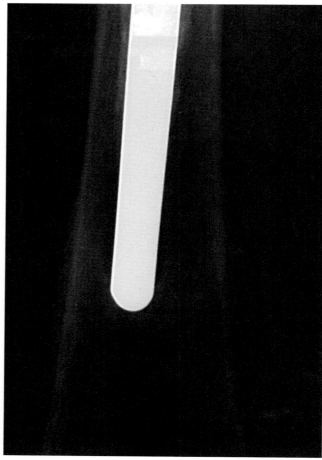

Fig. 1   Left, Anteroposterior (AP) radiograph of the pelvis in a 51-year-old man with ankylosing spondylitis who had bilateral cemented total hip arthroplasties 12 years previously. There is periosteal new bone formation medially in the proximal metaphysis of the left femur consistent with a low-grade infection. This patient had an infection requiring a Girdlestone resection arthroplasty. *Staphylococcus aureus* was isolated from the surgical tissue specimens. **Right,** An AP radiograph of the distal femur with a long-stem femoral prosthesis extending into the distal femoral metaphysis. There is periosteal new bone formation medially and laterally in the distal femoral metaphysis consistent with a septic process. The patient had a low-grade infection about the total hip. *Staphylococcus epidermidis* was isolated from the deep tissue specimens obtained at the time of surgery.

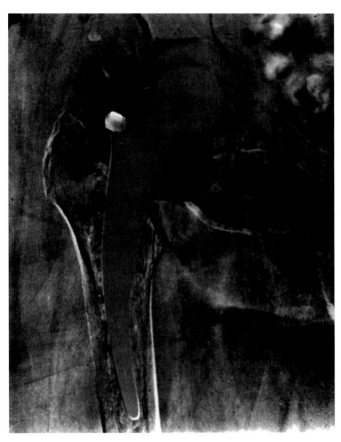

Fig. 2 Anteroposterior view of a subtraction arthrogram of a right total hip arthroplasty that reveals pocketing of the dye in the pseudocapsule and suggests the presence of a low-grade infectious process. *Staphylococcus epidermidis* was isolated from the aspirate recovered prior to the injection of the radiopaque dye.

to be identified and their pattern of antibiotic resistance delineated. If possible, the organism should also be characterized in regard to its ability to produce a glycocalyx slime or "biofilm" because this biofilm may influence the subsequent course of treatment. In addition, tuberculosis has become more common in the community at large and must be considered among potential pathogens, particularly in the patient who has a suppressed immune system. Some recent studies, however, question the efficacy of routine aspiration of the hip in patients with pain. It is essential to obtain fluid at the time of the aspiration.

Although arthrography can provide important information about the status of a painful hip replacement, routine arthrography of the hip is not cost-effective and can lead to the introduction of pathogenic organisms into a previously aseptic joint. Therefore, arthrography should be avoided unless there is suspicion of infection based on the medical history, physical examination, and preliminary laboratory results.

With the evolution of new diagnostic agents, scintigraphy has gradually become a more reliable technique in evaluation of the painful total hip replacement. Examination with [111]indium-labeled autologous leukocytes has superseded differential imaging with technetium and gallium. Indium-labeled leukocyte scintigraphy not only is more specific but also is more accurate in distinguishing aseptic from septic loosening. In a prospective study of 42 patients with suspected low-grade musculoskeletal infections, [111]indium scintigraphy correctly identified the presence or absence of sepsis in 88%, while technetium and gallium scintigraphy was accurate in only 62% ($p > 0.001$). In a canine total hip model, [111]indium scintigraphy was found to distinguish accurately among aseptic loosening, septic loosening, and a securely fixed prosthesis in 14 of 15 dogs, a rate of over 93%. Differential technetium and gallium scintigraphy was accurate in only 62% ($p > 0.001$).

Scintigraphy using technetium methyldiphosphonate-labeled leukocytes has been found effective in the evaluation of septic conditions such as abdominal abscesses. Unfortunately, the application of this diagnostic agent to the evaluation of the patient with a painful total hip arthroplasty has been disappointing. In a study of 29 hip arthroplasty patients who were subsequently treated surgically, this technique was found to be associated with an unacceptably high rate of false-positive images, particularly in the evaluation of patients with a resection arthroplasty who were being evaluated for a two-stage reconstruction.

Attempts to find more information-specific scintigraphic agents are ongoing. Two new scintigraphic agents for the diagnosis of sepsis are currently undergoing FDA-controlled evaluations in the United States. Theoretically, [111]indium labeled-IgG (a nonspecific immunoglobulin) can be used for the diagnosis of even low-grade sepsis (Fig. 3). Although this technique is not yet available in the United States, experience in Europe suggests that it will enhance the diagnosis of musculoskeletal infections.

Fortunately, the particular polyclonal antibody being used in the FDA study may obviate the problem encountered in Europe with an earlier version, which failed to differentiate adequately between aseptic loosening and sepsis. While [111]indium IgG scintigraphy will require further study to determine if it can accurately differentiate these two conditions, it does appear to hold promise in the diagnosis of a low-grade infectious process about orthopaedic implants. A second agent under evaluation is [99]technetium monoclonal imaging. The early experience suggests that it may be a more accurate diagnostic agent than [111]indium IgG imaging. However, [99]technetium monoclonal imaging will also need widespread investigation in a variety of different environments to determine its overall efficacy and cost-effectiveness.

Aerobic and anaerobic incubation of intraoperatively obtained tissue specimens, as well as frozen section and permanent pathology sections of the capsule, femoral, and acetabular interfaces, remain the most reliable documentation of infection. Some studies suggest that the white

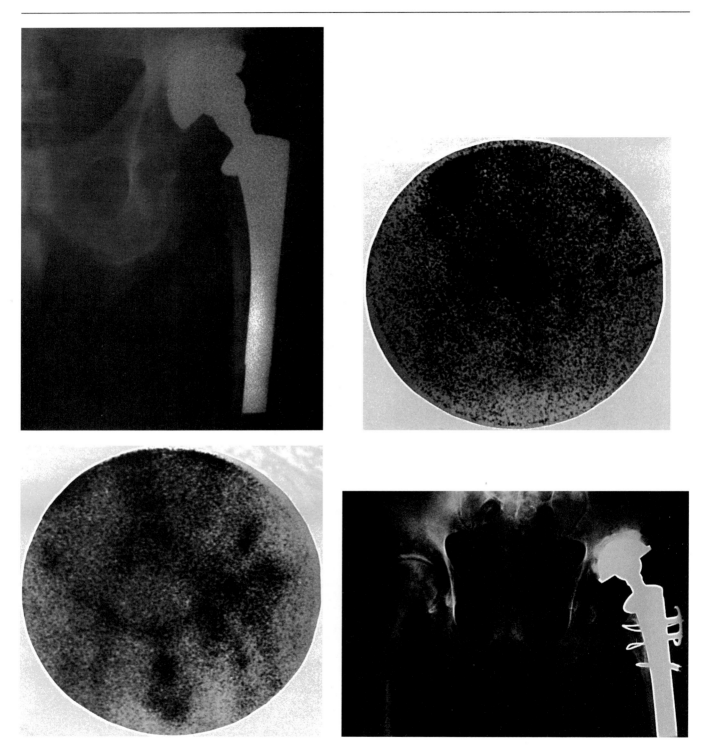

Fig. 3   A series of images in a 68-year-old who developed an enterococcal (Group D *Streptococcus* subsp *enterococcus*) infection of a well-fixed cementless AML total hip arthroplasty. **Top left,** Anteroposterior (AP) radiograph of the right hip. Group D *Streptococcus* subsp *enterococcus* was isolated from the preoperative aspirate. **Top right,** A ⁹⁹Tc white blood cell image revealed increased uptake in the ischium and iliac portion of the acetabulum, consistent with a persistent infection. **Bottom left,** The ¹¹¹In IgG image revealed increased uptake in the iliac portion of the acetabulum. Further debridement of the wound was performed. *Staphylococcus aureus* (β-lactamase positive), methicillin-resistant was recovered from the multiple surgical specimens submitted to the microbiology laboratory. **Bottom right,** Two-year follow-up following reconstruction with a second total hip arthroplasty.

blood cell count in the intraoperatively obtained joint fluid may be helpful in differentiating aseptic from septic loosening.

Treatment

In the past, antibiotic therapy alone has not been found effective in the eradication of peri-prosthetic infections. However, one recent report suggests that the combination of rifampin and a fluoroquinine (ofloxacin) may obviate the need for surgical debridement. Twenty-six of 37 patients given a 6-month course of the drugs were symptom-free 1 to 2 years later. However, in most patients with deep sepsis, two-stage reconstruction, including complete surgical extirpation of the prosthesis as well as all cement and infected bone, followed by appropriate antibiotic therapy and delayed reimplantation continues to be the generally accepted treatment. Four to 6 weeks of intravenous antibiotics are recommended.

The placement of antibiotic-impregnated methylmethacrylate beads as an adjuvant to the resection arthroplasty has been used with some success. A more recent modification of this technique involves the insertion of an antibiotic-impregnated methacrylate acetabular component, which articulates with a more orthodox femoral component that also is fixed temporarily with antibiotic-containing cement. As an interim procedure before permanent fixation of new prosthetic components, this technique offers much better function than resection arthroplasty.

The time to reimplantation of the prosthetic hip may vary from weeks to 12 or more months depending on the organism involved, the extent of the infection, and the state of health of the patient. Less virulent organisms, such as methicillin-sensitive, nonglycocalyx-forming staphylococci, are generally amenable to early reconstruction, whereas organisms such as enterococci and gram-negative bacilli such as *Pseudomonas aeruginosa* should not be considered for re-operation for at least 6 months or, preferably, 1 year. During the interim, the patient may be monitored with serial ESR or C-reactive protein levels. Repeat aspirations offer little information of value and are not generally recommended.

Reconstruction of the previously infected hip is usually undertaken using cement containing one or more heat-stable antibiotics. More recently, cementless reconstruction, which is more appropriate for the younger patient, has been shown possible if the ESR has returned to normal levels and the ^{111}indium scan is negative. Single-stage or direct exchange arthroplasty using antibiotic impregnated cement has been popular in Europe for some time, but has met with limited acceptance in North America. However, this technique may offer advantages in those infections involving a low-virulence, gram-positive organism that does not produce glycocalyx. Single-stage exchange may also need continued evaluation and study due to its cost-effectiveness.

Annotated Bibliography

Drancourt M, Stein A, Argenson JN, et al: Oral rifampin plus ofloxacin for treatment of staphylococcus-infected orthopedic implants. *Antimicrob Agents Chemother* 1993;37:1214–1218.

The treatment of *S. aureus* sepsis in 22 total hip and 15 total knee arthroplasty patients with 6 months of oral antimicrobial therapy consisting of rifampin and ofloxacin without concomitant surgical treatment was successful in 26 patients. Three patients experienced intolerance to the antibiotic regimen. Recurrent infections were encountered in eight patients. Unfortunately, follow-up was short (< 2 years) and may indicate suppression rather than eradication of the infectious process.

Duncan CP, Beauchamp C: A temporary antibiotic-loaded joint replacement system for the management of complex infections involving the hip. *Orthop Clin North Am* 1993;24:751–759.

A new technique, which uses a temporary prosthesis that acts as a local antibiotic delivery system, affords better pain relief and function than a resection arthroplasty. Revision surgery is also facilitated by maintenance of tissue tension and limb length.

Oyen WJ, Claessens RA, van Horn JR, et al: Scintigraphic detection of bone and joint infections with indium-111-labeled nonspecific polyclonal human immunoglobulin G. *J Nucl Med* 1990;31:413.

A new scintigraphic technique, ^{111}indium-labeled IgG, appears to be an excellent diagnostic tool for the identification of musculoskeletal infections. This study does, however, suggest that this technique may have difficulty differentiating a septic process from aseptic loosening if there is an inflammatory reaction to particulate debris.

20

Other Complications of Total Hip Arthroplasty

Neural and Vascular Injury

Neural and vascular injuries can occur during any phase of total hip arthroplasty. Positioning of the patient in preparation for surgery can cause these injuries, as can the surgical approach to the hip. Intraoperative injuries can be caused by retractor placement, hip reduction and dislocation, and fixation with cement or screws. Although uncommon, neural and vascular injuries can result in serious and debilitating problems.

A quadrant system has been described, which identifies the location of intrapelvic structures in relationship to a fixed point in the acetabulum. The quadrants are defined by drawing a line from the anterior superior iliac spine that divides the acetabulum into equal halves, and then by bisecting this line perpendicularly with another line at its midpoint. By using the quadrant system, orthopaedic surgeons can identify safe and dangerous zones for the transacetabular placement of screws and retractors, for drilling, or for estimating bone depth. Using the anterior quadrants for the placement of screws and anchoring holes or to help secure retractors may injure the external iliac artery and vein and the obturator nerve, artery, and vein, which lie opposite the anterior superior quadrant. The polar zone of the acetabulum can be violated during excessive reaming, injuring the external iliac vein and obturator nerve, artery, and vein. Within the posterior quadrants are the sciatic nerve and the superior gluteal nerve vessels; screws and anchoring holes can be placed relatively safely through the two posterior zones. Careful retraction of the sciatic nerve during retractor and screw placement lessens the likelihood of injury.

A clear understanding of the anatomy of the region is of critical importance in order to avoid the important neural and vascular structures and the significant complications that can result from their injury.

Vascular Injury

External Iliac Artery and Vein The external iliac artery is the anterior division of the common iliac artery. The external iliac vein is the continuation of the femoral vein from the inguinal ligament to the sacroiliac articulation, where it joins with the internal iliac vein to form the common iliac vein. The external iliac vein accompanies the artery along the anterior superior quadrant of the acetabulum. Injury of the external iliac artery is more common than injury of the external iliac vein.

Positioning the patient with preexisting atherosclerotic disease may result in limb ischemia, thrombosis, or distal limb infarction from a plaque embolism. For patients whose Doppler pressures are low or who have clinical evidence of ischemia, preoperative consultation with a vascular surgeon should be obtained.

These intrapelvic vessels can be injured during acetabular exposure by retractors placed over the anterior column, usually too far medially. Hip dislocation maneuvers may also cause injury to these vessels. Recurrent dislocation may cause thrombotic external iliac occlusion and pseudoaneurysm formation. Excessive reaming medially through the inner table of the acetabulum can injure the external iliac vein. Cement extruded into the pelvis through an anchoring hole or medial defect may cause occlusive injury to the external iliac artery as a result of heat of polymerization or of direct compression. Transacetabular screws, which are often required for cementless acetabular component fixation, can lacerate the external iliac vein, resulting in a large retroperitoneal hematoma. The posterior quadrant is safest for screw placement.

Delayed injury to the external iliac vessels also can occur. Socket migration and extruded cement can cause compressive occlusion. During acetabular revision, injury to the external iliac vessels can occur when cement extruded toward the iliac vessels through perforations in the anterior superior quadrant of the acetabulum catches on these vessels. When there is a likelihood that vessel injury will occur during revision surgery, preoperative evaluation should be performed using standard and oblique radiographs, arteriography, or contrast-enhanced computed tomographic (CT) scanning.

Common Femoral Vessels The portion of the femoral artery proximal to the branching of the deep femoral artery is known as the common femoral artery. The common femoral vein lies in the proximal two thirds of the thigh and is a direct continuation of the popliteal vein, which follows the course of the femoral artery. At the inguinal ligament it becomes the external iliac vein. The common femoral artery is lateral to the vein at the level of the inferomedial capsule and is more susceptible to injury. These vessels are reported to be the most frequently injured extrapelvic vessels during total hip arthroplasty. During preoperative positioning of patients with atherosclerotic disease in the lateral decubitus position, stabilizing the pelvis between the pubic symphysis and posterior sacrum can compress the femoral vessels. Retractor placement during the surgical approach often injures the femoral vessels. Injury can occur during the anterolateral approach when the retractor is placed too far medially over the anterior inferior acetabular margin. Osteophyte resection and resection of scarred capsule in the anterior inferior acetabulum have also resulted in injury to the femoral artery.

Postoperatively, ischemia can occur even in the absence of intraoperative hemorrhage. Additionally, traction on vessels during dislocation or reduction in patients with atherosclerosis can cause limb ischemia without intraoperative bleeding. Limb lengthening and surgical correction of a significant hip contracture can injure vessels tethered by scar tissue.

Profunda Femoris Vessels The profunda femoris vessels are rarely injured during total hip arthroplasty.

Obturator Vessels The obturator artery originates from the internal iliac artery. The obturator veins drain the hip joint and regional muscles, enter the pelvis through the obturator canal, and empty into the internal iliac or the inferior epigastric vein, or both. These vessels, along with the obturator nerve, most frequently traverse the lateral wall of the pelvis (quadrilateral surface). Injury can occur via the anterior inferior quadrant or by retractor placement under the transverse acetabular ligament into the superolateral aspect of the obturator foramen.

Superior Gluteal Vessels The superior gluteal artery branches from the posterior division of the internal iliac artery. The inferior branches of the superior gluteal vessels are approximately 2.5 cm to 4 cm superior to the superior lateral edge of the acetabulum and can be injured by proximal dissection during direct lateral, modified direct lateral, and anterolateral approaches to the hip.

Laceration of the gluteal artery has been caused by fixation screw placement in the area of the sciatic notch. Injury has also occurred when a pin retractor has been inserted into the direction of the notch. Injury to the inferior gluteal and internal pudendal vessels is unusual.

Neural Injury

The incidence of nerve palsy has been reported to range from 0% to 3% following primary total hip arthroplasty and from 2.9% to 7.6% following revision surgery. Sciatic nerve palsy (peroneal with or without tibial division) accounts for the majority of these lesions. Although some of these patients experience a return of function and do well, many are left with severe impairment and disability.

Neural injury is caused by compression, traction, and/or ischemia. Although the cause of neural injury may appear to be evident, two or more of these causes may have an additive effect. For example, while lengthening the limb by 2.5 cm may appear to be the cause of postoperative peroneal nerve palsy, prolonged retractor pressure or extensive perineural dissection may lower the threshold of the nerve's ability to tolerate subsequent lengthening. Significant neurologic damage may result from an acute stretch of only 6% of nerve length. Ischemic nerve damage is caused by compression and traction mechanisms, whereas primary ischemia can result from direct damage of the neurovascular supply. Compressive nerve injury may result from retractor placement or hematoma formation.

Sciatic and Peroneal Nerves The fibers of the sciatic nerve are spatially oriented as the nerve passes through the sciatic notch. The common peroneal nerve is located more laterally, and the fibers are more superficial and more susceptible to injury. Sciatic and peroneal nerve palsies are reported to be the most common peripheral nerve injuries occurring with total hip arthroplasty; the incidence ranges from 0.5% to 2.0%. These palsies occur more frequently with revision arthroplasty, with lengthening (with or without lateral displacement of the extremity), and in women. The known causes of sciatic (peroneal) nerve palsy following total hip arthroplasty have been summarized, and it was found that 22% were due to direct injury, 10% were due to postoperative dislocations, 20% were due to bleeding complications, and lengthening and lateral displacement of the extremity accounted for 50%.

The anatomic course of the sciatic nerve makes it vulnerable to injury during reconstructive surgery. The nerve can be injured by power reamers and posterior acetabular retractors. Posterior quadrant placement of acetabular screws is relatively safe, but placement of drill holes, especially in the sciatic notch area, should be accompanied by digital palpation.

Although there are varying reports of recovery from sciatic and peroneal palsies, some believe that the prognosis for recovery could be considered good unless the nerve had sustained severe damage. Patients who retained or regained some motor function postoperatively have a better recovery, in general. Objective hip score measurements of function may indicate a successful outcome, but patients may be generally dissatisfied with the outcome.

Femoral Nerve Palsy In a recently published report of femoral palsies after total hip arthroplasty, an incidence of 2.3% in a series of 440 consecutive procedures was reported. These palsies may occur in combination with sciatic palsies, and the clinical manifestations may be masked by the use of postoperative assistive walking devices. Most mechanisms of sciatic nerve injury also can cause femoral nerve injury. These include cement extravasation, lengthening or stretch, hematoma, and retractor placement. The use of anterior-superior and anterior-inferior screw placement may result in femoral nerve injury. As stated previously, the anterior quadrants are not safe and are not generally recommended for screw placement.

Retractor placement appears to be the major cause of femoral nerve lesions. Multiple studies have reported good recovery of the femoral nerve following nonoperative treatment; however, surgical decompression of hematomas involving the femoral triangle may be recommended to prevent further nerve compression. Patients with femoral nerve injuries secondary to anterior retractor placement do well. Obturator nerve palsies are a rare complication of total hip replacement.

Somatosensory evoked potentials (SSEP) have been used successfully in spinal surgery, and have recently been used in total hip arthroplasty to detect sciatic nerve compromise. The peroneal nerve is the most commonly injured peripheral nerve during total hip arthroplasty and is easily stimulated, intraoperatively.

In a study of 100 consecutive total hip arthroplasties in which SSEP monitoring was used the investigators reported an incidence of 2% of sciatic nerve palsy, as compared to a 2.6% rate with previously unmonitored patients. They concluded that SSEP monitoring was not indicated on a routine basis, but that monitoring could be of benefit to high-risk patients, such as those with congenital dislocation of the hip, those undergoing revision arthroplasty, and those with expected limb lengthening.

Femoral Fractures

Intraoperative Fracture

Overall, femoral fractures occurring with total hip arthroplasty are rare, with an incidence of approximately 0.1%. Understandably, fractures occur more frequently when the prosthetic device is uncemented or press fit. The incidence reported in the orthopaedic literature ranges from 3% to 28%. The wide variation in the reported incidence is due to the variety of prosthetic designs available and the instrumentation used to insert the prosthetic component. In contrast, the less-common femoral fractures during cemented procedures usually occur with dislocation or reduction.

Fracture during revision procedures usually occurs through weakened bone during dislocation or reduction of the hip or during preparation of the host bone for the new prosthetic device. Although long-stem components used to bypass stress risers in the femur will decrease the risk of postoperative fracture, such components are associated with an increased risk of intraoperative fracture. Curved, long-stem prostheses require over-reaming of the femur. Removal of the proximal lateral cement column before prosthetic extraction decreases the risk of trochanteric fracture. Nondisplaced fractures may be difficult to detect, but may be obvious when there is a sudden loss of resistance when inserting a cementless prosthesis. Many fractures are first detected on postoperative radiographs.

Several systems of classifying intraoperative fractures have been developed. Most systems propose three major categories: I, fracture of the proximal and lesser trochanter; II, fracture distal to the lesser trochanter but proximal to the isthmus or proximal to the prosthetic tip; and III, fracture distal to the prosthesis. These three categories can be further subtyped (displaced or nondisplaced).

For a type I proximal fracture, cerclage will usually suffice. If the fracture is longer, a second wire below the fracture may be advisable. Type II fractures can also be treated with cerclage, as can type III fractures or distal fractures. Type II or III fractures may require insertion of a longer stem to give further intramedullary fixation. With cemented arthroplasty, care must be taken to avoid cement penetration through the fracture site. Supplemental bone grafting has been recommended to help fracture healing, with more extensive grafting required for types II and III fractures. Postoperatively, a cast or a brace should be used in addition to protected weightbearing for patients with types II and III fractures.

No significant difference was found in the result of cementless total hip arthroplasty between those with type I fractures and those with no fractures who used the same prosthetic component. No significant difference was also found between types II and III fractures and the control. A series of intraoperative femur fractures was reported, in which 50% were recognized intraoperatively. Unrecognized fractures that extended to the tip of the prosthesis were treated with hip spica casting, if nondisplaced or incomplete; displaced fractures were treated with open reduction and internal fixation.

The Mayo Clinic experience reported a 6.3% incidence of intraoperative femur fracture in uncemented total hip arthroplasty (7% for revision procedures and 2% for primary). Most fractures were treated with application of Parham bands, and all were shown to have healed, radiographically. In all cases, protected weightbearing with support was used for 2 to 4 months. Loosening of the femoral component developed in a small number and required revision; in all cases of revision, the fracture was believed to be the significant cause. Thus, intraoperative fractures may lead to secondary loosening.

Prevention is the best treatment for intraoperative femoral fractures. The surgeon must obtain adequate exposure, avoid undue manipulative force, and carefully prepare the host femur. In situ osteotomy for severe ankylosis or protrusio acetabula should be performed using trochanteric osteotomy for exposure and bypassing cortical defects. Careful review of anteroposterior and lateral radiographs and proper templating are also important. Prophylactic wiring of the femur has been described in the literature, and healing reported in several series has been excellent. Bone grafting, either allograft or autograft, has been recommended for type II and type III fractures. In most cases, if the fracture is recognized, stabilized, and grafted and the patient protected from weightbearing, fracture healing can be expected in 2 to 4 months.

Postoperative Fracture

Postoperative femur fractures occur more frequently after revision arthroplasty and present different treatment problems to the orthopaedic surgeon. The incidence of postoperative fracture in revision total hip arthroplasty has been reported to be as high as 4.2%, in contrast to 0.1% in primary total hip arthroplasty.

Postoperative femur fractures usually occur through some defect in the bone. In most series, some type of trauma has usually been found to contribute to the postoperative fracture. Usually, such fractures occur through a stress riser. The use of longer stem femoral components has been advocated to reduce the fractures after perforation of the femur. The effects of stress risers on the femur have been studied, and it was found that bypassing a defect with an intramedullary stem extending two cortical bone diameters past the distal extent of the defect will restore the torsional strength of the intact femur in 84% of the cases. Bone grafts are required to help healing and, recently, cortical allograft struts have been found to be successful in enhancing both strength and union in revision total hip arthroplasty.

One classification of postoperative fractures identifies three types: type I, proximal to the tip of the prosthesis; type II, proximal and distal to the tip of the stem with the stem dislodged in the distal fragment; and type III, entirely distal to the tip of the stem.

Recommendations for the treatment of postoperative femur fractures depend on the status of the component at the time of the fracture. If loosening has occurred, revision with a long-stem prosthesis is the best treatment. If the fracture has not compromised the fixation of the stem but is displaced around the stem, open reduction and internal fixation are advocated without revision of the femoral component. With healing of the fracture, subsequent loosening may occur, thus indicating an elective revision procedure. Further distal fractures, such as supracondylar femur fractures below the stem, can be treated successfully using standard techniques based on the surgeon's experience and the fracture type.

As with intraoperative fractures, prevention is the best treatment. If cementing in a revision procedure, cement must be kept from the fracture site. Bone grafting is recommended in many instances, as is plate fixation with an Ogden or Dall-Miles plate, which allows the use of cables or bands and results in better internal fixation.

The results of 14 postoperative femoral fractures, five of which occurred through stress risers, have been reported. The results of type II fractures treated nonsurgically were all poor. Thus, revision is recommended using a long-stem component with internal fixation of the fracture, followed by postoperative immobilization if rigid fixation was not obtained intraoperatively. Type II fractures without prosthetic loosening could be treated nonsurgically, with late revision performed if loosening developed after union occurred. Type III fractures were treated successfully with a variety of techniques, with care taken to avoid stress risers between internal fixation devices and the femoral component.

The results of 31 postoperative femur fractures have been reported. Femoral loosening occurred in 75% of the cases. In seven cases, significant trauma led to fracture, and nine had stress risers. The majority of patients reported increasing hip pain before the fracture. Fourteen fractures were type I, 11 were type II, and six were type III. All of the type III fractures were treated with long-stem revision. Type II fractures can be treated nonsurgically, although late loosening occurred in 50% of the cases in the reported series.

Two other groups of authors reported the results of open reduction and internal fixation for postoperative femoral fractures in 10 and 6 cases, respectively; union occurred in all 16 cases. Thus, these authors recommend surgical treatment for postoperative fractures of the femur about total hip components.

In conclusion, review of the literature supports internal fixation with a plate and cables along with bone grafting or revision with a long-stem femoral component. Revision should be the treatment of choice if the fracture has compromised the original implant's stability, or if instability is anticipated after fracture healing. Nonsurgical treatment may be successful if the fracture is minimally displaced, although the literature supports the increased possibility of late loosening of the femoral component. If the fracture is entirely below the stem, treatment can be nonsurgical or surgical, based on the fracture itself and the surgeon's experience.

Dislocation

Dislocation is the most common complication of total hip arthroplasty; its incidence ranges from 3% to 5%. Dislocation is second only to prosthetic loosening as an indication for reoperation. Factors implicated as causes for dislocation include surgical approach, inadequate restoration of soft-tissue tension, prosthetic component design, and orientation of the components. It is generally agreed that the incidence of dislocation diminishes as surgical experience increases.

Surgical Approach

The posterolateral approach with the patient in the lateral position has a higher incidence of dislocation than the anterior and transtrochanteric approaches with the patient in the supine position. In the lateral decubitus position, the lumbar lordosis is flattened and the pelvis is flexed to 35°. Postoperatively, the pelvis extends and the acetabulum may be retroverted. Retroversion and detachment of the external rotators can lead to dislocation. Also, in the lateral position, excess abduction, greater than 60°, of the acetabular component, can occur as the pelvis is relatively adducted.

Restoration of Soft-Tissue Tension

Restoration of tissue tension was believed to be the most important factor in preventing dislocation after total hip arthroplasty. Seventy-five percent of patients with dislocation were found to have severe medical and neurological problems that resulted in poor tissue tension.

The incidence of postoperative dislocation is much higher among patients who have had prior total hip arthroplasties. Seventy-five percent of the dislocations in one series were revision cases, and 80% of the dislocations in another series were among patients with previous hip surgery.

Prosthetic Design

Prosthetic design has been implicated as an etiologic factor in dislocation. The effect has been assessed of prosthetic design on dislocation, and three modes of dislocation were identified: poor tissue tension, neck impingement, and impingement from bony prominences about the acetabulum. This remains germane today because of the use of acetabular extended labrums and skirted head/neck components. Impingement must be avoided as the labrum and the neck can lever the head out of the acetabulum in either extension and external rotation or flexion and internal rotation.

Orientation of the Components

It is generally agreed that the femoral component should be anteverted 15° to 20°, as is the anatomical neck of the femur. However, achieving proper orientation of the acetabular component is more complex. It has been reported that the prosthetic acetabulum was stable in 30° to 50° of abduction and 20° to 40° of flexion. The normal acetabulum is positioned in 50° of abduction and 40° of anteversion, which is significantly more abducted and flexed than recommended by most hip surgeons. Of course, the normal hip is stable in this position because the femoral head is much larger and the supporting capsular ligaments have not been distorted.

If malpositioned, the hip may be protected from dislocation for a few months postoperatively by soft-tissue and capsular healing. However, a study that indicates a late dislocation (5 to 10 years postoperatively) of 0.4% indicates that a malpositioned component will not be protected indefinitely by the capsule.

Management of Chronic Dislocation

Dislocation is painful. It increases morbidity, requires bracing and, frequently, reoperation. Multiple revision operations can increase the dislocation rate to 25%. Methods of treating the dislocated hip include closed reduction and hip abduction brace, spica cast, revision of one or both components, acetabular augmentation, or a constrained prosthetic system. Both the hip abduction brace and spica cast have been successful in preventing dislocation in 78% to 98% of the cases.

An 81% success rate was reported for the use of trochanteric advancement to manage chronic dislocation. Use of this procedure requires caution. It is difficult in patients who have had a previous anterolateral approach, because a portion of the abductor mechanism has been removed from the trochanter and, by removing the trochanter, all the problems inherent with trochanteric osteotomy must be dealt with.

Another technique in the management of recurrent dislocation is the use of large inside diameter acetabular cups with either bipolar or large unipolar heads (average head size = 45 mm). Stability was achieved in all of a small group of recurrent dislocations (eight patients).

In cases of marked extremity shortening, loss of musculature, weakness of any residual musculature, altered kinesiology, the elderly and/or disoriented patient, and the multiply-revised patient who has failed other attempts at treatment, constrained acetabular components have been used. Constrained prostheses diminish range of motion, may potentially disrupt the acetabular or femoral interface between the component and bone, and do not completely solve the problem of chronic dislocation. If redislocation occurs, reduction requires operative treatment.

Reviews of the operative correction of unstable arthroplasties have shown a 61% to 75% success rate in achieving stability following reoperation for dislocation after cemented total hip replacements. There have been reports in the literature of the displacement of uncemented acetabular components after dislocation and of disassembly of modular components following dislocation after attempts at closed reduction.

Causes of instability include component malposition, disruption of the trochanter and abductor mechanism, and impingement or are multiple and unknown. Reoperation rates for dislocation have been reported at 32%, 42%, and 44%. It was found that the success of the reoperation for dislocation was not associated with sex or age of the patient, number of previous operations, operative approach, leg-length discrepancy, increased head diameter, acetabular tilt, femoral anteversion, rehabilitation, or immobilization. Early instability (within the first 3 months) is usually due to soft-tissue laxity and can be treated by closed reduction and bracing. Late instability, although often due to malposition, trochanteric or abductor disruption, acetabular wear, or increased range of motion with weakened soft tissue, may require reoperation.

Heterotopic Ossification

After total hip arthroplasty, heterotopic bone forms in as many as 53% of patients. In as many as 7% of the cases the ossification can be severe, resulting in pain and decreased motion, particularly internal rotation. Heterotopic ossification is more likely to develop in patients who have formed ectopic ossification at a previous surgery on either the same or contralateral hip. Others at risk are those with hypertrophic osteoarthritis and active ankylosing spondylitis. Some reports have cited an increased incidence of bone formation from the transtrochanteric, anterior, and direct lateral approaches as compared with the posterolateral approach. The incidence of heterotopic ossification has been reported to range from 1% to 53% in general populations and to be as high as 90% in the high-risk groups.

Although several causes have been cited for the formation of heterotopic bone, its formation traditionally has been thought to be caused by trauma to and the resulting inflammation of muscle tissue; however, this actually results in myositis ossificans. Bony formations in soft tissues (other than the periosteum), in the absence of a well-defined cause, should be referred to heterotopic ossification. It is currently believed that primordial mesenchymal cells differentiate into osteoprogenitor cells that then modulate into osteoblastic tissue. This process has been noted to occur as soon as 16 hours postoperatively, with a peak response noted at approximately 32 hours.

Classification

The Brooker system is the most widely used system of classifying heterotopic bone formation. Class I is characterized by islands of bone within the soft tissues about the hip, and class II includes bone spurs in the pelvis or the proximal end of the femur, leaving at least 1 cm between the opposing bone surfaces. Class III consists of bone spurs that extend from the pelvis or proximal end of the femur, which reduce the space between the opposing bone surfaces to less than 1 cm. Class IV may be defined as radiographic evidence of ankylosis of the hip.

Prevention

Several methods of preventing heterotopic ossification have been advocated. It has been recommended that oral diphosphonates be administered 1 to 2 months preoperatively and continued 3 to 6 months postoperatively. Although the diphosphonates could inhibit mineralization of osteoid, they had no effect on the formation of the osteoid matrix. In addition, the delay in mineralization reverses when the treatment is discontinued. This agent has also been associated with gastrointestinal side effects.

A prophylactic effect of indomethacin in preventing the formation of heterotopic bone after total hip arthroplasty has been reported. Nonsteroidal, anti-inflammatory agents inhibit prostaglandin synthesis and may interfere with the inflammatory response that occurs after trauma, a phenomenon associated with the formation of heterotopic bone. The minimal dosage and treatment regimen required for preventing heterotopic ossification have not been determined. Data from a variety of clinical studies have indicated that both indomethacin and ibuprofen, as well as aspirin, are effective in lessening the severity of het-

erotopic bone formation after total hip arthroplasty. However, these agents may also have the adverse effect of inhibiting bony ingrowth into porous-coated, cementless prosthetic components. Moreover, the prophylactic use of warfarin for thromboembolism could place the patient at increased risk of bleeding when the nonsteroidal anti-inflammatory agents are also administered.

In 1981 radiotherapy was recommended as a preventive measure against heterotopic ossification. Initially, 10 doses were given over a 12-day course, providing a total of 2,000 rads. Treatment failures were attributed to a delay in the initiation of treatment beyond 5 days postoperatively. This study reported a 2% incidence of heterotopic ossification. In another study, hips were irradiated after ectopic bone was surgically removed; in this study, the incidence of heterotopic bone formation was 5%.

The use of irradiation in 1 or 2 fractions for a total of 700 to 800 rads has been advocated. This regimen was found to be as effective as the previously recommended protocol of 2,000 rads and 10 fractions, if the irradiation is delivered before postoperative day 4. Because radiotherapy may inhibit the bony ingrowth into porous-coated prostheses, the porous-coated prosthesis should be shielded from the primary radiation beam. Although the possibility exists of the late development of malignancy when radiation is used, no malignancy was found in a series of 90 patients followed for up to 8 years. Current recommendations are for a fraction of 700 rads to be delivered 1 to 4 days postoperatively.

If surgical resection of bone becomes necessary, resection should be delayed until 6 months after total hip arthroplasty. This delay will permit maturation of bone and development of a distinct fibrous capsule. The operative approach for resection should be chosen after review of the anteroposterior and lateral radiographs. During surgery, hemostasis should be meticulously controlled; this control will help avoid the formation of hematoma, which would increase the risk of recurrence. Because of the high incidence of recurrence noted in the literature, prophylactic radiotherapy should be used in such patients.

Annotated Bibliography

Neural and Vascular Injury

Schmalzried TP, Amstutz HC, Dorey FJ: Nerve palsy associated with total hip replacement: Risk factors and prognosis. *J Bone Joint Surg* 1991;73A:1074–1080.

A retrospective review of 3,126 consecutive hip replacements identified a 1.7% incidence of nerve palsy. All patients who had complete recovery of neurologic function had it by 21 months. The ability to walk decreased for all patients who had nerve palsy. Prognosis for neurologic recovery was related to the degree to which the nerve was damaged.

Wasielewski RC, Crossett LS, Rubash HE: Neural and vascular injury in total hip arthroplasty. *Orthop Clin North Am* 1992;23:219–235.

The authors review the quadrant system and caution against using the anterior quadrant for acetabular screw fixation. Complete review of the anatomy and etiologic factors in neural and vascular injuries are stated in this article, including SSEP monitoring in difficult revision and primary arthroplasties. Incidence of postoperative nerve palsy is given.

Femoral Fractures

Kavanagh BF: Femoral fractures associated with total hip arthroplasty. *Orthop Clin North Am* 1992;23:249–257.

This article reviews the principles of rigid fixation of both prosthesis and the fracture to achieve satisfactory results. Intraoperative and postoperative fractures of the femur are included. Methods of prevention are also highlighted.

Missakian ML, Rand JA: Fractures of the femoral shaft adjacent to long stem femoral components of total hip arthroplasty: Report of seven cases. *Orthopedics* 1993; 16:149–152.

Seven femoral shaft fractures adjacent to the distal aspect of long stem revision femoral components were evaluated from 2 to 12 years after fracture, average 6 years. Nonoperative treatment was used in four, and resulted in delayed union in two patients and malunion in two patients. Operative treatment resulted in no malunions and early recovery of function. Femoral shaft fractures adjacent to long stem total hip arthroplasties are difficult to manage. The complication rate is 71%.

Mont MA, Maar DC, Krackow KA, et al: Hoop-stress fractures of the proximal femur during hip arthroplasty: Management and results in 19 cases. *J Bone Joint Surg* 1992;74B:257–260.

Nineteen intraoperative hoop-stress fractures described as incomplete, linear, and minimally displaced were identified in a retrospective review of 730 consecutive primary uncemented and cemented total hip arthroplasties. Management included cerclage wiring in 12, bone graft and cerclage in two, further impaction in two, and the use of cement in three. Eighteen patients had an excellent or good result with an average HHS of 93. All but one patient had a stable fixation score according to Engh. Properly managed fractures of the proximal femur do not detract from the results of total hip arthroplasty.

Sharkey PF, Hozack WJ, Booth RE Jr, et al: Intraoperative femoral fractures in cementless total hip arthroplasty. *Orthop Rev* 1992;21:337–342.

In this series, no difference was found in clinical or radiographic results of cementless total hip arthroplasty between patients who had an intraoperative femoral fracture and patients who did not have this complication. All fractures were recognized intraoperatively. Initial stability of the implant was felt to be satisfactory for all cases.

Dislocation

Daly PJ, Morrey BF: Operative correction of an unstable total hip arthroplasty. *J Bone Joint Surg* 1992;74A:1334–1343.

Results of reoperation in 95 patients who had acute subluxation or dislocation following cemented total hip replacement were reviewed. Instability was classified as caused by malposition of the component, disruption of the trochanteric abduction mechanism, impingement, or multiple and unknown factors. Of the reoperations, 61% were successful in that there was no additional subluxation or dislocation. The authors concluded that the results of operative treatment for an unstable total hip replacement can be optimized when a precise determination of the cause of the instability is made and appropriate measures are applied.

Ekelund A, Rydell N, Nilsson OS: Total hip arthroplasty in patients 80 years of age and older. *Clin Orthop* 1992; 281:101–106.

The dislocation rate of this group of patients was 9.2%. Dislocations were common in patients operated on for complications from proximal femoral fractures, and the risk for recurrent dislocation was high.

Laughlin RT, Smith KL, Adair DM: Displacement of an uncemented acetabular component after dislocation of a total hip prosthesis: A case report. *J Arthroplasty* 1992; 7:303–307.

This is a case report of a patient in whom a noncemented acetabular component was dislodged after closed reduction of a dislocated total hip component. Reductions must be performed with care, under general anesthesia, with cementless component to prevent disruption of the interface. The authors recommended bicortical screw fixation to provide maximum contact and rigid fixation in the early postoperative period.

Heterotopic Ossification

Kjaersgaard-Andersen P, Ritter MA: Short-term treatment with nonsteroidal anti-inflammatory medications to prevent heterotopic bone formation after total hip arthroplasty: A preliminary report. *Clin Orthop* 1992;279:157–162.

This study demonstrated that treatment with either 650 mg of aspirin twice daily for 6 weeks or 25 mg of indomethacin 3 times daily for the first 14 postoperative days was sufficient to prevent the formation of severe heterotopic ossification after total hip arthroplasty.

Maloney WJ, Jasty M, Willett C, et al: Prophylaxis for heterotopic bone formation after total hip arthroplasty using low-dose radiation in high-risk patients. *Clin Orthop* 1992;280:230–234.

Use of 7.5 Gy over three fractions minimized the radiobiologic impact, whereas the use of precision shielding minimized the total volume of tissue treated. The authors felt this regimen is an effective means of preventing significant heterotopic ossification in high-risk patients while minimizing radiation exposure.

Maloney WJ, Krushell RJ, Jasty M, et al: Incidence of heterotopic ossification after total hip replacement: Effect of the type of fixation of the femoral component. *J Bone Joint Surg* 1991;73A:191–193.

The incidence of severity of heterotopic ossification after 65 consecutive primary uncemented total hip replacements was compared with that after 70 consecutive primary hybrid total hip replacements. Either none or only class I ectopic bone developed in 74% of the hips in the hybrid group compared with 40% of the hips in the uncemented group. None of the patients in the hybrid group needed reoperation for excision of ectopic bone, but 4% or 6% of the patients in the uncemented group needed such a reoperation because of severe limitation of motion.

Pellegrini VD Jr, Konski AA, Gastel JA, et al: Prevention of heterotopic ossification with irradiation after total hip arthroplasty: Radiation therapy with a single dose of eight hundred centigray administered to a limited field. *J Bone Joint Surg* 1992;74A:186–200.

A comparison was made between a single 800 cGy dose of limited-field radiation to 1,000 cGy of limited-field radiation in divided doses in patients at high risk for heterotopic ossification following total hip arthroplasty. A single-dose, limited-field radiation was effective for the prevention of heterotopic ossification without compromise of early fixation of uncemented implants.

Thomas BJ: Heterotopic bone formation after total hip arthroplasty. *Orthop Clin North Am* 1992;23:347–358.

This article reviews the etiology and treatment of heterotopic bone formation as well as surgical excision once performed.

Tozun R, Pinar H, Yesiller E, et al: Indomethacin for prevention of heterotopic ossification after total hip arthroplasty. *J Arthroplasty* 1992;7:57–61.

Twenty-nine hips were given 75 mg of indomethacin daily for 4 weeks after surgery with a minimum follow-up of 6 months. The indomethacin effectively prevented higher grades of heterotopic ossification, meaning greater than grade I following total hip arthroplasty. Two patients who were not included in the study had gastrointestinal bleeding and recovered after withdrawal of indomethacin.

Warren SB, Brooker AF Jr: Excision of heterotopic bone followed by irradiation after total hip arthroplasty. *J Bone Joint Surg* 1992;74A:201–210.

Twelve patients who had total hip arthroplasty had extensive excision of heterotopic ossification, followed by prompt, low-dose irradiation. Eleven of the 12 had excellent relief of pain, and all 12 gained an average of 45° of flexion and 25° of abduction.

21

Surgical Approaches to the Hip

The proper selection of a specific surgical approach to the hip should be based on the anticipated exposure requirements (femoral, acetabular, and iliac); the location of prior incisions; preoperative leg lengths and range of motion; soft-tissue tension and integrity; patient size; surgical goals; and the surgeon's familiarity with the involved anatomy, both normal and pathologic. All hip surgeons should be comfortable with use of the anterior, lateral, posterior, and transtrochanteric capsular approaches to the hip; more complicated extensile exposures are generally undertaken by the more experienced hip surgeons. The purpose of this chapter is to discuss surgical principles, pertinent anatomy, indications, advantages, limitations, and results of the more commonly used surgical approaches for simple and complex reconstructive hip surgery.

General Principles

For optimum exposure, all surgical approaches to the hip require positioning that provides rigid immobilization of the pelvis with free mobility of the lower extremity. This positioning allows a surgeon to improve his orientation and visualization of the patient's anatomy by simple changes in leg position and soft-tissue tension. The lateral decubitus position is used for all exposures except the anterior, ilioinguinal, medial, and anterolateral approaches. All incisions should be placed with the ability to make an extensile exposure, if needed, from the ilium to the distal femur. Large patients and "stiff" hips most often require an extended incision, extensive soft-tissue releases, and/or trochanteric osteotomy for adequate exposure. Cutaneous blood supply to the hip (unlike the knee) generally is favorable, but the risk of tissue necrosis can be minimized by following these principles: use straight incisions, avoiding curved proximal and distal incisions; incorporate old incisions where possible; avoid parallel incisions; and make skin bridges as broad as possible when incorporating old incisions or using parallel incisions.

Surgical Approaches

Anterior Iliofemoral Approach

This exposure involves a dissection between the sartorius and tensor fascia lata superficially, and the rectus femoris and gluteus medius more deeply. Structures at risk for injury include the lateral femoral cutaneous nerve, which usually crosses the sartorius 2 to 5 cm distal to the anterior superior iliac spine, and the ascending branch of the lat-

eral femoral circumflex artery, which overlies the rectus femoris muscle. The anterior approach permits excellent visualization of the inner and outer iliac tables, the anterior and superior acetabulum, and the anterior femoral head and neck. It also allows a hip to be dislocated anteriorly with minimal risk of injury to the femoral head blood supply. Disadvantages include poor visualization of the posterior and inferior acetabulum, poor femoral canal access, and a high incidence of heterotopic bone formation. This approach is most useful for pelvic osteotomies, open reduction of congenital dislocation of the hip (CDH) and pelvic fractures, hip joint debridements, resurfacing and cup arthroplasties, and in combination with other approaches for hip fusion and revision total hip arthroplasty (THA). As an isolated exposure, it has limited usefulness in primary and revision THA.

Ilioinguinal Approach

This approach (Fig. 1) is used in conjunction with other hip exposures (eg, posterolateral) to allow complete visualization of the acetabulum, medial pelvic wall, pubis, and anterior column of the hip. The main structures at risk for injury include the spermatic cord and round ligament medially, the contents of the femoral triangle (femoral nerve, artery, and vein), and the lateral femoral cutaneous nerve. Indications for use of the ilioinguinal approach with other hip exposures include: anterior column fractures, especially those involving the pubis; reconstruction of the medial acetabular wall; complex acetabular allografts; and severe cases of protrusio prosthetica. The ilioinguinal approach is best combined with the triradiate approach for maximum exposure of the acetabulum and anterior pelvis.

Anterolateral Approach

This approach is commonly used for resurfacing arthroplasty, primary and simple revision THA, open reduction of femoral neck fractures, and joint exploration and biopsy. This approach preserves the blood supply to the femoral head if anterior capsulotomy is performed proximally near the acetabular rim with preservation of the anterior inferior capsule. Dissection proximal to the greater trochanter must be limited to avoid injuring the superior gluteal nerve, which enters the tensor fascia lata and anterior gluteus medius. To improve exposure and avoid injury to the anterior abductors during retraction, either an anterior wafer of bone (with attached gluteus medius and minimus) can be osteotomized or trochanteric osteotomy can be performed. Other limitations include poor exposure of the structures posterior to the posterior

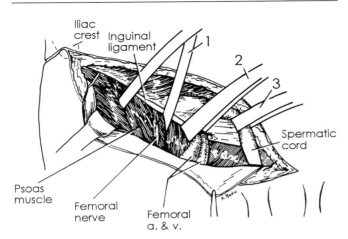

Fig. 1 The ilioinguinal approach isolates three windows: 1) psoas muscle and femoral nerve; 2) femoral artery and vein; and 3) spermatic cord or round ligament.

acetabular rim and limited exposure of the interior femoral canal distally unless trochanteric osteotomy is performed. Most studies demonstrate a lower incidence of postoperative dislocations with the anterolateral approach in THA when compared to the posterolateral and trochanteric osteotomy approaches.

Lateral Approach

This approach (Fig. 2) was popularized to assure proper orientation during THA and was recently modified for extensile exposure of the femur during revision THA. The hip is approached anteriorly after release of the anterior two thirds of the gluteus medius into the vastus lateralis, maintaining a continuous musculotendinous sleeve. As with the anterolateral approach, femoral head blood supply can be maintained by careful anterior-superior capsulotomy. When the gluteus medius tendinous insertion is atrophic, a wafer of bone from the anterior greater trochanter may be mobilized to create a musculo-osseous muscular sleeve for more secure reattachment of the tissues. Several studies suggest an increased incidence of abductor weakness, prolonged limp, and heterotopic bone when this approach is used. Abductor dysfunction can be minimized by splitting the abductors more anterior than originally recommended; by secure soft-tissue reattachment; and by limiting separation of the gluteus medius muscle fibers to no more than 4 cm above the superior acetabular rim, thus, avoiding injury to the superior gluteal nerve. Retention of the posterior fibers of the gluteus medius and the greater trochanter will interfere with the surgeon's ability to gain leg length, may limit access to the interior femoral canal distally, and provides poor exposure to structures posterior to the posterior acetabular rim (eg, for posterior column plating). Advantages to the lateral approach include preservation of femoral head blood sup-

ply; excellent exposure of the acetabulum and proximal femur in difficult cases without the associated risks of trochanteric osteotomy; ease of orientation during THA; and retention of the posterior soft tissues to lessen the incidence of postoperative posterior dislocation of the hip. These advantages make the lateral approach particularly useful in the elderly, noncompliant patient with a femoral neck fracture or the neurologically compromised patient (eg, polio or Parkinson's disease) undergoing hemiarthroplasty or THA. For the above reasons, the lateral approach is currently one of the most commonly selected exposures for primary and revision THA.

Posterolateral Approach

This approach provides posterior capsular exposure to the hip by splitting the gluteus maximus, releasing the external rotators, and retracting the posterior fibers of the gluteus medius and minimus anteriorly. Extended exposure during primary and revision THA can be accomplished easily by anterior capsulectomy or release of the gluteus maximus tendon insertion, which allows improved anterior and lateral retraction of the proximal femur. Nevertheless, exposure to the anterior column and internal canal of the distal femur may be limited unless trochanteric osteotomy is performed. Structures at risk include the sciatic nerve and branches of the medial femoral circumflex artery. The sciatic nerve is particularly vulnerable if it is scarred or displaced from previous surgery or developmental dysplasia.

Frequent injury to the posterior retinacular blood supply to the femoral head makes the posterior approach a poor selection for hip arthrotomy in which maintenance of femoral head viability is desired (eg, surface replacement arthroplasty, synovectomy, open reduction and internal fixation of femoral neck fractures). Data from several studies indicate an increased incidence of postoperative posterior dislocation when the posterolateral approach is compared to the anterolateral, lateral, and trochanteric osteotomy approaches during THA. This complication can be reduced significantly by careful repair of the posterior capsule and external rotators and strict adherence to hip precautions during the early postoperative rehabilitation phase. Decreased time of surgery, excellent exposure with minimal muscle damage, and fast rehabilitation make this approach particularly attractive for most types of primary and revision THA in the active, cooperative patient. Other indications include posterior column acetabular fractures, biopsy of the posterior femoral neck or acetabulum, and treatment of comminuted femoral neck fractures in young patients requiring internal fixation with muscle pedicle vascular supplementation.

Trochanteric Osteotomy Approach

Osteotomy of the greater trochanter (Fig. 3) can be accomplished easily through anterolateral, lateral, posterolateral, or triradiate incisions. The level and type of osteotomy should be determined after assessment of bone stock, tro-

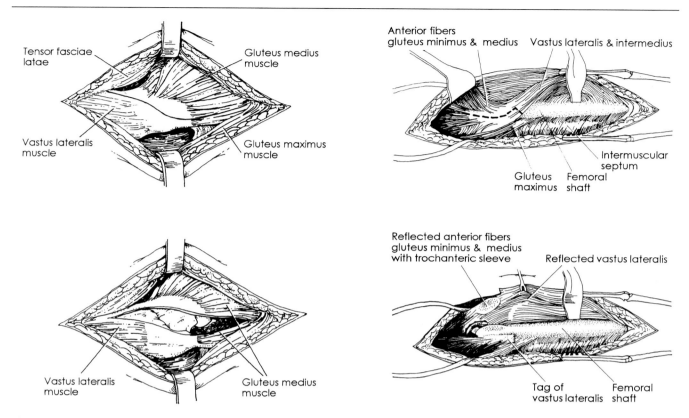

Fig. 2 Comparison of the direct lateral (**top and bottom left**) and extensile lateral approach (**top** and **bottom right**) without (**top right**) and with (**bottom right**) osteotomy of the anterior greater trochanter. The extensile lateral approach improves acetabular and femoral exposures for allografting.

chanteric size and position, the need for trochanteric advancement (eg, leg length adjustment), and the location of cement and prosthesis during revision THA. Anterior, lateral, and posterior exposure of the osteotomy plane prior to osteotomy will aid in mobilization of the trochanteric fragment. Branches of the medial and lateral circumflex arteries (cruciate anastomosis) will require hemostasis. This approach provides extensible exposure of the acetabulum and improves access to the distal femoral canal during primary and revision THA. Other advantages include preservation of the superior gluteal nerve and abductor muscle fibers; preservation of the femoral head blood supply during anterior capsulotomy and dislocation; and the ability to adjust abductor soft-tissue tensioning during limb lengthening or limb shortening. Disadvantages when compared to other approaches include increased blood loss and operative time; slower rehabilitation; and the complications of trochanteric nonunion, migration, and bursitis following inadequate fixation of the osteotomy. These complications not only compromise abductor function and clinical results, but may lead to hip instability if

the trochanteric fragment migrates proximally and anteriorly (Fig. 4). The incidence of trochanteric nonunion is particularly high after postoperative hip irradiation for heterotopic bone prophylaxis.

Modifications of the conventional Charnley trochanteric osteotomy have been described recently for THA to reduce the complications associated with conventional osteotomy. The anterior trochanteric slide (Fig. 3, *top right*) preserves an intact musculo-osseous muscular sleeve of gluteus medius, greater trochanter, and vastus lateralis; it also allows physiologic reconstruction of the hip's soft-tissue envelope and reduces the incidence of trochanteric nonunion and migration. Osteotomy of the anterior portion of the greater trochanter (Fig. 2, *bottom right*) maintains the continuity of the tendinous junction of the anterior half of the gluteus medius with the vastus lateralis; reattachment of the osteotomized fragment is simple and secure, reducing the incidence of nonunion and migration. Extended proximal femoral osteotomy (Fig. 3, *bottom*) appears promising in revision THA in which the trochanteric bed is severely compromised as a result of osteolysis or

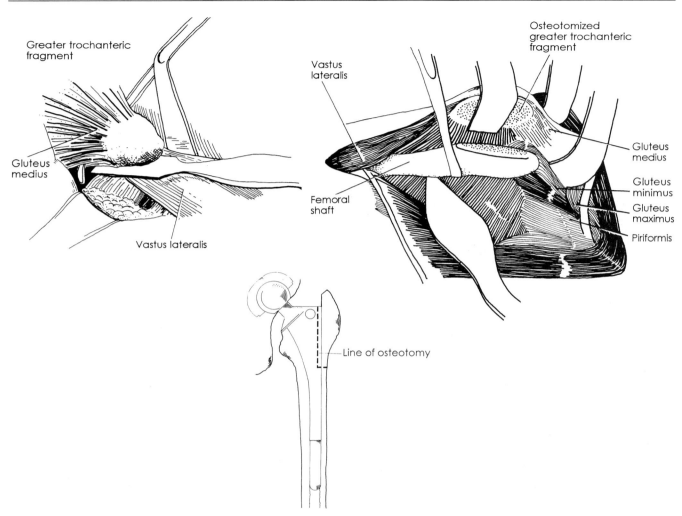

Fig. 3 Comparison of the conventional osteotomy (**top left**), the anterior trochanteric slide (**top right**), and the extended proximal femoral osteotomy (**bottom**) for extensible hip exposures. The anterior slide preserves an intact sleeve of gluteus medius, greater trochanter, and vastus lateralis. The extended proximal femoral osteotomy avoids problems associated with osteotomies of the greater trochanter and allows easier extraction of femoral components and bone cement.

prior cement; it also permits easy removal of extensively porous coated or longer cemented femoral stems. Current indications for trochanteric osteotomy include preservation of the femoral head blood supply by anterior dislocation of the hip for debridement, synovectomy, or surface replacement arthroplasty; significant limb lengthening or shortening during THA; and complex primary and revision THA. Trochanteric osteotomy is particularly beneficial for cases of severe protrusion, "high riding" CDH, hips with limited preoperative range of motion, conversion of long-standing resection arthroplasty to THA, and acetabuli requiring large segmental allografting.

Triradiate Approach

This approach (Fig. 5) eliminates the need for separate anterior and posterior approaches for complete exposure of the anterior and posterior acetabular columns. It also avoids the potential complication of ischemic necrosis of the hip abductors by injury to the superior gluteal vessels, which is possible when the extended iliofemoral approach is chosen. The triradiate approach combines the anterior, posterior, and trochanter osteotomy approaches, thereby allowing extensible exposure of the acetabulum, anterior and posterior columns, the internal iliac wall, the anterior aspect of the sacroiliac joint, and the outer aspect of the innominate bone. The superior angle of the skin incision

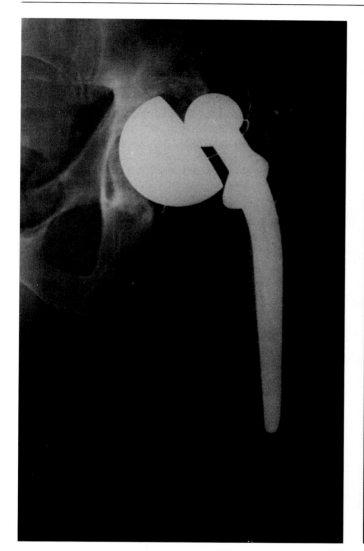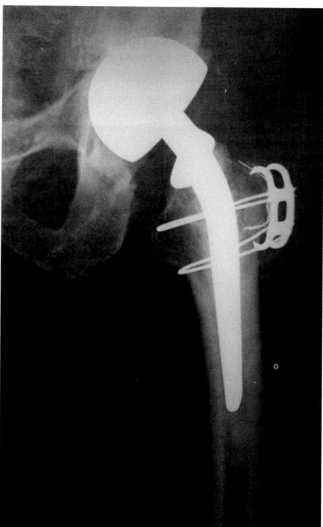

Fig. 4 Proximal and anterior migration of the greater trochanter may lead to impingement and instability (**left**). Repair has been performed with a cable grip system (**right**).

should be at least 120° to avoid skin necrosis (Fig. 5). This is often difficult when prior incisions are present. Great care must be taken to stay anterior to the tensor fascia lata, which receives its vascular supply posteriorly from the superior gluteal artery. The anterior column is exposed by detaching the sartorius and rectus femoris muscles. Improved exposure of the medial pelvic wall and pubis is accomplished by extending the anterior incision into an ilioinguinal exposure (the extensile triradiate approach; Fig. 5). The triradiate approach was originally developed to reduce and repair complex acetabular fractures. Other useful indications include tumor reconstruction, severe protrusio prosthetica, pelvic discontinuities associated

with THA, and complex acetabular allograft reconstruction, including whole acetabular allografts.

Medial Approach

The medial approach was developed for open reduction of CDH, and this approach still has particular use for CDH when the iliopsoas tendon blocks closed reduction. Structures at risk for injury include the anterior branch of the obturator nerve lying between the adductor longus and adductor brevis and the medial femoral circumflex artery adjacent to the medial aspect of the iliopsoas tendon. Besides CDH, this approach is also indicated for release of

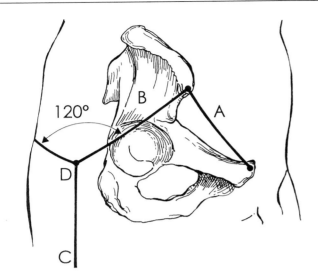

Fig. 5 The extensile triradiate approach incorporates the ilioinguinal exposure (limb A) with the triradiate exposure (limbs B, C, and D) for complex acetabular allograft reconstruction.

the iliopsoas tendon unit, biopsy of the proximal medial femur, and adductor tenotomy with obturator neurectomy.

Surgical Exposure in Revision Total Hip Arthroplasty

Exposure of the hip in revision THA presents special challenges to the reconstructive hip surgeon. Revision surgery usually requires improved exposure over primary surgery in order to safely remove scar tissue, particulate debris, and failed implants and cement. Extensible exposure of the pelvis, acetabulum, and femur is often required to manage fractures, discontinuities, bone deficiencies, and bone deformities. The surgical approach selected should allow flexibility for extension of the exposure as needed. The anterolateral and posterolateral approaches are the best alternatives because both offer excellent acetabular and femoral exposures; also, enhanced exposure is easily achieved through either approach by trochanteric osteotomy. Fewer surgeons today routinely use the conventional Charnley trochanteric osteotomy in revision surgery because of problems associated with union of the greater trochanter. Osteotomy of the anterior greater trochanter, anterior trochanteric slide, the extended proximal femoral osteotomy, the direct lateral approach, and the extensible lateral approaches all provide extensive exposure while reducing the problems associated with union of the greater trochanter. All approaches should allow exposure of the entire proximal femur and entire circumference of the acetabulum to permit careful implant removal and reconstruction. Complete removal of the scarred pseudocapsule is essential for this exposure, and circumferential subperiosteal stripping of the proximal 5 cm of the femur with release of the iliopsoas and gluteus maximus tendons may be required in more difficult cases.

When planning acetabular reconstructions, remember that plating or bone grafting of the posterior acetabular column is most difficult through the anterolateral or lateral approaches, even when the greater trochanter is osteotomized. Anterior column defects often require a secondary exposure through an ilioinguinal approach. Acetabular discontinuity and complex acetabular allografts (eg, whole acetabular allografts) require a triradiate or extensible triradiate exposure for optimum reconstruction. For difficult femoral reconstructions, femoral windows or osteotomies may be required for proper removal of bone cement and fully porous or long-stem cemented prostheses. The extended proximal femoral osteotomy appears particularly promising for these difficult revisions.

Annotated Bibliography

General Principles

Crenshaw AH: Surgical Approaches, in Crenshaw AH (ed): *Campbell's Operative Orthopaedics,* ed 8. St. Louis, MO, Mosby Year Book, 1992, pp 23–116.

Surgical approaches to the hip are described in anatomic detail.

Cuckler JM: Surgical approaches, in Steinberg ME (ed): *The Hip and Its Disorders.* Philadelphia, PA, WB Saunders, 1991, pp 88–105.

Surgical anatomy, indications, limitations, and structures at risk for various hip exposures are presented.

Surgical Approaches

Callaghan JJ, Dysnet SH, Savory CG: The uncemented porous-coated anatomic total hip prosthesis: Two-year results of a prospective consecutive series. *J Bone Joint Surg* 1988;70A:337–346.

Moderate or severe limp was present at 2 years in 28% of patients in whom the lateral approach was used compared to 0% at 1 year with the posterolateral approach. With the lateral approach, heterotopic bone was present in 80% (8% with grade 3 or 4).

Carlson DC, Robinson HJ Jr: Surgical approaches for primary total hip arthroplasty: A prospective comparison of the Marcy modification of the Gibson and Watson-Jones approaches. *Clin Orthop* 1987;222:161–166.

Comparable series of 37 cases each showed similar operative times, placement of implants, and complications including postoperative dislocations.

Dall D: Exposure of the hip by anterior osteotomy of the greater trochanter: A modified anterolateral approach. *J Bone Joint Surg* 1986;68B:382–386.

This approach provided excellent exposure with retention of good abductor function in 69 hips with 100% union of the osteotomized fragment.

Frndak PA, Mallory TH, Lombardi AV Jr: Translateral surgical approach to the hip: The abductor muscle split. *Clin Orthop* 1993;295:135–141.

A modification of the Hardinge lateral approach with a more anterior split of the gluteus medius and posterior split of the vastus lateralis is described to improve postoperative hip abductor function.

Glassman AH, Engh CA, Bobyn JD: A technique of extensible exposure for total hip arthroplasty. *J Arthroplasty* 1987;2:11–21.

This exposure was found to be particularly useful in difficult primary and revision surgeries where leg length is adjusted. Nonunion of the trochanter occurred in 10% of 90 patients but was not a source of pain.

Hardinge K: The direct lateral approach to the hip. *J Bone Joint Surg* 1982;64B:17–19.

This approach allows adequate access for orientation of total hip arthroplasty components.

Head WC, Mallory TH, Berklacich FM, et al: Extensile exposure of the hip for revision arthroplasty. *J Arthroplasty* 1987;2:265–273.

The authors describe a lateral approach with or without anterior trochanteric osteotomy for complex revision surgery. Abductor lurch or (+) Trendelenberg sign was present in 40 of 158 patients.

Krackow KA, Steinman H, Cohn BT, et al: Clinical experience with a triradiate exposure of the hip for difficult total hip arthroplasty. *J Arthroplasty* 1988; 3:267–278.

Indications and technique for the triradiate exposure are discussed.

Letournel E: Acetabulum fractures: Classification and management. *Clin Orthop* 1980;151:81–106.

The ilioinguinal approach for anterior column acetabular fractures is described.

Younger TI, Bradford MS, Magnus RE, et al: Extended proximal femoral osteotomy: A new technique for femoral revision arthroplasty. *J Arthroplasty* 1995;10:329–338.

The authors present the extended proximal femoral osteotomy to avoid the complications of trochanteric osteotomy. It also facilitates removal of femoral implants and cement when compared to trochanteric osteotomy approaches.

Mears DC, Rubash HE: Extensile exposure of the pelvis. *Contemp Orthop* 1983;6:21–31.

The triradiate exposure for complex acetabular fractures is presented.

Mostardi RA, Askew MJ, Gradisar IA Jr, et al: Comparison of functional outcome of total hip arthroplasties involving four surgical approaches. *J Arthroplasty* 1988;3:279–284.

Superior isokinetic strength in adduction, flexion, and extension was demonstrated with an anterior bone wafer technique when compared to other anterior capsular exposures.

Stiehl JB: Acetabular allograft reconstruction in total hip arthroplasty: Part II. Surgical approach and aftercare. *Orthop Review* 1991;20:425–432.

The extensile triradiate approach (combination ilioinguinal and triradiate exposure) is described for complex acetabular allograft reconstruction.

Turner RH, Mattingly DA, Scheller A: Femoral revision total hip arthroplasty using a long-stem femoral component: Clinical and radiographic analysis. *J Arthroplasty* 1987;2:247–258.

Trochanteric complications were encountered in 34% and symptomatic separation in 16% of 105 hips undergoing revision total hip arthroplasty through a trochanteric osteotomy.

22

Primary Cemented Total Hip Arthroplasty

Introduction

In order to understand the great variability in the published results of primary cemented total hip replacement, it is necessary to be familiar with the concept of "generations" in cementing techniques. First generation cementing technique refers to finger packing doughy cement into the unplugged femoral canal and acetabulum. In this era, the femoral components often had sharp corners with a narrow medial border and were not made of superalloys. Although some surgeons were able to achieve a satisfactory cement mantle using this method, in most hands, it resulted in an incomplete cement mantle with large defects. Second generation technique involved plugging the medullary canal, pulsatile (pressurized) lavage, and cement insertion in a retrograde fashion using a cement gun. The implants were made of superalloys and had a broad medial border. Third generation cementing includes second generation techniques plus porosity reduction, pressurization of the cement mantle, and surface modifications on the implants.

Another important factor in reviewing the published results of cemented arthroplasty is to be aware of how the author defines failure. Endpoints used to define a failed arthroplasty include revision surgery, clinical failure (a painful arthroplasty), and radiographic failure. The reported failure rate depends on how failure is defined. The mechanical failure rate for a particular implant can be defined by the percentage of cases in a given series requiring revision surgery plus the percentage of cases determined to be radiographically loose.

Radiographic Assessment

The definition of what constitutes a radiographically loose implant is not agreed on by all authors. However, most agree that a cemented femoral component is definitely loose if one of the following criteria are met: (1) implant subsidence on serial radiographs or change in implant position; (2) new metal–cement radiolucency (not present on the initial postoperative radiograph); (3) cement mantle fracture; and (4) implant fracture.

One commonly used radiographic assessment of cemented femoral component stability also defines probably and possibly loose components. Radiographs that demonstrate a continuous radiolucent line at the cement-bone interface are graded probably loose. If there is an incomplete radiolucent line occupying between 50% and 99% of the cement–bone interface, the implant is graded as possibly loose. In light of recent autopsy studies in which the remodeling at the cement-bone interface has been evaluated, these criteria as well as the definition of a radiolucent line need to be reevaluated. Arthrography and radionuclide studies have not provided any significant additional information on cemented femoral component stability.

A cemented acetabular component is definitely loose if implant migration can be demonstrated on serial radiographs. In addition, it has been demonstrated that over 90% of cemented acetabular components that have a complete cement–bone radiolucency, regardless of width, are loose at revision surgery. Arthrography, properly performed, may be helpful in further assessing the stability of cemented acetabular components, especially in the absence of serial radiographs.

Long-Term Results: First Generation Cementing

The initial published results of first generation cementing techniques in North America were disappointing. On the femoral side, radiographic loosening was reported in 20% to 24% of cases at 5 years. By 10 years, reported femoral loosening rates had increased to 30% to 40%. In one study of 100 consecutive Müller total hip replacements followed for 10 years, 20 patients with 22 arthroplasties had died without having a revision and 25 arthroplasties had been revised (19 for aseptic loosening of one or both components). The overall femoral loosening rate was 40%. Femoral osteolysis was often associated with aseptic loosening. In another study, the femoral failure rate of Charnley low friction arthroplasties went from 24% at 5 years to almost 30% at 10 years.

The time course for aseptic loosening using first generation techniques was different for the femur and the acetabulum. Whereas relatively short-term results (5 years) on the femoral side demonstrated high failure rates, the cemented acetabular failure rates at the same time interval were low. In one study, the average time from surgery to the beginning of cemented acetabular component migration was reported to be 5 years. This was determined by examining serial radiographs. Use of more sensitive techniques, such as roentgenographic stereophotogrammetry, would likely demonstrate earlier migration. By 10 years, however, the reported rate of aseptic loosening with cemented acetabular sockets increased dramatically. At 10 to 14 years following surgery, socket loosening has been reported in several studies to be greater than 25%. The investigators who followed 100 consecutive Müller implants reported a 29% acetabular failure rate at 10 years.

In the long-term follow-up study of Charnley hip replacements noted above, the acetabular failure rate increased from 6.5% at 5 years to 11.3% at 10 years. This same group of patients were reviewed at 15 years, and in that report, the authors redefined their criteria for loosening. The probability of loosening for one or both components was calculated at 32% at 15 years. The probability of failure defined as revision or symptomatic loosening of one or both components was 12.7% at 15 years.

Despite the use of first generation cement technique, some investigators have reported excellent long-term clinical results. Three hundred and thirty Charnley prostheses inserted from 1970 to 1972 were followed for a minimum of 20 years. Eighty-three patients with 98 hips were still living at the 20-year follow-up. The mechanical failure rate (revised and radiographically loose, but not revised) was 13% of all 322 acetabular components and 6% of all 322 femoral components. In the surviving patients, the mechanical failure rate was 22% for the 98 acetabular components and 7% for the 98 femoral components. The excellent long-term clinical results presented in this study can be attributed to the expert handling of bone cement, which resulted in technically satisfactory cement mantles despite finger packing of the cement.

Contemporary Cement Technique

Cement is most commonly used on the femoral side, therefore, the discussion on contemporary use of bone cement will focus on cementing femoral components. The general principles apply to cementing of acetabular components as well. The goal in femoral cementing is to optimize the cement–bone interface, obtain a cement mantle free of mantle defects with a minimum 2-mm thickness, and insert the femoral component so that it is centered in the cement mantle in a neutral alignment.

Canal Preparation

To optimize the cement–bone interface, preparation of the femoral canal is important. First, the femoral canal must be plugged. Plugging allows for greater intrusion pressure and better filling. The femoral canal can be plugged with bone cement, bone, or commercially available plastic plugs. The plug should be placed 2 to 4 cm distal to the level of the tip of the femoral component. This placement automatically extends the cement mantle an equal distance, which has been shown to be an important factor in cemented femoral component fixation.

Loose cancellous bone can be removed with a curette. When preparing the femoral canal for a cemented component, reamers should not be used. By removing stable cancellous bone, reaming creates a smooth endosteal surface, which in turns decreases the interfacial shear strength between cement and bone.

Pressurized lavage is used to clean the femoral canal. This serves two purposes. First, removal of marrow, fat, and blood improves the interface between bone and cement. One study compared interfacial shear strength and cement intrusion into unprepared trabecular bone, bone prepared with irrigation, and bone prepared with pressurized lavage. Pressurized lavage led to a significant increase in the depth of cement penetration and interfacial shear strength when compared to unprepared bone. Second, adequate lavage significantly reduces the risk of clinically significant fat and marrow emboli. The canal is dried using suction and dry and adrenaline soaked sponges. Spinal anesthesia has also been shown to decrease bleeding from the cancellous bone of the femoral canal, as have hydrogen peroxide and iced saline.

Cement Preparation

There is an ongoing controversy concerning the benefit of porosity reduction. Cement fails in fatigue, and it has been estimated that the hip is loaded approximately one million times a year during gait. Laboratory testing has demonstrated that centrifugation decreases the pore size in cement to 200 to 400 μm in diameter. As a result, data from studies have demonstrated a 24% increase in ultimate tensile strain of standard test specimens and a 136% increase in tension-compression fatigue strength. Data from similar studies have shown that porosity reduction can improve the fatigue life of bone cement by a factor of five. Similar benefits have been demonstrated with vacuum mixing.

In vitro models have been studied to examine the effects of porosity reduction in the face of surface imperfections. Most authors have demonstrated a beneficial effect of porosity reduction. Centrifuged Simplex P bone cement (Howmedica, Rutherford, NJ) was able to withstand significantly more cycles before failure at all strain levels tested when compared to uncentrifuged test specimens. Vacuum mixing also reduces porosity and improves the mechanical properties of cement. The increase in strength demonstrated with porosity reduction appears to be independent of surface conditions. One study, which did not show a beneficial effect in terms of increased strength, was undertaken to evaluate the effect of notching the specimen. In the presence of the notch, there was no difference between specimens with or without porosity reduction. However, there may have been problems with the methods of this study. Specimens used in this study were 26 × 90 mm. The exothermic reaction in a specimen of this size would be expected to increase the temperature to the boiling point of the monomer.

Cement Insertion and Pressurization

Cement is inserted in a retrograde fashion using a cement gun. Following insertion, the cement mantle is pressurized. The strength of the cement–bone interface is directly related to the depth of penetration of cement into bone. In turn, the depth of penetration is related to the intrusion pressure. It is technically easy to obtain high intrusion pressures in the diaphysis, but it is more difficult to obtain similar pressure in the proximal femur (metaphyseal region). Three commercially available cement pressurization systems were evaluated in a recent study. The use of all three systems resulted in average peak cement pressures at the cement–bone interface, including the proximal region of the femur, of over 30 psi with in vitro testing. One of the systems was then evaluated intraoperatively. In ten primary cases, the average peak intrusion pressure in the proximal femur was 32 psi ($\pm$ 10). In revision cases, the average peak intrusion pressure was significantly less (19 $\pm$ 9 psi).

Stem Centralization and Cement Mantle Thickness

Many contemporary cemented stems are designed to be used with stem centralizers. The purpose of these devices is to aid in centering the stem within the canal to ensure a more uniform cement mantle, avoiding areas where the mantle becomes thin or nonexistent. Radiographic studies have been undertaken to evaluate the effectiveness of stem centralizers in achieving these goals. In one study, femoral stems with a distal centralizer were more neutrally aligned and had thicker cement mantles in Gruen zone 5 when compared to controls.

The ideal cement mantle thickness is not known. Finite element and strain gauge studies have shown that there is a high stress and strain concentration in the distal cement mantle around the tip of the stem and to a lesser extent in the proximal cement mantle. Attention to cement mantle thickness, especially in these areas of high stress, is appropriate. Finite element studies have shown that by increasing cement mantle thickness over 2.5 mm around the tip of the stem, there is a marked reduction in cement mantle strain. Autopsy studies examining the integrity of the cement mantle have noted that fractures rarely occur in mantles greater than 2 mm thick. Numerous clinical studies have demonstrated the association of thin cement mantles and mantle defects with mechanical failure. Based on this information, it seems prudent to obtain a mantle thickness of at least 2 mm.

Long-Term Results: Second Generation Cementing

Improved cementing has led to an enhancement in the long-term fixation of cemented femoral components. In a study from the Massachusetts General Hospital, 117 cemented total hip replacements, in which the Harris Design II femoral stem (Howmedica, Rutherford, NJ), a medullary plug, and a cement gun were used, were followed up for a minimum of 5 years. One femoral component was revised and a second was definitely loose and not revised, for a mechanical failure rate of 1.7%. The authors of a similar retrospective study of 251 patients at the Mayo clinic who were followed up for a minimum of 5 years after insertion of the Harris Design II femoral stem with use of an intramedullary plug, a cement gun, and pulsatile lavage, reported 98% excellent results. Only three femoral components and one acetabular component were defi-

nitely loose. There were no revisions and no reoperations. In a matched pair study from the Brigham and Women's Hospital, first and second generation techniques by the same group of surgeons were compared. In this study, the T-28 implant (Zimmer, Warsaw, IN) was used. At 4 years following surgery, the femoral failure rate with use of first generation cementing was 21%. With use of second generation cementing there was no definite femoral loosening.

In an 11-year radiographic review, the authors from the Massachusetts General Hospital followed the same group of patients previously reported at 5 years. In 105 hips, only three femoral components were definitely loose; this represents a statistically significant reduction in the rate of aseptic loosening of cemented femoral components. However, the rate of acetabular loosening was unchanged. Between the 5- and 11-year reviews, the acetabular loosening rate increased 20 fold. Of the 43 definitely loose acetabular components at 11 years, only two were loose at the 6-year review.

Improved longevity with second generation cementing has not been reported for all stem designs. One hundred and ten consecutive Exeter stems (Howmedica, Rutherford, NJ) with a matte stem surface were reviewed at a minimum of 5 years after surgery. The cementing technique included canal plugging, pressurized lavage, a cement gun, and pressurization of the cement. At last follow-up, 15 femoral components were definitely loose, eight were suspected to be loose, and eight additional femurs demonstrated osteolysis in the absence of loosening. The authors concluded the late complication rate with the matte-surfaced Exeter stem was unacceptably high.

Cemented Total Hip Replacement in the Younger Patient

The early 5-year reports on cemented total hip replacement in the young patient were also disappointing. At an average of 5.5 years after surgery in a group of patients who were less than 30 years of age, 21% of the patients in one study had undergone revision surgery and 58% had loosened components. In another study, only 72% of patients less than 45 years old at surgery had a satisfactory result at 5 years. By 9 to 10 years after surgery, the percentage of patients with a satisfactory result had decreased to 58%. Both of these studies reported on the results of first generation cementing. Results have been reported of two more recent studies with longer-term follow-up of cemented total hip replacement, which was performed by a single surgeon. At 12 to 18 years after surgery in a group of patients who were less than 50 years old, 30% of the acetabular components and 23% of the femoral components had been revised; 75% of the implants were still in place. However, 39% of the unrevised acetabular components and 29% of the unrevised femoral components had evidence of radiographic loosening. In a 16- to 21-year follow-up study of 84 Charnley total hip replacements, only 13% of the acetabular components and 2% of the femoral components had been revised. However, 37% of the remaining acetabular components were radiographically loose, but only 5% of the remaining femoral components were loose.

Improved cementing technique has led to improvements in long-term results in femoral component survival for young patients that are similar to those reported for older patients. Using second generation techniques, no femoral components were revised in 44 patients who were younger than 50 years old at 10 to 14.8 years after surgery. Only one component was definitely loose radiographically. In contrast, 11 patients had undergone revision for loose acetabular components and 11 more patients had evidence of radiographic loosening of their acetabular components. This represents a mechanical failure rate of 50% for the cemented acetabular components compared to a mechanical failure rate of only 2% for the cemented femoral components.

Factors Related to Failure

Technical factors in terms of cementing technique are important for long-term survival. In one study, the initial postoperative radiographs were retrospectively evaluated to predict femoral failure. Failed femoral components were compared to successful components. On the initial postoperative radiograph, there was a statistically significant greater incidence of femoral cement–bone radiolucencies indicative of incomplete filling in the failed group. In addition, when femoral cement–bone radiolucency, collar–calcar contact, femoral metal–cement radiolucency, femoral cement mantle adequacy, cement distal to the stem tip, and femoral component stem position were analyzed together, worse radiographic findings were noted in the failed femoral group ($p < 0.006$). In a review of patients who required revision surgery for mechanical failure, loosening was associated with varus positioning in 50% of the cases. In 34% of the cases, an inadequate cement mantle was associated with mechanical failure. These studies demonstrate the importance of technique for long-term survival of cemented femoral components.

Clinical factors have also been evaluated as potential risk factors for mechanical failure of cemented total hip replacements. In one study from Stanford, the type of prosthesis, the preoperative Harris hip score, and the surgeon did not correlate with the need for revision. Increased weight was associated with an increased risk of failure. Only 8% of patients less than 68 kg required revision compared to 15% of patients weighing more than 68 kg at 12 years following surgery. Many of the failures in the under-68-kg group occurred in the first 2 years and could be attributed to technical errors. If those were excluded, only 3.4% of the under-68-kg group required revision. There was a decreased risk of failure with increasing age. Females did better than males, and patients with trauma did poorer than a comparable osteoarthritic population. The use of regression tree analysis demonstrated that patients who weighed less than 75 kg had the best outcome, with a 90% chance of survival at 12 years.

Mechanisms of Failure

Autopsy studies have demonstrated that the mechanisms of failure of cemented femoral and acetabular components appear to be different. Much attention has been paid to the soft-tissue membrane that forms at the cement–bone interface; on the femoral side, this membrane occurs late in the loosening process. Mechanical factors are responsible for the initiation of femoral failure. Debonding at the cement–metal interface occurs early. Finite element studies have shown that when debonding occurs at the metal–cement interface, high peak stresses in the cement mantle result; these stresses are highest proximally and around the tip of the stem. The result is fracture of the cement mantle. Most fractures occur proximally and are associated with thin cement mantles, mantle defects, and pores in the cement. Biologic processes then become important. As a result of debonding and cement fracture, stability is compromised and particulate polymeric debris can gain access to the endosteal bone. Debris stimulates a foreign body reaction, which causes bone resorption and results in the soft-tissue membrane commonly seen at revision surgery.

In contrast, the initial events in the acetabular loosening process are biologic. Wear debris (primarily polyethylene) induces three-dimensional bone resorption, which begins circumferentially at the mouth of the acetabulum, extends toward the dome of the acetabulum, and results in loosening. Unlike on the femoral side, cement–bone radiolucencies are indicative of fibrous tissue formation. The extent of the soft-tissue membrane correlates with implant stability. This correlation supports the concept that a complete cement–bone radiolucency around a cemented acetabular component, regardless of width, is good evidence that the component is loose. It also explains why changes, such as metal backing and improved cement technique, that improve the mechanical environment around a cemented cup have little effect on the longevity of cemented acetabular components.

Several important points help explain the differing mechanisms of loosening for the femur and acetabulum. The first is the issue of access of particulate debris to the cement–bone interface. In the proximal femur, the interdigitation between trabecular bone and cement probably acts as a barrier for migration of debris along this interface. The same interdigitation between cement and bone is not seen around the mouth of the femur. Next, the geometries of the femur and acetabulum are obviously different. The ratio of the circumference of the mouth of the acetabulum to the total surface area of the acetabular cement–bone interface is much larger than the ratio of the circumference of the mouth of the femur to the total surface area of the femoral cement–bone interface. Therefore, even if access for particulate debris in the two regions was equivalent, resorption beginning circumferentially at the mouth of the acetabulum and extending 2 cm toward the dome would have a greater destabilizing effect than resorption beginning at the mouth of the femur and extending 2 cm distally. Finally, the loading environments of the femoral and acetabular components are quite different. High shear and torsion forces are present on the femoral side. In contrast, relatively benign compressive forces are present on the acetabular side. These factors likely explain the differences in the rates and mechanism of loosening of cemented acetabular and femoral components as well as the clinical function of loose components.

Skeletal Remodeling

Following insertion of a cemented femoral component, in vitro testing has demonstrated a marked reduction in stress and strain in the proximal femur. Osteoporosis in the proximal medial femoral cortex following cemented femoral replacement has been attributed to stress shielding. The adaptive bone remodeling theory predicts resorptive remodeling would occur as a result of stress shielding and the process would continue until bone mass decreased to restore normal strain patterns. Detailed strain analyses of whole femoral autopsy specimens following cemented total hip arthroplasty have demonstrated that marked strain (and stress) shielding persists and that the normal strain relationships were never restored, even 17 years after surgery. In the absence of normalization of the strain pattern, finite element analysis has predicted complete loss of bone. However, this was not seen clinically and it is likely that factors other than mechanical play a role that results in preservation of a minimum bone mass.

Analysis of cross sections through the femoral specimens further elucidated the biologic response to these well-fixed specimens. Host bone was in intimate contact with the cement mantle over most of the cement–bone interface (Fig. 1). Fibrous tissue was found only rarely. Densification of bone at the cement–bone interface was a common finding. The outer cortex was often thinned and relatively osteoporotic when compared to the contralateral intact femur (Fig. 1, *top right*). The inner cortex was indistinguishable from the cement mantle on clinical radiographs because of the presence of barium in the cement (Fig. 1, *top left*). Between the inner and outer cortices, a second medullary canal forms (Fig. 1, *top right*). Formation of the second medullary canal has also been described in animal experiments. The second medullary canal is seen as a radiolucency between the outer cortex and cement on clinical radiograph and may be misinterpreted as representing fibrous tissue formation.

Osteolysis

Much of what has been learned about the biologic reaction to bone cement comes from analysis of tissue from revision surgery. Many investigators have described the membrane at the cement–bone interface in failed cases. The soft-tissue membrane typically consists of abundant macrophages and giant cells consistent with a foreign body reaction. The bone resorption or osteolysis that is associated was incorrectly referred to as cement disease. It is now clear that osteolysis can and does occur in the absence of bone cement. It is difficult to separate the biologic effects of particulate polyethylene and polymethylmethacrylate (PMMA) by analyzing material obtained at revision surgery.

Focal femoral osteolysis in stable femoral reconstructions has been examined at autopsy. A detailed analysis of the cement mantle in the area of osteolysis showed focal cement fragmentation that resulted in generation of particulate debris. Data from clinical studies have indicated that focal femoral osteolysis occurs in areas of thin cement mantles or mantle defects. In addition, polyethylene debris has been found in these focal osteolytic lesions. It has been postulated that polyethylene from the hip articulation gains access to the endosteal surface via a debonded metal–cement interface.

The biologic effects of bulk and particulate PMMA have been studied directly in vivo and in vitro. Animal study data have shown that bulk cement is well tolerated. In one report, at 1 to 42 weeks after surgery, canine diaphyseal PMMA implants resulted in no evidence of cell death or inflammation. In another study, using a rabbit model, data demonstrated that new bone can be deposited on bone cement, filling gaps between cement and bone.

In cell culture studies, particulate PMMA was found to stimulate production of interleukin-1, tumor necrosis factor, and prostaglandin E2. All of these substances have been implicated in bone resorption. When conditioned media from these cultures are added to limb bone assays, bone resorption as measured by radioactive calcium release results.

The role of the immune system in the biologic response to particulate debris is debated. It has been demonstrated that the typical foreign body response results when immunodeficient mice are challenged with cement particles. In addition, lymphocytes in culture do not appear to respond to particulate cement. Results of these studies suggest that the immune system does not play a significant role in the response to wear debris. In immunohistochemical studies, however, lymphocytes were identified in the soft-tissue membrane around failed implants (up to 10% of the cells present). These cells may be important in modulating the biologic response to wear debris.

Design Issues

Metal-Backed Acetabular Cups

Metal backing of cemented acetabular components was introduced to allow exchange of worn polyethylene without the need for complete acetabular revision. Finite ele-

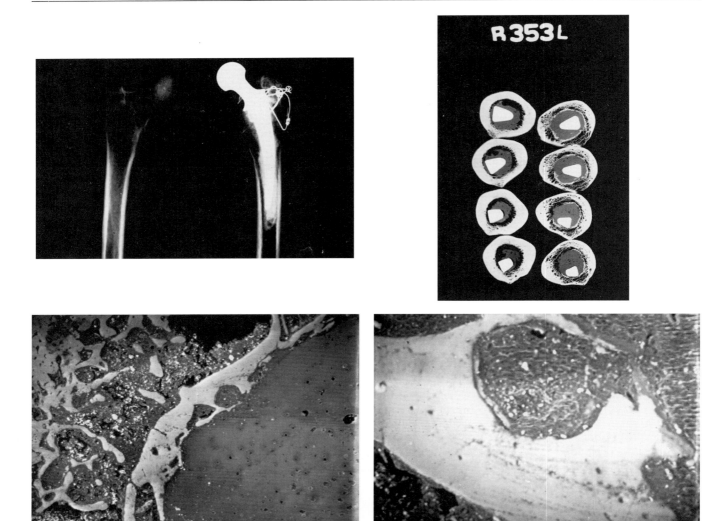

Fig. 1 **Top left,** Radiographs of bilateral femora harvested at autopsy 15 years after surgery. **Top right,** Cross-sectional radiographs taken through diaphyseal sections. The left side represents the control femur in which a cemented femoral component was placed in the laboratory for a comparison. The right side represents the implant which had been cycled in vivo for 15 years prior to death. Note the cortical remodeling including the formation of the inner cortex around the cement mantle and the formation of the second medullary canal between the inner and outer cortex. **Bottom left,** Scanning electron micrograph of the cement–bone interface highlighting the inner cortex. Note osteointegration at the cement–bone interface. **Bottom right,** High-powered scanning electron micrograph again noting the osteointegration between cement and bone. There are no gaps and no intervening fibrous tissue at this interface.

ment analysis predicted that the increased stiffness afforded by metal backing would cause a decrease in the stresses in the cement and cancellous bone. Data from subsequent strain gauge analysis in which metal-backed and all polyethylene acetabular components were compared demonstrated a decrease in the peak strains in the cement mantle with metal backing. Based on the improvement of the mechanical environment of the bone–implant composite, it was predicted that metal backing would result in a delay of cemented acetabular loosening.

Recent clinical studies have shown no benefit in long-term survival of metal-backed acetabular components. In a recent 11-year radiographic review of cemented total hip replacement, the all-polyethylene acetabular components had a loosening rate of 39% compared to 53% for the metal-backed components. The difference was not statistically significant. In this study, the patients in the metal-backed and all-polyethylene groups were not matched. The patients in the metal-backed group were younger, heavier men. Another study compared two comparable groups of patients who differed only in the type of acetabular component implant: 138 patients had a metal-backed acetabular component and 100 patients had an all-polyethylene acetabular component. Failure was assessed using three different criteria: radiolucency at the cement–bone interface, migration greater than 5 mm, and revision. The metal-backed acetabular components showed an increased failure rate using all three criteria for failure.

The failure of metal backing to improve clinical results can be explained by the mechanism of loosening of cemented acetabular components. As noted above, analysis of autopsy specimens reveals acetabular loosening to be primarily a biologic process. Therefore, factors that improve the mechanical environment are not likely to have a marked effect on longevity.

Collar

Many biomechanical studies have been performed supporting the use of a collar in cemented hip arthroplasty. In these in vitro and finite element studies, the collar has been shown to increase load transfer to the proximal femur and reduce strain in the proximal medial cement mantle. Results of these studies also show that a collar helps to pressurize the cement mantle and reduce implant micromotion.

Data from clinical studies have shown that with modern instrumentation collar-medial neck contact can be achieved in 90% of cases and maintained in 88% of those cases. There has only been one randomized, prospective clinical study to examine the effects of a collar. In that study, identical cemented stems with and without a collar were implanted. There was a higher incidence of femoral loosening in the collarless group.

Proponents of collarless stems feel it is difficult to obtain and maintain collar–calcar contact clinically. In addition, they cite the potential for debris generation secondary to micromotion between the collar and cement and/or calcar as a possible detriment.

Metal–Cement Interface

A variety of surface finishes and textures have been used for cemented femoral components. In addition, the femoral component has been precoated with PMMA to enhance the strength of the metal–cement interface and prevent debonding. In vitro testing has shown that precoating strengthens the metal–cement interface, even in the presence of contaminants such as blood.

Opponents of precoating favor a polished stem secondary to concerns with precoating. These concerns include increased generation of particulate debris secondary to fretting if the precoated interface fails. Opponents also raise the possibility of a deleterious effect on the cement–bone interface as a result of strengthening the metal–cement interface in the long-term situation.

Cemented Total Hip Replacement: Special Problems

Fracture of the Acetabulum

Degenerative changes in the hip joint have been reported in up to 57% of patients who have had fracture of the acetabulum. The risk of secondary degenerative changes increases with displacement and involvement of the weight-bearing surface. Avascular necrosis can be associated with acetabular fracture and has been reported in up to 40% of cases.

A recent report reviewed 55 primary total hip replacements in 53 patients whose average age was 56 years at surgery and who were followed up for an average of 7.5 years. The incidence of femoral failure was similar to that for routine hip replacements in patients with osteoarthritis. However, the cemented acetabular failure rate was four to five times higher.

Sickle-Cell Hemoglobinopathy

Sickle-cell hemoglobinopathies have been linked to osteonecrosis of the femoral head. Sickling can result in occlusion of the small vessels in the femoral head, which may produce infarction. Collapse of the femoral head and secondary degenerative joint disease result. Complication rates in these patients undergoing total hip replacement are high. One study in which 14 hips were reviewed at a mean of 6.5 years following surgery had a reported complication rate of 100%. The authors reported an increased blood loss, increased transfusion requirements, and prolonged hospitalization. In another more recent study, 35 primary total hip replacements (17 cemented, 18 uncemented) were reviewed at a mean of 7.5 years following surgery. The average age at the time of surgery was only 30 years. The overall revision rate was 40% (59% for the cemented group and 22% for the uncemented group). The infection rate in the series as a whole was 20%.

The authors concluded that the risk-to-benefit ratio in patients with sickle-cell hemoglobinopathy is high. Recommendations include a preoperative hematology consultation, preoperative transfusion to achieve a hemoglobin A level of greater than 50%, perioperative antibiotics, hydration and oxygenation to prevent crisis, and caution in the use of bone cement because of the high failure rates.

High loosening rates may be related to bone remodeling and bone quality. The chronic anemia related to sickle-cell hemoglobinopathy results in marrow proliferation. In the proximal femur, this proliferation results in canal widening. In addition, there is often associated cortical thinning. The high infection rates may be related to a deficiency in the immune system in these patients. Sickle cell patients also are functionally asplenic secondary to autoinfarction of the spleen.

Developmental Dislocation of the Hip

Total hip replacement for neglected developmental dislocation of the hip presents several technically challenging issues. Bone stock for acetabular reconstruction is poor. Historically, when the acetabulum has been cemented, it was reconstructed at the true hip center, which often necessitated the use of bulk structural grafts. Concerns over late graft failure as well as the introduction of cementless acetabular components have presented the option of reconstruction using a high hip center. The high hip center does not appear to be a mechanical disadvantage as long as the hip center is not displaced laterally. Because the acetabular volume in the these patients is small, small acetabular components are often required. Twenty-two millimeter heads should be used to maximize polyethylene thickness. On the femoral side, deformity of the proximal femur and small intramedullary canal may result in the need for special or custom femoral components. Careful preoperative planning is important to ensure an adequate selection of implants at surgery.

Limb lengthening is often required in an attempt to equalize limb lengths. Lengthening greater than 2 cm has been associated with a greater incidence of trochanteric nonunion. In addition, with limb lengthening, there is an increased risk of nerve palsy. In the largest reported series of nerve palsies after total hip replacement, the incidence of palsy in patients with developmental dysplasia or dislocation was 5.2%.

A recent study reported on 34 cemented total hip replacements in 28 patients for neglected congenital dislocation of the hip followed up for 5.6 to 14 years (mean 9.4 years). The overall success rate was 71%. Radiographic loosening occurred in three femoral components and was attributed to poor cementing. Eight sockets were loose radiographically. There was an increased incidence of socket loosening associated with marked acetabular deficiency. In another long-term study (8 to 16.5 years), six revisions in 29 cemented hip arthroplasties were reported for dysplasia or dislocation. Four of the six failures, however, were for a fractured Trapezoidal-28 (Zimmer, Warsaw, IN) stem. The two remaining revisions were for femoral loosening in one case and acetabular loosening in the other.

Juvenile Rheumatoid Arthritis

Patients requiring total hip replacement for juvenile rheumatoid arthritis often have polyarticular involvement and are severely disabled. The local anatomy in these patients is often abnormal secondary to soft-tissue contractures and bony deformity. Hypoplasia of both the acetabulum and femur is common, and special or custom implants may be required.

Although short-term results of cemented total hip arthroplasty in this patient population were encouraging, longer-term studies have reported high failure rates. In one report of 96 primary cemented total hip arthroplasties in 54 patients at a minimum of 5 years after surgery (mean 11.5 years), revision surgery was performed in 25% of patients, and 17 additional patients had evidence of radiographic loosening. In another report, 62 cemented hip replacements in 34 patients were followed up for 2 to 11 years (mean 6 years). Although only two patients required revision (one loose acetabular component and one broken femoral stem), 26% of the acetabular components and 8% of the femoral components demonstrated progressive radiolucencies or migration.

In general, these reports include surgeries performed over many years so the cement technique may have changed during the course of the study. Although patients with juvenile rheumatoid arthritis are young, the relatively high failure rates are higher than might be expected considering their low body weight and activity level. Factors such as poor bone quality and highly vascular bone, which may compromise cement technique, have been cited as possible causes of the high failure rate in this patient population. Position of the acetabular component has also been cited as a factor in aseptic loosening. In one study, 42% of 26 acetabular components placed more than 5 mm superior or medial to the normal hip position developed extensive cement-bone radiolucencies.

Ankylosing Spondylitis

Ankylosing spondylitis has been traditionally felt to be a risk factor for the development of heterotopic bone following total hip arthroplasty. The reported rates of ectopic bone formation vary from 4% to 61.7%. In one recent large study, clinically important heterotopic bone developed in 11% of cases. All of these patients had either previous hip surgery, a postoperative infection, or complete ankylosis preoperatively. The authors concluded that routine prophylaxis for uncomplicated total hip arthroplasty was not necessary.

Annotated Bibliography

Long-Term Results

Kavanagh BF, Dewitz MA, Ilstrup DM, et al: Charnley total hip arthroplasty with cement: Fifteen-year results. *J Bone Joint Surg* 1989;71A:1496–1503.

Three hundred thirty-three cemented Charnley total hip arthroplasties were followed up for 15 years. Data were available for 166 of the 170 patients who were still alive. At 15 years, the probability of no revision was 89%. The probability of loosening of one or both components was 32%.

Mulroy RD Jr, Harris WH: The effect of improved cementing techniques on component loosening in total hip replacement: An 11 year radiographic review. *J Bone Joint Surg* 1990;72B:757–760.

At a minimum of 10 years following surgery using second generation techniques, only 3% of the femoral stems were definitely loose. In contrast, 42% of the acetabular components were definitely loose.

Rockborn P, Olsson SS: Loosening and bone resorption in Exeter hip arthroplasties: Review at a minimum of five years. *J Bone Joint Surg* 1993;75B:865–868.

Using second/third generation cementing techniques, the authors report a 14% incidence of definite femoral component loosening using the matte-surface Exeter stem. In addition, another 7% of the stems were suspected to be loose and 7% had osteolysis in the absence of loosening.

Schulte KR, Callaghan JJ, Kelley S, et al: The outcome of Charnley total hip arthroplasty with cement after a minimum twenty-year follow-up. *J Bone Joint Surg* 1993; 75A:961–975.

Three hundred twenty-two cemented Charnley total hip replacements were followed up for a minimum of 20 years or until the patient died. Of the 98 hips in patients surviving at least 20 years, 85% had retained their original prosthesis. At 20 years, the mechanical failure rate of the femoral component was 7%.

Cement Technique

Bannister GC, Young SK, Baker AS, et al: Control of bleeding in cemented arthroplasty. *J Bone Joint Surg* 1990; 72B:444–446.

The effects of anesthesia, blood pressure, freezing saline, saline at room temperature, and adrenaline solution on bleeding from cancellous bone were measured. Spinal anesthesia reduced bleeding an average of 44%, freezing saline an average of 24%, and the remaining factors an average of 14% each.

Davies JP, Harris WH: In vitro and in vivo studies of pressurization of femoral cement in total hip arthroplasty. *Arthroplasty* 1993;8:585–591.

In vitro testing of three commercially available cement pressurization systems showed all three systems produced average peak cement intrusion pressures of over 30 psi. Intraoperative testing using pressure transducers in the proximal femur demonstrated average peak intrusion pressures of 32 psi in primary cases (N = 10) and 19 psi in revision cases (N = 5). A pressure of at least 15 psi was obtained in nine of ten primary cases and three of five revision cases.

Davies JP, O'Connor DO, Burke DW, et al: The effect of centrifugation on the fatigue life of bone cement in the presence of surface irregularities. *Clin Orthop* 1988;229: 156–161.

The authors performed in vitro tests to examine the effect of surface irregularities on the fatigue life of centrifuged and uncentrifuged cement. They concluded porosity reduction significantly extended the fatigue life, even in the presence of sharp notches.

Majkowski AJ, Miles AW, Bannister GC, et al: Bone surface preparation in cemented joint replacement. *J Bone Joint Surg* 1993;75B:459–463.

The authors compared the effect of various techniques of bone preparation on cement intrusion and shear strength of the bone–cement interface. The mean penetration of cement increased from 0.2 mm in unprepared bone to 4.8 to 7.9 mm in bone prepared with pressurized lavage. Similarly, the interfacial shear strength increased from 1.9 MPa to 26.5 to 36.1 MPa.

Cemented Total Hip Replacement in the Younger Patient

Barrack RL, Mulroy RD Jr, Harris WH: Improved cementing techniques and femoral component loosening in young patients with hip arthroplasty: A 12-year radiographic review. *J Bone Joint Surg* 1992;74B:385–389.

Forty-four patients who had a cemented femoral component inserted using second generation techniques were followed up for an average of 12 years (10 to 14.8). At the time of the index procedure all patients were younger than 50 years old. None of the patients had undergone revision for femoral loosening and only one femoral component was definitely loose based on radiographic criteria. In contrast, 11 patients had undergone revision surgery for aseptic acetabular loosening and 11 additional patients had radiographic evidence of acetabular loosening.

Collis DK: Long-term (twelve to eighteen-year) follow-up of cemented total hip replacements in patients who were less than fifty years old. *J Bone Joint Surg* 1991;73A: 593–597.

Fifty-one cemented total hip replacements were done in 43 patients who were younger than 50 years old at the time of surgery, and were followed up 12 to 18 years postoperatively. Thirty-seven patients (44 hips) were available for follow-up. Thirteen hips required revision (only one before 6 years). In these 12 revisions, five were for loosening of both components, five for femoral loosening only, and three for acetabular loosening only. The overall rate of survival at 15 years was calculated to be 69%.

Failure

Harrigan TP, Kareh JA, O'Connor DO, et al: A finite element study of the initiation of failure of fixation in cemented total hip components. *J Orthop Res* 1992;10:134–144.

A three-dimensional linear finite element model was constructed and verified. Both single limb stance and stair climbing loads were examined. The authors concluded that the out of plane forces in stair climbing posed the greatest risk for cement–metal debonding and crack initiation.

Jasty M, Maloney WJ, Bragdon CR, et al: The initiation of failure in cemented femoral components of hip arthroplasties. *J Bone Joint Surg* 1991;73B:551–558.

The most common early finding of mechanical failure of autopsy femora with cemented femoral components was debonding at the metal-cement interface.

Schmalzried TP, Kwong LM, Jasty M, et al: The mechanism of loosening of cemented acetabular components in total hip arthroplasty: Analysis of specimens retrieved at autopsy. *Clin Orthop* 1992; 274:60–78.

Analysis of autopsy pelvises with cemented acetabular components demonstrated the loosening was the result of particulate debris induced bone resorption that progressed from the acetabular margins toward the dome of the acetabulum.

Schurman DJ, Block DA, Segal MR, et al: Conventional cemented total hip arthroplasty: Assessment of clinical factors associated with revision for mechanical failure. *Clin Orthop* 1989;240:173–180.

Multiple clinical factors were assessed to determine their association with failure. Cox proportional hazard analysis indicated weight and age were important variables associated with failure. Regression tree analysis showed patients less than 75 kg had the best chance of long-term survival (90% at 12 years).

Skeletal Remodeling

Jasty M, Maloney WJ, Bragdon CR, et al: Histomorphological studies of the long-term skeletal responses to well fixed cemented femoral components. *J Bone Joint Surg* 1990;72A:1220–1229.

Femora retrieved at autopsy after total hip arthroplasty demonstrated that the cement-bone interface was intact in these well-fixed specimens. Fibrous tissue intervened only rarely. Densification of bone occurred at the cement-bone interface forming the so-called inner cortex. The outer cortex was thinner and more osteoporotic when compared to contralateral intact specimens.

Maloney WJ, Jasty M, Burke DW, et al: Biomechanical and histologic investigation of cemented total hip arthroplasties: A study of autopsy-retrieved femurs after in vivo cycling. *Clin Orthop* 1989;249:129–140.

Eleven whole femoral specimens were harvested at autopsy in patients who had previously undergone cemented total hip arthroplasty. Strain gauge studies demonstrated that even 17 years following surgery, the strains in the proximal femur did not normalize. Excellent stability was demonstrated on mechanical testing in these clinically well-functioning implants.

Biologic Response to Bone Cement and Osteolysis

Herman JH, Sowder WG, Anderson D, et al: Polymethylmethacrylate-induced release of bone-resorbing factors. *J Bone Joint Surg* 1989;71A:1530–1541.

In this murine limb bone assay resulting in bone resorption, mononuclear cells were cultured in the presence of bone cement. Unfractionated blood mononuclear cells and surface adherent cells stimulated by particulate polymerized and nonpolymerized cement produced interleukin-1, tumor necrosis factor, and prostaglandin E2. The conditioned medium was added to a murine limb bone assay resulting in bone resorption.

Horowitz SM, Gautsch TL, Frondoza CG, et al: Macrophage exposure to polymethylmethacrylate leads to mediator release and injury. *J Orthop Res* 1991;9:406–413.

Polymethylmethacrylate (PMMA) particles in cell culture stimulated macrophages to release inflammatory mediators. Cell death as measured by lactate dehydrogenase release was also noted.

Jasty M, Jiranek W, Harris WH: Acrylic fragmentation in total hip replacements and its biological consequences. *Clin Orthop* 1992;285:116–128.

Mice with varying immunologic deficiencies were challenged with subcutaneous injections of PMMA powder. Immunocompetent mice, mice deficient in T cells, mice deficient

in T and B cells, and mice deficient in T, B, and natural killer cells were studied. Regardless of the immunodeficiency, the mice responded by forming a granuloma consisting of macrophages and giant cells.

Maloney WJ, Jasty M, Rosenberg A, et al: Bone lysis in well fixed cemented femoral components. *J Bone Joint Surg* 1990;72B:966–970.

Twenty-five cases of focal osteolysis associated with stable cemented femoral components were identified. In eight of 11 cases in which serial radiographs were available for review, the lesions had progressed. Mechanical testing of three autopsy specimens with focal femoral osteolysis documented that the implants were stable. Analysis of the cement mantles in the areas of osteolysis demonstrated fragmentation and generation of particulate debris.

Design Issues

Harris WH: Is it advantageous to strengthen the cement-metal interface and use a collar for cemented femoral components of total hip replacements? *Clin Orthop* 1992;285:67–72.

Evidence for using a collared femoral component and strengthening the metal-cement interface is presented.

Ling RS: The use of a collar and precoating on cemented femoral stems is unnecessary and detrimental. *Clin Orthop* 1992;285:73–83.

The rationale for the use of a collarless, non-precoated cemented femoral stem is presented.

Ritter MA, Keating EM, Faris PM, et al: Metal-backed acetabular cups in total hip arthroplasty. *J Bone Joint Surg* 1990;72A:672–677.

Cemented metal-backed acetabular components had a significantly higher rate of failure when compared to all-polyethylene components. The authors concluded that metal backing of acetabular components is not recommended.

Special Problems

Fracture of the Acetabulum

Romness DW, Lewallen DG: Total hip arthroplasty after fracture of the acetabulum: Long-term results. *J Bone Joint Surg* 1990;72B:761–764.

The rates of cemented acetabular loosening were four to five times higher in patients with a history of previous acetabular fracture compared to routine total hip arthroplasties for osteoarthritis from the same institution.

Sickle-Cell Hemoglobinopathy

Acurio MT, Friedman RJ: Hip arthroplasty in patients with sickle-cell hemoglobinopathy. *J Bone Joint Surg* 1992;74B:367–371.

Twenty-five cemented total hip arthroplasties in 25 patients were reviewed at 2 to 18 years after surgery. The overall complication rate was 49%. Twenty percent of the patients developed postoperative infections. By a mean of 7.5 years after surgery, 40% of the patients had undergone revision.

Developmental Dysplasia and Dislocation

Anwar MM, Sugano N, Masuhara K, et al: Total hip arthroplasty in the neglected congenital dislocation of the hip: A five to 14-year follow-up study. *Clin Orthop* 1993; 295:127–134.

Thirty-four cemented total hip replacements were performed in 28 patients and were followed up for 5.6 to 14 years. Three femoral components were loose at last follow-up and were attributed to poor cementing. Marked acetabular deficiency was associated with acetabular loosening.

Garvin KL, Bowen MK, Salvati EA, et al: Total hip arthroplasty in congenital dislocation and dysplasia of the hip. *J Bone Joint Surg* 1991;73A:1348–1354.

Twenty-three cemented hip arthroplasties were followed up an average of 14 years. At final follow-up evaluation, seven hips were rated excellent, nine good, and one poor. In addition, there were six revisions. Four of the revisions were for fractured Trapezoidal-28 stems.

Juvenile Rheumatoid Arthritis

Witt JD, Swann M, Ansell BM: Total hip replacement for juvenile chronic arthritis. *J Bone Joint Surg* 1991;73B: 770–773.

In a minimum 5-year follow-up study, the mechanical failure rate of 96 primary cemented total hip arthroplasties in 54 patients was 43%. Twenty-five percent of the hips had been revised by an average of 9.5 years. Seventeen additional hips had radiographic signs of loosening.

Ankylosing Spondylitis

Kilgus DJ, Namba RS, Gorek JE, et al: Total hip replacement for patients who have ankylosing spondylitis: The importance of the formation of heterotopic bone and of the durability of fixation of cemented components. *J Bone Joint Surg* 1990;72A:834–839.

Clinically important heterotopic bone developed in 11% of cases. All of these patients had a previous hip surgery, a postoperative infection, or complete ankylosis preoperatively.

23

Cementless Primary Total Hip Replacement

It is estimated that approximately 196,500 primary total hip replacements were performed during 1993 in the United States alone and that of these, slightly greater than 60% were performed without cement.

Historic Perspectives

The development and popularization of cementless total hip replacement is often attributed to dissatisfaction with the results of first generation cemented arthroplasty. However, by the time Charnley published his landmark monograph on acrylic cement in 1970, the results of 158 cementless total hip arthroplasties had already been reported, porous-coated stainless steel hips were being implanted in the United States, and large-scale clinical trials of cementless arthroplasty were beginning in Europe. The short-term results of 500 cases in which "poro-metal" implants without cement were used were reported by 1974. In the United States, the first large series of cementless femoral components was initiated in 1977, several years before major studies demonstrated high rates of aseptic loosening of cemented components. In 1983, the fully porous-coated femoral component used in that series became the first to be approved by the United States Food and Drug Administration for general use without cement. Thus, cementless and cemented arthroplasty actually evolved contemporaneously, and continue to do so.

Successive generations of cementless stems can be identified. First-generation cementless stems were designed and implanted with little knowledge of the factors governing biologic fixation. Instrumentation was crude, implant inventories were severely limited, and pore sizes were often suboptimum. In addition, many first-generation stems were manufactured with rudimentary techniques, resulting in high incidences of stem breakage and porous coating loss.

The second generation of cementless stems benefited from efforts to improve immediate- and long-term fixation. Expanded implant inventories were developed, based on detailed scientific analysis of femoral anatomy. Superalloys and modularity were introduced, pore sizes were optimized, coating techniques were refined, and surgical techniques improved. Femoral component "fit-and-fill" improved dramatically, and biologic fixation became more predictable.

Third generation cementless stems comprise a more heterogeneous group. Design innovations include features to reduce osteolysis (improved bearing surfaces, circumferential porous coating), thigh pain (flexible/split distal stems), and stress shielding (limited porous coating, decreased stem stiffness), and to improve hip biomechanics (variable offset and anteversion). Custom stems represent yet another effort to create implants more mechanically compatible with the individual patient.

Early cementless acetabular sockets included metallic or all polyethylene cone shaped designs with a single post driven into the ilium, polyethylene sockets with "magic pegs," cylindrical porous cups, and a wide variety of different threaded rings and "screw sockets" fabricated of polyethylene, metal, and ceramic. In the United States, the earliest cementless sockets were porous-coated hemispheric designs with fixed spikes or pegs and factory inserted polyethylene liners. Threaded sockets enjoyed brief popularity during the mid 1980s, but have now been largely abandoned in the United States. Current designs are once again generally hemispheric, include options for secondary fixation (screws, spikes, peripheral fins), and have modular polyethylene inserts.

Biologic Fixation

Under appropriate conditions, bone and/or fibrous tissue can grow either into or onto the surface of prosthetic components. This phenomenon, known as biologic fixation, has been repetitively observed in both animal and human studies, and is the basis for cementless fixation of hip implants.

The same studies have helped to identify the requirements for bone ingrowth fixation. These requirements include a suitable implant surface in close apposition to adequate bone and immediate mechanical implant stability. The various surfaces suitable for biologic fixation are discussed in chapters on bone ingrowth and cementless implant design. Clinically, achieving immediate implant stability at the time of surgery is the single most important factor in the subsequent development of bone ingrowth fixation. The maximum amount of micromotion compatible with bone ingrowth in humans is still unknown. One group of investigators, using a canine tooth model, found that motion of less than 28 μm did not prevent bone ingrowth, whereas motion of greater than 150 μm resulted in a fibrous interface. In a similar study, it was found that interface micromotion up to 40 μm was compatible with bone ingrowth. Clinically, the stability achievable at the time of surgery is determined by interactions among bone quality, implant design, and surgical technique.

Clinical Application of Cementless Total Hip Replacement

Indications for Cementless Total Hip Replacement

Few topics in orthopaedic surgery are more controversial than the choice of implants for total hip replacement. The choice of cemented versus cementless prostheses has been the subject of intense debate. The first question to be addressed is whether or not an individual is a suitable candidate for either type of arthroplasty. The initial suggestion was to reserve total hip replacement for individuals 60 years of age and older, unless some generalized condition provided "built-in restraints" limiting the patient's activities. This recommendation was reinforced by the disastrous results of cemented hip replacement in young patients when first generation techniques were employed.

The possibility of extending the indications for total hip replacement to a much younger population was a major force in the development of cementless arthroplasty, and some substantiation for that belief is now available. The results of 173 arthroplasties using cementless femoral components in patients 40 years of age or younger have been reported. At mean follow-up of 4.6 years there was a 3.5% mechanical failure rate. Pain and walking scores were 5.9 and 5.8, respectively, and no revisions were required in those patients followed up 5 to 12 years postoperatively. For a subgroup of these patients in whom only AML stems (DePuy, Warsaw, IN) were used, a mechanical failure rate was reported of 5.7% at an average follow-up of 7.5 years, although 17% demonstrated some evidence of proximal femoral or periacetabular osteolysis. In a series of 44 patients (average age 43 years) with avascular necrosis in whom the PCA (Howmedica, East Rutherford, NJ) prosthesis had been implanted, only one stem (2.3%) required revision at a follow-up of 4 to 6 years, although 14% showed migration, as did one (2%) of the acetabular components. It would appear that if biologic fixation can be achieved, late aseptic loosening is less likely with cementless than with cemented components in young patients. However, other problems, such as osteolysis, may prove to be equally as problematic as aseptic loosening. Current recommendations regarding the treatment of young patients with end-stage hip disease might be summarized as follows: For very young patients (less than 40 years old), whose activity is not limited by systemic disease, nonreplacement alternatives should still be considered. For those patients in whom total hip replacement is selected, cementless technique is recommended after careful counseling regarding potential problems of osteolysis and the possible need for revision, the desirability of avoiding impact loading activities, and the need for careful yearly follow-up evaluation.

For patients 50 years of age or less, several studies suggest near equivalent performance of cementless and second-generation cemented femoral arthroplasty. The author of a recent review of this subject emphasized two points. The first was that with either method, technique must be optimal. The second was that, notwithstanding improvements in the preparation and delivery of cement, the results of cemented acetabular arthroplasty in young patients are still unacceptable. Therefore, cementless acetabular components are recommended in this age group.

Selecting the most appropriate mode of femoral implant fixation is perhaps most difficult for patients between the ages of 50 and 65 years. The published results of hybrid total hip replacement using modern cementing techniques for patients older than 50 have been extremely favorable. The results have been reported of an ongoing longitudinal study of 171 patients with mean age of 57.4 years in whom second-generation cementing techniques were utilized. Femoral failure rates at 3.3, 6.2, and 11 years follow-up were 1.1%, 1.7%, and 3%, respectively.

Little has been written specifically about cementless total hip replacement in this particular age group. However, it is important to note that several studies have failed to show a decline in the incidence of bone ingrowth fixation with increasing age. In an analysis of the survivorship of 959 primary total hip replacements using cementless stems, including 307 performed in patients 65 years of age and older, no significant differences were found in the survivorship probability when patients were analyzed according to age. In a separate study, the same authors found no difference in the incidence of thigh pain for younger versus older patients when extensively porous-coated stems were used. It must be recognized that there is considerable variability in "physiologic age" and bone quality for patients between the ages of 50 and 65. Hence, the choice of implant fixation should be individualized, based on both clinical and radiographic evaluation. For physiologically young patients—those in good general health who are still quite active and/or heavy—and especially those who have unilateral lower extremity impairment, cementless femoral fixation may be considered. The final decision should, however, be based on careful radiographic evaluation of bone quality. Dorr has described the "calcar isthmus" as the narrow, funnel-shaped outlet of the distal metaphysis at the level of the mid lesser trochanter. He furthermore defined the calcar-canal ("C-C") ratio, which is derived by dividing the diameter of the femoral canal 10 cm distal to the mid lesser trochanter by the calcar isthmus measurement. If this ratio exceeds 75%, cement rather than cementless prostheses designed for metaphyseal fixation are recommended.

For patients over the age of 65, there is general consensus that cemented femoral component fixation is preferred. While good results have been reported following the use of cementless implants in this age group, two factors must be considered. The first is that with advancing age, the femoral canal is known to enlarge. Hence, canal filling with cementless stems requires the use of larger, stiffer implants, thereby increasing the potential for stress shielding and possibly thigh pain. Secondly, at the time of this writing, the cost of cementless femoral implants is considerably greater than that of cemented components. Results of preliminary studies have indicated that significant cost savings may be realized without compromise of clinical results when cemented as opposed to cementless femoral components are used in this age group. Although there currently is limited information regarding the long-term performance of cementless acetabular components, it appears that their fixation at 10 years will prove superior to that of cemented cups. Hence, cementless acetabular components are recommended for elderly patients with life expectancies greater than 10 years.

Preoperative Planning

The goals of cementless total hip replacement are a pain-free, stable joint, a good range of motion, and a normal gait. Success in achieving these goals is in large part determined by the technical adequacy of the procedure, including the appropriate selection of implants. This process begins with careful planning of both the intraosseous and extraosseous aspects of each case.

A pain-free hip requires optimum implant fixation, which depends on achieving immediate mechanical implant stability at the time of surgery. This, in turn, depends on maximum "fit-and-fill" of cementless components, ie, intraosseous considerations. Because the anatomy of the femoral canal is highly variable, no single implant is optimum for every case. The surgeon should, therefore, be familiar with several different designs of femoral component. In general, both the anatomy of the acetabulum and the design of contemporary acetabular components are less variable. A noteworthy exception commonly encountered in primary interventions is congenital dysplasia.

Hip stability and range of motion as well as a normal gait depend on restoring the normal hip biomechanics. This restoration requires consideration of leg length, femoral offset, and anteversion, ie, the extraosseous aspects of the reconstruction.

Preoperative planning requires a minimum number of appropriate radiographs. These include an anteroposterior (AP) view of the pelvis, which shows both hip joints, a separate AP view of the femur, which extends well beyond the isthmus, and a Lowenstein lateral view of the femur. Additional views may be required in certain special situations. Specific measures are taken to minimize and control for magnification. The thigh must be closely applied to the film cassette. When significant flexion contracture exists, the patient is sat up until the femur can be placed flat. In the presence of an external rotation contracture, a standard AP radiograph will underestimate the medial to lateral dimension of the metaphysis. Therefore, a posteroanterior view of the femur is obtained by first placing the patient prone and then elevating the normal side of the pelvis to an angle equivalent to the contracture. This internally rotates the affected thigh and places the coronal plane of the femur parallel to that of the film cassette. A magnification marker should always be used, taped to the thigh at the level of the femur. These devices generally feature radiopaque markers separated by a known distance. The distance between the markers is then measured on the radiograph and the magnification factor is calculated using the following formula:

$$\frac{(\text{measured distance}) - (\text{actual distance})}{\text{actual distance}} = \text{magnification}$$

Templating is performed next. All major manufacturers supply clear templates depicting the dimensions of the femoral component in both the AP and lateral projections, and acetabular components in the AP projection. These templates are available with varying degrees of magnification, typically 110%, 115%, and 120%. The set of templates with a magnification factor that most closely matches the calculated value above should be chosen. Templating is begun on the acetabular side, using the AP pelvic radiograph, which establishes the center of rotation of the prosthetic joint. The template should closely approximate the subchondral plate, should be completely contained, and ideally should be inclined between 40° and 50° from the horizontal as determined by the interteardrop line. Its center should be the mirror image of the contralateral hip if it is normal. In cases of acetabular dysplasia in which a false acetabulum is present, several choices exist. In mild cases, the socket may be contained in a "high" position, 1 to 2 cm above anatomic without undue compromise of hip biomechanics. In severe cases, this may not be possible, and the surgeon can then plan femoral head autografting of the false acetabulum or the use of an oblong cup to fill the defect. In either case, an attempt is made to return the head center to the anatomic position. It must be acknowledged that structural autografts are subject to resorption and collapse, with reported rates of subsequent component loosening in the range of 8% to 19% at 2 to 5 year follow-up. No data are as yet available regarding the use of oblong cups.

Provisional intraosseous templating of the femoral component is performed. Because significant disproportion may exist between the dimensions of the metaphysis and the femoral isthmus, it may be difficult to simultaneously achieve component fit and fill in both areas. It is, therefore, essential that the design rationale of the femoral component being contemplated for use be fully understood. Specifically, "anatomic" proximally porous-coated stems are critically dependent on proximal fit and fill. Therefore, metaphyseal sizing is given priority. In contrast, for extensively porous-coated straight-stemmed prostheses, canal filling within the femoral isthmus is given priority. Stated differently, it is best if that portion of the stem bearing the ingrowth/ongrowth surface provides a substantial amount of the initial implant stability.

Preoperative planning to establish optimum extraosseous relationships is performed next. With the availability of modular femoral heads, the surgeon can choose a preferred level of femoral neck resection and, subsequently, correct leg length with various lengths of heads. The level of neck resection determines the depth of seating of the femoral component and, therefore, the component size required. This is especially true for those implants designed for metaphyseal filling. Various combinations of neck resection and femoral head length can be combined to yield the same leg length, but each results in a different amount of femoral offset. Proper offset is important in reestablishing the abductor moment arm, proper muscle tension, and avoidance of impingement. Cases of coxa valga can be addressed by combining a high neck resection, a larger femoral component, and a shorter prosthetic head. In cases of coxa vara, a low neck cut, a smaller femoral component, and a long prosthetic head may be combined to restore both leg length and offset. However, the consequences of this technique should be carefully considered. Sacrifice of the femoral neck results in diminished torsional stability of the implant. The use of a longer head and neck segment also increases the stresses placed on the prosthetic neck. Adequate femoral head length may require a "skirt" about the base of the head, which can lead to reduced range of motion, impingement, and dislocation. Finally, the need for a long head may exclude the possibility of using a ceramic component, particularly if a 26- or 28-mm diameter is preferred. Hence, it is recommended that in extreme cases of coxa vara, an implant with adequate inherent offset be selected.

After the level of neck resection and implant size are determined, the center of rotation of the prosthetic femoral head is marked. If the disease process has resulted in even minor distortion of anatomic relationships, this mark will not coincide with the templated center of the acetabular component. Assuming that the acetabular component is placed at the normal anatomic hip center, the effect of a particular femoral component size and position on leg length and offset can be assessed by measuring the vertical and horizontal distances between the templated component centers. As an example, in a typical case of osteoarthritis, the femoral head center may be displaced cephalad and lateral, with resulting limb shortening and increased offset. After appropriate templating, the center of the prosthetic femoral head will be at a position lateral and

cephalad to the center of the prosthetic acetabulum. After "reduction" of the hip, the leg will be lengthened by an amount equal to the vertical distance between the templated component centers, and the offset will be reduced by an amount equal to the horizontal difference (Fig. 1).

Surgical Technique

The outcome of cementless hip replacement is highly dependent on the technical adequacy of the procedure. Compared to cemented implants, there is considerably greater diversity in the design of cementless components. All share the requirement that a tight fit of the components be achieved at the time of surgery. Bone preparation as well as the recommended tolerances between the implant and the bone vary significantly among different designs. Many manufacturers deliberately undersize trial implants relative to the actual implants, and the degree of undersizing is implant specific. Hence, surgical protocols have been developed for each implant system, and these should be strictly followed. Despite this specificity, there are some general principles to which the surgeon should adhere, regardless of the specific implant being used.

Exposure to the hip is discussed in a separate chapter. There is no single approach to the hip that is best for cementless arthroplasty. In general, the surgeon should use the approach with which he or she has the most experience and confidence. However, the approach used should lend itself to extensile exposure in case complications such as femoral fracture occur.

Acetabular arthroplasty begins with complete, circumferential exposure of the acetabulum. Many manufacturers provide aiming guides to facilitate proper orientation of acetabular components. These usually require positioning in reference to objects external to the patient such as the

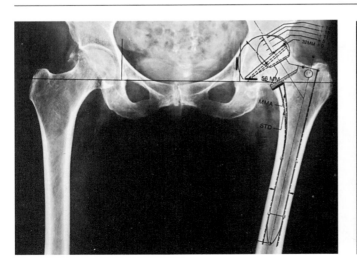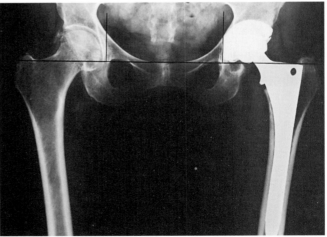

Fig. 1 Preoperative templating. **Left,** the femoral head has been displaced in a cephalad and lateral direction. The centers of rotation of the templated components do not coincide **(right).** Postoperatively, leg length and offset have been restored.

floor. Hence, their utility is decreased by minor changes in the patient's position on the operating room table. It is more reliable to use internal bony landmarks as references to component position. These landmarks include the lateral wing of the ilium, the root of the pubis, the ischium, and the inferior aspect of the true medial wall of the acetabulum (the "teardrop"). Peripheral osteophytes that obscure visualization of these landmarks should be carefully trimmed. Medial "curtain osteophytes" over the acetabular fossa should also be removed. Some remnant of the pulvinar (haversian gland) is invariably present and is removed to expose the true acetabular floor. An acetabulum whose shape deviates significantly from a hemisphere can be detected by comparing the AP versus the superoinferior dimensions. Minor deviations can be compensated by thinning of walls in one dimension (usually AP). Extreme cases require methods similar to those described above for acetabular dysplasia. Various types of acetabular reamers are available. The most common is the "cheese grater" design. It is recommended that reamers be available in 1-mm increments to allow the surgeon to select the degree of desired underreaming depending on bone quality and to allow one set of reamers to be used for components from different manufacturers. Commonly, bone in the superolateral aspect of the acetabulum has become sclerotic as a result of the arthritic process, and tends to deflect reamers inferiorly. This situation is remedied by using a much smaller reamer or a high-speed burr directed into the sclerotic area prior to further attempts at expanding the cavity.

Mechanical, strain gauge, and finite element studies have shown that sacrifice of the subchondral plate of the acetabulum results in substantial weakening of the socket. It is therefore recommended that incremental reaming be continued only until a hemispheric contour is achieved, all cartilage remnants are removed, a uniform petechial bleeding surface is attained, and the acetabular component can be well contained. As the appropriate amount of reaming nears completion, considerable resistance is often encountered (particularly in osteoarthritic patients with good bone quality) as the reamer engages the acetabular rim. Great care must be exercised during acetabular preparation in patients with rheumatoid arthritis or osteoporosis, because the subchondral plate may be easily violated. Acetabular cysts should be evacuated and packed with morselized autogenous bone from either the femoral head or metaphysis. Care is exercised to avoid interposition of this graft between areas of healthy bleeding acetabular surface and the implant. Acetabular components are generally available in 2 or 3 mm incremental sizes. Underreaming of the acetabular bed by 1 to 2 mm and occasionally 3 mm is recommended, depending on the manufacturer.

The nominal size of the acetabular component may not be the actual size of the prosthetic component. Some manufacturers deliberately oversize components relative to their stated size. Some minor variation (in the range of 0.5 mm) can also occur as a result of the porous coating process. Likewise, reamers may not actually be their stated

size. Repetitive sharpening results in a smaller reamer. This occurs most commonly in centers where high volumes of joint replacements are performed, or alternatively, when well-used "loaner sets" are brought in for a particular case. The most reliable means of avoiding underreaming or overreaming are to use radius gauges to measure both the reamers and the prosthetic components prior to their use, and to be thoroughly familiar with the manufacturer's sizing nomenclature. The acetabular component is impacted in the anatomic position, perhaps with slight exaggeration of inherent anteversion, particularly if a posterior approach has been used. Initial implant stability is tested by gently toggling the attached impaction device.

The use of adjunctive fixation devices and particularly screws to augment initial acetabular component stability is controversial. The potential benefits of screws were demonstrated in a canine study as early as 1981. Results of two recent studies have demonstrated superior in vitro mechanical stability of cups fixed with screws versus lugs or spikes, or no adjunctive fixation. At least two human retrieval studies have demonstrated significantly more bone ingrowth adjacent to lugs, spikes, and screws than in other areas. In one of these, an average of 50% more bone ingrowth was noted in areas adjacent to screws than in other areas. No complications associated with the use of screws were revealed in separate clinical studies from three different centers of 271 total hip replacements in which one design of acetabular component was used and followed up between 2 and 6 years postoperatively. On the other hand, concern has been raised about the potential problems that screws could cause, including breakage, migration, difficulty in removal, stress shielding, fretting between the shell or impingement on the polyethylene liner leading to metallic or polyethylene wear debris, and damage to vital neurovascular structures during insertion. Apart from the screws themselves, the holes provided for their insertion lessen the amount of porous surface available, may cause cold flow of polyethylene, and have been found to be sites of accumulation of polyethylene wear debris. Furthermore, these holes represent potential avenues for the migration of debris of other origins into the periacetabular bone. Also, in vitro studies exist which demonstrate that the most important contribution to initial acetabular component stability is an interference fit of the cup at its periphery. Some clinical studies have failed to demonstrate any benefit from screw fixation, and multiple reports of screw breakage, fretting, and penetration of vital structures exist.

It seems appropriate to suggest that, if possible, cementless components be inserted using 1 to 2 mm of press fit without screws. It has been suggested that approximately 90% of primary procedures can be accomplished in this fashion. It is also important to emphasize that no number of screws can compensate for poor surgical technique and lack of inherent press-fit stability. When screws are used, the surgeon should be thoroughly familiar with the medially-situated vital structures at risk during insertion. Safe zones for screw insertion, in the posterior superior and posterior inferior aspects of the acetabulum, have been described. The use of screws in the anterior quadrants of the acetabulum is to be avoided. Adjunctive fixation devices fixed to the acetabular shell may be of some value and avoid many of the potential problems of screws. However, they render cup insertion more difficult and may prevent complete seating of the component.

Polyethylene inserts are available in diameters to accommodate varying head diameters. Whenever possible, the thickest polyethylene liner (smallest inner diameter) should be used. Wear studies suggest that linear and volumetric wear are minimized with the use of a 28-mm diameter insert. Built up rims or lips, adjustable to the position of maximum instability, may be very useful in certain circumstances. However, they may serve as sites of impingement and create instability in the opposite direction. In addition, data from at least one report demonstrate osteolysis as a result of polyethylene wear debris generated from femoral neck impingement against such a lip. Conformity and fixation of modular liners varies considerably among manufacturers. Designs in which areas of the liner are exceedingly thin or unsupported should be avoided. Likewise, designs that permit micromotion between the shell and the outer aspect of the liner may lead to problems with debris generation. These concerns warrant careful scrutiny when selecting among the many cups available.

Despite the wide variety of different femoral component designs available, most stems, whether modular or monolithic, fall into one of two broad categories. The first is the anatomic type of stem that is proximally porous coated, is designed for metaphyseal fit and fixation, and generally has a curved stem to conform to the anterior bow of the femur. The second is the straight stem design, which may be proximally or extensively coated. Proximally coated straight stems are designed to fill the metaphyseal region and attain axial stability there. The distal, straight portion of the stem may be either cylindric or tapered, and has different proposed roles depending upon the design and manufacturer. Some degree of distal stability or toggle control is attributed to all. Tapered designs also provide for some axial stability. Flutes incorporated into stems with a cylindrical distal configuration can also contribute to immediate torsional stability. Extensively porous-coated straight stem designs prioritize fit and fill in the femoral isthmus over proximal metaphyseal filling. The surgical preparation of the femoral canal for straight-stemmed implants varies according to the intended function of the distal stem.

Preparation for femoral component insertion begins with transection of the femoral neck. Several manufacturers provide implant-specific neck resection guides. The level of the neck resection should be approximated at the time of templating. Both categories of femoral components described above require broaching of the proximal femoral metaphysis. Exceptions to this include certain modular designs that use a milling device to prepare the metaphysis. Broaching of the femoral canal should begin with the smallest available broach and proceed until metaphyseal filling is achieved. It is emphasized that broaches are designed for the removal of cancellous bone. They are ineffective and dangerous when used to remove endosteal cortical bone. Rotational orientation must be maintained when impacting broaches. A sequence of repetitive insertion and withdrawal of the broach is recommended, as is frequent irrigation of the femoral canal.

Broaching of the femur in preparation for the insertion of straight-stemmed prostheses is generally preceded by axial reaming with either tapered or cylindrical reamers. The entry point of the reamers is critical. It is, therefore, suggested that a pilot hole be created first, generally at the former point of insertion of the piriformis tendon in the trochanteric fossa. The smallest available reamer should be gently inserted to its full depth by hand, using it as a canal finder. The femoral isthmus should control the direction of the reamer. A pilot hole placed too far medially or an overhanging greater trochanter will direct reaming into varus. Successively larger reamers are passed by hand until resistance is met. Preoperative planning gives the surgeon certain expectations as to which size of reamer will first engage the endosteum. If resistance is met using a much smaller reamer than anticipated, the surgeon must suspect a problem, such as improper pilot hole positioning. If the discrepancy is not immediately resolved by redirecting the reamer, intraoperative radiographs should be obtained in two planes prior to proceeding with power reaming. Otherwise, eccentric reaming or even distal cortical perforation may occur. As stated above, the extent of distal reaming varies with the specific implant system used. Proximally coated stems without distal flutes are generally inserted line-to-line or slightly undersized relative to the prepared canal. On the other hand, when an extensively porous-coated stem or one with distal flutes is to be inserted, the distal canal is generally underreamed by 0.5 to 1.0 mm relative to the distal stem diameter. Reaming of the distal canal is followed by preparation of the metaphysis with either broaches or a milling device. As is true for the acetabular reamers and components, the actual dimensions of femoral reamers and components may vary from their stated sizes. It is, therefore, recommended that both reamers and implants be measured intraoperatively using either specially designed hole gauges, vernier calipers, or a gas-sterilized dial micrometer.

Depending on the design, proximally porous-coated stems without distal flutes can generally be inserted by hand to a depth of 1 or 2 cm short of full seating, and then gently tapped in the remaining distance. In sharp contrast, extensively coated and fluted stems may require a surprising amount of force to fully seat. Those unfamiliar with the insertion of such devices are urged to observe several procedures performed by a surgeon familiar with their use before attempting this alone.

Following impaction of the femoral component, some authors advocate testing implant stability in torsion, using the equivalent of a wrench attached to the stem. Others regard this as unnecessary because the surgeon generally gets an impression of the degree of implant stability during impaction. Vigorous testing of implant stability in torsion does pose some risk of femoral fracture. Any evidence of instability at the time of surgery is an absolute indication for stem removal. Under these circumstances, it is recommended that the surgeon consider using one size larger stem. The use of cement in such circumstances should be undertaken with great caution. The usual preparation of the femoral canal for a cementless device, especially if it involves reaming of the femoral canal, effectively removes all cancellous bone, rendering cement interdigitation impossible.

Intraoperative Femoral Fractures

The reported incidences of intraoperative femoral fracture complicating total hip replacement are higher for cementless versus cemented stems. Ranges of 0.1% to 3.2% have been cited for cemented femoral arthroplasty versus 4.1% to 27.8% for series of cementless stems. A review of more recent studies of cementless arthroplasty reveals incidences of intraoperative fracture between 2% to 10.5% (Table 1). The possible reasons for the higher incidence of fracture with cementless versus cemented stems are several. One is the very nature of cementless arthroplasty, which demands an immediate, tight fit of the stem at the time of surgery. Second is the diversity in the design and surgical techniques recommended for each cementless stem. In contrast, techniques for the implantation of cemented stems are substantially similar regardless of the manufacturer or design. Finally, there is a definite learning

Table 1. Intraoperative femoral fractures and cementless THR

Year of Study	Design*	No. of Hips	Incidence of Fracture
1989	AML	1,318	3%
1989	Custom	156	7%
1992	Harris-Galante	82	3.8%
1992	Harris-Galante	69	2.9%
1992	Harris-Galante	100	6%
1992	Harris-Galante	122	7.4%
1992	PCA	100	2%
1992	HA Omnifit	436	7.3%
1993	S-Rom	48	10.5%

*AML (DePuy, Warsaw, IN); Custom (Techmedica, Camarillo, CA); Harris-Galante (Zimmer, Warsaw, IN); PCA (Howmedica, East Rutherford, NJ); HA Omnifit (Osteonics, Allendale, NJ); S-Rom (Joint Medical Products, Stamford, CT)

curve associated with the use of any particular cementless stem, which may be more prolonged than that associated with cemented stems. This learning curve is, in part, supported by the reduced incidences of fractures noted in the more recent literature compared to earlier studies, although improvements in stem design and instrumentation might also be partially responsible for this trend. One group reported an overall incidence of intraoperative fracture of 7.4% (9/122). However, when studied chronologically, all fractures occurred during the first 50 cases and none occurred during the subsequent 72. Another group reported two fractures in their first 100 cases; both occurred during the first 50 procedures.

The treatment of intraoperative fractures depends first on when they are recognized, and second on the type of fracture and the design of stem being used. Fractures have been classified according to their location (Fig. 2). Proxi-

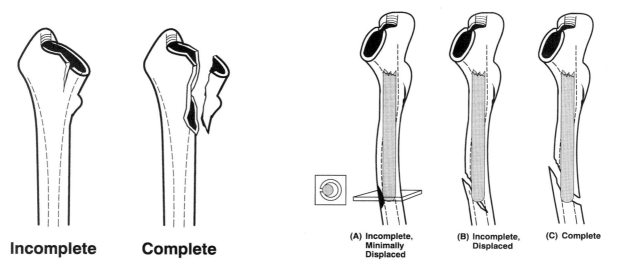

Incomplete   **Complete**

(A) Incomplete, Minimally Displaced   (B) Incomplete, Displaced   (C) Complete

Fig. 2 Classification of femoral fractures. **Left,** proximal fracture patterns. **Right,** distal fracture patterns. (Reproduced with permission from Schwartz JT Jr, Mayer JG, Engh CA: Femoral fractures during non-cemented total hip arthroplasty. *J Bone Joint Surg* 1989;71A:1135–1142.)

mal fractures may be incomplete, representing small fissures or cracks, or complete, in which case a portion of the metaphysis is displaced from the remaining femur. Distal fractures are either incomplete (some cortical continuity remains) or complete. Fractures incurred during preparation for, or implantation of proximally coated metaphyseal filling implants are most likely to occur proximally. Because the immediate and long-term stability of such implants depends on the integrity of the metaphysis, these fractures should be fixed if discovered at the time of surgery. The implant is removed, after which the fracture is completely exposed and cerclage wired. The implant is then reinserted. Immediate implant stability can generally be restored in this fashion. Nonetheless, two cases have been reported in which proximal fractures were treated in this fashion and subsequent stem subsidence occurred. Therefore, it is recommended that these patients remain nonweightbearing for 6 weeks or until fracture healing is noted. If immediate stability of the proximally coated stem cannot be restored despite cerclage wire fixation, the surgeon may wish to consider the use of a distally porous coated or fluted stem. Proximal fractures discovered postoperatively are generally treated with nonweightbearing and serial radiographic evaluation. Implant subsidence in the early postoperative period is a strong indication for subsequent surgery.

Distal fractures may occur in association with either proximally or extensively coated stems. Incomplete, minimally displaced fractures are usually longitudinal fissures of the anterior femoral cortex that follow the use of a straight-stemmed implant. These are more likely to go undetected at the time of surgery. Thankfully, most can be treated with nonweightbearing for 6 weeks. Callus recognized at the stem tip at 6 week follow-up is sometimes the only evidence that such a fracture has occurred. Incomplete displaced distal fractures are more serious. If the implant is stable, the surgeon has the choices of spica cast immobilization or open reduction and internal fixation with or without exchange to a long-stem prosthesis. Complete distal fractures should be treated with immediate open reduction and internal fixation. In most cases, properly treated intraoperative femoral fractures have no deleterious effect on the final outcome of the arthroplasty.

Results of Cementless Arthroplasty

The term "cementless," when applied to either acetabular or femoral components, encompasses vast assortments of different designs, the performances of which cannot be expected to be equivalent. In addition, a cementless acetabular component might be (and commonly is) used in combination with a cemented stem, or vice versa. In such hybrid arthroplasties, the relative contributions of each component to postoperative pain or limp is not always certain. With these considerations in mind, the radiographic results of cementless acetabular and femoral components will be presented separately, and where feasible, according to design. Clinical results will emphasize series in which both components were inserted using cementless technique.

Radiographic Results: Acetabulum

Criteria for the radiographic evaluation of cementless implant fixation have been established by noting changes about implants on clinical or specimen radiographs and correlating these findings with subsequent histologic examination of the bone-implant interface. These criteria are based on assessment of implant migration, interface appearance, and (for femoral components), adaptive remodeling of the surrounding bone.

For acetabular components, implant migration or the lack thereof is the most important parameter of stability. An optimum appearance is defined as no implant migration on serial radiographs, and nonprogressive radiolucency in no more than one zone. Stable implants also show no progressive migration, but have minimum (eg, < 2 mm), nonprogressive radiolucencies in two or more zones. The hallmark of an unstable implant is progressive migration. Widening radiolucencies are also predictive of impending failure. Because of the loading conditions and the large volume of cancellous bone in the acetabulum, adaptive remodeling about acetabular components is limited. Densification in zone 1 has been regarded by some as indicative of bone ingrowth, but this has not been substantiated histologically. Acetabular components should also be assessed for eccentric wear of the polyethylene liner, migration or breakage of adjunctive screws, and osteolysis in the periprosthetic bone. All-polyethylene and various threaded cups are designs which showed promising early results, were widely embraced, and subsequently failed in a high percentage of cases.

Polyethylene Cups   The Ring all-polyethylene UPM cup (Downs Brothers, Surrey, UK), introduced in 1979, incorporated a Freeman osseous peg and was intended to improve on earlier metal-on-metal designs while incorporating the metal-on-polyethylene couple introduced by Charnley. Ring reported no loosening of this design among 164 cases followed up at 1 to 3 years. Subsequently, the results were reported of 1,402 arthroplasties with the same cup that were followed up for 2 to 7 years, with only six (0.43%) requiring revision. Despite an increasing rate of failure after 5 years and a 14% incidence of polyethylene-induced osteolysis, it was concluded that polyethylene bearing directly on bone in the acetabulum appears to be quite satisfactory. However, others subsequently reported catastrophic failure of eight such cups 3 to 8 years postoperatively as a result of polyethylene wear at the external cup surface. Similarly, another author reported no aseptic loosening of 250 RM isoelastic all-polyethylene cups fixed with pegs or pegs and screws at 1 to 5.5 years. In a subsequent follow-up of 445 RM cups (Robert Mathys, Bettlach, Switzerland), progressive loosening was noted beyond 6 years, with 28% having failed at 9 years. Significant osteolysis was present in 21%. The author concluded that polyethylene should never come into direct contact with bone.

Threaded Cups Like all-polyethylene cups, various threaded designs demonstrated promising early results. A review of 491 threaded cobalt-chromium (CoCr) cups of truncated ellipsoid design indicated no evident loosening or migration 4 years after surgery. Among 136 Endler all-polyethylene or titanium alloy conical threaded cups, 0.7% loosening was reported at 3- to 5-year follow-up. Only 0.9% loosening was reported among 415 ceramic threaded cups at a maximum follow-up of 8 years. In subsequent studies, 33.3% (34/102) of Endler threaded cups (Ruhr-chemte AG, Oberhausen, Germany) were loose at mean follow-up of 57.4 months, 16.1% (115/714) of Bi-Metric titanium threaded cups (Biomet, Warsaw, IN) were revised at 2 to 5 years, and 24.6% of Mittlemeier threaded ceramic cups (Osteo AG, Selzach, Switzerland) had migrated between 24 and 52 months. In a study of a different design of threaded ceramic cup, 46% failed between 10 and 14 years. A review of the implantation of 130 threaded titanium cups of two different designs indicated combined rates of instability of 10% at 1 year and 21% at 2 years. The rate of loosening of those same cups now exceeds 50% at 6-year follow-up.

Porous Acetabular Components Porous-coated acetabular components were first used without cement in the early 1970s, and a subsequent report of 531 cases in which these cylindrical poro-metal sockets were used indicated 4% had migrated at 1.5-to 5-year follow-up. Twenty years later, the author of a comprehensive review of the state of acetabular arthroplasty indicated that uncemented porous-coated acetabular components currently represent the state of the art in total hip arthroplasty. Considerable clinical data exist to support this view. A review of the contemporary literature (Table 2) reveals rates of loosening and/or revision for various designs of porous acetabular components in the range of 0 to 6% at 2- to 7-year follow-up. The cups in these studies had beaded, plasma-sprayed, or fiber-mesh surfaces.

Component migration or lack thereof is the most critical determinant of implant stability. The long-term significance of minimal (eg, < 2 mm), nonprogressive radiolucencies adjacent to porous-coated acetabular components is uncertain. Such lucencies have been noted in one or more zones in up to 60% of cases in the studies reviewed, with no apparent adverse effect on intermediate-term (5-year) stability or clinical performance. Both acetabular anatomy and the metallic density of porous cups renders detection of such radiolucencies difficult on plain radiographs. Contact radiographs of sectioned autopsy specimens commonly reveal radiolucencies when none were visible on plain films. Histologic examination of such interfaces demonstrates fibrous tissue at the bone—implant interface, which could potentially allow the ingress of osteoclasts and subsequent loosening, as has been demonstrated for cemented acetabular components. However, at present, stable fibrous fixation as evidenced by nonprogressive radiolucencies appears compatible with excellent clinical performance and, thus far, is not predictive of subsequent loosening.

Recently, various bioactive calcium-phosphate ceramics have been applied to cementless cups in hopes of enhancing their fixation. In one series, the addition of hydroxyapatite (HA) coating to threaded cups appeared to produce better clinical and radiographic results than those for an identical threaded cup without HA. In a study in which 285 smooth HA-coated cups were compared to 132 porous cups, three (1%) of the HA cups had migrated at 3 years, as compared to none of the porous-coated cups. The effect of HA or other calcium-phosphate compounds applied to a porous surface is presently unknown.

Radiographic Results: Femoral Components

Criteria for the radiographic evaluation of cementless femoral component fixation have been developed and are summarized pictorially in Figure 3. Bone ingrown components show no migration (subsidence, tilting, or rotation), the absence of radiolucencies adjacent to the ingrowth surface, endosteal hypertrophy (spot welds) at the junction of the smooth and coated portions of the stem, and a variable amount of stress-induced atrophy above the termination

Table 2. Results of porous-coated cementless cups

Year of Study	Design*	No. of Hips	Follow-up	Revision/Loosening
1992	Harris-Galante	69	2 to 5 years	0%/0%
1992	Harris-Galante	122	3 to 6 years	0%/0%
1992	Harris-Galante	100	2 to 5 years	0%/0%
1993	Harris-Galante	66	2 to 4.3 years	0%/0% (among primaries)
1993	Optifix	40	2 to 4.3 years	0%/0%
1993	PCA	100	5 to 7 years	2%/6%
1988	PCA	70	mean 30 months	0%/0%
1990	AML	285	mean 4.8 years	0%/0%
1992	Omnifit	132	2 to 3 years	0%/0%

*Harris-Galante (Zimmer, Warsaw, IN); Optifix (Richards, Memphis, TN); PCA (Howmedica, East Rutherford, NJ); AML (DePuy, Warsaw, IN); Omnifit (Osteonics, Allendale, NJ)

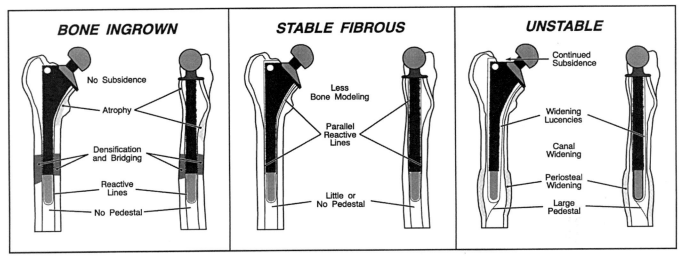

Fig. 3 The radiographic features of different modes of cementless femoral component fixation. (Reproduced with permission from Engh CA, Glassman AH, Suthers KE: The case for porous-coated hip implants: The femoral side. *Clin Orthop* 1990;261:63–81.)

of the porous coating. Reactive lines may be present adjacent to the distal, uncoated portion of the stem. Implants with stable-fibrous fixation show either no migration or minimal migration, which subsequently stabilizes (usually within the first year), parallel, nonprogressive reactive lines adjacent to the ingrowth surface, lack of spot welds, and minimal or no proximal atrophy. Unstable stems demonstrate progressive migration, and/or widening reactive lines/radiolucencies surrounding the stem, pedestal formation at the stem tip, and hypertrophy beneath the collar. Widening of the intramedullary canal or debonding of the ingrowth surface may also occur.

The earliest experiences with cementless femoral stems were in Europe and England. The first use of a smooth, straight, CoCr stem was in 1964. Of 164 hips, ten (7.3%) developed aseptic loosening and two of these (1.2%) required revision 1 to 3 years postoperatively. Among 116 Ring prostheses (Downs Brothers, Surrey, UK) followed up a mean of 8 years, 23% loosened and 11% required revision. The Mittlemeier ceramic hip (Osteo AG, Selzach, Switzerland) was also CoCr but incorporated macrotexturing to improve fixation. The early (Mark I) design was curved, with transverse ribs, and loosened in 22% of cases. The Mark II design was straight, had longitudinal ribs, and a lateral fin. In a series of 851 such stems, 8.9% were loose at 6 years. In another study of the same stem, 26% were revised for loosening at a mean of 39.6 months. Macroporous stems were introduced between 1972 and 1974. Of 499 Judet poro-metal stems (Benoist-Girard, Paris, France) followed up for 2 to 6 years, aseptic loosening developed in 4.6%. No loosening was reported among 207 Lord Madreporic stems (S.A. Benoist-Girard, Paris,

France) at 5- to 7-year follow-up. Both stems featured roughnesses cast into their entire lengths and suffered a significant incidence of late stem fracture. The ability of smooth titanium alloys to become osseointegrated prompted development of the Zweymuller stem (Sulzer Brothers Ltd, Winterthur, Switzerland). Over 40,000 of these titanium alloy (aluminum-vanadium or aluminum-niobium) stems were implanted in Europe. Of 136 such stems followed up for 3 to 5 years, 1.5% were revised for loosening and another 5.1% were loose. Subsidence, presumably to a position of greater stability, was regarded as a self-locking mechanism and occurred in 22%.

Composite stems of various designs underwent clinical trials in Europe and North America, with disappointing results. To reduce the stiffness mismatch between the stem and the femur, all had a metallic core covered by a lower modulus polymeric surface. The Isoelastic stem (Robert Mathys, Bettlach, Switzerland), covered with polyacetyl resin, was the first such design. Excessive flexibility resulted in interface micromotion and subsequent loosening. Stems coated with Proplast (Vitek, Inc., Houston, TX), a spongy composite of Teflon and carbon fibers, suffered from coating fragmentation, loosening, and pain; a 36% failure rate was reported at mean follow-up of 37 months. Porous polysulfone-coated stems were abandoned for similar reasons.

During the late 1960s and early 1970s, active research into porous-coating technology progressed. In Canada, methods were developed for porous coating CoCr stems using powder-made sintered beads. Titanium-fiber mesh ingrowth surfaces were developed at the same time. Subsequently, titanium beaded surfaces, plasma-sprayed titanium, and plasma-sprayed calcium phosphate ceramic coatings were introduced. The majority of contemporary cementless stems have one of these surface treatments. The radiographic results obtained using several representative designs of such stems are summarized in Table 3. Rates of revision for aseptic loosening in these series range between zero and 3.8% and for loosening without revision between zero and 9% at 2- to 13-year follow-up. The highest rates of loosening were reported for series of titanium stems with discrete regions of porous coating in the form of patches or pads. All have been superseded by circumferentially coated designs, which have had improved results at short-term follow-up. The average follow-up for all series presented is approximately 5 years, considerably less than the 10 years generally felt necessary to assess the durability of cemented stems. However, the fixation of cementless stems is determined within the first few months after surgery and is radiographically evident by 2 years. Although it is pos-

sible, late aseptic loosening of ingrown stems has not been documented except in cases of severe osteolysis.

Clinical Results

Equitable comparisons among different series of total hip replacements, whether cementless or cemented, are difficult for several reasons. Patient populations are not always comparable, various femoral and acetabular components are sometimes used within the same series, and a standardized evaluation protocol has not been universally adapted.

When composite hip scores are used, the overall clinical results of cementless and cemented primary arthroplasty are comparable. Among five separate studies involving 422 Harris-Galante femoral components (Zimmer, Warsaw, IN), the mean Harris hip score was 90.8 at 2 to 6 years. The average Harris score for 100 PCA prostheses followed up 5 to 7 years was 92. For 436 HA-Omnifit stems (Osteo-

Table 3. Radiographic results of cementless stems

Year of Study	Design*	Design Features	No. of Hips	Follow-up	Revision for Aseptic Loosening	Unstable, Unrevised
1992	Harris-Galante	Ti-Straight Stem CP-Ti Fibermesh Pads	100	2 to 5 years mean 37 months	1%	0%
1992	Harris-Galante	Ti-Straight Stem CP-Ti Fibermesh Pads	122	3 to 6.2 years	3.8%	9%
1994	Multilock	Ti-straight stem, CP-Ti fibermesh coating (circumferential)	176	mean 2 years	0%	0%
1990	APR-I	Ti-curved stem, cancellous patch porous coating	200	mean 49 months	2%	3/5%
1994	APR-II	Ti-curved stem, circumferential cancellous porous coating		awaiting data		
1993	PCA	CoCr, curved stem sintered beads	100	5 to 7 years	1%	5%
1994	AML	CoCr, straight stem, sintered beads, extensively coated	166	6 to 13 years mean 41 months	0.6%	1.9%
1994	Omniflex	Ti-straight stem Ti bead pads, modular	88	2 to 5 years	3.4%	6.8%
1992	Omnifit	Hydroxyapatite coated straight stem	430	3 to 5 years	0.46%	0%
1993	S-Rom	Ti-straight stem Ti beaded spout, modular	48	3 to 6 years	0%	0%
1994	Mallory-Head	Ti-straight stem plasma sprayed	121	mean 6.7 years	3.3%	0%

*Harris-Galante and Multilock (Zimmer, Warsaw, IN); APR-I and APR-II (Intermedics Orthopedics, Austin, TX); PCA (Howmedica, East Rutherford, NJ); AML (DePuy, Warsaw, IN); Omniflex and Omnifit (Osteonics, Allendale, NJ); S-Rom (Joint Medical Products, Stamford, CT); Mallory-Head (Biomet, Warsaw, IN) nics, Allendale, NJ), the average score was 95 at 3 years. However, composite scores obscure problem areas if the reasons for deducted points are not identified. Among the various parameters for assessing clinical results, pain is most directly influenced by the choice of implant fixation. Range of motion is not. Multiple factors, including pain, affect walking and overall function. Decreased performance in either category for reasons other than pain (eg, systemic disease, surgical approach, hip biomechanics) is not directly related to the choice of cementless fixation.

Groin or buttock pain with weightbearing or active straight leg raising is usually attributed to the acetabular component. Such pain has been reported infrequently in association with porous-coated acetabular components, with incidences ranging between 0 and 5.7%. In a comparison of 285 porous and 130 threaded acetabular components, groin and/or buttock pain correlated positively with implant fixation. Pain was present in 2.8% of cases with porous cups, all of which were radiographically stable. In contrast, 25.4% of cases with threaded cups were symptomatic and 21% were unstable. Other authors have noted surprisingly little pain in the presence of radiographic instability of cementless and cemented cups, suggesting that the acetabulum may be less sensitive to pain than the proximal femur.

Thigh and/or knee pain is generally attributed to the femoral component, and several distinct types can be distinguished. Start-up pain upon initiation of weightbearing is associated with instability of the femoral component, whether cemented or cementless. In a study comparing cemented versus cementless femoral components, thigh pain was noted in five (20%) of the cementless stems. Of these, three required revision for aseptic loosening and two others were radiographically unstable. Study results have consistently demonstrated that implant fixation is the most important determinant of clinical results.

Of particular concern is thigh pain in association with radiographically stable cementless stems. Such pain typi-

cally occurs after prolonged weightbearing and is described as a dull ache or a tired feeling. It is frequently interpreted by patients as muscle soreness. Proposed mechanisms for such pain relate to the observation that, unlike cemented stems, cementless implants may be rigidly fixed to the femur proximally and mobile distally. Relative motion between the distal, unfixed stem and the surrounding femur could result in irritation of the endosteum, producing so-called end-of-stem pain. Larger, stiffer stems, which induce larger excursions between the stem tip and the femur, accentuate this phenomenon. Observations supporting this theory are as follows: (1) Thigh pain commonly diminishes with time and frequently is accompanied by cortical thickening in the region of the stem tip. (2) When two identical stem designs with varying degrees of porous coating were compared, proximally coated stems were associated with a significantly higher incidence of thigh pain than extensively coated stems during the first 3 years postoperatively. (3) A 40% incidence of thigh pain was reported when a proximally porous-coated modular femoral component with a solid (stiff) distal stem was used. When the distal stem was made more flexible by the introduction of a longitudinal split in the coronal plane (clothespin design), only 4.7% of patients experienced thigh pain.

Stable cementless femoral components may be fixed by fibrous tissue rather than bone ingrowth. Radiographic stability of such implants has been maintained as long as 16 years postoperatively. Although the clinical results are also usually satisfactory, they are substantially less good than those obtained with bone ingrown stems. In a review of 307 cementless stems, the incidences of pain and limp were 10% and 16%, respectively, for cases with bone ingrown stems. Corresponding incidences for cases with stable-fibrous fixation were 28% and 46%.

The reported incidences of thigh pain in several series in which cementless femoral components were used are summarized in Table 4. It is important to note that some

Table 4. Thigh pain after cementless THR

Year of Study	Design*	No. of Hips	Follow-up	Incidence	Pain Designation
1987	AML	307	2 to 5 years	14%	Any thigh pain
1994	AML	166	mean 9.5 years (6 to 13 years)	12%	Mild activity-related thigh pain
1988	PCA	50	2 years	16%	Activity-related thigh pain
1993	PCA	100	5 to 7 years	15%	Activity-related thigh pain
1992	Harris-Galante	69	mean 44 months (2 to 5 years)	45%	Episodic thigh pain
				17.9%	Slight/mild thigh pain
				1.5%	Moderate pain
				1.5%	Severe pain
1994	Multilock	176	2 years	4.5%	Activity-related thigh pain
1992	HA-Omnifit	320	2 years	2.2%	Activity-related thigh pain
	HA-Omnifit	142	3 years	4.2%	Mild to moderate "limb" pain
				1.4%	Activity-related thigh pain
1994	Mallory-Head	105	2 years	2%	Mild thigh pain
				1%	Moderate thigh pain
1993	S-ROM	48	3 to 6 years	6.3%	Thigh pain, not otherwise specified

*AML (DePuy, Warsaw, IN); PCA (Howmedica, East Rutherford, NJ); Harris-Galante and Multilock (Zimmer, Warsaw, IN); HA-Omnifit (Osteonics, Allendale, NJ); Mallory-Head (Biomet, Warsaw, IN); S-Rom (Joint Medical Products, Stamford, CT)

authors record a positive response for thigh pain if any discomfort is experienced whereas others exclude slight (episodic, nonactivity related) pain. Also, the method of inquiry may influence the results. It is generally held that self-administered patient questionnaires are more valid than direct questioning by the operating surgeon.

Problems/Drawbacks of Cementless Total Hip Replacement

Stress Shielding Because implants affixed to or within bone carry part of the normal load on the bone, the bone experiences less stress, ie, is stress shielded. The physiologic response of bone, in accordance with Wolff's law, is adaptive remodeling. This manifests radiographically as bone resorption in some areas and hypertrophy in others. All intramedullary devices, including cemented and cementless prosthetic femoral hip stems, induce stress shielding. This phenomenon is more pronounced with cementless components, because of the requirement that they be canal filling without the use of low modulus cement as a grout. Hence, larger, stiffer stems are required. Plain radiographic evaluation was used in the earliest clinical studies of stress shielding. The degree of bone resorption appeared to stabilize without further progression beyond the second postoperative year. Newer techniques, which provide more accurate quantitative assessment of changes in bone density, indicate that further minor resorptive changes of the proximal femur, on the order of 1% to 2% of bone mineral content per year, may continue for 5 years or more postoperatively.

Among the factors influencing stress shielding after cementless hip replacement are the mode of implant fixation, the stem stiffness, and the level of porous coating. In a study of 411 stems with various porous coating levels and stem diameters, stress shielding was absent in or mild in 81.8%, second degree (moderate) in 14.1%, and third degree (severe) in 4.1%. Bone ingrown stems demonstrated a higher incidence and greater degree of stress shielding than either stable-fibrous or unstable stems. Moderate and severe stress shielding were 2.5 times as likely to occur in cases with bone ingrown stems as in those without. Among cases with bone ingrowth, stem stiffness was the most important determinant of stress shielding; moderate and severe stress shielding were five times more likely in stems with diameters of 13.5 mm or larger than in smaller, less stiff stems. Porous coating level was also an important determinant; extensively porous-coated stems were twice as likely to demonstrate moderate and severe stress shielding as proximally coated stems.

Although stress shielding occurs with all designs of cementless stems, reporting has been inconsistent. In two sequential studies of a proximally porous-coated anatomic design fabricated of CoCr, 66% of the first 50 cases had some loss of proximal femoral bone density at 2 years, as did 67% of the first 100 cases. The degree of stress shielding had progressed in 10% of patients at 3 years, 8% at 4 years, and 10% at 5 years. In a study of 69 proximally porous-coated titanium alloy stems, 16% demonstrated grade 3 or 4 (corresponding to moderate and severe) stress shielding at a mean follow-up of 44 months. In another study of 122 stems of the same design, loss of proximal cortical density extending slightly distal to the lesser trochanter was noted in 92% of patients. In a review of 100 40% hydroxyapatite-coated titanium stems, 30% of cases demonstrated calcar round-off and slight cortical thinning in the upper 1 cm of the femur. Twenty percent showed more pronounced thinning and osteoporosis in the upper part of the calcar (> 1 cm), which still appeared progressive at 2 years. In a preliminary study of 50 stems using dual-energy x-ray absorptiometry, loss of bone mineral content varied between 5% and 20%, with three cases (6%) showing up to 50% loss.

To date, no adverse effect on clinical results has been ascribed to stress shielding. Attempts to reduce stress shielding have been directed toward reducing stem stiffness and limiting the amount of porous coating. Stem stiffness is determined by both the modulus of elasticity and stem geometry. Titanium alloy has, as a material property, a lower modulus compared to that of cobalt-based alloys. However, much of this advantage is lost when stems with bulky, metaphyseal-filling geometries are used. Stress shielding is confined to that portion of the femur above the distal limit of the ingrowth surface. Partially coated designs limit the distal extent of stress shielding, but the degree of proximal bone loss may be substantial. Low modulus composite materials are currently under investigation. These, when combined with alterations in proximal stem geometry, may result in reduced stress shielding in the future.

Difficulty of Removal The difficulty of removing ingrown cementless components was once considered a relative contraindication to their use. Methods for the safe removal of these implants have now been developed. Successful removal with minimal bone stock damage requires careful preoperative planning, special instrumentation, and proper technique.

The removal of well-fixed cementless components may be indicated for malposition leading to recurrent dislocation or excessive leg lengthening, osteolysis, infection, or persistent pain. Mechanically stable (bone or stable-fibrous tissue ingrown) implants require interface access and division prior to their removal. For femoral components, the method of accomplishing this varies with the extent of the porous coating and the degree of femoral canal filling. For proximally coated and undersized, extensively porous-coated stems, the interface is divided with specially designed thin osteotomes or thin cutting tools on high speed pneumatic drills. A trochanteric osteotomy is recommended to improve interface access. For bone ingrown, extensively porous-coated, canal-filling stems, the stem is transected using tungsten-carbide cutting tools passed through an anterior cortical window. Following proximal interface division, the upper portion of the stem is extracted. The remaining distal stem is then cored out using specially designed hollow trephines. In a series in which these techniques were used, 70 cementless stems were successfully removed. Two minor femoral fractures were incurred. The removal of well-fixed cementless acetabular components is accomplished with a series of curved osteotomes passed in the bone-implant interface.

Heterotopic Ossification   Femoral and acetabular preparation for cementless component implantation generates a considerable volume of particulate bone. Seeding of the periarticular soft tissue with this debris was once believed to increase the risk of heterotopic ossification (HO) as compared to that with cemented arthroplasty. To date, however, both the overall incidence of HO and of clinically significant HO are similar for cemented and cementless hip replacement. Without specific prophylaxis, overall incidences of HO as high as 43% to 45% have been reported following cementless total hip replacement. Clinically significant HO (Brooker grades 3 and 4) is considerably less common, in the range of 1% to 27%, and of bridging HO, 1% to 18%.

Intraoperatively, measures to prevent HO are similar for cemented and cementless total hip replacement and include copious lavage, meticulous hemostasis, and atraumatic technique with minimal muscle retraction. The accepted methods of postoperative HO prophylaxis require special consideration when used following cementless arthroplasty. Pharmacologic prophylaxis with nonsteroidal anti-inflammatory drugs and low-dose radiation therapy inhibit not only HO formation but also bone ingrowth. Of these, low-dose radiation is preferred, as it represents the only method of prophylaxis that can be applied locally as opposed to systemically. Rectangular radiation portals can be adjusted to include only the periarticular soft tissue while excluding the interface between bone and the ingrowth surface. Single-dose therapy with an administered dose in the range of 600 to 800 cGy is most often recommended.

Wear/Osteolysis   Osteolysis from particulate wear debris has superseded issues of thigh pain, stress shielding, and difficulty of implant removal as the single most worrisome aspect of cementless total hip replacement. Regardless of particle composition (metal or polyethylene) or the mechanism of its production, debris generation and osteolysis are time dependent phenomena. Incidences of osteolytic lesions in the range of 2.8% to 9.3% have been reported at 2-year follow-up. In a study of 115 replacements with minimum follow-up of 6 years, 27.8% of patients demonstrated osteolysis and all were asymptomatic. The application of cementless technique to increasingly younger populations with long life expectancies is, therefore, of particular concern.

Space limitations dictate that only the most clinically relevant aspects of osteolysis, over which the surgeon has some control, be discussed here. Prevention begins with careful screening of potential candidates for total hip replacement. Nonarthroplasty alternatives should be con-

sidered in young, active individuals. Patients unwilling to accept certain activity limitations are poor candidates. Total hip replacement is intended to enable relatively painless performance of activities of daily living rather than a return to work or competitive sports that involve repetitive impact loading.

To date, polyethylene wear debris has been the most commonly documented cause of clinically significant osteolysis. Multiple mechanisms for the generation of polyethylene wear debris exist. The most important association is inadequate polyethylene thickness. An absolute minimum of 8 and preferably 10 mm is recommended. Polyethylene thickness is determined by the outer diameter of the acetabular component shell, the thickness of the shell, and the diameter of the inner bearing surface. Shell outer diameter is largely determined by patient anatomy. Nonetheless, the largest component consistent with preservation of the subchondral plate should be used. Stability should depend on circumferential rim contact rather than screw fixation. Excessively thick-walled shells should be avoided. Studies indicate that both linear and volumetric wear of the polyethylene liner are minimized with the use of a 28-mm femoral head. Assuming a minimum acceptable metallic shell wall thickness of approximately 3 mm, a polyethylene thickness of 8 mm cannot be achieved with a 28-mm femoral head for acetabular components smaller than 50 mm. Hence, a 26-mm or even 22-mm head is required. With regard to surgical technique, vertical orientation of the acetabular component increases peak stresses in the superolateral aspect of the polyethylene liner and is positively correlated with an increased rate of cold flow and wear.

Femoral head material is an important determinant of polyethylene wear. Titanium femoral heads have been associated with the generation of metal debris and increased abrasive wear of polyethylene and are no longer recommended. CoCr is currently the most widely used material, and recent studies confirm acceptable tolerances of sphericity and surface smoothness for most commercially available heads. Ion implantation of CoCr bearing surfaces appears to increase their surface wettability and reduce the friction at articulations with polyethylene. In simulated wear testing, nitrogen ion implantation of CoCr femoral heads resulted in a 58% reduction in polyethylene wear as compared to untreated heads. However, the in vitro service life of such treatments is limited to approximately 5 years, after which the wear properties revert to those of untreated CoCr. Hence, alumina or zirconia ceramic heads, despite being considerably more expensive (usually by a factor of two to three) may be preferred in young or active patients. Studies performed in Japan indicate that wear rates of alumina ceramic-polyethylene couples are one half to one twentieth those of metal-polyethylene couples. In simulated wear testing, zirconia ceramic femoral heads were associated with a 61% reduction in polyethylene wear as compared to CoCr heads.

Small, focal areas of osteolysis of the proximal femoral neck or acetabular margins are almost universally present in series of cases with follow-up beyond 3 years. Of greater concern are distal osteolytic lesions of the femoral shaft, which have been reported mostly in association with titanium femoral components with discrete areas of porous coating in the form of pads or patches. Such distal lesions were reported in 8% of stems of this design at mean follow-up of 54 months. They are rarely found in association with circumferentially coated femoral implants, which suggests that such coatings may serve the important barrier function of limiting the migration of wear debris. In analogous fashion, "blow hole" lesions adjacent to the central dome hole of cementless acetabular components have been noted. The possibility that vacant screw holes may serve as portals for the migration of wear debris has been discussed. Thus, femoral components should have circumferential ingrowth surfaces. Cementless acetabular components should be fixed without screws if possible, and should have a minimum number or no holes in their dome.

Recently, attention has focused on fretting and corrosion at the metal-to-metal couples of modular femoral components, particularly CoCr heads on titanium alloy trunnions. Similar findings, although less marked, have been noted in CoCr-CoCr modular head couples. The implication is that motion occurs at the head–taper junction as a result of suboptimum taper tolerances. The significance of these findings is presently uncertain. Unfortunately, such problems are likely to escape the attention of most orthopaedists unless widespread problems become clinically manifest.

Careful yearly radiographic evaluation for the presence of osteolytic lesions or wear, evidenced as femoral head eccentricity, is imperative. Treatment depends on multiple factors, including the extent and location of the lesions and patient age, health, and activity level. Small proximal femoral lesions or marginal acetabular lesions in sedentary or frail patients may be carefully observed. Large lesions, which jeopardize component fixation or pose the risk of femoral fracture, are indications for revision surgery. The discovery of component design flaws subsequent to their implantation (such as inadequate polyethylene support or fixation) is reason for more frequent radiographic evaluation.

Summary

The most widely accepted indication for primary cementless total hip replacement is end-stage arthritis in carefully selected, young, active individuals. Cementless acetabular components are also preferred in older patients with life expectancies beyond 10 years. There is currently evidence that biologic fixation can be predictably achieved in a high percentage of patients with a variety of different femoral components. No single stem design is optimum for all patients. Porous hemispheric acetabular components are preferred.

Clinical results are largely determined by the quality of implant fixation. Nonetheless, a certain number of patients continue to experience thigh pain in the presence of well-fixed components. In the majority of cases, this pain is mild and not limiting. Although it has not been associated with clinical problems, stress shielding remains a concern. The removal of well-fixed cementless components, especially extensively porous-coated stems is difficult but possible. Special instruments and techniques are required. The principle concern surrounding cementless arthroplasty is wear debris induced osteolysis. Major contributing factors are component design and bearing surface composition, as opposed to cementless fixation itself.

Annotated Bibliography

General

Callaghan JJ: Total hip arthroplasty: Clinical perspectives. *Clin Orthop* 1992;276:33–40.

The current status of total hip arthroplasty is reviewed. Specific attention is given to the choice of cementless versus cemented arthroplasty in various age groups, based on the available results using contemporary designs and techniques for each. Cementless implants are indicated in most patients younger than 65. Concerns regarding cementless implants include thigh pain and limp, intraoperative femoral fractures, and the long-term durability of the bone-implant interface.

Spector M: Historical review of porous-coated implants. *J Arthroplasty* 1987;2:163–177.

A comprehensive review of the history of biologic fixation.

The development of contemporary cementless orthopaedic implants is traced, citing important laboratory and clinical studies.

Acetabular Arthroplasty

Incavo SJ, DiFazio FA, Howe JG: Cementless hemispheric acetabular components: 2–4 year results. *J Arthroplasty* 1993;8:573–580.

Results of 106 cases using two designs of porous hemispheric acetabular components are reviewed. No component migration or screw breakage occurred in primary cases. Radiolucent lines were common, particularly in zones I and III, and occurred in 45% of cases with one design and in 60% of cases with the other. The significance of these radiolucencies is uncertain.

Keating EM, Ritter MA, Faris PM: Structures at risk from medially placed acetabular screws. *J Bone Joint Surg* 1990;72A:509–511.

In both articles, intra-pelvic structures at risk during the insertion of screws for the adjunctive fixation of cementless acetabular components were identified using cadavers or intraoperative examination. These include the internal iliac vein, the external iliac vein and artery, and the obturator nerve, artery, and vein. Their relationships to the acetabulum are described. "Safe zones" for screw insertion include the posterior-superior and posterior-inferior quadrants. Screw placement in the anterior half of the acetabulum should be avoided.

Morscher EW: Current status of acetabular fixation in primary total hip arthroplasty. *Clin Orthop* 1992;274:172–193.

The results and problems associated with various designs of cementless acetabular components are reviewed. Porous-coated components are recommended, without the use of adjunctive screw fixation if possible.

Wasielewski RC, Cooperstein LA, Kruger MP, et al: Acetabular anatomy and the transacetabular fixation of screws in total hip arthroplasty. *J Bone Joint Surg* 1990;72A:501–508.

Femoral Arthroplasty

D'Antonio JA, Capello WN, Jaffe WL: Hydroxylapatite-coated hip implants: Multicenter three-year clinical and roentgenographic results. *Clin Orthop* 1992;285:102–115.

Four hundred thirty-six HA-coated femoral components were used in combination with either HA-coated, porous, or bipolar cups. Harris hip scores averaged 96 in 142 cases with three year follow-up. Two (.46%) stems required revision for loosening. Mild to moderate limb pain was present in 4.2% of cases at 3 years. Three (1%) of HA-coated cups and none of the porous cups migrated.

Engh CA, Bobyn JD, Glassman AH: Porous-coated hip replacement: The factors governing bone ingrowth, stress shielding, and clinical results. *J Bone Joint Surg* 1987;69B: 45–55.

The factors influencing bone ingrowth, stress shielding, and clinical results are discussed. Three hundred and seven cases using porous-coated femoral components are reviewed. The most important determinant of clinical success was implant fixation, which in turn was dependent on the quality of initial implant fit. Ninety-three percent of canal-filling stems become bone ingrown versus 69% of undersized stems. Pain and limp with a press fit stem were 9% and 13%, respectively. Corresponding figures for

undersized stems were 23% and 34%. Histologic study of 11 retrieved specimens demonstrated bone ingrowth in 9.

Glassman AH, Engh CA: The removal of porous-coated femoral hip stems. *Clin Orthop* 1992;285:164–180.

Techniques for the removal of cementless femoral stems are described. Regardless of design, mechanically stable stems require interface access and division. For extensively porous-coated implants, a method involving stem transection and distal stem removal with a hollow trephine is described. Experience with 70 stem removals is presented. Minor proximal femoral fractures occurred in two.

Heekin RD, Callaghan JJ, Hopkinson WJ, et al: The porous-coated anatomic total hip prosthesis, inserted without cement: Results after five to seven years in a prospective study. *J Bone Joint Surg* 1993;75A:77–91.

Results of the first 100 cases using a single design are reviewed. Ninety-four stems demonstrated bone ingrowth, one was stable-fibrous, and five were unstable with one revision pending. Six percent of acetabular components migrated and 2% were revised. Thigh pain varied between 18% at 1 year and 16% at 7 years. Limp diminished from 28% at 2 years to 11% at 5 years, suggesting gradual recovery after the direct lateral approach.

Schwartz JT Jr, Mayer JG, Engh CA: Femoral fractures during non-cemented total hip arthroplasty. *J Bone Joint Surg* 1989;71A:1135–1142.

A 3% incidence of femoral fractures was noted among 1,318 consecutive cementless total hip replacements. Fractures were classified as proximal or distal. The mechanisms and treatment of both are described. Properly treated fractures had little impact on the outcome of the arthroplasty.

Stress Shielding

Engh CA, Bobyn JD: The influence of stem size and extent of porous coating on femoral bone resorption after primary cementless hip arthroplasty. *Clin Orthop* 1988;231:7–28.

Four hundred eleven primary total hip replacements with one design of CoCr femoral component but various levels of porous coating and stem diameter were studied. Three degrees of stress shielding were described. Second and third degree (significant) stress shielding were more likely when the stem was canal-filling and/or bone ingrown. Stem stiffness and porous coating level were the most important determinants of stress shielding; significant stress shielding was five times more likely when stems 13.5 mm in diameter or larger were used, and twice as likely for extensively coated versus proximally coated stems. Stress shielding did not progress beyond 2 years on plain radiographs.

24

Cemented Revision of Total Hip Arthroplasty

With the passage of time since the first total hip arthroplasty (THA) and the increasing numbers of hip prostheses implanted each year since, revision THA has become an increasingly frequent procedure. Because of loosening, prosthetic failure, "cement disease," "cementless disease," polyethylene wear, and other causes of primary prosthetic replacement failure, revision THA has become increasingly complex. A variety of issues confront the surgeon faced with performing a total hip revision: whether or not to use cement for fixation; what type of prosthesis to use; whether or not to use bone graft and the type of bone graft best suited to the case; and whether or not the patient can survive the surgery and/or comply with the rehabilitation necessary for recovery from the revision performed. Factors that affect the surgeon's decision-making process are the age, health, and activity level of the patient; the type of prosthesis being revised and its condition at the time of revision; the degree of bone loss; and the reason for the revision.

Results

The clinical and radiographic results of cemented revision have been well documented over the past decade and are accepted as being significantly inferior to the results of primary THA. One report on revision THA reported a 32% deep infection rate as well as a significantly higher incidence of other complications. Failure rates have ranged from 3% to 60%, with follow-up ranging from 2 to 10 years. Radiographic loosening has been reported as high as 50% with only 4.5 years of follow-up if revision was done for component loosening. Other complications include dislocation (4% to 10%), femoral shaft perforation or fracture (4% to 13%), trochanteric nonunion (6% to 8%), and infection (generally in the range of 2% to 4%).

Clinical results can be satisfactory despite the higher incidence of loosening, failure, and other complications. In one series of 145 cases, 90% of patients felt they were better or much better at final follow-up after revision. In another series of 166 patients, 77% had no or slight pain at final examination (mean 4.5 years). In this series, now updated to a mean 11-year follow-up, 50% have no or slight pain, yet 90% of patients still feel they are doing satisfactorily. Eighty-six percent of patients in a single surgeon's series had little or no pain at 7 years. Thus, although cemented revision obviously has a poorer clinical outcome than cemented primary THA, a functional result that improves the patient's condition can be obtained and maintained for a period of time. There is a wide range of outcomes following cemented revison THA that is evident with review of different series. This range is attributable to the wide variation in the state of the hip at the time of revision, the age of patient, the quality of bone, the number of previous hip arthroplasties, and the technique of revision.

In one series, patients revised for prosthetic fracture had the best results both clinically and radiographically. Patients revised for dislocation or acetabular loosening more frequently required use of a cane or other support aid for ambulation and were less able to walk long distances and climb stairs than patients revised for femoral loosening or stem fracture. The highest incidence of pain after revision was in those patients revised for acetabular loosening. Patients who underwent multiple revisions of the same hip also had poorer clinical outcomes in two different series when compared to first time revisions. Some of these diagnosis-related differences in outcomes can be attributed to the soft-tissue envelope of the hip joint. Multiple surgical procedures lead to increased scarring and loss of contractile muscle tissue, which compromise the patient's ability to climb stairs and walk. Similar scarring can lead to soft-tissue contracture with limited range of motion diminishing function. These deficits are reflected in the decreased hip scores (Harris, Mayo clinical scores) seen in revision series. In one series, the mean Mayo Hip Scores (a combined clinical and radiographic score with 100 points maximum) were 73.2 for revision for recurrent dislocation, 66.9 for acetabular loosening, 76.2 for femoral loosening, and 80.9 for femoral prosthetic fracture. These differences were not only due to differences in the clincial outcomes of the revisions but were also influenced by the radiographic results.

For revisions performed for component loosening, the incidence of probable radiographic loosening was 50% at mean 4.5 years in this same series. This high incidence of loosening following revision for loosening is related to bone quality at the time of revision. Bone loss resulting from loosening of components leads to poorer fixation of the components during the revision. In a biomechanical study done on canine bone, a cemented revision model was created. The investigators showed a decrease in the bone–cement interface shear strength with each subsequent cementing of a prosthesis in the bone (20% of primary THA with first revision, 6.8% of primary THA with second revision). These data raise the issue of whether or not a satisfactory bone–cement bond can be created at revision of a previously cemented prosthesis. The high incidence of radiographic loosening after cemented revision is noted in multiple series from the United States and abroad. Failure rates of first revisions with cement are variously reported as 9% at mean 4.5 years, 14% at mean 3.4 years and then 29% in the same patients at mean 8.1 years, 36% at 4 years, and so forth. In cases with poor bone stock at the time of revision, the results with cement are worse according to one series from New York. In another series, the chief mode of failure of the revised femoral component in loosening was bone-cement interface loosening, which illustrates the problem with cement bonding to the sclerotic bone of the revised femur.

In the case of second or third revisions, the failure rates are even higher (25% at 3.5 years for revision two and 33% at 3 years for revision three). Clinical and radiographic results were worse in the multiple revision patients, and the results varied by reason for revision as they did for first time revisions. Multiple revisions for acetabular loosening had increasingly poor outcomes and occasionally resulted in component removal without reconstruction due to lack of bone stock. Use of supplememental fixation with roof rings, allografts, and mesh were frequently necessary to allow insertion of a cemented acetabular component. In one study of 21 patients with allograft reconstruction of the acetabulum for bone deficiency in primary THA, there were two cases of progressive loosening at the bone cement interface, one nonunion, and one graft collapse by 3.5 years. However, other studies have shown graft failure at 7 to 10 years, where incorporation had been suspected at shorter follow-up. In revision cases, incorporation of the graft is less predictable, and the use of uncemented acetabular reconstructions with or without grafts has become more popular and appears to have a better success rate (see next chapter).

The use of long-stem femoral components became popular as part of an effort to gain improved fixation with cement despite proximal bone loss. Use of long-stem femoral components may improve the results of cemented revision. Two studies both confirm the decrease in progressive femoral bone–cement interface radiolucencies seen with cemented long-stem femoral revisions. The failure rate in one series was 12% with average follow-up of 6.7 years. In the other series, there was a 50% decrease in the incidence of probable radiographic loosening of the femoral component when compared to short-stem femoral revisions with cement at the same institution with similar follow-up. The re-revision rates for femoral loosening, however, were similar for short (4%) and long stems (6%). However, patients who received long-stem implants tended to have worse bone stock or femoral perforations and so may have been expected to have a poorer outcome. Nonetheless, use of a long-stem implant with cement may improve the duration of survival of the revision. In the long-term study, the authors found that the time to failure of the long-stem revision was greater than 5 years, which indicates that a minimum 5-year survival without femoral revision might be expected with a cemented long-stem femoral revision.

One problem with the above mentioned studies is that they represent the first revisions performed at the various centers and by the different authors. It is well documented that in primary hip arthroplasty the results of first generation cementing techniques have been significantly surpassed by second and third generation techniques. The use of long-stem femoral components for revision came later in the 1970s and represented an improvement on the technique of femoral revision. The improved results reflect the advance gained by knowledge of how the first short-stem revisions fared with respect to loosening over time. In addition, with revisions performed in the late 1970s and early 1980s, some of the advances in primary cement technique, such as thorough cleansing of the femoral canal, cement injection guns, pressurization of the cement, and plugging of the distal canal, came into use. One group of investigators found that use of "modern" techniques did not significantly improve the rate of failure of the cemented revision: 16% failed at a mean follow-up of 3.6 years with a re-revision rate of 8.6%. This was not significantly different from a failure rate of 14% at mean 3.4 years from the same institution with "primitive" cement techniques.

Another group of investigators, however, reported significant improvement in the results of cemented femoral revision with the use of modern cement techniques. They achieved a 2% re-revision rate for the femur, 5% for the acetabulum, and 9% femoral loosening with 6-year follow-up. With 10- to 11-year follow-up, there has been an increase in the incidence of failure as expected but it is still better than in the early studies of revision without modern technique. Reports of two other studies of revisions performed around 1980 with modern techniques have also documented improved success. In one, the 14-year survival was 85%, although the range of follow-up was 5 to 14 years and the patient population was elderly. In the other, the 5-year survival was 95%, which is similar to that seen with long-stem femoral revision, but the 10-year survival was only 77%. Progressive loosening over time leads to an increased rate of failure.

The increased rate of failure over time is especially significant in the younger, more active patient. In a study from Sweden, the results of cemented hip revision in young patients were significantly poorer, with higher rates of loosening and failure. All patients were less than 55 years of age and follow-up was 4 years. The incidence of mechanical failure was 36% with 14 of 67 patients undergoing second revision and an additional 10 patients with probable radiographic loosening. Another long-term follow-up study of revision with early cement techniques and short stems showed a significantly higher probability of failure based on revision in younger patients compared to older patients. In this study, femoral cement technique was evaluated and rated with a scoring system that rewards a complete cement mantle of at least 2 mm in thickness, a good distal cement plug (at least 2 cm), and good cancellous bone removal. There was little correlation between failure and cement technique using this rating system. However, there was a correlation between ability to achieve a good bone–cement interface without complete femoral bone–cement radiolucency and long-term survival. The majority of cases of femoral component loosening in this series occurred by bone–cement interface failure rather than by other modes of failure involving cement fracture or fatigue. Failure also correlated with poor bone stock at the time of revision. Revision efforts with modern cement technique should be directed at improving the bone–cement interface bonding. If the surgeon feels a good bone–cement interface cannot be achieved because of bone stock problems or other considerations, then other fixation methods should be considered.

It is well documented that the incidence of complications following revision surgery is increased compared to primary THA. Similarly the incidence of revision is decreased in the elderly population of THAs as a result of concern regarding the ability of the patient to undergo revision. In a study from England, 57 revision THAs were performed in patients over 80 years of age. At 2.3-year mean follow-up, 21 patients felt their outcome was excellent, 25 satisfactory, and 10 were unhappy with the result. All received a cemented Charnley prosthesis. American Society of Anesthesiology ratings were used to evaluate the patients' medical status. Class 3 patients had a 41% chance of developing a moderate or major complication compared to 20% for class 1 or 2 patients. No class 1 or 2 patients had a major complication. Three of 22 class 3 patients developed a major complication. Of the complications, there were five trochanteric nonunions, two cemented acetabular loosenings, and three recurring dislocations. Perhaps trochanteric osteotomy should be avoided in this age group. Nonetheless, with proper patient selection octagenarians can undergo successful revision.

Complications

Complications of revision are increased compared to primary THA. However, the complications are not necessarily related to the method of revision, cemented or uncemented, but rather to the revision itself. In one study, uncemented femoral revisions were compared to cemented femoral revisions. There was not a significant difference in the incidence of complications in the two groups with the exception of intraoperative fracture of the proximal femur, which was more common due to the aggressive rasping and seating of the press-fit prosthesis. Prophylactic cerclage fixation of the weak proximal femur may help reduce this risk.

Dislocation after revision is increased (6% to 10% for revision, 2% to 4% for primary). The incidence of dislocation after revision was higher if the revision was performed for recurrent dislocation. In one study seven of 35 hips revised for recurrent dislocation dislocated again; five of these seven patients experienced recurrent dislocation (three or more episodes) and four were revised a second time. In another study, 12 of 45 patients dislocated after their second revision (seven with three or more episodes). Multiple revisions for dislocation were successful in eliminating instability in only two of eight cases.

The incidence of medical complications was not increased in one series of revisions when compared to the same patients after their primary THA. Heterotopic bone formation has been seen more frequently after revision (absent 35%, mild 48%, moderate 12%, severe 5% in one series). If significant heterotopic bone is removed at the time of revision, then consideration should be given to prophylactic irradiation of the hip. Trochanteric nonunion is more common in revision, ranging from 5% to 15%. A variety of new devices are available for better fixation of the trochanter; however, the bone stock is poorer at revision, and this compromises healing. A multiple wire technique appears to provide the best results. Others have tried a long osteotomy starting well distal to the trochanter on the lateral cortex of the femur. This osteotomy creates a window laterally that can be used to facilitate cement removal.

Femoral shaft fracture is more common with revision than with cemented primary THA, as might be expected. Frequently, the femoral cortex is perforated while removing cement. This perforation may predispose the patient to postoperative fracture and was a cause of postoperative fracture of the femur in two series. Bone grafting any perforations and bypassing them with the stem, if possible, should reduce the risk of fracture. Deep infection is also more common after revision, with infection rates in the range of 1% to 3% most common (some series have even higher rates). Superficial infection is also increased, and wound healing problems have been reported between adjacent incisions. If a previous incision is close to the intended new incision (less than two inches) and is less than 3 years old, it is probably better to use the old incision and perhaps lengthen it to gain the exposure desired. A midline lateral incision over the distal one half of a posterior incision (Southern exposure) has been used, which deviates from the old incision as proximal on the greater trochanter as possible, without encountering wound healing problems. However, caution should be used in changing incisions.

Technical Considerations

A variety of techniques exist for the surgical approach to the hip for THA. For revision in general, a wider exposure is needed and extra dissection and time are required to gain satisfactory exposure to the acetabulum and femur for component removal and bone grafting or insertion of supplemental fixation as required. Many surgeons prefer to use a transtrochanteric approach to the hip for revision. This gives excellent exposure but adds a risk of trochanteric nonunion, which may lead to weakness, instability, and/or reoperation. Of 18 reoperations other than revision in one series of 166 revisions, 11 were for trochanteric problems—nonunion or wire breakage and pain. In that same series, trochanteric nonunion was noted radiographically in 20 of 153 cases with trochanteric osteotomy (13.1%). In some cases in which limited work will be needed on the hip and exposure is relatively simple (small patient with minimal scarring), a posterolateral or antero-lateral approach may be sufficient for revision. However, for most surgeons and most cases a more extensive approach is required.

The Hardinge or direct lateral approach has been effective in allowing excellent access to the hip and avoiding the problems of trochanteric osteotomy. The anterior half of the approach may be all that is needed in many cases, leaving the posterior portion of the abductor tendon and vastus muscles intact on the femur and reflecting only the anterior half from the femur. The capsule can then be excised if still remaining or the capsular scar tissue can be "carved" off the underside of the tendon and muscle to gain mobility and exposure of the acetabulum and femur. It is important to free up the femur so that it can be elevated from the depth of the wound for access in removing cement from the canal and to gain in visibility of both the acetabulum and the femoral canal. This can be done by removing the capsule or scar tissue from the back of the proximal femoral neck and intertrochanteric region. If this additional dissection does not give adequate exposure to the femur or acetabulum, then the posterior sleeve of the abductor and vastus can be removed from the femur, thereby skeletonizing the proximal aspect of the femur. This procedure gives additional exposure, which should allow extensive acetabular and femoral reconstruction. Closure should be accomplished by suturing the anterior and posterior sleeves to the femur through drill holes placed at regular intervals along the length of the dissection. In the area where the abductor tendon merges with the vastus, there is a relatively thin layer of tissue that will not hold adequately by itself. Several heavy sutures should be directed superiorly to this area to anchor the abductors to the proximal femur. The repair can be reinforced by sewing the anterior and posterior sleeves of muscle and tendon to each other. A nonabsorbable number 5 suture works well for the repair to the bone. Release of the iliopsoas tendon can be done, if necessary, in continuity with the anterior sleeve, which allows reattachment of the hip flexor with the muscle closure after the reconstruction has been completed. This approach has obviated the need for trochanteric osteotomy in many hands.

Cement can be removed in a variety of ways. New methods include the use of ultrasonic chisels to remove the cement in pieces. One technique involves cleansing of the existing cement mantle after femoral component removal and the insertion of new cement with a threaded rod in the center. A slap hammer is attached to the threaded rod and the cement (new and old bonded together) is removed in 1-cm segments. These new techniques have had successes and failures as have the old techniques of femoral cement removal with osteotomes and high speed drills. Cannulated Gray drills and reamers can be used effectively to remove femoral cement with considerably less expense than the first two techniques mentioned. The surgeon must be careful not to leave any cement in the femoral canal. This can be checked with radiographs or with a reverse

hook type osteotome scraped from distal to proximal in the femoral canal. Retained "cementophytes" can deflect rasps and reamers and cause perforation of the femoral shaft. For the acetabulum there has been little change in the technique of cement removal. Large curved osteotomes can be passed around metal-backed components, working around the dome until the prosthesis is loose. It is helpful to use two osteotomes at once from anterior and posterior, working each one farther in a little bit at a time. Consideration may need to be given to retroperitoneal exposure of cement lying inside the pelvis.

The most important consideration in the longevity of the cemented revision is the quality of the bone–cement interface bond achieved at revision. It is difficult to obtain a "white-out" at the bone–cement interface if the cancellous endosteal bone of the femur has been lost due to loosening of a previous cement mantle. The same is true of a loose press fit prosthesis, which has developed an envelope of sclerotic bone around the stem. This "plate" of sclerotic bone must be broken down through reaming or rasping prior to cementing the new component. The sclerotic bone characteristic of most revision femurs is difficult to prepare for cementing. An attempt should be made to roughen the bone using high speed drills or burrs or sharp curettes. Special effort must be made to dry the canal prior to introducing cement (use of 1:250,000 dilute epinephrine solution may help). There must be a good distal plug in the canal to achieve adequate pressurization. A bony sling at the tip of the previous prosthesis may suffice, but often these are too proximal for the new prosthesis or do not completely occlude the canal. A large Silastic plug often works the best and should be used even if a long or mid-length stem is inserted. Distal to the isthmus, a cement plug should be considered. Any perforations in the femur should be plugged prior to cementing. A cement gun and a proximal seal will help in increasing injection pressure. Cement that is early or very liquid, although good for primary cemented THA, may not be best for revision. It may be advantageous to take the cement a little later for revision to allow good pressurization in a dry canal. On the acetabular side, if cement is to be used the bony surface should be dry. Multiple 3.2-mm drill holes will give better cement fixation in sclerotic as well as normal bone as shown in studies for primary THA in the early 1970s. Defects through the inner table of the acetabular wall should be covered with thin bone grafts or with cancellous chips packed into the holes. An acetabular component with an overhanging rim can help in pressurization of the cement.

Frequently, more extensive bone grafting is required to repair areas of bone loss. A variety of techniques exist for this. A recent study has found that cemented revision without bone grafting but with second-generation cement techniques was successful in 29 cases with focal femoral osteolysis with 86% of components well fixed at an average of 8.5 years and only 2 of 29 cases with recurrence of osteolysis. The use of morcellized bone grafts packed into femoral defects with cementation of a new polished stem on top of the grafts has become popular. Bone healing has been demonstrated at 3 to 5 years with maintenance of stable fixation of the femoral component. Similar techniques have been tried on the acetabulum. Morcellized grafts are reamed into the defects with acetabular reamers on reverse and covered with vitallium mesh; the new component is cemented onto the construct. Results with this technique have been variable, with some long-term success that is mostly on an anecdotal basis. Current trends would favor use of an uncemented cup in this situation. Bipolar components placed into an acetabular bed with defects filled with morcellized bone grafts have likewise had variable success. Failure rates of 20% at 2 to 5 years are reported. However, cases that were done using this technique usually had extensive bony defects and were not considered candidates for reconstruction with an uncemented cup in the mid 1980s. One important finding of the follow-up studies on the bipolar was that the component must have solid rim fixation around the acetabular margins or it will migrate through the morcellized grafts. Revision to a fixed acetabular component may be necessary in the future, but at the time of re-revision the grafts were generally well incorporated and the second revision was fairly straightforward. Failure of a fixed porous acetabular component in the same setting had a higher incidence of graft failure as well, necessitating more grafting at second revision.

For more significant defects, allografts may be required both on the acetabular and femoral sides. For major allograft reconstruction of the femur with the prosthesis in the allograft fixed to the distal femur, cement is usually used to fix the prosthesis in the allograft. A long step cut may be used to fix the allograft to the host distal femur if the proximal host femur has been removed. It is easier to place the allograft into the shell of the host femur and crush the host femur around the allograft with cables. Satisfactory fixation can usually be obtained with this method. Frequently, strut grafts can be used to reinforce the host femur if there are thin or perforated areas around or near the tip of the new cemented femoral component. It is generally recognized that femoral cortical defects should be bypassed by the stem. A biomechanical study has recommended bypassing the defects by two bone diameters. Use of additional bone graft to the defect or a strut over the defect is advisable.

The prosthesis to be used should be selected according to the needs of the case. Because the data with long-stem revisions seem to show better results, it may be preferable to use a mid-length stem (8 in) if cementing the revision of a short-stem prosthesis. This will usually bypass the previous cement plug and most areas of lysis. If the femur is perforated, a long stem (10 in) may be necessary, depending on the location of the defect in the cortex. If a long stem is to be used, it will likely need to be curved to get around the bow of the femur. Usually, this is not a problem with the mid-length stem. In revision situations it is better to have greater femoral head offset to laterally displace the femur so as to prevent impingement and dislocation in adduction. This is due to the gradual mediali-

zation of the socket caused by loosening and revision. A medially built up acetabular component that laterally displaces the center of rotation of the hip is advantageous in this situation.

The rehabilitation necessary after revision depends on the patient's preoperative condition both medically and physically and on the nature of the revision performed. If cement is used with minimal bone grafting, then weight-bearing as tolerated can be begun using a walker or crutches initially and shifting to a cane. If the Hardinge approach has been used, minimal protection is necessary unless the repair was tenuous. For reconstructions with bone grafting for the acetabulum or for femoral perforations, the patient should continue protected weightbearing for 6 to 12 weeks, depending on the stability of the reconstruction and the healing. For major allograft reconstructions, prolonged protected weightbearing is recommended, with adjustments based on radiographic union of the graft to host bone.

Muscle rehabilitation can begin isometrically in the immediate postoperative period. However, progressive resistive exercises for the abductors should be delayed for 6 weeks to allow healing of the muscle repair. Use of underwater treadmills or pool exercises can be very helpful in the revision setting to rehabilitate the patient. The patient must be told to expect a prolonged period of rehabilitation in order to regain good strength and function, especially in the multiply revised hip.

Conclusion

Blanket statements regarding revision THA cannot be made because so many variables influence the results. Based on studies of cemented revision with long-stem femoral components and with modern cement techniques, a satisfactory 10-year result can be expected in most cases. For patients who are over 75 to 80 years of age at the time of revision, this may be the last revision the patient will require. Similarly, this revision may outlive the patient with a limited life expectancy. When an uncemented femoral revision is attempted but stable fixation cannot be achieved at surgery, cemented revision with a mid-length stem or perhaps impaction bone grafting (Ling technique) may be indicated. Based on the literature, a cemented mid- or long-stem prosthesis should give more predictable fixation with longer survival than a cemented short-stem prosthesis. On the acetabular side, the trend has been toward uncemented fixation with or without bone grafts as needed for revision. This trend is especially good for cases of hip dysplasia or loss of acetabular bone stock due to loosening or other causes that have a higher rate of failure of cemented revision. In revision, effort should be made to improve the bone stock for the future, especially in the young patient. For this reason, uncemented reconstruction of the acetabulum and femur with bone grafting where needed is preferable. An effort should be made to lateralize the femur to improve the abductor lever arm and decrease impingement of the femur against the acetabulum (reducing the risk of dislocation). One way to do this is with an uncemented, lateralized acetabular prosthesis with a thicker medial wall.

The surgeon performing revision total hip arthroplasty should be able to widely expose the hip, remove the components without doing excessive damage to the bone (although this risk exists in the best of hands), reconstruct the hip with allografts and bone grafts, with cement or without cement, and successfully rehabilitate the patient after the surgery. Careful follow-up is required at regular intervals after revision as for primary THA (4 to 6 weeks, 3 months, 6 months, 1 year, 2 years, then every 2 years thereafter). Patients' expectations should be downgraded as the results of revision are not the same as the results of primary THA.

Annotated Bibliography

Allan DG, Lavoie GJ, McDonald S, et al: Proximal femoral allografts in revision hip arthroplasty. *J Bone Joint Surg* 1991;73B:235–240.

Seventy-eight proximal femoral allograft revisions with use of large proximal femoral allografts and cortical struts were successful in 85% at 36 months. Small calcar grafts were more frequently resorbed (50%) although 81% were felt to be successful.

Callaghan JJ, Salvati EA, Pellicci PM, et al: Results of revision for mechanical failure after cemented total hip replacement, 1979–1982: A two to five year follow-up. *J Bone Joint Surg* 1985;67A:1074–1085.

Review of revisions performed with "modern" cement techniques showed a mechanical failure rate of 16% at 3.6 years (mean follow-up) and a re-revision rate of 8.6%.

Estok DM II, Harris WH: Long-term results of cemented femoral revision surgery using second-generation techniques: An average 11.7-year follow-up evaluation. *Clin Orthop* 1994;299:190–202.

Thirty-eight cemented femoral revisions performed with second generation technique were reviewed at a minimum ten years of follow-up. 10.5% of hips were revised and an additional 10.5% were radiographically loose.

Izquierdo RJ, Northmore-Ball MD: Long-term results of revision hip arthroplasty: Survival analysis with special reference to the femoral component. *J Bone Joint Surg* 1994;76B:34–39.

One hundred forty-eight cemented and cementless revisions at a mean age of 67 had 95% 10-year survival to re-revision. Some patients were revised for sepsis. Radiologic survival was 90.5% at 10 years.

Jasty M, Harris WH: Salvage total hip reconstruction in patients with major acetabular bone deficiency using structural femoral head allografts. *J Bone Joint Surg* 1990;72B:63–67.

Thirty-eight revisions with major acetabular allografts and cemented cups were reviewed at 4 years with 0% failure and at 6 years with 32% failure. Twelve components became loose with six requiring re-revision. All allografts united but evidence of some bone resorption was present in 23 of 38 hips.

Kavanagh BF, Ilstrup DM, Fitzgerald RH Jr: Revision total hip arthroplasty. *J Bone Joint Surg* 1985;67A:517–526.

One hundred sixty-six cemented revisions followed a mean of 4.5 years had 50% radiographic loosening if revised for loosening. There was re-revision for symptomatic loosening in 8 of 210 hips in the series and re-revision for other reasons in 7 of 210 hips. Patient satisfaction was good in 90%. Mean age at revision was 61.8 years.

Kavanagh BF, Fitzgerald RH Jr: Multiple revisions for failed total hip arthroplasty not associated with infection. *J Bone Joint Surg* 1987;69A:1144–1149.

Forty-five patients with two revisions and seven patients with three revisions were followed a mean of 3.5 years after the second revision and 3 years after the third. Eight of 45 acetabular components and 13 of 45 femoral components were loose after second revision. Eleven of 45 were considered mechanical failure after the second revision and two of seven after the third.

Kershaw CJ, Adkins RM, Dodd CA, et al: Revision total hip arthroplasty for aseptic failure: A review of 276 cases. *J Bone Joint Surg* 1991;73B:564–568.

Between 1977 and 1986, 276 cemented revisions were done with "modern" technique: 12 re-revisions for loosening, two for sepsis, four for other causes. Five-year survival was 95%; 10-year survival was 77%. Results were improved compared to early or "primitive" techniques.

Marti RK, Schuller HM, Besselaar PP, et al: Results of revision of hip arthroplasty with cement: A five to fourteen-year follow-up study. *J Bone Joint Surg* 1990;72A:346–354.

Survival at 14 years in a group of 60 cemented revision total hip arthroplasties was 85%. With 5 to 14 years follow-up, 4 of 60 were re-revised for loosening and 11 were loose radiographically.

Murray WR: Acetabular salvage in revision total hip arthroplasty using the bipolar prosthesis. *Clin Orthop* 1990;251:92–99.

At average follow-up of 2.9 years, 29 of 106 bipolar revisions had failures, although 14 of these were successfully reconstructed with a cementless fixed acetabulum.

Pellicci PM, Wilson PD Jr, Sledge CB, et al: Long-term results of revision total hip replacement: A follow-up report. *J Bone Joint Surg* 1985;67A:513–516.

Previously reported follow-up was lengthened to 8 years. Failure rate increased from 14% at 3 years to 29% at 8 years. Most new failures related to progressive loosening of hips with radiolucencies at initial follow-up interval.

Pierson JI, Harris WH: Cemented revision for femoral osteolysis in cemented arthroplasties: Results in 29 hips after a mean 8.5-year follow-up. *J Bone Joint Surg* 1994;76B:40–44.

Twenty-nine cemented revisions with osteolysis prerevision

were followed an average of 8.5 years. Osteolysis had recurred in two cases (6.9%) and 85% of components remained well fixed. There was 10% femoral re-revision.

Raut VV, Wroblewski BM, Siney PD: Revision hip arthroplasty: Can the octogenarian take it? *J Arthroplasty* 1993;8:401–403.

Fifty-seven revision hip arthroplasties in patients over the age of 80 were followed a mean of 2.3 years. For patients in good health (American Society of Anesthesiologists class 1 or 2), there was a 20% risk of developing a major or moderate complication. Class 3 patients had a 41% risk of complications. Mortality of 1.8% and 82.5% successful results were reported.

25

Cementless Revision Total Hip Arthroplasty

Introduction

Revision of the failed total hip arthroplasty is becoming an increasingly more common procedure for the total joint surgeon; an incidence as high as 30% of total joint replacements has been reported. Revision arthroplasty is increasing in frequency and complexity because more people are outliving the "life expectancy" of the prostheses and because more young, very active people are undergoing total hip replacements so they can remain active and productive members of society.

Results of early and long term revision with cemented prostheses have been very discouraging. At 2 to 5 years, re-revision rates are 4% to 9% and loosening rates are 12% to 29%. The long-term results have continued to be less than encouraging. A re-revision rate of 19% and a loosening rate of 29% were reported at an average follow-up of 8.1 years, and acetabular failure rates of 53% and a femoral failure rate of 24.2% were reported at a minimum 10 year follow-up. When "modern cementing" technique was used the combined mechanical and radiographic failure rate was 20% at 10-year follow-up. The continuing barrage of disappointing cemented revision results has continued to increase interest in cementless revision techniques. This chapter presents an overview of this broad and still controversial area.

Preoperative Evaluation

The initial and probably most important clinical finding to the patient is pain. The first step in the evaluation of this pain is to ensure that it is intrinsic to the hip joint and not related to some other pathology, such as disk herniation, spinal stenosis, vascular problems, and so forth. The pain that typically has been described as associated with component loosening is the so-called start-up pain that occurs suddenly with the initiation of activity. It can occur in the groin, thigh, or both. The advent of cementless prostheses has blurred the diagnostic usefulness of activity-related thigh pain in the initial postoperative period (up to 2 years) because up to 40% of patients can have this pain with a stable prosthesis and, on occasion, may require revision of a bony ingrown prosthesis as a result of intractable thigh pain. A painful prosthesis may also result from infection; this pain is described as occurring more at rest and at night. However, there may be great overlap in the patient's symptoms, particularly if the prosthesis is loose and infected. Therefore, clinical symptoms can lead to a degree of suspicion regarding the reason for pain, but cannot give a definitive answer.

The laboratory results of a white blood cell (WBC) count and differential WBC count have not proven useful in ruling out infection during evaluation of the painful hip. The erythrocyte sedimentation rate has been felt to provide information regarding possible infection, particularly if it is persistently elevated or increasing, and the C-reactive protein level may be more sensitive, especially if it exceeds 20 mg/l.

The features to look for in radiographic evaluation of the painful prosthesis include loosening, possible infection, and lysis without loosening. Loosening is best determined with the use of sequential radiographs. The classic signs of loosening of a cemented prosthesis have been migration and circumferential radiolucencies of 2 mm or more. A recent suggestion that radiolucent lines are not as important as once thought emphasizes the importance of evaluating migration. Migration of the femoral prosthesis in the cement mantle is a definite sign of femoral loosening. On the acetabular side, a radiolucent line in two zones is suggestive of probable loosening, whereas a line in all three zones is consistent with component loosening in 94% of cases. A scoring system has been developed for assessing the stability of cementless prostheses. This system is based on the presence or absence of reactive lines adjacent to the porous surface, the presence of spot welds, pedestal formation, calcar hypertrophy/atrophy, implant migration, interface deterioration, and particle shedding. The components are classified as ingrown, stable fibrous, or unstable based on these criteria.

Plain radiographs can also be useful in the evaluation of a possible infected prosthesis. Signs suggestive of infection include rapid, early development of continuous radiolucencies greater than 2 mm, endosteal scalloping, periosteal lamination, focal lysis, and extensive nonfocal lysis.

Possibly the most important feature to look for is osteolysis with or without component loosening. Lytic lesions can lead to secondary component failure, interface deterioration, fractures about the prosthesis, and catastrophic bone loss, which requires allograft reconstruction. Thus, annual radiographic follow-up of all total joint replacement patients is mandatory to try and prevent catastrophic failures.

The use of isotope scans in the diagnosis of loose or infected prostheses has met with mixed results. The technetium Tc 99m polyphosphonate bone scan probably has no place in the diagnosis of infection of total hip replacements. It did not provide additional information with regard to loosening and serial radiographs were more effective in detecting loosening. Bone scanning was felt to be useful only when radiographs are inconclusive. The use of gallium scans or indium labeled WBC scans may be more efficacious in diagnosing infection. A report of 40 possible infected prostheses showed 18 confirmed positive scans and only two false-positive results.

The most important test in the diagnosis of infection is the culture of an organism from the joint. This test has led to the routine aspiration of all hips by many. However, it has been reported that the chance of a positive result is quite low on routine aspiration, and a high false-negative result has been reported in many series. Aspiration should be reserved for clinically or radiographically suspicious cases. A recent review noted there was an improvement in the sensitivity and specificity when fine needle aspiration was combined with radiometric culture.

The most important intraoperative measure has been shown to be the cell count of the fluid present in the hip joint; a cell count greater than 25,000 is diagnostic. The second important test is the pathologic examination of tissue obtained from the hip joint. Although it has been shown not to be foolproof, a cell count of greater than 10 polymorphonuclear leukocytes per high power field is presumptive of an acute inflammatory process and infection. The most accurate indication of infection continues to be the cultures obtained at the time of revision. The best policy is to combine all modalities available, use clinical judgment, and, if necessary, await the final culture results prior to implanting the revision prosthesis.

Preoperative Planning

Preoperative templating and planning are second in importance only to the technical aspects of the reconstruction itself. In this stage, decisions are made regarding the degree of acetabular and femoral bone loss, and reconstructive options are planned. This step ensures that all required prostheses, grafts, and instruments will be available in the operating room and that no unnecessary surprises will occur.

The most important aspect of preoperative planning is the closest possible determination of the exact patterns of bone loss that will be found intraoperatively. Numerous attempts have been made to classify acetabular and femoral bone loss in order to standardize reporting protocols and to assist the surgeon in planning the reconstruction. The American Academy of Orthopaedic Surgeons acetabular classification system is essentially divided into segmental and cavitary defects and whether they are located centrally or peripherally. These defects can occur singularly or in combination, and they can be combined with problems of pelvic discontinuity and arthrodesis. The femoral classification is similar, with segmental, cavitary, and combined defects and their location on the femoral shaft, but it also has classifications of malalignment, femoral canal stenosis, and femoral discontinuity. The two classification systems are descriptive, but are cumbersome to incorporate into a treatment plan.

A classification system based on readily available plain radiographs has been developed for the femur and the acetabulum. It is based on clinically recurring patterns of bone loss and the technique that will be required to reconstruct the hip, based on the amount of host bone available for component fixation and long-term stability. This classification requires no special and expensive studies. Acetabular defects are broken down to three main groups. The type I defect has only minor cavitary defects and a supportive rim. The three type II defects have varying degrees of medial and superior bone loss, but continue to have a supportive rim. The two type III defects have severe acetabular bone stock loss, which requires an allograft to partially support the cup in type IIIA and to totally support the cup in type IIIB. The advantage of this system is that objective criteria, which are based on the degree of superior migration, the amount of ischial lysis, the degree of medial tear drop lysis, and the integrity of Kohler's line, have been developed to give an extremely accurate assessment of bone loss and intraoperative reconstructive options. The femoral classification is based on the degree of bone loss in the metaphysis and the diaphysis and the ability of the diaphysis and/or metaphysis to support a prosthesis. The type I defect has an intact and supportive metaphysis and diaphysis. The type II defects have a nonsupportive metaphysis, but an intact and supportive diaphysis. The type III defect involves the diaphysis and isthmus but still allows for distal diaphyseal support in most cases.

The use of more expensive methods to evaluate the remaining host bone stock has also been reported. This methodology usually involves a computed tomography (CT) scan and some type of computed reconstruction. These methods give excellent assessment of the acetabular bone stock in particular, but are quite costly and time consuming, and they may not be required if good quality plain radiographs are assessed adequately and systematically.

The next step in preoperative planning is the selection of the revision implants and the possible bone graft that may be required. This is the most controversial area in cementless hip replacement, whether revision or primary. The bone grafts will be discussed in more detail later in the chapter, but the basic choices are no graft, cancellous graft, structural support grafts, and total acetabular replacement grafts.

The femoral prostheses can be divided into two main groups, distal fixation prostheses and proximally stabilized prostheses. The prostheses that rely on distal fixation and stability consist of a straight stemmed component with varying degrees of coating available. The proponents of this design generally suggest using the more extensively coated prosthesis in the revision setting. These stem designs are generally made of a cobalt-chromium alloy, which has the theoretical disadvantage of being stiffer and allowing more stress shielding.

The proximally coated devices are generally of a curved or anatomic proximal design and rely on proximal support for fixation. Some proximally fixed devices have a straight contour and also incorporate various sleeves or flutes for distal rotational stability. These prostheses are generally manufactured from a titanium alloy that has the theoretical advantages of improved bone ingrowth, decreased stiffness, and subsequent improved proximal load transfer. This alloy has the disadvantages of being very notch sensitive, thus limiting the extent of coating possible, and being very wear sensitive, which virtually eliminates it as a bearing surface in total hip replacements.

The modularity of some revision prostheses has been increased in recent years; this allows "customization" of the prosthesis intraoperatively. Modular implants must be approached with caution. It has been shown that fretting and corrosion occur at all modular interfaces, whether the modules are made of similar or dissimilar metals. Thus, there is a potential for increased debris formation with the increase in modularity. The tissue response to cobalt-chromium and titanium alloy particles has been examined. In general, the cobalt-chromium particles demonstrated a toxic effect to the periprosthetic tissue. The titanium particles demonstrated an increased inflammatory response, with increased release of prostaglandin E2, interleukin-I, and other inflammatory mediators implicated in osteolysis.

The acetabular component used in revisions is less controversial; most have a hemispherical design and titanium alloy construction. The main differences occur in the type of secondary fixation present in the cup design, ie, peripheral screws, dome screws, and anti-rotation pegs. Adequate polyethylene thickness and good tolerance with the metal shell must be ensured. Other problems are the possible access to the prosthesis–bone interface of poly wear debris through the remaining empty screw holes and possible fretting and debris generation by dome screws.

Surgical Technique

The technical success of revision total hip arthroplasty depends greatly on adequate exposure of the femur and acetabulum. The generally advocated basic approaches are posterior, transtrochanteric, and anterolateral. The posterior approach is probably the most popular among revision hip surgeons. The trochanteric osteotomy can be added to this approach to improve acetabular and femoral exposure. However, there is an increase in dislocation rate with this approach compared with the anterolateral approaches. Some feel the anterolateral approaches have better acetabular exposure with the combined benefit of a lower dislocation rate. Others feel there is an increased risk of heterotopic ossification and abductor muscle weakness with this approach. No difference in the muscle strength between the direct lateral approach and the transtrochanteric approach was found after 2 years. Good muscle function was reported after a modified translateral approach, and the use of an extensive anterolateral approach has been reported.

The use of the trochanteric osteotomy has fallen somewhat into disfavor recently because of high reported complication rates, including trochanteric nonunion and migration, trochanteric bursitis, and debris generation from fixation wires. There have been two recent advances in the technique to decrease the complications. An extended trochanteric osteotomy with union of all osteotomies and no significant complications has been reported, and an extended proximal femoral osteotomy that extends through one third the circumference of the femur has been described. The osteotomy can be carried down as far as 20 to 22 cm distal to the tip of the greater trochanter. All these osteotomies healed with no significant complications. These two techniques greatly improve femoral canal access, and are fixed with cerclage wire or cable fixation in the shaft of the femur, thus avoiding the complications encountered in trochanteric osteotomy fixation.

Many techniques have been described for removing well-bonded cement or well-fixed cementless prostheses. The availability of the implant specific or universal femoral and acetabular extraction devices is imperative and can save much time and frustration. Many types of cement and cementless osteotomes are available to break down the bone cement and bone implant interfaces prior to extraction of the prosthesis. The availability of a high speed burr is also useful in interface dissection. The high speed burrs, combined with fluoroscopy, have also been advocated in cement removal, but this method has a relatively high perforation rate and distal canal access is still necessary for optimum cement removal. Cortical windows have been advocated to improve distal access, but their use requires that a longer prosthesis be inserted to bypass the created defect. A technique of segmental cement extraction has been described in which new polymethylmethacrylate is used to bond to the old cement and remove it in 1.5- to 2.5-cm segments. Low complication rates were reported for the use of ultrasonically driven tools in the removal of femoral bone cement. Another technique is to use the extended proximal femoral osteotomy to allow direct exposure to the distal cement mantle and plug so that the plug can be drilled under direct vision and the cement sequentially removed with cement taps.

A technique for removal of well-fixed cementless prostheses has been reported, which involves creation of an anterior cortical window with sectioning of the stem followed by trephining of the distal extent of the stem for removal. A cortical window technique for the removal of a well-fixed precoated cemented stem has also been described, as well as a modified cementless stem removal technique that employs the extended proximal femoral osteotomy combined with the technique of stem sectioning and then trephining out the distal portion of the stem.

Removal of a well-fixed acetabulum can be difficult, time consuming, and potentially destructive to acetabular bone stock if great care is not used in the extraction. It is important to perform a circumferential exposure of the acetabular component to allow removal. The high speed burr is again useful in starting the interface dissection. A series of curved osteotomes have been developed that allow dissection around the cup. An alternative involves the use of osteotomes or a burr to section the polyethylene cup or the metal shell of a cementless prosthesis; the cup is then removed in pieces, thereby preserving acetabular bone stock. The use of a pneumatic compression wrench has been described, which repetitively torques the prosthesis and creates sheer forces at the cement–bone or implant–bone interfaces. Universal clamps and extractors are available to grasp the cups or to screw into the polyethylene to aid in acetabular component removal. Patience is required, and no attempt should be made to "force" a component out until the entire interface is freed or a large portion of the acetabulum may be removed with the prosthesis.

Acetabular Reconstruction

Acetabular reconstruction can be technically demanding if there is osteolytic bone loss secondary to polyethylene wear debris and/or if the patient did not have symptoms until there were large defects. Continued annual follow-up for the life of the total hip replacement patient will minimize these problems.

Most acetabulae to be reconstructed have cavitary defects that are associated with a supportive acetabular rim and sufficient host bone available to ensure bony ingrowth or at least stable fibrous fixation of a noncemented acetabular prosthesis. Cancellous nonsupportive autograft, or more commonly allograft, can be used to fill these defects, with excellent long-term results.

Results of the use of a fiber metal-backed noncemented acetabular component in revision were recently reviewed. Evaluation of 129 of 138 consecutive revisions treated with a Harris-Galante (Zimmer, Warsaw, IN) acetabular prosthesis and nonstructural grafting to cavitary defects indicated that, at an average follow-up of 44 months, all of the grafts had united and no components had failed. Four patients required re-revision of the acetabulum due to infection or postoperative instability.

In a review of 316 acetabular revisions with an average follow-up of 5.1 years, 247 patients had been treated with a porous-coated hemispheric acetabular component and peripheral screw augmentation with only cancellous allograft to treat cavitary defects. The acetabular rim was intact and supportive in all cases; there were no failures and no re-revisions secondary to loosening in this series. Good results have been reported for noncemented acetabular components and nonstructural grafting techniques in other series.

The controversy in cementless acetabular revision begins when the acetabular rim is deficient and no longer able to support a prosthesis in its anatomic position without a support allograft, a change in prosthesis type, or placing the head center superiorly. Initial results for the use of femoral head allografts to treat acetabular bone stock showed no failures at 4.5 years follow-up. However, by 10 years follow-up 47% of the acetabular components were loose. In this series, no difference was found between femoral head grafts just bolted to the side of the ilium and those that were contained within the acetabulum. The use of allografts is thus advocated only in cases where girdlestone arthroplasty is the alternative. Early results were good for 54 hips that were placed with a "high hip center;" ie, the mean head center was placed 32 mm superior to the mean anatomic hip center. The theoretical biomechanical disadvantages are overcome by the lack of lateral displacement of the hip center. However, an increased risk of dislocation may require excision of the anterior inferior iliac spine, a portion of the anterior column, and a part of the ischium. The trochanter will require advancement to restore abductor tension, and a long head-neck segment or a calcar-replacing prosthesis will be required to allow appropriate leg length and prevent excessive shortening.

The use of bipolar prostheses with acetabular bone grafts has not met with many good results. In a review of 81 hips with a mean follow-up of 16 months, the majority showed migration that worsened with time. The clinical results were better than the radiographic results. When bipolar cups and morselized bone grafts were used, 11 of 18 hips had an unsatisfactory result at 35 months after surgery, with 55% of these showing complete resorption of the graft at an average of 24 months. Bipolar components and acetabular grafts cannot be routinely recommended for use at this time.

There have been reports of improved results with grafts other than femoral heads. Solid acetabular grafts, 18 of which were fresh frozen allografts, were used in 38 hips, with an average follow-up of 9.5 years. In five of the acetabulae that required re-revision, the allograft was solidly incorporated radiographically, and this was confirmed at the time of surgery. When shelf acetabular grafts in which male femoral heads were used as graft material were placed in 22 hips, the majority of patients showed union of the graft, with only two showing significant resorption. Acetabular implant migration was present in three cases, but in two of these the component was a bipolar prosthesis.

Of 45 hips that required a support allograft, with an average follow-up of 5.1 years, nine patients received femoral head grafts and 36 were treated with distal femur allografts. The defects in these patients left a nonsupportive acetabular rim and 40% to 60% host bone available for ingrowth with a porous-coated prosthesis. In all cases, osseous union of the grafts was determined. Two of the nine femoral head grafts failed with migration of the component of greater than 4 mm, and none of the distal femur grafts failed.

The success of distal femoral allografts in reconstruction of the failed acetabulum is based on several important factors. At least 50% host bone must be present for ingrowth of a porous-coated prosthesis. The distal femurs should be selected for their shape and size. The shape maximizes rigid fixation and surface contact with the host bone. The graft must be large enough to ensure that after reconstruction there is sufficient allograft remaining to prevent early collapse and migration, which occur in smaller femoral head grafts. The grafts should be placed to ensure correct orientation of the trabeculae, and only fresh frozen grafts should be used to ensure minimal change in graft structural support. The graft should be shaped into a modified "number 7" so that it hangs into and locks into the superior acetabular defect and is buttressed against the remaining ilium. The graft should be secured to the ilium with multiple 6.5 cancellous screws that are oriented in an oblique fashion along the lines of stress of the graft. The graft should be reamed such that maximal contact is ensured between the porous surface of the component and the remaining host bone. Adherence to these factors should allow for early component stability and later fixation through ingrowth from the remaining host bone.

Acetabular components with superior augments incorporated into the cup have been developed for use as an alternative to bone grafting in the severely deficient acetabulum. These components can either be off the shelf components or they can be a custom-designed prosthesis based on computed tomography (CT) scans and computer reconstruction of the acetabulum. They have the attractive advantage of decreasing time in surgery because time-consuming allograft shaping and fixation are not required. However, these components are based on radiographic examination of the defect and may not give an exact fit at the time of surgery, in which case they must be abandoned or possibly cemented in place.

Although cementless fixation of the acetabular component in revision surgery should probably be strived for in all cases, cementless fixation is inappropriate for occasional defects. In defects with less than 50% host bone, the use of support distal femur allografts and porous-coated prostheses has led to a failure rate of 70% at 5.1 years. In these severe defects some form of major structural allograft and/or a reconstruction ring will be required along with a cemented all polyethylene acetabular component. A review of 42 failed hip arthroplasties with massive acetabular bone loss, which was treated with a Burch-Schneider anti-protrusio cage fixed to the ilium and ischium, showed 76% with no migration at an average of 5 years, five hips re-revised for aseptic loosening, and five failures secondary to infection.

The alternative to the placement of a reconstruction ring is to treat the defect with a major structural allograft and a cemented prosthesis into the allograft. A technique to deal with this problem involves the use of whole cadaveric hemipelvis allograft to treat the severe defects present. The host bone is resected to allow placement of the hemipelvis graft, which is secured superiorly to the ilium and inferiorly to the ischium. The fixation is augmented with a pelvic reconstruction plate or a reconstruction ring to ensure that fixation extends from host bone above to host bone below. Six of 14 true acetabular allografts have required reoperation due to fracture or fragmentation of the graft. The subsequent reconstruction was greatly simplified by the restored bone stock present. Five of these six

reoperated allografts have adequate hip scores at a minimum of 2 years after reoperation.

An acetabular transplant procedure has been described in which the hemipelvis graft is cut and shaped to fit and lock into the existing defect with very minimal resection of host bone. The graft is buttressed against the host ilium and initially fixed with cancellous screws. The fixation is augmented with a pelvic reconstruction plate that extends from host ischium inferiorly to host ilium superiorly. A report of 14 patients with 2 years follow-up indicated a high initial anterior dislocation rate secondary to excessive anteversion of the graft and poor abductor function. All dislocations have responded to conservative treatment with bracing and short-term immobilization. The early results have been quite promising.

Femoral Reconstruction

Revision of failed cemented or cementless femoral components can be fraught with problems and complexity if there is osteolysis from polyethylene wear debris. Although most patients have severe symptoms before these defects are large, some do not react until there is massive proximal femoral bone loss or even fractures about the prosthesis secondary to the osteolysis.

The basic aims of femoral revision are to obtain satisfactory initial component stability to allow bony ingrowth for long-term success and to replace existing bony defects with component augments or allografts, depending on the severity of femoral bone loss. Most surgeons currently would employ bone grafting to replace significant femoral deformities so long as component stability can be obtained. In those cases in which no component can be made stable with present fixation methods, a total femoral replacement as used in tumor surgery may be the only viable option. Fortunately, these are few and far between.

The type of implant that can be employed in femoral revision depends on the intrinsic support available from the host femur. In most revisions there will be some degree of metaphyseal bone damage. If the metaphyseal bone damage is only moderate or mild, then a proximally or distally fixed device could be used with a presumed equal chance of success. As the femoral bone stock loss extends past the metaphysis and into the diaphysis, the use of a purely proximally stabilized device becomes less successful. In these cases, a distally fixed device or a proximally coated device with supplemental distal rotational stability will be required. In rare cases in which the femoral bone loss progresses distally below the isthmus, purely cementless techniques become less appropriate, and bone grafts with combined cement and cementless fixation or purely cemented fixation must be used.

Proximally fixed and coated devices have had good success in the femur that provides intact proximal rotational stability. However, when the proximal femur cannot support a prosthesis, the prosthesis must provide some method of distal rotational stability in order to obtain proximal ingrowth and long-term success. Good initial results have been reported for use of a proximally one third coated prosthesis that also incorporates distal flutes to provide initial rotational stability when the proximal femur cannot.

Proximally coated devices with increased modularity of the proximal femoral component have recently become popular. There are two basic designs: one has a modular proximal sleeve and the other incorporates modular proximal pads and stem extensions. Good early results have been reported for the S-ROM prosthesis (Joint Medical Products, Stamford, CT), which uses a proximal porous-coated sleeve and a stem with distal flutes for augmented distal stability. If a primary type of stem could be used in revision total hip arthroplasty, the re-revision rate was 6.8% at 2 to 6 years of follow-up. However, in cases with more proximal bone loss that required a long, curved calcar-replacing revision prosthesis, the re-revision rate rose to 16.1%. The second prosthesis has a titanium stem and multiple modular proximal pads to "customize" it on the operating table in order to optimize proximal contact and ingrowth. This prosthesis also has multiple straight and curved stem extensions to augment proximal fixation distally. Longer study is necessary to determine the usefulness of this prosthesis and to look for any of the feared complications that increased modularity and potential increases in metal, particularly titanium, wear debris may bring.

The use of a true custom femoral component provides a prosthesis that matches the defects present proximally and, therefore, ensures excellent proximal fixation. However, this use requires CT scans and computer-designed prostheses that increase the expense and production time. Another problem is what to do with the custom component if intraoperative findings do not exactly match the preoperative radiographic findings or if an intraoperative complication precludes its use. When custom femoral prostheses were used in 47 revision total hip replacements, 19% of patients had intraoperative proximal femoral fractures that required wire fixation and one patient required traction and a redesigned prosthesis because the first did not fit and no conventional prosthesis could be used. In all cases, particulate graft was used proximally and 34% required structural graft for bony deficiencies, but not to support the prosthesis. At 30 months follow-up there has been one re-revision for failure due to pad separation and one separation that has not required re-revision. Other clinical results have been good.

An extensively coated, distally fixed prosthesis can be used in any femur, provided there is sufficient diaphyseal bone left to provide rotational and axial stability of the prosthesis. When an extensively porous coated femoral component was used in 174 revision total hip arthroplasties, the re-revision rate was 5.7% and the radiographic failure rate was 1.1% for a mechanical failure rate of 7.4% at 7.4 years follow-up. A survivorship analysis of 90.6% at the ninth year was reported. Clinical evaluation showed the pain level was improved in 89.1% of the hips, the walking status in 82.8%, and the functional level in 88.5%.

An extensively coated femoral prosthesis was used in 297 cementless femoral revisions that were followed up for a mean of 5.2 years. There have been no failures in 136 patients in whom the metaphysis was intact and supportive. The remaining 161 patients had proximal femoral bone loss that left the proximal femur nonsupportive and required bone grafting along with the extensively coated stem. There were five re-revisions and two radiographic failures with migration of 4 mm or greater in this group. The mechanical failure rate was 3.4%. The canal fill was less than 75% in all failed stems, and there was less than 4 cm of diaphyseal fixation due to long straight stems with three-point fixation. The remaining stems had an average canal fill of 88% and an average diaphyseal fixation of at least 4 cm. The five re-revised stems were changed to more canal filling and curved extensively porous-coated stems; all have done well.

Bone stock deficiencies present in the femur are generally replaced by allograft bone, although the option of augments to the prosthesis, such as calcar-replacing prostheses or custom replacing prostheses, is available. A report on proximal femoral allografts in revision hip surgery indicates that in calcar grafts of 3 cm or less, 10% resorbed between one third and one half, 40% resorbed more than one half of the graft, and the prosthesis subsided in 43%. Based on these results, the authors recommended that calcar grafts of less than 3 cm not be used; however, most surgeons now would use a calcar-replacing type of prosthesis for these defects.

In a report on the use of femoral strut allografts to restore proximal femoral bone stock in revision total hip arthroplasty using a proximal one third coated prosthesis, 106 patients were followed for an average of 2.8 years. Graft union occurred in 98% at an average time to union of 7.3 months. This method was found to be reliable for augmenting proximal femoral deficiencies if the graft was not used to support the prosthesis.

The results were reviewed of 113 femoral revisions with an extensively porous-coated prosthesis. These included 18 cases of calcar grafts and 95 cases of cortical strut grafts to augment proximal femoral deficiencies. Mean follow-up was 4.75 years. Eleven of the 18 calcar grafts resorbed. Radiographic evidence of strut graft incorporation and improvement of proximal femoral bone stock was present in 92.6% of cases despite the use of a distally fixed, extensively porous-coated prosthesis. In the seven struts that failed, the prosthesis was undersized, and in five cases prostheses were revised to a more canal filling prosthesis with good results. The authors felt the use of an extensively coated femoral prosthesis and cortical strut augmentation allografts was a good method to restore proximal femoral bone loss.

A technique of intramedullary allografting to the expanded femoral canal has been described. If the deficiency is confined to the proximal femur, an allograft is shaped as a truncated cone to fit into the proximal femoral deformity and the S-ROM femoral component (Joint Medical Products, Stamford, CT) is cemented into the allograft with the distal flutes press fit to the remaining diaphysis of the host femur. In the event of more severe proximal femoral deformity, an allograft proximal femur is machined to press fit into the remaining distal host femur with a butt joint allograft–host junction, and the femoral prosthesis is again cemented into the allograft femur. In both of these reconstructions, the fixation of the graft to host bone is augmented with cerclage wire. Early results were good, with an average of 50 months follow-up.

In another report on the use of large segment proximal femoral allografts to deal with severe proximal femoral deformities, 40 allografts were followed up for an average of 33.6 months. The overall success rate was 85%. Three unstable nonunions responded to subsequent grafting, and one smaller graft fragmented. Three patients underwent resection for infection and one for recurrent dislocations. The authors recommend the graft be cemented to the prosthesis and the prosthesis then be press fit into the remaining femur with a host–graft step cut junction and autograft to the junction. If the prosthesis requires cementing into the distal host femur, every effort should be made to exclude cement from the host–graft junction. The authors also recommended avoiding placing holes in the graft as would be required with plate fixation.

A recently reported technique involves cementing the proximal portion of a modular prosthesis into the allograft and press fitting the distal stem to the host bone. The host–allograft junction is created with a butt joint. At a mean follow-up of 22 months, all but two of 30 allografts united to the host bone at the host–allograft junction.

Cement fixation of the stem to the allograft was recommended in a report on an allograft prosthetic composite technique in tumor resections that has also been used in revision arthroplasty cases. Two techniques were used. In one, a short prosthesis was used with double plate and screw fixation of the graft to host bone with a butt joint. In the other, a longer stem was cemented into the graft, with a single plate fixing the junction to augment any stability provided by the stem extending into the host femur. In four cases, there were three allograft fractures below the stem, two nonunions, and one dislocation for a 100% complication rate. Although higher than reported in most larger series, this rate stresses the complexity and possible disastrous outcomes.

The use of custom-made segmental femoral replacement prostheses has also been advocated for revision in which there is severe proximal femoral deformity. Twenty-five of 36 patients with severe proximal femoral bone loss were followed for an average of 11 years. Overall survivorship was 73%, with a high rate of dislocations (22%) and a high rate of acetabular loosening (24%). The authors recommend limiting the use of these prostheses in the elderly and the inactive patient.

Early results have been reviewed for use of a composite fixation method with a custom segmental replacement prosthesis that has a porous-coated modular segment at the prosthesis–host junction. The stem is cemented into the distal host femur for initial implant stability, then autogenous bone grafts are placed over the porous-coated region to achieve extracortical bone bridging from the distal host femur and bony ingrowth for long-term implant stability. Seven patients treated with this prosthesis for femoral revision had good results and no loosening at 25 months average follow-up. A larger series with increased follow-up will be required to assess the true value of this prosthesis in revising the severely proximally deficient femur.

A recent review of the use of a low modulus, composite, plastic porous-coated canine femoral prosthesis indicated that bone ingrowth occurred with equal frequency, quality, and quantity to that in conventional stems with the same coating. There will obviously need to be much more work on this intriguing possibility before it may be available for use in revision surgery.

Complications

In general, revision total hip arthroplasty has a higher complication rate than primary surgery in all classes of complications including sciatic nerve injury, dislocation, infection, heterotopic ossification, and thromboembolic problems.

Probably the most feared and the most distressing complication to the patient is sciatic nerve injury. In 3,126 cases of total hip arthroplasty, the incidence of postoperative neuropathy was 1.3% in primary surgery and 3.2% in revision surgery. Limb lengthening of greater than 2.5 cm only partly accounted for the increase. Other possible causes were felt to be scarring, the distorted anatomy present about the hip, and the relative immobility of the nerves and soft tissues. All patients that regained full neurologic function had done so by 21 months after surgery. The patients who had a partial injury or some return of function while still hospitalized had a good recovery, but all patients with severe dysesthesias had a poor neurologic recovery.

A report on 23 cases of sciatic nerve monitoring during revision total hip arthroplasty describes a simple method of intraoperative monitoring using somatosensory evoked potentials (SSEP). No postoperative neurologic complications were found with lengthening of up to 43 mm. SSEP monitoring should probably be considered in all cases in which significant lengthening (greater than 2.5 cm) is planned and in all difficult revision total hip replacements.

The infection rate in revision total hip arthroplasty is at least double the rate in primary hip replacement surgery because of the longer operating time and the larger surgical exposure, which result in the risk of increased direct contamination. The larger exposure also leads to increased volumes of devascularized bone and soft tissue and larger dead space, with an increased risk of bacterial colonization. The use of appropriate soft-tissue handling combined with perioperative prophylaxis and an appropriate operating room environment must be followed to try and prevent this severe complication.

Dislocation rates after revision total hip arthroplasty are reported to be at least double the primary dislocation rate and in some series are reported to be as high as 22%. This disparity is accounted for by the lack of adequate soft tissue and hip abductor function that may be present in the revision case, particularly in the revision that requires large segment allograft for severe proximal femoral deformity in which abductor function is poor. However, in some series, lower instability rates have been reported in those cases in which fixation of the abductors to the graft was possible. The use of a trochanteric osteotomy and a subsequent trochanteric nonunion can lead to an increase in postoperative dislocations, which has been reported to be as high as a sixfold increase (to 18%) with a nonunion and proximal migration of the trochanter of greater than 1 cm. In the cases of severe soft-tissue loss and instability, the patient may require prolonged immobilization in a brace or hip spica cast. Early results have been encouraging for use of a capture type of acetabular prosthesis for severe instability. This type of prosthesis should probably be reserved as a last-ditch effort because of the increased stresses placed on the cup fixation and potential increased rate of acetabular loosening.

The loss of femoral bone stock in the multiply revised femur can lead to increased postoperative femoral fracture. Postoperative fracture rates as high as 4.2% have been reported for revisions. Prevention is the best treatment. Care should be taken during surgery to prevent stress risers created by femoral perforations or defects caused by eccentric reaming. If a defect is created, it is important to bypass it with a longer stem extending two cortical diameters distal to the defect or by using extramedullary bypasses with cortical strut allografts. It has been reported that in the unstable fracture about a prosthesis, the best results have been obtained with operative fixation. There were no significant complications at 26 months follow-up after compression plating in 10 patients. One nonunion required subsequent revision to a long-stemmed extensively porous-coated prosthesis. Revision to an extensively porous-coated prosthesis in 17 patients was reported to have good results and no nonunions.

Heterotopic ossification has been reported to occur to some degree in up to 60% of total hip arthroplasties. The patients at greatest risk for this complication are those who have a previous history of heterotopic ossification. It is important to ensure that the heterotopic bone is mature prior to any revision or resection of the bone. This can be done most effectively with serial serum alkaline phosphatase levels, which parallel the bone activity. Meticulous surgical technique must be used to ensure complete removal of heterotopic bone and hemostasis must be used to prevent postoperative hematoma formation. An intraoperative radiograph should be performed to ensure complete removal. Postoperative prophylaxis is essential to prevent recurrence. The only clinically proven method of prophylaxis is a single dose of postoperative treatment at currently suggested levels of 600 to 700 rads in the first 48 hours postoperatively. It is important to shield the prosthesis and the trochanter if a cementless stem or a trochanteric osteotomy are used. Indomethacin has not been proven as a method of prophylaxis to prevent recurrence post-resection.

Thromboembolic complications are possibly the most common. Reported incidences of deep venous thrombosis have been as high as 70% and of pulmonary embolism, as high as 19.7%. Some form of prophylaxis is necessary for prevention of these possibly fatal complications; however, there is no clear-cut choice for the best method of prophylaxis. The best available options at this time include low dose coumadin, adjusted dose heparin, or low molecular weight heparin. All have shown some degree of effectiveness, but none have given convincing evidence of being definitely more effective than any other. The length of prophylaxis is also controversial, with reports varying from 3 to 4 weeks duration to a full 3-month course being recommended by some.

Annotated Bibliography

Callaghan JJ: Total hip arthroplasty: Clinical perspective. *Clin Orthop* 1992;276:33–40.
  This provides a good overview of the field of total hip arthroplasty and presents a review of the results of cemented and cementless primary and revision total hip arthroplasty.

Callaghan JJ: The clinical results and basic science of total hip arthroplasty with porous-coated prostheses. *J Bone Joint Surg* 1993;75A:299–310.

This provides a review of the different types of porous-coated implants available with a review of the basic science of cementless total hip fixation and a review of the clinical results.

Preoperative Evaluation

Engh CA, Massin P, Suthers KE: Roentgenographic assessment of the biologic fixation of porous-surfaced femoral components. *Clin Orthop* 1990;257:107–128.
  Radiographic criteria are provided to evaluate the femoral

prosthesis postoperatively. Then the prostheses are classified as bony ingrown, stable fibrous ingrowth, or unstable based on these radiographic criteria.

Harris WH, Barrack RL: Developments in diagnosis of the painful total hip replacement. *Orthop Rev* 1993;22: 439–447.

This provides a review of the use of diagnostic tests in the evaluation of the painful total hip arthroplasty. The criteria to evaluate loosening on radiographs, arthrograms, and arthroscintigraphy are reviewed. This also reviews the results of routine aspirations and suggests that this should be used more selectively to improve the yield in preoperative evaluation.

Harris WH, Barrack RL: Contemporary algorithms for evaluation of the painful total hip replacement. *Orthop Rev* 1993;22:531–539.

This reviews the results of nuclear medicine scans in the evaluation of the painful total hip. The intraoperative assessment of the failed total hip includes the use of frozen sections, Gram stains, and mechanical testing. Algorithms to the evaluation and diagnostic work-up of the painful total hip arthroplasty are provided.

Lieberman JR, Huo MH, Schneider R, et al: Evaluation of painful hip arthroplasties : Are technetium bone scans necessary? *J Bone Joint Surg* 1993;75B:475–478.

Technetium bone scans were found to provide little information in the routine evaluation of the painful total hip. The authors felt that serial radiographs provided more useful information and that bone scans should be reserved for those cases in which the plain radiographs are inconclusive.

Roberts P, Walters A-J, McMinn DJ: Diagnosing infection in hip replacements: The use of fine-needle aspiration and radiometric culture. *J Bone Joint Surg* 1992;74B:265–269.

Seventy-eight patients were treated with a fine-needle aspiration combined with a radiometric culture technique. The authors found this to be a reliable method of determining infection of hip prostheses. The sensitivity was 87% and the specificity was 95%.

Preoperative Planning

Collier JP, Mayor MB, Jensen RE, et al: Mechanisms of failure of modular prostheses. *Clin Orthop* 1992;285: 129–139.

The authors describe design characteristics that have led to the early failure of acetabular components. Modular femoral components of dissimilar alloys were susceptible to corrosion. All modular connections are at risk of disassociation and fretting.

Collier JP, Surprenant VA, Jensen RE, et al: Corrosion between the components of modular femoral hip prostheses. *J Bone Joint Surg* 1992;74B:511–517.

In a study of 139 modular tapers, no corrosion was found in 91 tapers with the same alloy used for head and stem, but in 25 of 48 tapers with dissimilar alloys there was definite corrosion present. The corrosion was time dependent, with none if the stem was implanted less than 9 months and in all implanted more than 40 months.

D'Antonio J, McCarthy JC, Bargar WL, et al: Classification of femoral abnormalities in total hip arthroplasty. *Clin Orthop* 1993;296:133–139.

This classification system of femoral deformities is based on segmental, cavitary, and combined defects. It was designed to give a standard nomenclature system, but is cumbersome and does not give a treatment plan to aid the surgeon.

Friedman RJ, Black J, Galante JO, et al: Current concepts in orthopaedic biomaterials and implant fixation. *J Bone Joint Surg* 1993;75A:1086–1109.

This is a review which was taken from three chapters in *Instructional Course Lectures 43,* of the use of orthopaedic biomaterials, including the systemic and remote-site effects and the local responses to these materials. It also reviews new methods for the enhancement of the bone–prosthesis interface and of long-term implant fixation.

Haynes DR, Rogers SD, Hay S, et al: The differences in toxicity and release of bone-resorbing mediators induced by titanium and cobalt-chromium-alloy wear particles. *J Bone Joint Surg* 1993;75A:825–834.

The tissue response to titanium and cobalt-chromium particulate debris was investigated. Cobalt-chromium was found to be more toxic to periprosthetic tissues. The titanium particles were found to cause release of more inflammatory mediators implicated in osteolysis.

Surgical Technique

Glassman AH, Engh CA: The removal of porous-coated femoral hip stems. *Clin Orthop* 1992;285:164–180.

The authors describe a technique for the removal of a porous-coated femoral prosthesis. This involves the use of a cortical window and the sectioning of the stem to remove the proximal portion of the stem. The distal portion of the stem can then be removed with a specially designed trephine.

Pierson JL, Jasty M, Harris WH: Techniques of extraction of well-fixed cemented and cementless implants in revision total hip arthroplasty. *Orthop Rev* 1993;22:904–916.

Several techniques are described for the removal of well-fixed cemented and cementless hip prostheses. The authors also describe the various methods available for the removal of bone cement.

Schurman DJ, Maloney WJ: Segmental cement extraction at revision total hip arthroplasty. *Clin Orthop* 1992;285: 158–163.

A new method of segmental cement extraction that involves the insertion of new cement into the old cement mantle is described. An extractor rod is then screwed into the cement mantle and the cement is removed in 1.5- to 2.5-cm segments.

Younger TI, Bradford MS, Magnus RE, et al: Extended proximal femoral osteotomy. *J Arthroplasty* 1995;10:1–10.

An osteotomy technique for removal of distally fixed cemented and cementless femoral components is described that allows for excellent cement and component removal and optimal revision component implantation, thereby minimizing the risk of intraoperative fracture. There was a high rate of osteotomy healing.

Acetabular Reconstruction

Berry DJ, Muller ME: Revision arthroplasty using an anti-protrusio cage for massive acetabular bone deficiency. *J Bone Joint Surg* 1992;74B:711–715.

The use of an antiprotrusio cage in the reconstruction of 42 failed total hip arthroplasties is described. The failure rate due to loosening or infection was 24% at a mean follow-up of 5 years.

Gross AE, Allan DG, Catre M, et al: Bone grafts in hip replacement surgery: The pelvic side. *Orthop Clin North Am* 1993;24:679–695.

The use of allograft bone in the reconstruction of acetabular deficiencies in primary and revision arthroplasties and the use of morsellized bone in contained defects and of structural allografts in noncontained defects are described.

Harris WH: Management of the deficient acetabulum using cementless fixation without bone grafting. *Orthop Clin North Am* 1993;24:663–665.

The use of a cementless acetabular component and a high hip center in the reconstruction of the failed total hip arthroplasty is described. This author feels that the use of structural bone grafts is not necessary with this technique.

Huo MH, Friedlaender GE, Salvati EA: Bone graft and total hip arthroplasty: A review. *J Arthroplasty* 1992;7:109–120.

This is a review of the types of bone grafts available and of the bone banking procedures. It also reviews the literature on the results of both acetabular and femoral allograft reconstructions.

Kwong LM, Jasty M, Harris WH: High failure rate of bulk femoral head allografts in total hip acetabular reconstructions at 10 years. *J Arthroplasty* 1993;8:341–346.

The results of the use of femoral head allografts with cemented acetabular components in acetabular reconstruction are described. The authors found a 47% failure rate at a mean follow-up of 10 years with the use of femoral head grafts and condemned the use of all bulk allografts based on these results.

Padgett DE, Kuff L, Rosenberg A, et al: Revision of the acetabular component without cement after total hip arthroplasty: Three to six-year follow-up. *J Bone Joint Surg* 1993;75A:663–673.

The results of 138 consecutive acetabular revisions with a cementless hemispheric acetabular component were reviewed. The authors reported good results with only a 5% re-revision rate at an average follow-up of 44 months.

Paprosky WG: Allograft reconstruction in massive acetabular defects. *Tech Orthop* 1993;7:44.

Using a classification system that had previously been reported, this describes the surgical technique for acetabular allografting. It gives guidelines based on the type of defect as to which type of reconstruction will be necessary and gives the results of 177 acetabular reconstructions at a mean of 5.1 years.

Paprosky WG, Magnus RE: Principles of bone grafting in revision total hip arthroplasty: Acetabular technique. *Clin Orthop* 1994;298:147–155.

A series of 316 acetabular revisions with 69 support allografts were followed an average of 5.1 years. Biologic fixation of a porous-coated cup and a distal femoral support graft was possible if 40% to 50% host bone was available for ingrowth. If less than 40% host bone was available, total acetabular transplant and cemented acetabular fixation was required.

Femoral Reconstruction

Allan DG, Lavoie GJ, McDonald S, et al: Proximal femoral allografts in revision hip arthroplasty. *J Bone Joint Surg* 1991;73B:235–240.

Seventy-eight proximal femoral allografts were followed for a mean of 36 months. The large fragment and cortical strut allografts were successful in 85%, but 50% of calcar grafts less than 3 cm showed significant resorption and should be abandoned.

Bargar WL, Murzic WJ, Taylor JK, et al: Management of bone loss in revision total hip arthroplasty using custom cementless femoral components. *J Arthroplasty* 1993;8:245–252.

The authors describe 47 revisions with a porous custom-designed femoral prosthesis with an average follow-up of 30 months. There was only one re-revision, and there was a 19% incidence of proximal femoral fracture requiring cerclage wire; 15% had subsided more than 3 mm.

Cameron HU: The two- to six-year results with a proximally modular noncemented total hip replacement used in hip revisions. *Clin Orthop* 1994;298:47–53.

The results of 91 revisions with 29 primary type stems and 62 long curved revision calcar-replacing stems are presented. The re-revision rate of the primary type stem is 6.8%, but when there was sufficient proximal bone loss to require the long revision prosthesis, the re-revision rate increased to 16.1% at relatively short follow-up.

Chandler H: Intramedullary grafting of the expanded femoral canal in total hip replacement. *Tech Orthop* 1993;7:33.

Seventeen patients with an intramedullary structural graft were followed for a mean of 50 months. Nine metaphyseal grafts were impacted into the host femur and all of these united. Seven smaller allograft femurs were impacted into the host diaphysis and five of these united. The two that did not unite were due to not providing a butt joint and relying on press fit for stability. The femoral prosthesis was cemented into all grafts.

Chandler H, Clark J, Murphy S, et al: Reconstruction of major segmental loss of the proximal femur in revision total hip arthroplasty. *Clin Orthop* 1994;298:67–74.

A long-stemmed modular prosthesis, cemented into an allograft proximal femur and then press fit into the host femur, was used in 30 hips. The follow-up was a mean of 22 months, with only 2 nonunions of graft to host bone. Authors were encouraged but stressed the short-term follow-up.

Head WC, Wagner RA, Emerson RH Jr, et al: Revision total hip arthroplasty in the deficient femur with a proximal load-bearing prosthesis. *Clin Orthop* 1994;298:119–126.

One hundred and seventy-four patients were treated with a calcar replacement proximally porous-coated femoral prosthesis and onlay cortical strut allografts. The grafts united in 98%. There have been six re-revisions for femoral failure. The prosthesis must be supported primarily and not by the struts.

Lawrence JM, Engh CA, Macalino GE: Revision total hip arthroplasty: Long-term results without cement. *Orthop Clin North Am* 1993;24:635–644.

The authors reviewed 174 revisions treated with an extensively porous-coated femoral prosthesis and with an average of 5 years follow-up. There was a 5.7% re-revision rate and a mechanical failure rate of 6.7%. The pain level, walking status, and functional level improved in 80% to 90% of patients.

Malkani AL, Sim FH, Chao EYS: Custom-made segmental femoral replacement prosthesis in revision total hip arthroplasty. *Orthop Clin North Am* 1993;24:727–733.

The long-term results of a segmental proximal femoral replacement prosthesis have shown a high rate of dislocations and acetabular loosening, with a survivorship of 73% at 11 years. The authors also report good early results in 46 hips treated with a second generation modular proximal femoral replacement prosthesis, with only two dislocations and no aseptic loosening at short-term follow-up.

Pak JH, Paprosky WG, Jablonsky WS, et al: Femoral strut allografts in cementless revision total hip arthroplasty. *Clin Orthop* 1993;295:172–178.

This reports on 113 femoral revisions with an extensively porous-coated femoral prosthesis and cortical strut allografts. At a mean follow-up of 4.75 years, 87 of 95 cortical struts showed evidence of incorporation, but 11 of 18 calcar grafts resorbed. The cortical struts were found to incorporate with a well-fixed extensively porous-coated prosthesis and to augment the femoral bone stock.

Complications

Frankel A, Booth RE Jr, Balderston RA, et al: Complications of trochanteric osteotomy: Long-term implications. *Clin Orthop* 1993;288:209–213.

The results of 58 trochanteric nonunions in 1,162 patients are reported. The pain and function scores in the nonunion group were lower. The nonunion group had a 17% incidence of a Trendelenburg gait and had a threefold increase in re-revision rate.

Kennedy WF, Byme TF, Majid HA, et al: Sciatic nerve monitoring during revision total hip arthroplasty. *Clin Orthop* 1991;264:223–227.

Intraoperative somatosensory evoked potentials are monitored during revision total hip arthroplasty. A decrease in amplitude response provides a reliable intraoperative assessment of possible impairment to sciatic nerve function during the revision procedure, particularly if leg lengthening is anticipated. There were no sciatic nerve injuries with lengthening of 6 to 43 mm.

Morrey BF: Instability after total hip arthroplasty. *Orthop Clin North Am* 1992;23:237–248.

This reviews the risk factors for dislocation post total hip replacement, with prior surgery, trochanteric nonunion, and posterior approach being most significant. The results of surgical treatment are also reviewed. The author stresses that a clearly definable cause should be found in order to plan the appropriate surgical treatment.

Schmalzried TP, Amstutz HC, Dorey FJ: Nerve palsy associated with total hip replacement : Risk factors and prognosis. *J Bone Joint Surg* 1991;73A:1074–1080.

In 3,126 hip arthroplasties the incidence of nerve injury was 1.7%. Primary arthroplasties for congenital dislocation or dysplasia and revision arthroplasties were significant risk factors. The cause was unclear in 57%. The prognosis for recovery was related to the degree of nerve damage. No patient with severe dysesthesias had a good recovery of neurologic function.

Serocki JH, Chandler RW, Dorr LD: Treatment of fractures about hip prostheses with compression plating. *J Arthroplasty* 1992;7:129–135.

Femur fractures about a hip prosthesis were treated with open reduction and compression plating. Nine of ten fractures healed at an average of 5 months with no significant complications other than one nonunion.

Swayze OS, Nasser S, Roberson JR: Deep venous thrombosis in total hip arthroplasty. *Orthop Clin North Am* 1992;23:359–364.

The incidence, pathogenesis, and diagnosis of deep venous thrombosis and pulmonary embolism after total hip arthroplasty are reviewed. The options for prophylaxis are also reviewed, and the recommended options include warfarin, adjusted dose heparin, low-molecular–weight heparin, or dextran in younger patients.

Thomas BJ: Heterotopic bone formation after total hip arthroplasty. *Orthop Clin North Am* 1992;23:347–358.

The possible etiologies of heterotopic ossification are reviewed along with the most used classification systems. The use of prophylaxis with diphosphonates, anti-inflammatory medications, and radiotherapy are described. Anti-inflammatories and radiation therapy were the most effective. The timing and planning of operative resection and postoperative prophylaxis after resection are discussed.

26

Anatomy and Biomechanics of the Knee

Introduction

Understanding of the anatomy and related biomechanics of the knee joint has increased significantly in the past 10 years. Anatomic structures of the knee have been meticulously delineated by many researchers, and the biomechanics of the knee joint has been studied in great detail, with emphasis on the role of the individual structures that make up the joint. Major contributions have addressed many of the clinical issues related to the normal knee joint, the arthritic knee joint, and knee joint replacement.

Motion of the Knee

Kinematics is the study of the geometry of motion and is a subdivision of dynamics. An understanding of the kinematics of the knee joint is important in the study of human locomotion in general as well as in the diagnosis of joint diseases and the design of prosthetic devices.

The motion of the knee joint is polycentric and has been described anatomically by many investigators. More specifically, the motion at the knee joint can be classified as having six degrees of freedom—three translations: anterior/posterior, medial/lateral, and inferior/superior and three rotations: flexion/extension, internal/external, and abduction/adduction. The motions at the knee joint are determined by the shape of the articulating surfaces of the tibia and femur and the orientation of the four major ligaments of the knee joint. Flexion is defined as the movement of the posterior aspect of the leg towards the posterior aspect of the thigh. Flexion at the knee joint can be defined as either active or passive and depends on the position of the hip joint. When the hip joint is extended, the hamstring muscles lose their efficiency at flexing the knee joint. During active flexion, the knee can attain 120° and 140° when the hip joint is flexed. Passively, the knee joint can flex to 160°.

Articular Surfaces

The articular surfaces at the knee joint consist of the curved surfaces that form the lateral and medial condyles of the distal portion of the femur and are in contact with the lateral and medial tibial plateaus of the proximal portion of the tibia. The medial tibial condyle is biconcave, whereas the lateral condyle is concave in the frontal plane and convex in the sagittal plane. The femoral condyles are convex in both the frontal and sagittal planes. Studies of femorotibial articulation have shown that the medial com-

partment has an average of 1.6 times greater contact area than the lateral compartment.

Knee flexion/extension involves a combination of rolling and sliding. Motions of the articular surfaces relative to one another are determined predominantly by the geometry of the surfaces and the orientation of the four major ligaments (anterior and posterior cruciate and medial and lateral collateral ligaments) crossing the knee joint. Because the lateral femoral condyle has a larger radius of curvature than the medial femoral condyle, it rolls a greater distance than the medial condyle during the first 15° to 20° of knee flexion. This asymmetry in the radii of curvature of the condyles imposes an internal rotation of the tibia with respect to the femur during flexion. Beyond 20° of flexion, sliding motion begins on both condyles. Extension of the knee joint produces a coupled external rotation of the tibia with respect to the femur; this rotation has been described as the screw-home movement of the knee.

The Menisci and Their Function

The meniscal cartilages are interposed between the femoral condyles and the tibial articular surfaces. They are crescent shaped, with the lateral meniscus being more of a full circle and the medial meniscus nearly semicircular in form. Both menisci are thicker at the periphery and become very thin toward the center (Fig. 1). Thus, on cross-section,

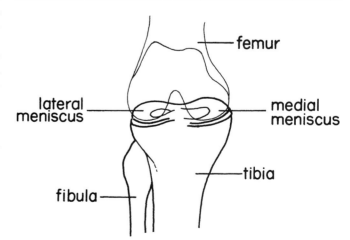

Fig. 1 Proximal portion of the tibia and distal portion of the femur with locations of the menisci in the knee joint.

they have a wedge-like appearance. Although both menisci are unattached centrally, they have very complex attachments at the periphery. The medial meniscus is firmly attached to the medial collateral ligament, whereas the lateral meniscus is not attached to the lateral collateral ligament. Thus, the lateral meniscus can move more freely on the condyle during flexion and extension of the knee, and the medial meniscus is moderately constrained.

Load-bearing is an important function of the menisci. Strong evidence exists that the menisci support a large fraction of the load on the knee; they distribute this load between the medial and lateral surfaces of the knee joint. Experimental studies have shown that in the absence of the menisci, the load-bearing area approximates 2 cm^2, and that it increases to 6 cm^2 on each condyle when the menisci are present. These data have important implications in the transfer of stress to the underlying cartilage. When the effective area of load-bearing is increased, the stress transferred to the cartilage is reduced, and when, in the absence of the menisci, the effective area of load-bearing is reduced, the stress transferred to the cartilage is increased. The sharing of the load between the menisci and the amount of exposed cartilage in either the medial or lateral compartment depends on the relative stiffness of the meniscus and the cartilage.

Collateral Ligaments and Their Function

The medial collateral ligament (MCL) is made up of two layers—the superficial MCL and the deep MCL. The MCL has both vertical and oblique fibers. The anterior or vertical fibers of the superficial MCL originate primarily at the medial epicondyle of the femur and consist of heavy, vertically-oriented fibers running distally to an insertion on the medial surface of the tibia (on average 4.6 cm inferior to the tibial articular surface), immediately posterior to the insertion of the pes anserinus. The posterior oblique fibers originate from the femoral epicondyle and are attached to the tibia immediately inferior to the posterior tibial articular surface and to the medial meniscus. During flexion of the knee, the superficial vertical fibers of the MCL remain taut while the oblique fibers are relaxed. In extension of the knee, the anterior fibers are relaxed while the posterior fibers are tensed. The deep fibers of the MCL extend from the femur to the midpoint of the peripheral margin of the medial meniscus and the tibia. Anteriorly, the deep ligament is separated from the superficial ligament by a bursa. Posteriorly, the layers of the deep and superficial ligament blend near their attachment (Fig. 2).

The primary function of the MCL is to restrain valgus rotation of the knee joint. Data from several cadaveric studies have indicated that sectioning the superficial MCL resulted in a significant increase in valgus rotation at knee flexion angles of 0° and 45°. Data also indicated that sectioning the deep medial or posterior oblique ligaments or the posterior capsule did not increase the instability. External rotation, which resulted from an applied external rota-

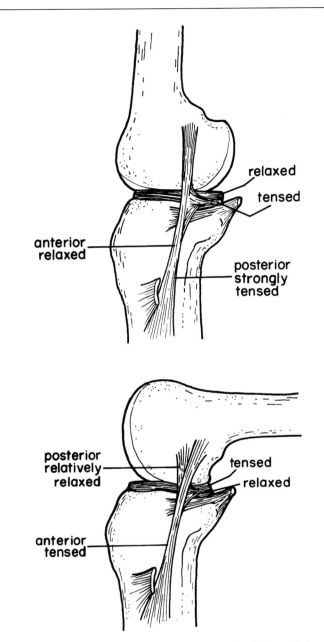

Fig. 2 **Top,** At full extension, the posterior margin of the medial collateral ligament (MCL) is tense while the anterior border is relatively relaxed. **Bottom,** In flexion, the posterior oblique fibers of the MCL become tense along with the anterior border of the MCL. The proximal posterior fibers are relatively relaxed.

tional moment, increased significantly with loss of the superficial MCL. Similarly, sectioning of other medial structures did not affect the external rotation instability.

The origin of the lateral collateral ligament (LCL) is at the lateral epicondyle of the femur, anterior to the origin of the gastrocnemius. The LCL forms a cordlike structure that runs beneath the lateral retinaculum to insert into the head of the fibula, and it blends with the tendon of the insertion of the biceps femoris. The function of the LCL is opposite to that of the MCL; the LCL restrains against varus rotation as well as resisting internal rotation. The LCL is taut in extension but is relaxed in flexion; thus, in flexion there is a greater degree of rotation laterally than medially. Data from cadaveric studies have indicated that the LCL is the primary restraint against varus moments at all degrees of knee flexion.

Cruciate Ligaments and Their Function

The anterior cruciate ligament (ACL) attaches to the posterior portion of the medial surface of the lateral femoral condyle in the form of a segment of a circle. It is oriented slightly oblique to the vertical, with the anterior side straight and the posterior side convex. The tibial attachment of the ACL is in a wide depressed area in front of and lateral to the anterior tibial spine. The average length of this ligament is 38 mm with an average width of 11 mm (Fig. 3).

The primary function of the ACL is to resist anterior displacement of the tibia on the femur when the knee is flexed. Data from experimental cadaveric studies have shown that at 90° of knee flexion, the ACL provides 85.1% ± 1.9% of the anterior restraining force. A secondary function of the ACL is to resist varus or valgus rotation of the tibia, especially in the absence of the collateral ligaments. The ACL also resists internal rotation of the tibia. Between 10° and 30° of knee flexion, internal rotation is limited by the ACL. Upon further flexion of the knee, the ACL slackens, and restraint to internal rotation is provided by anterolateral and posteromedial capsular structures.

The posterior cruciate ligament (PCL) originates at the lateral aspect of the medial femoral condyle and inserts at the most posterior aspect of the intercondylar area of the tibia. Its femoral attachment is shaped like a segment of a circle, horizontally directed, with the upper boundary of attachment horizontal and the lower boundary convex and parallel to the lower articular margin of the condyle. The average length of the PCL is 38 mm and its average width is 13 mm (Fig. 4).

The main function of the PCL is to resist posterior translation of the tibia relative to the femur. Data from cadaveric studies have shown that the PCL provides a mean 95% of the total restraining force against posterior translation at 90° of flexion, with similar results at 30° of flexion. Sectioning of the PCL results in increased external rotation of the tibia with increasing knee flexion.

Retention of the PCL in total knee replacement has been shown biomechanically to provide normal kinematic rollback of the femur on the tibia. Normal rollback is necessary for adequate flexion motion and normal muscle function. Passive kinematics of the knee can be increased

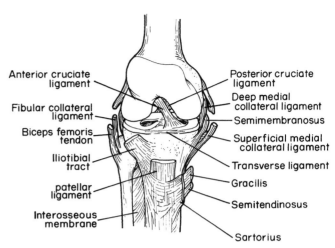

Fig. 3 Anterior view of the proximal portion of the tibia, distal portion of the femur, and accompanying soft-tissue structures.

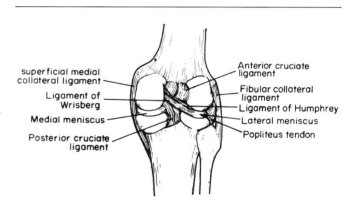

Fig. 4 Posterior view of the proximal portion of the tibia, distal portion of the femur, and accompanying soft-tissue structures.

through the rollback of the femur on the tibia, thus preventing the impingement of the femur on the posterior portion of the bony tibia with flexion. Between full extension and 90° of flexion, rollback mechanically changes the position of the tibiofemoral contact by approximately 14 mm. In effect, this amount of rollback represents an approximately 40% change in the lever arm of the quadriceps mechanism with flexion. Studies have shown that patients with PCL-retaining total knee designs demonstrated better stair climbing ability than patients with PCL-sacrificing or substituting total knee designs.

Knee Stability

Knee stability results from a complex interaction among ligaments, muscles, and other soft-tissue restraints; the geometry of the articulating surfaces; and the tibiofemoral reaction forces during weightbearing activities. These factors are all interdependent and allow for normal motion of the knee while limiting motion beyond a certain point.

Joint Surface

The articular surface of the femur has been described as a segment of a pulley. The two femoral condyles are convex in both planes and form the two lips of the pulley, which extends anteriorly to the pulley-shaped patellar surface. The neck of the pulley is formed anteriorly by the central groove on the patellar surface and posteriorly by the intercondylar notch. The articular surface of the medial femoral condyle is larger than that of the lateral femoral condyle.

The tibial surfaces in the frontal plane comprise two curved concave parallel gutters that are separated by a blunt eminence running anteroposteriorly. The lateral and medial condyles lie in each of the gutters and are separated by a blunt anteroposterior eminence that contains the two intercondylar tubercles. The tibial tubercles or spines, as they are sometimes called, contribute to stability by resisting side-to-side translation of the femur on the tibia (Fig. 5). In the sagittal plane, the medial condyle of the tibia is concave superiorly, and the lateral condyle is convex superiorly. Thus, the medial condyle is biconcave and

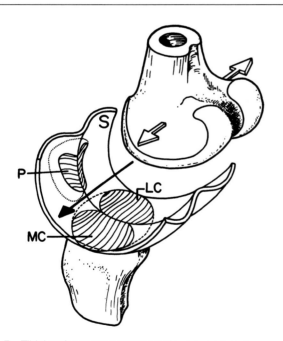

Fig. 5 Tibial surfaces are comprised of two curved and concave parallel gutters separated by a blunt eminence running anteroposteriorly. LC is lateral condyle, MC is medial condyle, P is patella and S is surface. The bottom arrow is the transverse axis of the tibia and the top arrow is the intercondylar axis. (Reproduced with permission from Kapandji IA: The knee, in Kapandji IA (ed): *The Physiology of the Joints: Annotated Diagrams of the Mechanics of the Human Joints,* ed 2. Edinburgh, Scotland, Churchill Livingstone, 1970.)

the lateral condyle is concave in the frontal plane and convex in the sagittal plane.

Cadaveric studies have shown that the geometric conformity of the condyles is the most important factor for decreased laxity under load-bearing conditions. Under these conditions, the anteroposterior, rotatory, and mediolateral movements of the femur on the tibia require that the femur must ride upward on the tibial curvature. This motion of the femur on the tibia has been called the "uphill principle."

The Menisci

The menisci have been shown to provide little resistance to medial-lateral movements of fully-extended cadaver knees under a compressive load. However, the menisci seemed to exert some stabilizing effects for both anterior-posterior and rotational displacements near full extension under a compressive load.

Although varus-valgus instability of the unloaded knee has been shown to increase after bilateral meniscectomy, varus-valgus stability of the loaded knee is unaffected by bicondylar meniscectomy.

Rotatory laxity in the cadaveric knee under loads varying from 0 to 100 kg has been evaluated. Rotatory laxity was noted to be quite variable, which was attributed to specimen variability. In approximately half of the bilateral meniscectomized cadaver knees tested, rotatory laxity increased by 14% for an applied torque of 5 kg·cm.

Loading and Stability

The effect of joint loading on stabilization of the knee joint has been studied extensively. When a tibiofemoral compressive force is applied across the knee joint, there is decreased joint laxity, and tibial translations and rotations resulting from the application of a given force or moment are decreased. It has been suggested that joint loading protects the ligaments of the knee joint from traumatic external loads by dynamically stabilizing the joint if the muscles are active prior to load application.

Dynamic loading of the knee joint has been shown to influence the progression of degenerative joint disease. Candidates for a high tibial osteotomy (HTO) for treatment of medial gonarthrosis have been shown to exhibit external loading (adduction moments) during presurgical gait that could be related to postoperative clinical outcome. The following example shows the interaction between muscle forces, ligaments, and external loading in providing dynamic stability to the knee joints of patients with lateral gonarthrosis during level walking.

The model of the knee joint used to study dynamic stability during gait of normal subjects and patients with varus deformities included the quadriceps, hamstring, and gastrocnemius muscles; a changing contact point between the tibia and femur; and the anterior and posterior cruciate and medial and lateral collateral ligaments. Input to the model consisted of knee flexion angle, external flexion/extension and abduction/adduction moments, and axial

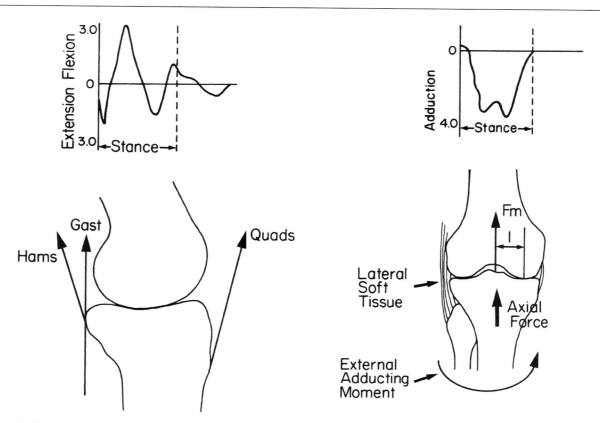

Fig. 6 **Left,** The external flexion moment was resisted by the quadriceps muscle group. The external extension moment was resisted by either the hamstring or gastrocnemius muscle groups. **Right,** The external adducting moment was resisted by the minimum sagittal plane muscle force (Fm) and axial load acting over (I). Pre-tension in the lateral soft tissues would maintain equilibrium if the muscle force was insufficient. (Reproduced with permission from Schipplein OD, Andriacchi TP: Interaction between active and passive knee stabilizers during level walking. *J Orthop Res* 1991;9:113–119.)

and anterior-posterior loads. The external flexion/extension (Fig. 6, *left*) and abduction/adduction (Fig. 6, *right*) moments acting at the knee joint are for normal level walking at a speed of 1 m/s. The flexion/extension moment (Fig. 6, *left*) pattern at the knee joint is biphasic in nature, tending to produce extension at heel-strike, flexion through midstance, extension in late stance, and flexion prior to toe-off. This moment pattern represents the net muscle activity of the flexor and extensor muscle groups at the knee. The presence of apparent muscle activity antagonistic to the primary function of balancing the external moment would require an incremental increase in the activity of the extensor or flexor muscles. For example, the model indicates that at heel strike, the net external moment tends to extend the knee as would occur at heel strike during normal walking. Myoelectric activity measurements consistently show that both extensor and flexor muscle activity is present. Thus, if a person were to balance the external moment tending to extend the joint, only flexors would be present. The abduction/adduction moment pattern (Fig. 6, *right*) at the knee produces an abduction moment at heel

strike and quickly reverses to a moment that produces adduction at the knee for the remainder of stance phase.

The model predicted that the contributions of both active and passive forces were necessary to balance the adduction moment during stance phase (both in patients that were candidates for HTO and in normal subjects during level walking) and, thereby, to produce a knee with dynamic lateral stability (no lateral joint opening). For the normal group with no antagonistic muscle force, it was not possible to balance the adducting moment; this imbalance resulted in lateral joint opening. Antagonistic muscle activity or lateral soft-tissue pre-tension was necessary to stabilize the knee without lateral joint opening (Fig. 7).

The HTO candidate group had a higher adducting moment than the normal subjects. The model predicted that 65% of the HTO candidate group had lateral joint opening when no antagonistic muscle activity or passive soft tissue pre-tension was present. The HTO candidate group relied on lateral soft-tissue pre-tension to maintain equilibrium for a lower percentage of time during stance phase than did the normal group.

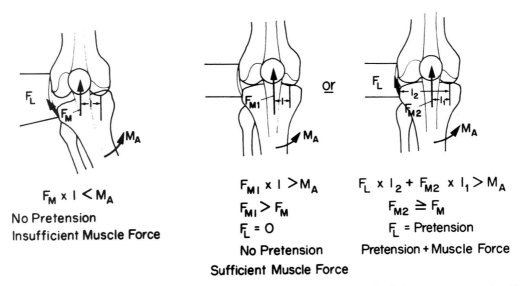

$$F_M \times I < M_A$$

No Pretension
Insufficient Muscle Force

$$F_{MI} \times I > M_A$$
$$F_{MI} > F_M$$
$$F_L = 0$$

No Pretension
Sufficient Muscle Force

$$F_L \times I_2 + F_{M2} \times I_1 > M_A$$
$$F_{M2} \geqq F_M$$
$$F_L = \text{Pretension}$$

Pretension + Muscle Force

Fig. 7   The knee joint was predicted to remain closed laterally if either pretension in the lateral soft tissues was present and/or increased muscle force resulting from antagonistic muscle groups. The distances I and I_1 are equal to 20 mm; I_2 equals 60 mm. F_L is soft tissue force; F_{m2} F_{m1}, F_{m2} are muscle forces; M_A is adducting moment. (Reproduced with permission from Schipplein OD, Andriacchi TP: Interaction between active and passive knee stabilizers during level walking. *J Orthop Res* 1991;9:113–119.)

Results of this study were consistent with those of previously reported studies in that the flexors and extensors, in addition to axial loads, are capable of stabilizing the knee joint against an adducting moment. Dynamic instability (lateral joint opening) of the knee can be delayed by increasing the compressive force acting at the knee through an increase in the quadriceps and hamstring forces.

Ligamentous Stability

The ligamentous structures provide stability to the knee through their ability to resist externally applied forces at the joint and, thus, limit motion. The orientation of the ligaments is such that rotational and translational displacements can be resisted for almost all directions of applied external force. Individual ligaments have fiber orientations that can resist more than one direction of external force. The roles of individual ligaments in providing ligamentous stability are extremely complicated because no one structure acts alone in resisting an applied external force. In addition, the presence of "coupled" motion at the knee implies that motions due to externally applied forces occur in more than one plane simultaneously.

The LCL acts primarily as a stabilizer against a varus moment in resisting varus rotation. It also acts as a stabilizer against external rotation of the tibia.

The PCL acts primarily as a stabilizer against posterior translation of the tibia. After serial cutting, no other structure at the knee joint accounts for more than 2% additional secondary stabilizing restraint against posterior

translation. The PCL's secondary function is to stabilize the knee against valgus rotation of the knee at full extension. The stabilizing effects of the PCL are maximum against external rotation at 30° of knee flexion and diminish with further flexion.

The retention of the PCL in total knee replacement can influence passive range of motion and rollback; the PCL also provides stability to the knee by transferring forces to the bone via the ligaments, rather than relying on the constraint provided by the prosthesis. During level walking and stair climbing, the predominant shear force tends to push back on the tibia. In the presence of the PCL, this shear force is reduced on the bone-prosthesis interface.

The ACL's primary function is to stabilize the tibia against an anterior displacement. At 90° of knee flexion, the ACL provides 85% of the anterior restraining force. The remaining ligamentous structures offer little restraint to anterior displacement. The ACL also provides rotatory stability to the knee joint in resisting internal rotation.

Recent studies have illustrated how the knee adapts to loss of the stability-providing function of the ACL after injury. Sixteen patients with unilateral deficiency of the ACL and ten healthy subjects used as a control were analyzed during level walking, stair climbing (ascending and descending), and jogging. The greatest changes in parameters measured in the gait laboratory occurred during level walking. The majority of the patients with ACL-deficient knees had changes in the flexion/extension moment pattern at the knee joint (Fig. 8). The external moment at the knee must be balanced by an internal moment, which is

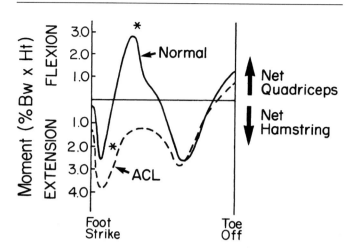

Fig. 8 Patients with an anterior cruciate ligament deficiency primarily had an external extension moment throughout stance phase for level walking as indicated by the dashed line. The solid line indicates the normal biphasic pattern. The asterisks indicate the times during stance phase when the moments about the knees of the control subjects and the patients were significantly different. (Reproduced with permission from Berchuck M, Andriacchi TP, Bach BR, et al: Gait adaptations by patients who have a deficient anterior cruciate ligament. *J Bone Joint Surg* 1990;72A:871–877.)

generated by the muscles crossing the knee. The changes in the ACL-deficient knees were reflected by a reduction in the magnitude of the external flexion moment at the knee joint during the midstance of the gait cycle. This reduced moment was reflected as a decrease in the demand placed on the quadriceps muscles and has been termed a "quadriceps avoidance" gait. Of the patients tested who had ACL-deficient knees, 75% had the quadriceps avoidance pattern and 25% had a normal biphasic flexion/extension pattern.

Results obtained during jogging and stair climbing did not indicate that the quadriceps avoidance pattern was a result of muscle weakness. The magnitude of the flexion/extension moment at the knee during jogging was 4.5 times that during level walking, and it was substantially larger during stair climbing. During jogging, the patients had a 25% reduction in the quadriceps moment, whereas during stair climbing, patterns and magnitudes of the quadriceps moment were essentially the same for patients and normal subjects.

It is hypothesized that patients with an ACL-deficient knee walk with a quadriceps avoidance pattern to prevent anterior displacement of the tibia. Contraction of the quadriceps produces an anteriorly directed force on the tibia when the knee is near full extension. As the knee is flexed, the pull by the patellar mechanism is reduced as the knee approaches 45° of flexion. Beyond 45° of flexion, the pull by the patellar mechanism reverses from a force on the tibia that is anteriorly directed to one that is posteri-

orly directed. This adaptation in patients with ACL deficiencies minimizes the demands placed on the quadriceps during level walking in which the knee is near full extension (approximately 20° maximum flexion during stance phase). However, during activities, such as jogging (the knee is flexed approximately 40°) and stair climbing (the knee is flexed approximately 60°), the pull by the patellar mechanism is directed posteriorly, acting as a secondary restraint to anterior displacement of the tibia.

This example indicates the importance of maintaining muscle mass after injury about the knee. Rehabilitation of the quadriceps and strengthening of the hamstrings has been recognized as a mechanism for stabilizing the knee in the absence of the ACL.

Patellofemoral Mechanics

The patella is roughly triangular when viewed anteriorly, it is wider superiorly and tapers inferiorly. The articular surface of the patella consists of seven facets, which are divided vertically into approximately equal thirds on the lateral and medial sides. The seventh or odd facet lies along the extreme medial border of the patella. The articular surfaces formed by the femur and the patella do not conform exactly. The contact area varies as a function of knee flexion, starting from distal and moving proximal with increasing knee flexion. The odd facet is in contact with the femur in the intercondylar notch at knee flexion angles between 120° and 135°.

The patellofemoral joint has been described as having five mechanical functions: (1) it increases the effective lever arm of the quadriceps; (2) it provides functional stability under load by providing the opposing articular surface of the trochlea; (3) it allows the transmission of the quadriceps force to the tibia through the quadriceps mechanism; (4) it provides a bony shield to the trochlea and the condyles of the distal femur when the knee is flexed; and (5) it cosmetically improves the appearance of the knee in flexion, eliminating exposure of the femoral condyles. This section examines the motion of the patellofemoral joint, contact areas, force transmission, and stability.

Motion

The motion of the patellofemoral joint can be characterized as gliding and sliding. During flexion of the knee, the patella moves distally on the femur while turning on itself about a transverse axis. This movement is governed by its attachments to the quadriceps tendon, ligamentum patellae, and the anterior aspects of the femoral condyles.

Three-dimensional (3-D) tracking of the patella has been analyzed by correlating patellar motion with respect to the topography of the trochlear surface of the femur and the retropatellar surface. Patellar motion between 0° and 120° of knee flexion was measured in ten fresh-frozen cadaveric specimens. Loads to reproduce static lifting were applied to the quadriceps muscle group of each specimen.

Results from this study demonstrated that the complex 3-D motion of the patella was governed by the trochlear topography. Variations between specimens were attributed to abnormalities in trochlear topography.

Contact Areas

The contact areas of the patellofemoral joint determine the ability of the patella to transmit to the trochlear surface load resulting from activity of the quadriceps muscles. Contact between the patella and the trochlear surface is initiated between 10° and 20° of knee flexion along a narrow band across the medial and lateral facets of the inferior margin of the patella. With increasing knee flexion, the contact areas move proximally on the patella extending from the ridge separating the medial from the odd facet to the lateral border of the lateral facet. The area in contact increases with increasing knee flexion. At approximately 90° of flexion, the articular surface of the patella contacts the lower part of the femoral trochlea. Beyond 90° of flexion, the tendinous band of the quadriceps shares in load transmission from the extensor mechanism. After 120° of knee flexion, the articular surface of the patella is in contact with the femoral condyles.

Forces and Force Transmission

The muscles and ligaments of the patellofemoral joint are responsible for producing extension of the knee. The patella acts as a pulley in transmitting the force developed by the quadriceps muscles to the femur and the patellar ligament. It also increases the extensor lever arm of the quadriceps muscle force relative to the instant center of rotation of the knee.

The force transmission of the patellofemoral mechanism has been shown to be a function of knee flexion. As the knee flexes, the patellofemoral joint reaction force (PFJRF) increases. This increasing PFJRF is distributed over a greater area between the patella and the femoral articulating surface, because the patellofemoral articulating area also increases as a function of knee flexion. With increasing knee flexion, the extensor lever arm increases in the range of 30° to 70° of knee flexion, thus increasing the mechanical advantage of the quadriceps. The ratio of the forces in the patellar tendon to forces in the patellar ligament also changes as a function of knee flexion (Fig. 9). Between 0° to 15° of knee flexion the ratio of the forces changes little from unity. Between 15° and 80° of knee flexion, the ratio decreases by approximately 40%. Beyond 80° of knee flexion to 120° the ratio increases slightly. The change in the ratio between the forces in the patellar tendon and the forces in the patellar ligament as a function of knee flexion is due primarily to the geometry of the patellofemoral mechanism.

Forces acting on the retropatellar surface depend on both the magnitude of the quadriceps force and the angle

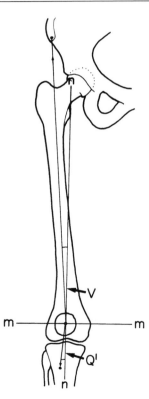

Fig. 10 The Q-angle is composed of a proximal part, V, related to the valgus angle, and a distal part, Q'(Q = V + Q'). The proximal angle is measured here between lines from the anterior-superior iliac spine to the center of the patella and the tibial axis (n-n). Line m-m was drawn parallel to the tibiofemoral joint line. (Reproduced with permission from Hvid I: The stability of the human patello–femoral joint. *Eng Med* 1983;12:55–59.)

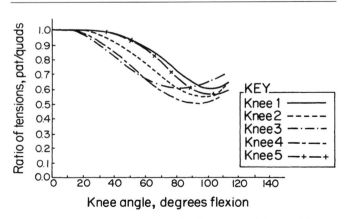

Fig. 9 The ratio between the patellar ligament and the quadriceps tendon at different angles of knee flexion for the five knees tested. (Reproduced with permission from Ellis MI, Seedhom BB, Wright V, et al: An Evaluation of the ratio between the tensions along the quadriceps tendon and the patellar ligament. *Eng Med* 1980;9:189–194.)

of knee flexion. The magnitude of the retropatellar force is relatively low when the knee is near full extension and increases as the knee flexes in the range between 0° and 40°. The retropatellar force reaches its maximum at knee flexion angles between 60° and 90°. The location of the retropatellar force with respect to the patella changes with knee flexion. At full extension, the retropatellar force is located distally on the patella, and it moves proximal with increasing knee flexion. The magnitude of the retropatellar force and its location on the patella are important considerations in total knee replacement. Analysis of failed patellar components has indicated that the shear component of the retropatellar force is the predominant factor leading to failure. A shift from normal in patellar kinematics will cause eccentric loading, which can increase the shear forces responsible for failure.

Stability

Stability of the patellofemoral joint is governed by both anatomic and biomechanical factors. Stability is provided by the articulating surfaces of the trochlea and the patella

as well as by the muscles that form the quadriceps mechanism.

The biomechanics of the patellofemoral joint has been examined using cadavers to investigate the ways stability is provided to the knee joint. The quadriceps muscle does not act in a straight line from the head of the femur to the center of the patella. Instead, it acts along a line parallel to the long axis of the femur. The angle formed between the lines joining the anterior superior iliac spine to the center of the patella and the center of the patella to the tibial tuberosity is defined as the Q-angle (Fig. 10). Stability to the flexed knee is provided between the articulating surfaces of the patella and the femoral trochlea. However, when the knee is fully extended, there is little contact between the patella and the femoral trochlea. Thus, during the early part of flexion (0° to 30°) stability is provided by the vastus medialis obliquus fibers of the quadriceps muscle. The Q-angle is greatest during the early part of knee flexion. It decreases with increasing knee flexion because of internal rotation of the tibia with respect to the femur.

Annotated Bibliography

Motion of the Knee

Blankevoort L, Huiskes R, de Lange A: Helical axes of passive knee joint motions. *J Biomech* 1990;23:1219–1229.

Finite helical axes for passive knee motion were determined in vitro for four knees. The three dimensional patterns of the helical motion were found to be reproducible and consistent for a flexion motion with an internal torque of 3N·m and an external torque of 3 N·m.

Lafortune MA, Cavanaugh PR, Sommer HJ, et al: Three-dimensional kinematics of the human knee during walking. *J Biomech* 1992;25:347–357.

Three-dimensional kinematics of the tibiofemoral joint were studied during level walking. Markers were fixed in the femur and tibia by means of intracortical traction pins. Motion between the tibia and femur was resolved with respect to a joint coordinate system for five subjects.

Articular Surfaces

Insall JN: Anatomy of the knee, in Insall JN, Windsor RE, Scott NW, et al (eds): *Surgery of the Knee,* ed 2. New York, NY, Churchill Livingstone, 1993.

A detailed description of the anatomy of the knee joint is provided along with a description of the motion and function of the ligaments.

Main WK, Scott WN: Knee anatomy, in Scott WN (ed): *Ligament and Extensor Mechanism Injuries of the Knee: Diagnosis and Treatment.* St. Louis, MO, Mosby Yearbook, 1991, pp 13–32.

A comprehensive description of the anatomy of the knee and function of individual structures.

The Menisci and Their Function

Renstrom P, Johnson RJ: Anatomy and biomechanics of the menisci. *Clin Sports Med* 1990;9:523–538.

The structure and shape of the menisci are optimal for weightbearing and shock absorption. The menisci maintain knee joint stability and congruity resist capsular and synovial impingement during knee motion, support the screw home mechanism and distribute load over a large area of the articular surface. It is the recommendation of this study, because of the roles the menisci play, to preserve the menisci when performing knee surgery.

Collateral Ligaments and Their Function

Gollehon DL, Torzilli PA, Warren RF: Abstract: The role of the posterolateral and cruciate ligaments in human knee stability: A biomechanical study. *Trans Orthop Res Soc* 1985;10:270.

This abstract describes a biomechanical study of the role of posterolateral and cruciate ligaments. The LCL provides restraint against varus and external tibial rotation at all angles of knee flexion and provides restraint against posterior translation at 0° and 30° of knee flexion.

Shapiro MS, Markolf KL, Finerman GA, et al: The effect of section of the medial collateral ligament on force generated in the anterior cruciate ligament. *J Bone Joint Surg* 1991;73A:248–256.

In the presence of an anteriorly directed force to the tibia of an intact knee, the force generated in the anterior cruciate ligament increased. This force was maximum near the middle part of the range of tibial rotation and minimum with external rotation of the tibia. Upon sectioning of the medial collateral ligament, the force generated in the anterior cruciate ligament did not change due to straight anterior tibial pull near the middle part of the range of tibial rotation.

Cruciate Ligaments and Their Function

Amis AA, Dawkins GPC: Functional anatomy of the anterior cruciate ligament: Fibre bundle actions related to ligament replacements and injuries. *J Bone Joint Surg* 1991;73B:260–267.

The authors studied the fiber bundle anatomy of the anterior cruciate ligament. The bundles identified consisted of the anteromedial, intermediate and the posterolateral bundle. Their contributions in resisting anterior subluxation in flexion and extension and tibial rotation were measured and reported in this manuscript.

Bassette GC, Hunter RE: The anterior cruciate ligament: A review. *Orthopedics* 1990;13:551–562.

This review article describes current knowledge of the anterior cruciate ligament. It addresses gross anatomy, vascular anatomy, and nerve supply; histology, biomechanics, mechanism of injury, diagnosis, associated pathology, natural history of the anterior cruciate deficient knee, treatment with functional bracing, operative treatment, extra-articular reconstruction, intra-articular and combined reconstruction, and rehabilitation.

Fuss FK: The restraining function of the cruciate ligaments on hyperextension and hyperflexion of the human knee joint. *Anat Rec* 1991;230:283–289.

The anterior and posterior cruciate ligaments each contain different fiber bundles that are taut at different angles of knee flexion. Fibers that are taut in extreme positions serve as restraints for hyperextension and hyperflexion.

Grood ES, Stowers SF, Noyes FR: Limits of movement in the human knee: Effect of sectioning the posterior cruciate ligament and posterolateral structures. *J Bone Joint Surg* 1988;70A:88–97.

Limits of movement for anterior-posterior tibial translation, internal and external rotation, and varus and valgus angulation were experimentally determined from 0° to 90° of knee flexion. Limits were measured in the intact knee and after serial cutting of the posterior cruciate ligament, lateral collateral ligament, popliteus tendon at its femoral attachment, and the arcuate complex.

Noyes FR, Stowers SF, Grood ES, et al: Posterior subluxations of the medial and lateral tibiofemoral compartments: An in vitro ligament sectioning study in cadaveric knees. *Am J Sports Med* 1993;21:407–414.

This article reports an in vitro cadaveric study that examined the abnormal increases in posterior subluxation of the medial and lateral tibial plateaus after sectioning the posterolateral structures and posterior cruciate ligament. Upon sectioning the posterior cruciate ligament and posterolateral structures, statistically significant increases in posterior translation of both the medial and lateral tibial plateaus occurred at 30° and 90° of flexion.

Takai S, Woo SL, Livesay GA, et al: Determination of the in situ loads on the human anterior cruciate ligament. *J Orthop Res* 1993;11:686–695.

Information provided by this study describes the function of the anterior cruciate ligament in response to external loading of the intact knee.

Knee Stability

Joint Surface

Bruns J, Volkmer M, Luessenhop S: Pressure distribution in the knee joint: Influence of flexion with and without ligament dissection. *Arch Orthop Trauma Surg* 1994;113:204–209.

The biomechanical factors influencing the patterns of pressure distribution at the articular surface and the subchondral bone are suggested to be the most important in the pathogenesis of osteoarthritis and osteochondritis dissecans at the knee joint. A cadaver model was used to investigate the patterns of pressure distribution on the femoral condyles of weightbearing knee joints.

The Menisci

Ihn JC, Kim SJ, Park IH: In vitro study of contact area and pressure distribution in the human knee after partial and total meniscectomy. *Int Orthop* 1993;17:214–218.

The study reports the contact area and pressure distribution after partial or total meniscectomy. By measuring the contact area after meniscectomy they showed that the meniscus performs a load transmitting function in the knee joint. The degree of stress concentration in the contact area was increased when part or all of the meniscus was removed. The changes in the contact area of the opposite side (intact) were minimal after partial meniscectomy but significant after total meniscectomy.

Thompson WO, Fu FH: The meniscus in the anterior cruciate-deficient knee. *Clin Sports Med* 1993;12:771–796.

Meniscectomy is implicated as a primary factor in the premature development of osteoarthritis of the knee joint. In the anterior-cruciate-deficient knee the menisci have been shown to enhance the knee's stability in anteroposterior, varus-valgus and internal-external directions in vitro.

Loading and Stability

Goh JC, Bose K, Khoo BC: Gait analysis study on patients with osteoarthritis of the knee. *Clin Orthop* 1993;294:223–231.

The study examined biomechanical changes that occur after high tibial osteotomy in 30 patients with osteoarthritis of the knee and 11 normal age-matched subjects. The study indicated that there was an overall improvement in the gait parameters measured following surgery. Of the surgically treated knees with good or excellent clinical results, 57% had abnormal load distributions. This abnormal loading may lead to deterioration of the joint in the future.

Hsu RWW, Himeno S, Coventry MB, et al: Normal axial alignment of the lower extremity and load-bearing distribution at the knee. *Clin Orthop* 1990;255:215–227.

Based on a mathematical model, the load-bearing distribution at the knee joint was studied using the geometry of the knee obtained from roentgenogram from 120 normal subjects. The authors observed that female subjects had a higher peak joint pressure and a greater patellotibial Q angle.

Schipplein OD, Andriacchi TP: Interaction between active and passive stabilizers during level walking. *J Orthop Res* 1991;9:113–119.

The interaction between dynamic (muscular) and passive (ligamentous) restraints effecting lateral stability of the knee was studied in both normal subjects and patients with varus deformities of the knee. Model results indicated that in normal subjects the midstance adduction moments would cause lateral knee joint opening if either antagonistic muscle force and/or pretension of the lateral soft tissues were not present at the knee. The patient group compensated for the higher than normal midstance phase adducting moment by walking with a style of gait that demanded more muscle force (increased flexion-extension moment at the knee).

Ligamentous Stability

Berchuck M, Andriacchi TP, Bach BR, et al: Gait adaptations by patients who have a deficient anterior cruciate ligament. *J Bone Joint Surg* 1990;72A:871–877.

This gait study examined 16 unilateral ACL deficient patients and 10 healthy control subjects during level walking, ascending and descending stairs, and jogging. During level walking, the maximum moment that tends to flex the knee was reduced by 140%. During jogging this moment was reduced by 30% and was not changed during descending stairs, and was slightly increased during ascending stairs. Results from this study are explained in terms of altering one's gait to avoid anterior displacement of the proximal end of the tibia that is normally produced when the quadriceps are contracted while the knee is in nearly full extension (ie, during level walking).

Johansson H, Sjolander P, Sojka P: Receptors in the knee joint ligaments and their role in the biomechanics of the joint. *Crit Rev Biomed Eng* 1991;18:341–368.

Knee joint ligaments contain Ruffini, Pacinian, Golgi, and free-nerve endings that provide the central nervous system with information about movement and position as well as noxious events. The primary muscle spindle afferent nerves participate in the regulation of muscular stiffness; the receptors in the knee joint probably contribute to the preparatory adjustment of the stiffness of the muscles around the knee joint and, thereby, to the overall joint stiffness and the functional joint stability.

Noyes FR, Schipplein OD, Andriacchi TP, et al: The anterior cruciate ligament-deficient knee with varus alignment: An analysis of gait adaptations and dynamic joint loadings. *Am J Sports Med* 1991;20:707–716.

The forces and moments were measured during level walking at the knee joint for 32 ACL-deficient patients. The majority of the patients had an abnormally high adduction moment at the affected knee. The adduction moment showed a statistical significant correlation to high medial tibiofemoral compartment loads and high lateral soft-tissue forces. The paper points out that any combination of conditions leading to higher medial joint forces is associated with factors leading to more rapid degeneration of the medial compartment in patients with ACL deficiencies, varus deformity and lax lateral ligaments.

Patellofemoral Mechanics

Motion

Ahmed AM, Chan KH, Shi S, et al: Correlation of patellar tracking motion with the articular surface topography. *Trans Orthop Res Soc* 1989;14:202.

The study correlated the three-dimensional (3-D) tracking motion of the patella with the topographies of the trochlear surface of the femur and of the retropatellar surface in ten fresh-frozen cadaver knees. Results of the study indicate that the 3-D tracking motion is governed by the trochlear topography. This motion is altered in the knees with severe aberrations in the quadriceps tension, soft-tissue structures or in knees with abnormal retropatellar topography.

Hehne HJ: Biomechanics of the patellofemoral joint and its clinical relevance. *Clin Orthop* 1990;158:73–85.

This study analyzes the patellofemoral joint based on experimental determinations of pressure distributions on the patellar cartilage and vectoral calculations of forces acting on the patellar mechanism. The contact areas on the articulating surface of the patella change as a function of knee flexion. The lateral to medial ratio of contact areas, pressing forces, cartilage areas and bone mass was found to always be 1.6:1. The mean pressure was found to be the same in both facets.

Lengsfeld M, Ahlers J, Ritter G: Kinematics of the patellofemoral joint. *Arch Orthop Trauma Surg* 1990; 109:280–283.

A mathematical computer model of the patellofemoral joint was used to study kinematics. The model revealed the changing contact between the articulating surfaces of the patella and the femoral trochlea. Implications of these results were discussed in terms of surgical internal fixation of patella fractures.

Contact Areas

Hefzy MS, Yang H: A three-dimensional anatomical model of the human patello-femoral joint, for the determination of patello-femoral motions and contact characteristics. *J Biomed Eng* 1993;15:289–302.

The purpose of the study was to develop a three-dimensional mathematical model of the patellofemoral joint, for the purpose of studying patellar motion and contact characteristics.

Forces and Force Transmission

Ahmed AM, Burke DL, Hyder A: Force analysis of the patellar mechanisms. *J Orthop Res* 1987;5:69–85.

This study experimentally evaluated the force analysis of the patellar mechanism assuming the patellofemoral joint is frictionless. The force ratio between the ligamentum patellae and the rectus femoris was measured in ten specimens during simulation of leg raising against a resistance and static lifting. The ratio increases with increasing knee flexion up to 30°, decreases up to 90°, and increases beyond 90°.

Buff HU, Jones LC, Hungerford DS: Experimental determination of forces transmitted through the patello-femoral joint. *J Biomech* 1988;21:17–23.

Tensions in the quadriceps tendon and the infrapatellar ligament were measured in eight cadaveric knees using a load cell. The ratio between the tensions in the quadriceps tendon and infrapatellar ligament ranged from 1.55 at 70° of flexion and decreased to 0.86° at 10° of flexion. The patellofemoral joint reaction force for extension against resistance was maximum at 60° of knee flexion.

Kaufman KR, An KN, Litchy WJ, et al: Dynamic joint forces during knee isokinetic exercise. *Am J Sports Med* 1991;19:305–316.

Forces in the tibiofemoral and patellofemoral joints during isokinetic exercise were analyzed using an analytical biomechanical model. During extension exercises, the loads in the patellofemoral joint can be as high as 5.1 body weight, which are 10 times higher than during straight leg raises. The results from this study indicate that isokinetic exercise should be used cautiously in patients with knee lesions.

Skyhar MJ, Warren RF, Ortiz GJ, et al: The effects of sectioning of the posterior cruciate ligament and the posterolateral complex on the articular contact pressures within the knee. *J Bone Joint Surg* 1993;75:694–699.

Measurements of the articular contact pressures in ten cadaveric knees with intact ligaments and sequentially sectioned posterior cruciate ligament and the posterolateral complex were obtained using film and a model that simulated nonweightbearing resistive extension of the knee. Patellofemoral pressures increased with the sectioning of the posterior cruciate ligament and the posterolateral complex compared to the intact knee.

Stability

Anouchi YS, Whiteside LA, Kaiser AD, et al: The effects of axial rotation alignment of the femoral component on knee stability and patellar tracking in total knee arthroplasty demonstrated on autopsy specimens. *Clin Orthop* 1993;287:170–177.

A cadaver study that examined knee stability, patellar tracking, and patellofemoral contact points with a femoral component positioned in 5° internal, 5° external or neutral rotational alignment of the femoral component referenced on the posterior femoral condyles. The study showed that internal rotation of the femoral component in the knee with perpendicular resection of the tibia causes undesirable changes in knee stability, patellar tracking, and patellofemoral contact points. The study also showed that neutral positioning produces similar but less negative effects on knee stability and patellar kinematics. However, it was shown that external rotation improves both patellar tracking and knee stability characteristics.

Heegaard J, Leyvraz PF, Van Kampen A, et al: Influence of soft structures on patellar three-dimensional tracking. *Clin Orthop* 1994;299:235–243.

The human patella moves along a complex path during flexion of the knee joint resulting from combined actions of the articular contact and soft-tissue stabilization. The present study characterizes the role of these soft-tissue structures on patellar kinematics. The study suggests that control of patellar motion is governed by the transverse soft-tissue structures near extension and by the patellofemoral joint geometry during further flexion.

Classic Bibliography

Motion of the Knee

Beer FP, Johnston ER (eds): *Vector Mechanics for Engineers: Dynamics,* ed 5. New York, NY, McGraw-Hill, 1988.

Fischer O, Braune CW (eds): *Der Gang Des Menschen.* Leipzig, Belgium, BG Teubner, 1901.

Freudenstein F, Woo LS: Kinematics of the human knee joint. *Bull Math Biophys* 1969;31:215–232.

Kapandji IA (ed): *The Physiology of the Joints: Annotated Diagrams of the Mechanics of the Human Joints,* ed 2. Edinburgh, United Kingdom, Churchill Livingstone, 1970, vol 2.

Townsend MA, Izak M, Jackson RW: Total motion knee goniometry. *J Biomech* 1977;10:183–193.

Articular Surfaces

Hallen LG, Lindahl O: The "screw-home" movement in the knee-joint. *Acta Orthop Scand* 1966;37:97–106.

Kettelkamp DB, Jacobs AW: Tibiofemoral contact area: Determination and implications. *J Bone Joint Surg* 1972;54A:349–356.

The Menisci and Their Function

Brantigan OC, Voshell AF: The mechanics of the ligaments and menisci of the knee joint. *J Bone Joint Surg* 1941;23:44–66.

Iseki F, Tomatsu T: The biomechanics of the knee joint with special reference to the contact area. *Keio J Med* 1976;25:37–44.

Walker PS, Erkman MJ: The role of the menisci in force transmission across the knee. *Clin Orthop* 1975;109:184–192.

Walker PS, Hajek JV: The load-bearing area in the knee joint. *J Biomech* 1972;5:581–589.

Collateral Ligaments and Their Function

Grood ES, Noyes FR, Butler DL, et al: Ligamentous and capsular restraints preventing straight medial and lateral laxity in intact human cadaver knees. *J Bone Joint Surg* 1981;63A:1257–1269.

Seering WP, Piziali RL, Nagel DA, et al: The function of the primary ligaments of the knee in varus-valgus and axial rotation. *J Biomech* 1980;13:785–794.

Warren LA, Marshall JL, Girgis F: The prime static stabilizer of the medial side of the knee. *J Bone Joint Surg* 1974;56A:665–674.

Warren LF, Marshall JL: The supporting structures and layers on the medial side of the knee: An anatomical analysis. *J Bone Joint Surg* 1979;61A:56–62.

Cruciate Ligaments and Their Function

Butler DL, Noyes FR, Grood ES: Ligamentous restraints to anterior-posterior drawer in the human knee: A biomechanical study. *J Bone Joint Surg* 1980;62A:259–270.

Girgis FG, Marshall JL, Monajem A: The cruciate ligaments of the knee joint: Anatomical, functional and experimental analysis. *Clin Orthop* 1975;106:216–231.

Kennedy JC, Grainger RW: The posterior cruciate ligament. *J Trauma* 1967;7:367–377.

Lipke JM, Janecki CJ, Nelson CL, et al: The role of incompetence of the anterior cruciate and lateral ligaments in anterolateral and anteromedial instability: A biomechanical study of cadaver knees. *J Bone Joint Surg* 1981;63A:954–960.

Knee Stability

Hsieh H-H, Walker PS: Stabilizing mechanisms of the loaded and unloaded knee joint. *J Bone Joint Surg* 1976;58A:87–93.

Johnson RJ, Pope MH: Knee joint stability without reference to ligamentous function, in McCollister Evarts CM (ed): American Academy of Orthopaedic Surgeons *Symposium on Reconstructive Surgery of the Knee.* St. Louis, MO, CV Mosby, 1978, pp 14–25.

Markolf KL, Bargar WL, Shoemaker SC, et al: The role of joint load in knee stability. *J Bone Joint Surg* 1981; 63A:570–585.

Markolf KL, Mensch JS, Amstutz HC: Stiffness and laxity of the knee: The contributions of the supporting structures. A quantitative in vitro study. *J Bone Joint Surg* 1976;58A:583–594.

Seebacher JR, Inglis AE, Marshall JL, et al: The structure of the posterolateral aspect of the knee. *J Bone Joint Surg* 1982;64A:536–541.

Shoemaker SC, Markolf KL: In vivo rotatory knee stability: Ligamentous and muscular contributions. *J Bone Joint Surg* 1982;64A:208–216.

Wang C-J, Walker PS: Rotatory laxity of the human knee joint. *J Bone Joint Surg* 1974;56A:161–170.

Patellofemoral Mechanics

Ahmed AM, Burke DL, Yu A: In-vitro measurement of static pressure distribution in synovial joints: Part II. Retropatellar Surface. *J Biomech Engin* 1983;105:226–236.

Ellis MI, Seedhom BB, Wright V, et al: An Evaluation of the ratio between the tensions along the quadriceps tendon and the patellar ligament. *Eng Med* 1980;9: 189–194.

Huberti HH, Hayes WC: Patellofemoral contact pressures: The influence of q-angle and tendofemoral contact. *J Bone Joint Surg* 1984;66A:715–724.

Hungerford DS, Barry M: Biomechanics of the patellofemoral joint. *Clin Orthop* 1979;144:9–15.

Hvid I: The stability of the human patello-femoral joint. *Eng Med* 1983;12:55–59.

Matthews LS, Sonstegard DA, Henke JA: Load bearing characteristics of the patello-femoral joint. *Acta Orthop Scand* 1977;48:511–516.

27

Evaluation of the Patient With an Arthritic Knee: History, Examination, Structured Assessment, and Radiologic Evaluation

Overview

The principal reason for evaluating a patient with knee arthritis is clearly to establish the patient's overall medical status, local knee joint status, and the outcomes of care delivered. Patient history, physical examination, and review of previous medical records supplemented with radiographic and laboratory evaluations form the foundation for subsequent decision making and care delivery.

Local knee joint pathology varies substantially, and accurate delineation of the type of knee arthritis can significantly impact the outcomes of treatment. Although patients with posttraumatic arthritis have an increased likelihood of revision surgery following knee arthroplasty, patients with rheumatoid arthritis who undergo knee arthroplasty are more likely to experience a late infection.

Disease severity also impacts outcomes. For example, patients with unicompartmental disease and better range of motion, who are treated with unicompartmental arthroplasty, will have better postoperative range of motion than those treated by tricompartmental arthroplasty. Patients with osteoarthritis who are undergoing revision surgery have a higher likelihood of complications than those undergoing primary arthroplasty.

The average patient receiving knee replacement in the United States is over 65 years of age. Older patients expect treatment of their arthritis despite having more medical comorbidities. This makes the assessment of therapeutic risks and benefits for treatment more difficult. A corollary of increased medical complexity is that there is increased potential for both complications and less optimal outcomes.

In addition to different medical conditions, each person presents with individual values about health as well as different knee-specific concerns. These different value systems can substantially affect therapeutic decisions for that person. Surgical judgment requires knowledge of the therapeutic interventions that will address a specific set of patient's needs and expectations. The relative risks and the potential benefits for each set of therapeutic options must be determined for each patient and a plan of action established. Maximization of patient satisfaction and quality of health care requires (1) sufficient baseline medical information, (2) knowledge of therapeutic options, (3) communication, (4) shared decision making, and (5) excellent execution of the treatment plan.

Because of the complexity of the medical process, it is not surprising that the performance of knee replacement in the United States is quite variable. This variation is being carefully evaluated in light of a projected annual expenditure of over $3.5 billion on knee replacement. The establishment of accountability for medical decisions, actions taken, and treatment outcomes is becoming increasingly important in the current health reform climate.

Currently, the measurement process is being used to provide the foundation for outcomes determination and assurance of health-care system quality. Multiple clinical measures have historically been proposed for patient assessment. Because these clinical scoring methods have not undergone rigorous scientific validation studies to prove their validity and because clinical scores should be obtained by trained, independent, and blinded observers, their continued use as a measure of outcomes is problematic.

Several patient-based outcome-assessment tools, which can be completed by the patient or by a nonmedical assistant, have undergone rigorous validation processes. Large-scale efforts are being made to construct normative scales for patients with differing demographic and medical characteristics. Moreover, specific tools have been developed and have undergone testing for assessment of patients with knee arthritis.

Evaluation Process

History

Arthritis of the knee is a common medical condition, with the prevalence of moderate to severe knee arthritis related to both gender and age. Of the male population between 55 and 64 years of age, 1% suffers from knee arthritis. This increases to 2% for males between 65 and 74 years of age. Women in the 55- to 64-year age range are affected at comparable rates to their male counterparts (0.9%). However, knee arthritis becomes increasingly common (6.6%) in women between 65 and 74 years of age. Untreated, knee arthritis is usually painful, functionally limiting, and progresses over time.

The history of a patient with knee arthritis will be dominated by complaints of knee pain on weightbearing. The pain may be localized to a single compartment or it may be diffuse. For joint replacement surgery to be considered, the pain is usually so severe that it interferes with the patient's activities of daily living (ADL) and significantly reduces the patient's quality of life. Other symptoms of knee dysfunction include giving way and joint locking.

Difficulties with ADL may be assessed by questioning the patient about performance in recreational sports; ability to walk, climb stairs, work, carry a package, and care for himself or herself; and ability to perform bent knee activities. Sleep patterns and sexual functioning may be disrupted. Patients may describe a general feeling of exhaustion that is secondary to their knee arthritis. Ultimately, social interactions may be reduced due to a patient's inability to function physically without pain. Left untreated, the patient may need general societal supports, such as home assistance or entry into an extended care facility.

Examination of the Patient With an Arthritic Knee

Examination of a patient with an arthritic knee can include inspection, palpation, physical maneuvers, and auscultation. The skin around the knee should be examined visually to identify previous traumatic wounds, surgical incisions, local infection, and superficial vascular status. The typical patient being considered for surgery will have an intact skin envelope. Patients with multiple previous incisions are at increased likelihood of postoperative wound-healing problems. Active local infection is a contraindication to joint replacement surgery and may necessitate other surgical or medical interventions.

Ideally, soft-tissue deficiencies will be identified early in the treatment process and preoperative plans for coverage made. The use of the gastrocnemius muscle as a local rotation flap has been advocated for treatment of preoperative soft-tissue defects and of postoperative patients with wound-healing problems.

Palpation will allow identification of points of tenderness and is helpful for disease localization and assessment of the vascular status. Palpation will usually reveal joint-line tenderness consistent with underlying articular cartilage or meniscal pathology. The distal pulses should be palpated to help determine the limb's ability to withstand a surgical insult. If the patient's vascular status is questionable, supplemental arterial Doppler and/or transcutaneous oxygen determinations should be considered.

Physical maneuvers are performed to assess sagittal range of motion, frontal plane stability, sagittal plane stability, presence of joint crepitus, and muscular and neurologic status. The sagittal range of knee motion has direct functional correlates to and is important in the prediction of post-knee replacement motion. For consistency and to allow objective standardization of knee impairment, a goniometer should be placed parallel to the long axis of the femur and the lower leg. The relationship of the goniometer arms to the limb segments should remain constant. The center point of the goniometer normally will move distally along the femoral axis as the knee flexes. Allowing translation of the goniometer center compensates for the normal posterior motion of the femorotibial contact point. For impairment determination and surgical goal setting, both maximal flexion and maximal extension should be recorded.

Expression of frontal plane instability in terms of degrees of motion will allow direct comparison of stability between patients regardless of body size. Careful identification of significant ligament pathology before surgical treatment will allow for the timely acquisition of knee replacement components that can provide intrinsic stability.

Quadriceps muscle status is important because patients with knee arthritis and quadriceps muscle deficiencies may obtain a 50% reduction in pain with exercise. Many surgeons believe that preoperative patient education and rehabilitative preparation will facilitate postoperative recovery.

Joint crepitus and auscultation have limited utility. Crepitus identified with motion is a nonspecific finding, which can be indicative of scar tissue, osteophytes, cartilage surface defects, intra-articular loose bodies, or meniscal pathology. Auscultation is helpful principally in identification of vascular anomalies, and it may be positive as a nonspecific evaluation tool in the delineation of patellofemoral arthritis.

Comorbidity Impacts

General medical assessment of the patient about to undergo major joint surgery is important because accurate identification of baseline medical comorbidities is needed for risk stratification. The 30-day mortality after knee replacement is low. However, mortality is directly associated with increasing age, male gender, and the number of associated medical problems recorded on the chart. Optimization of the patient's medical state before surgery should help reduce perioperative complications.

Social factors may also play a role in the patient's outcome from surgery. Individuals receiving workers' compensation appear to be at increased risk for less optimal outcomes from osteotomy and subsequent knee replacement surgery.

Active systemic bacterial or fungal infections are contraindications to joint replacement surgery. Remote local infections, such as a urinary tract infection, should be identified and properly treated.

The surgeon should always be cognizant of the potential for systemic viral infections, such as hepatitis or human immunodeficiency virus (HIV). The surgical team should be particularly wary and should always use universal precautions to minimize the risk of inadvertent transmission. Inadequate ability to identify and treat these infectious agents may accelerate the patient's demise and render the effectiveness of surgical interventions moot.

Structured Assessment (Outcomes Evaluation)

Error in the health information transfer process and in the recording of valid information has been recognized. Patient records may be missing, illegible, inaccurate, and incomplete. This problem has been approached increasingly by physicians, social scientists, psychologists, and engineers. These interested people have carefully constructed instruments and tools to improve the quantitative assessment of health status. Computer-based technologies and process-control techniques are now being used to improve the quality of the medical record and the medical decision-making process. Preliminary results have shown that these approaches can both improve quality of musculoskeletal care and reduce costs.

The resultant health assessment process is most analogous to the formal academic testing process. Validated instruments are completed by the patients and/or their lay companions. Several major research efforts have been made to incorporate these tools into the measurement of health status change associated with medical procedures.

However, there are both good and bad questions for acquiring health information. The assessment tools must ask logical questions (face validity) and provide similar results when administered at different times (test-retest reliability) and by different people (interobserver reliability). The test being administered must be sensitive enough to detect changes in the disease process and in the treatments given (sensitivity or responsiveness). The overall process must be efficient to be clinically useful.

Increasingly, surgeons have validated patient outcome assessment tools available to them for use in their practices. For general health status assessment, the Medical Outcomes Study Short Form 36 (SF-36) is achieving broad usage. For documentation of the disease-specific impacts of hip and knee osteoarthritis, the Western Ontario and McMasters Universities Osteoarthritis Index (WOMAC) has been found to be reliable and sensitive. Its usefulness has been demonstrated in patients undergoing hip replace-

ment, and it is now being used by the Indiana University Knee Replacement Patient Outcome Research Team (PORT). These published tools can accurately characterize, in a reliable and reproducible fashion, the patient's general health status, local knee status, and response to treatment.

Assessment has resulted in an increased understanding of the impact of knee arthritis on the patient's quality of life. The principal documented problems encountered by patients with knee arthritis are pain and inability to take part in physical activity. Additional functional deficits have been noted in recreational activities, sleep, and even emotional behavior.

Serial patient assessments, using general health status instruments, have demonstrated that several surgical techniques improve the patient's quality of life (Fig. 1). Through the combined use of the general health tools, patient utilities (a tool used to assess the "value" that a person places on different health states), and decision modeling, preliminary evidence from a few university centers has shown that joint replacement surgery is among the most effective health-care processes used to improve quality of life.

Radiographic Assessment of Knee Arthritis

Conventional radiographic views for the assessment of the patient with knee arthritis include the standing anteroposterior (AP) view of both knees, the lateral radiograph, and the patellofemoral view. Tunnel and oblique views are helpful for evaluation of patients with loose bodies, osteochondritis dissecans, fractures, and osteophytes. Long bone alignment films or segmental radiographs are worthwhile for detection of frontal plane malalignments and are helpful for preoperative planning.

The extent of knee arthritis can be classified radiographically through the use of standing AP radiographs with the knee in extension. Both the Ahlback and the Kellgren and Lawrence classification systems rely on such films. Standing radiographs are particularly helpful to demonstrate advanced knee arthritis. However, the standing technique lacks sensitivity in the demonstration of early knee osteoarthritis when compared to arthroscopic findings.

Alternative plain radiographic techniques have been proposed to address the diagnostic limitations of standing, extended knee, weightbearing AP radiographs. A standing, 45° posteroanterior weightbearing radiograph can improve the sensitivity of the radiographic technique in the detection of articular cartilage degeneration. However, the 45° view is unable to detect early (Outerbridge Grade 0, I, or II) articular cartilage change. Furthermore, the practical implementation of this technique can be difficult, especially in the elderly. If maximum sensitivity (100%) in the radiographic demonstration of articular cartilage change is required, stress radiographs with the knee in a flexed position (20°) should be considered.

As the prevalence of patients with knee replacements

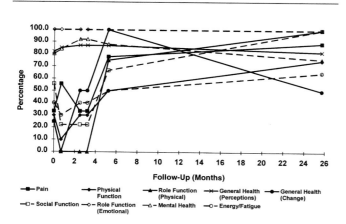

Fig. 1 Anecdotal demonstration of SF-36 changes in one patient after knee replacement for posttraumatic arthritis. (Reproduced with permission from Heck DA, Marmor L, Gibson A, et al: Unicompartmental knee arthroplasty: A multicenter investigation with long-term follow-up evaluation. *Clin Orthop* 1993;286:154–159.)

increases, the need for fluoroscopically positioned views is increasing. Conventional radiographic assessment of radiolucent lines is unreliable because small positioning errors can obliterate the bone-prosthesis interface. Fluoroscopic positioning of the knee is the only routine imaging procedure that allows for the accurate delineation of radiolucencies about the complex geometries of knee replacement components.

More sophisticated imaging modalities for the differential diagnosis of knee arthritis are of occasional benefit and include technetium bone scanning, indium white blood cell scanning, computed tomography scanning, and magnetic resonance imaging scanning. Their roles are limited in routine assessment and they should not be used exclusively. Cost-effectiveness studies to demonstrate the incremental benefits of advanced imaging investigations over the clinical evaluation by a trained orthopaedist alone or in combination with conventional radiographs are lacking.

Annotated Bibliography

American Medical Association: *Guides to the Evaluation of Permanent Impairment,* ed 3. Chicago, IL, American Medical Association, 1990.

This AMA publication provides the physician with specific, detailed methods for the examination and quantitative assessment of permanent impairment. It is of particular value in providing the entire medical community with a common language for patient examination.

Brandt KD, Fife RS, Braunstein EM, et al: Radiographic grading of the severity of knee osteoarthritis: Relation of the Kellgren and Lawrence grade to a grade based on joint space narrowing, and correlation with arthroscopic evidence of articular cartilage degeneration. *Arthritis Rheum* 1991;34:1381–1386.

This report demonstrates the difficulties in the use of standing radiographs to detect early osteoarthrosis. Both the Kellgren and Lawrence grade and the proposed grading system are problematic.

Cleary PD, Greenfield S, McNeil BJ: Assessing quality of life after surgery. *Control Clin Trials* 1991;12(suppl 4): 189S–203S.

The authors have used patient-based assessment tools to determine the impact of cholecystectomy, total hip replacement, trans-urethral resection of the prostate, and coronary artery bypass surgery on activities of daily living. For both basic and intermediate activities of daily living, patients undergoing THR showed the greatest change.

Heck DA, Partridge CM: *Patient-Based Assessment in Primary and Revision Knee Replacement.* Proceedings of the American Academy of Orthopaedic Surgeons 61st Annual Meeting, New Orleans, LA. Rosemont, IL, American Academy of Orthopaedic Surgeons, 1994, p 242.

Using the SF36, a patient-based assessment tool, patients at a single university center were found to have substantial improvements in the global health domains of pain, physical function, and energy/fatigue. Patients undergoing revision KR had comparable improvements in pain, but lesser levels of functional improvement.

Mattsson E, Bronstrom L-A: The physical and psychosocial effect of moderate osteoarthritis of the knee. *Scand J Rehabil Med* 1991;23:215–218.

This report documents the severe effect that knee arthritis has on a patient's life. It provides a framework to allow demonstration of the impact of treatment on this otherwise inexorable disease.

Mintz CA, Pilkington CA, Howie DW: A comparison of plain and fluoroscopically guided radiographs in the assessment of arthroplasty of the knee. *J Bone Joint Surg* 1989;71A:1343–1347.

The need for fluoroscopically positioned radiographs to delineate radiolucencies in the evaluation of knee arthroplasties was demonstrated. This technique is particularly helpful in the patient with unexplained pain and to increase the sensitivity of detection of osteolysis.

28

Nonprosthetic Management of the Arthritic Knee

Synovectomy

Synovectomy may be used to treat synovial proliferative disorders of the knee, most commonly rheumatoid arthritis. Indications for surgery include chronic synovitis that causes pain and swelling despite 6 months of appropriate medical management, good range of motion, and the radiographic appearance of a near normal or minimally damaged joint. The results of synovectomy are superior when it is performed early in the disease process, and standing radiographs should demonstrate preservation of articular cartilage. More advanced joint destruction characteristic of stage III or IV rheumatoid arthritis is not well suited for this procedure.

Surgical synovectomy of the knee may be performed using either open or arthroscopic techniques. Either a single incision or two parapatellar incisions have traditionally been used in open techniques. Studies demonstrate that a number of synovectomized knees may eventually require total knee arthroplasty. This indication favors the use of a single anterior midline incision to minimize possible wound or exposure problems at arthroplasty.

Recently, arthroscopic techniques have become increasingly popular. Improved arthroscopic instrumentation and techniques have reduced the time required for surgery and allowed for satisfactory removal of synovium.

Arthroscopic synovectomy is performed using a multiple portal technique. Large-diameter, motorized synovial resectors are used to remove the superficial layer of synovium down to the plane between the synovium and subsynovial tissues. The menisci and cruciate ligaments are preserved. The posterior synovium may be removed using additional posterior portals, both medially and laterally as needed. The improved motorized instrumentation has reduced operating time. Early range of motion with or without the use of continuous passive motion is encouraged postoperatively. Clinical results are similar to those reported for open synovectomy with less surgical and postoperative morbidity and with more rapid restoration of knee motion and return to function. Additionally, arthroscopic synovectomy may be performed on an outpatient basis, thereby reducing the need for hospitalization, which is required for open synovectomy.

Radioisotope techniques of synovectomy have been investigated as nonsurgical alternatives. Good initial results with radiation synovectomy have been reported in 80% of knees. Investigation of radiation synovectomy is continuing, although the benefits of radiation techniques may be less evident when contrasted to the benefits of arthroscopic synovectomy rather than those of open surgical synovectomy.

Arthroscopic Debridement for Degenerative Arthritis

Arthroscopic debridement is associated with both limited morbidity and swift postoperative recovery; therefore, its role in the surgical treatment of the arthritic knee has expanded. Clinical success rates for arthroscopic debridement procedures are reported to be between 60% and 70% at up to 5-year follow-up. Improvement in painful symptoms is more common than complete resolution of such symptoms. Techniques of arthroscopic debridement vary greatly. Arthroscopic debridement with joint lavage, removal of unstable meniscal fragments and loose articular cartilage, and minimal shaving appears to offer maximum benefit with minimal morbidity. More extensive arthroscopic procedures, such as abrasion arthroplasty and arthroscopic debridement with drilling of exposed condylar bone, do not appear to offer any additional benefit in the treatment of degenerative arthritis of the knee. A microfracture technique to manage chondral defects has been reported recently, with early optimism. Joint lavage with removal of loose debris and proteolytic enzymes is probably an important aspect of any arthroscopic procedure for osteoarthritis.

Arthroscopic debridement is particularly well suited for older patients with mild to moderate unicompartmental or tricompartmental degenerative disease. Inferior results can be expected in patients who have more advanced degenerative changes associated with loss of articular joint space, significant angular deformity, and rest pain. The 45° posteroanterior standing radiograph may be helpful in the preoperative evaluation, particularly in suspected lateral compartment disease.

Osteotomy

Despite the clinical success and durability of total knee arthroplasty over the past decade, there remains a role for osteotomy in the surgical management of the arthritic knee. The goal of knee osteotomy is to realign the mechanical axis of the limb, thereby shifting weightbearing forces from the diseased to a more normal compartment.

The mechanical axis of the limb is defined by a straight line drawn from the center of the femoral head through the center of the knee to the center of the ankle mortise. A normal mechanical axis is a straight line and defined as 0°. The tibiofemoral angle of the lower extremity is defined by the angle created by a line drawn down the longitudinal axis of the femur and a line drawn down the longitudinal axis of the tibia. A normal tibiofemoral angle is approximately 5° to 7° of valgus angulation. These angles may be determined from full length, three-joint weightbearing radiographs.

In the normal knee, approximately 60% of the weight-bearing forces are transmitted through the medial compartment. In the knee with single compartment degenerative changes, the altered limb alignment redistributes more load to the affected compartment; the additional load may accelerate the degenerative process. Progression of unicompartmental arthritis in the knee and the associated increase in angular deformity may affect the ligamentous support of the knee. Laxity of the contralateral soft tissue and ligaments may contribute to widening of the contralateral compartment joint space as well as to a thrusting of the knee on weightbearing. Assessment of this laxity is important in both surgical indications and preoperative planning for a proposed osteotomy.

The goal of osteotomy is to transfer joint forces from the arthritic compartment to the more normal compartment, thereby relieving pain and attempting to preserve what remains of the involved articular surface. In medial tibiofemoral osteoarthritis with a varus deformity, an upper tibial valgus osteotomy may be selected. In lateral tibiofemoral osteoarthritis with a valgus deformity, a varus-producing distal femoral osteotomy is the preferred choice.

Varus Deformity

Upper tibial osteotomy is a useful and reliable operation for varus gonarthrosis. Surgical indications for corrective osteotomy have been altered over the past decade because of the long-term clinical success of total knee arthroplasty.

Tibial osteotomy is well-suited for the younger, heavier, active patient with mild to moderate medial compartment osteoarthritis. It is particularly well-suited for patients involved in heavy labor or aggressive athletic activities. One study demonstrated that patients over the age of 60 years at the time of osteotomy did less well than patients under this age. In addition, the acceptance of the appearance of the lower extremity following valgus tibial osteotomy is an important selection criteria.

Relative contraindications to the procedure include limited range of motion (flexion less than 90° or fixed flexion contracture of 15°), advanced patellofemoral arthritis, and anatomic varus deformity greater than 10°. Varus deformities greater than 15° are frequently associated with lateral tibial subluxation or increased medial-tibial bone loss, both of which are associated with inferior results. Inflammatory arthritides involve all of the knee compartments and are a contraindication to osteotomy about the knee. Arthroscopic assessment of the knee prior to osteot-

omy, to confirm the indications, does not appear to be of prognostic value.

Preoperative Assessment A relationship between clinical improvement after osteotomy and postoperative alignment has been demonstrated. Although there is no consensus on the ideal postoperative alignment, most would favor over-correction of the tibiofemoral axis to 7° to 10°. Preoperative full length, three-joint weightbearing radiographs allow determination of the tibiofemoral angle and mechanical axis and allow for calculation of the desired correction to be achieved during surgery. A recent technical note describes a preoperative method for calculating the desired correction. This method results in a mechanical axis passing through 30% to 40% of the width of the lateral tibial plateau as advocated by many (Fig. 1). Ligament laxity may alter these determinations.

Gait analysis has demonstrated a relationship between preoperative gait and the clinical outcome of upper tibial osteotomy in which the procedure is successful in those patients who walked with a decreased magnitude of the knee adduction moment preoperatively. Although gait analysis allows a more quantitative approach to patient selection, the lack of availability of this method has limited its usefulness.

Surgical Technique A wedge or dome osteotomy may be performed through the cancellous bone of the upper tibia proximal to the tibial tubercle. A dome-shaped osteotomy allows for greater angular corrections. The closing-wedge osteotomy is performed 2 cm distal to the joint line and inclined medially and distally. This technique allows for the natural medial slope of the upper tibia. Several techniques in which a medially based opening-wedge tibial osteotomy is used have been reported.

The fibula may exert a tethering effect and prevent osteotomy closure. Satisfactory solutions include fibular head excision with lateral soft-tissue repair or simple division of the superior tibiofibular joint. Fibular shaft osteotomy appears unnecessary.

Multiple techniques of osteotomy fixation have been reported. Simple cast immobilization or cast bracing, with or without staples, as well as internal fixation with plates have all been reported as successful. External fixation techniques have been associated with both an increased risk of infection and nerve palsy. Rigid internal fixation of the osteotomy allows for early range of motion. Although both longitudinal and transverse skin incisions have been described, the future possibility of total knee arthroplasty should be considered in selection of surgical exposure. Transverse incisions have not posed a problem for future arthroplasty. Intraoperative fluoroscopy is a useful adjunct in performing the osteotomy and securing internal fixation.

Clinical Results Numerous reports attest to the effectiveness of upper tibial osteotomy in relieving pain and

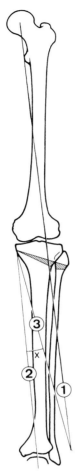

Fig. 1 A full-length weightbearing radiograph is obtained. Line 1 is the predicted mechanical axis from the center of the femoral head passing through a portion of the lateral tibial plateau, which is measured to be between 30% and 40% of the lateral plateau width and extrapolated to the level of the projected position of the center of the ankle. Line 2 runs from the medial corticoperiosteal hinge or pivot point where the arms of the osteotomy will meet down to the center of the ankle. Line 3 runs from the medial pivot point to the projected position of the center of the ankle. The angle X subtended by lines 2 and 3 is the desired amount of correction. (Reproduced with permission from Miniaci A, Ballmer FT, Ballmer PM, et al: Proximal tibial osteotomy: A new fixation device. *Clin Orthop* 1989;246: 250–259.)

improving function. Despite 5-year success rates of 80% to 90%, clinical results with tibial osteotomy deteriorate with time. For large series, 61% good results were reported for an average follow-up of 10 years and 63% good results for 95 knees at average follow-up of 8.5 years.

The association of undercorrection of deformity with decreased survivorship and early deterioration of good results emphasizes the importance of accurate surgical technique. Considerable risk of osteotomy failure is re-

ported if the anatomic alignment is not corrected to at least 8°.

A number of complications following tibial osteotomy have been reported. The reported rate of nonunion ranges from 0 to 3%. Treatment may require bone grafting, compression fixation, and revision of the osteotomy if correction has been lost. Technical errors that result in creation of a thin proximal fragment may be associated with avascular necrosis of the fragment or intra-articular tibial fracture.

Compartment syndrome may follow upper tibial osteotomy; therefore, prophylactic anterior compartment fasciotomy and wound drainage are advocated by some authors. Reports of peroneal-nerve palsy are more commonly associated with osteotomy of the proximal third of the fibula or the use of external fixation.

Fortunately, vascular injuries are uncommon. Although the frequency of deep-venous thrombosis and pulmonary embolism is low, further studies regarding prophylaxis are required.

Total Knee Arthroplasty After Upper Tibial Osteotomy   A large proportion of patients undergoing upper tibial osteotomy will eventually require total knee arthroplasty. A successful arthroplasty after tibial osteotomy is technically more demanding than a primary total knee arthroplasty. In one comparative study of 21 knees with an average follow-up of 2.9 years, 81% of patients with a previous upper tibial osteotomy achieved a satisfactory result compared with 100% of a matched control group without previous osteotomy. In a study of 45 total knee arthroplasties following previous tibial osteotomy, clinical results were similar to those reported for patients who required a revision arthroplasty for failed primary total knee arthroplasty. In a review of 35 patients, clinical results were comparable to those of primary total knee arthroplasty. Indications for upper tibial osteotomy should reflect these findings.

The surgical technique for knee replacement is often affected by the previous osteotomy. Patella infera is not uncommon, making surgical exposure and patellofemoral mechanics more problematic. Careful planning is needed before arthroplasty. Problems with the tibial resection may be encountered, which include possible central peg impingement and anterior tilting of the tibial articular surface. Management of bone defects with either metal augmentation or bone graft techniques as well as the possibility of an offset tibial stem may be required.

Valgus Deformity

The pathomechanics of genu valgum result in mechanical overloading of the lateral compartment and, in time, a superolateral tilting of the joint line in the coronal plane. Additionally, stretching of the medial collateral ligament may contribute to joint instability. Upper tibial osteotomy for a valgus deformity will increase joint obliquity and predispose the knee to mediolateral subluxation. A distal femoral osteotomy may be indicated if the angle between the anatomic femoral axis and the tibial mechanical axis is greater than 12° of valgus or when the tibial plateau deviates from the horizontal by more than 10°. Distal femoral varus osteotomy allows correction of the superolateral tilt of the joint while minimizing medial laxity.

Similar to tibial osteotomy, distal femoral osteotomy is better suited for the younger, heavier, active patient with mild to moderate lateral compartment osteoarthritis who is capable of managing the demanding postoperative rehabilitation. Tricompartmental arthritis, severe patellofemoral disease, or associated joint instability with medial thrust clinically are contraindications to the procedure. Inflammatory arthritis is also a contraindication for distal femoral osteotomy; less than satisfactory results have been reported for a small number of patients with rheumatoid arthritis. Flexion contractures of less than 20° and knee flexion greater than 90° are important clinical prerequisites.

Although there is no clear consensus regarding surgical technique, most favor a medial closing-wedge osteotomy.

The desired correction should render the transcondylar axis perpendicular to the tibiofemoral axis neutral (0°) or slightly varus. A variety of incisions have been described and used successfully. An anterior midline incision allows for adequate exposure of the distal femur for osteotomy and does not compromise a future total knee replacement. Early postoperative range of motion is encouraged to minimize joint stiffness if adequate bone quality is present and good internal fixation is achieved. Adequate internal fixation is critical to success: staples are inadequate. Restricted weightbearing with crutches extends from 4 to 12 weeks, depending on the rate of osteotomy healing and stability of fixation. Resumption of full activity usually occurs between 3 and 6 months after osteotomy.

Several recent series report clinical success similar to that of upper tibial osteotomy at 4 years. Reported complications included nonunion and failures of fixation. Although the series of patients were small, results following distal femoral varus osteotomy did not appear to deteriorate over time in several studies. However, longer follow-up will be needed to fully determine the longevity of results.

Annotated Bibliography

Synovectomy

Ogilvie-Harris DJ, McLean J, Zarnett ME: Pigmented villonodular synovitis of the knee: The results of total arthroscopic synovectomy, partial arthroscopic synovectomy, and arthroscopic local excision. *J Bone Joint Surg* 1992;74A:119–123.

Twenty-five patients with pigmented villonodular synovitis (PVNS) of the knee were followed for an average of 4.5 years (2–104) after arthroscopic treatment. Good improvement with no recurrence was noted in five patients with localized lesions managed with local resection. Eleven patients with diffuse PVNS underwent complete arthroscopic synovectomy with only one recurrence. Improvement in pain, range of motion, and function was observed in all patients. In the remaining nine patients with diffuse PVNS, a partial synovectomy was performed. The disease recurred in five of nine.

Smiley P, Wasilewski SA: Arthroscopic synovectomy. *Arthroscopy* 1990;6:18–23.

No surgical complications were encountered in 25 knees with inflammatory arthritis that underwent arthroscopic synovectomy. Gradual deterioration of good results from 96% to 57% were noted from 6 months to 4 years follow-up. Clinical results correlated well with radiographic results.

Arthroscopic Treatment of the Degenerative Knee

Bert JM, Maschka K: The arthroscopic treatment of unicompartmental gonarthrosis: A five-year follow-up study of abrasion arthroplasty plus arthroscopic debridement and arthroscopic debridement alone. *Arthroscopy* 1989;5:25–32.

A comparative study of 126 patients revealed superior clinical results with arthroscopic debridement alone in patients who had advanced unicompartment degenerative disease. The results of abrasion arthroplasty plus arthroscopic debridement were unpredictable. Radiographic evidence of joint-space widening with abrasion arthroplasty was not predictive of symptom relief.

Ogilvie-Harris DJ, Fitsialos DP: Arthroscopic management of the degenerative knee. *Arthroscopy* 1991;7:151–157.

Patients who underwent 441 arthroscopic procedures for degenerative arthritis of the knee were followed for 2 to 8 years. Best results were obtained after resection of unstable flap tears of the meniscus in association with mild degenerative changes. Results were better in normally aligned knees.

Rand JA: Role of arthroscopy in osteoarthritis of the knee. *Arthroscopy* 1991;7:358–363.

At 5 years following arthroscopic partial meniscectomy and limited debridement in a series of 131 patients, 67% were improved. A second group of 28 patients with exposed condylar bone were treated with abrasion arthroplasty. Only 39% were improved at 3.8 years and 57% underwent subsequent total knee arthroplasty at 3 years. Abrasion arthroplasty yielded unpredictable results, offering no advantage to arthroscopic partial meniscectomy and limited debridement.

Proximal Tibial Osteotomy

Coventry MB, Ilstrup DM, Wallrichs, SL: Proximal tibial osteotomy: A critical long-term study of eighty-seven cases. *J Bone Joint Surg* 1993;75A:196–201.

Statistical and survivorship analysis of 87 proximal tibial osteotomies followed for 10 years revealed a considerable risk of osteotomy failure if the alignment is not overcorrected to at least 8° of valgus angulation and if the patient is substantially overweight. Sixty-seven percent of knees were less painful at follow-up. Survival rate was 94% at 5 years and was similar at 10 years when valgus angulation of 8° or more was obtained.

Hernigou P, Medevielle D, Debeyre J, et al: Proximal tibial osteotomy for osteoarthritis with varus deformity: A ten to thirteen-year follow-up study. *J Bone Joint Surg* 1987;69A:332–354.

Of 93 knees treated with proximal tibial opening wedge osteotomy, 45% demonstrated good to excellent results at 10 to 13-year follow-up. Although results deteriorated with time, accurate preoperative radiographic measurements and postoperative alignment were associated with longer relief of symptoms.

Hoffmann AA, Wyatt RWB, Beck SW: High tibial osteotomy: Use of an osteotomy jig, rigid fixation and early motion versus conventional surgical technique and cast immobilization. *Orthop Clin* 1991;271:212–217.

Fifteen patients (19 knees) underwent high tibial osteotomy (HTO) using standard surgical technique and cast immobilization. This group was compared to a group of 20 patients (21 knees) with HTO using an oblique osteotomy surgical jig with rigid internal fixation with an L-buttress plate. Postoperatively these patients were started on immediate continuous passive motion and 50% weightbearing. Forty-two percent of patients with standard HTO technique had associated complications compared with a single complication in the second group consisting of a nondisplaced tibial intra-articular fracture. The osteotomy jig with internal fixation technique, which allowed early range of motion, provided satisfactory clinical results with somewhat increased precision of correlation when compared to the standard surgical technique.

Katz MM, Hungerford DS, Krackow KA, et al: Results of total knee arthroplasty after failed proximal tibial osteotomy for osteoarthritis. *J Bone Joint Surg* 1987;69A:225–233.

A comparative study was performed of 21 patients undergoing total knee arthroplasty after a failed proximal tibial osteotomy for osteoarthritis and 21 patients with a primary total knee arthroplasty for osteoarthritis. The groups were well matched; in 81% of patients with a previous osteotomy good to excellent results were demonstrated at 2.9 years compared to 100% of patients with a primary arthroplasty at 2.8 years. Technical challenges in restoring the failed osteotomy to total knee arthroplasty are discussed.

Mont MA, Antonaides S, Krackow KA, et al: Total knee arthroplasty after failed high tibial osteotomy. *Clin Orthop* 1994;299:125–130.

Seventy-three total knee arthroplasties (TKA) in 67 patients after a high tibial osteotomy were reviewed at follow-up 73 months average (24–132). This group of patients were then compared to two comparison groups following primary TKA without high tibial osteotomy (HTO). Thirty-six percent of the study group had either a fair or poor result or required additional surgery. Factors associated with a worse outcome in the HTO patients included ($p < 0.01$): (1) workers' compensation patient, (2) history of reflex sympathetic dystrophy after HTO, (3) less than 1 year or no period of pain relief after HTO, (4) multiple surgeries before HTO, and (5) occupation as a laborer.

Prodromos CC, Andriacchi TP, Galante JO: A relationship between gait and clinical changes following high tibial osteotomy. *J Bone Joint Surg* 1985; 67A:1188–1194.

Correlation between clinical results of osteotomy and preoperative gait analysis revealed the best results were achieved when the preoperative adduction moment was low. The overall geometry and alignment did not correlate with dynamic loading occurring during gait nor with associated clinical results.

Distal Femoral Osteotomy

Edgerton BC, Mariani EM, Morrey BF: Distal femoral varus osteotomy for painful genu valgum: A five- to 11-year follow-up study. *Clin Orthop* 1993;288:263–269.

An 8-year study of 23 patients treated with distal femoral varus osteotomy for painful lateral compartment osteoarthritis revealed 71% good to excellent results. The complication rate was 63% and was primarily due to inadequate osteotomy fixation with staples. No tendency for a good result to deteriorate with time was noted.

Healy WL, Anglen JO, Wasilewski SA, et al: Distal femoral varus osteotomy. *J Bone Joint Surg* 1988;70A:102–109.

Of 23 knees that underwent distal femoral osteotomy, 83% demonstrated good or excellent results at 4 years while 93% of the 15 knees with osteoarthritis had a good or excellent result. Three of four knees with rheumatoid arthritis failed. Average preoperative tibiofemoral angle of 18° valgus was corrected to an average 2° valgus.

29

Unicompartmental Total Knee Arthroplasty

Introduction

Despite almost two decades of controversy, the status of unicompartmental knee replacement remains uncertain. In the early 1970s, there were several reports of early discouraging results with unicondylar arthroplasty, and its role was questioned except, perhaps, in lateral compartment disease. During the next 10 years, more favorable results began appearing. These results were largely the result of refined surgical technique and the narrowing of patient selection to candidates ideally suited for the procedure.

The concept of unicompartmental total knee replacement is attractive as an alternative to tibial osteotomy or tricompartmental replacement in the elderly osteoarthritic patient who has unicompartmental disease confirmed at arthrotomy. Unicompartmental arthroplasty has a higher initial success rate and fewer early complications than osteotomy. Any internal derangement can be relieved at the time of arthrotomy. Intra-articular debridement can lead to an improvement in range of motion. Patients with bilateral disease can have both knees operated on during the same anesthetic with full recovery within 3 months of surgery. Osteotomies in the same patient should probably be spaced from 3 to 6 months apart, and as much as a year from the time of the initial procedure may be required to achieve full recovery.

Compared to tricompartmental arthroplasty, unicompartmental replacement has the advantage of preserving both cruciate ligaments, thereby yielding a knee with nearly normal kinematics. A study of 42 patients with a bicompartmental or tricompartmental arthroplasty on one side and a unicompartmental replacement on the other showed that more patients preferred the unicompartmental side because it felt more like a normal knee and had better function.

Another potential advantage over tricompartmental replacement is the preservation of bone stock in the patellofemoral joint and opposite compartment. Theoretically, this preservation should make revision easier to perform should it become necessary. Until recently, however, this theoretic advantage had not been supported by studies of revision of unicompartmental replacements. Results of revision were not superior to those seen after revision of bicompartmental or tricompartmental replacement, and deficient bone stock in the femoral condyle or tibial plateau often had to be augmented with bone graft or special components. These deficiencies may have been the result of early surgical techniques or prostheses that invaded the bone stock unnecessarily. More modern techniques in which surface replacements are used on the femoral and tibial sides have made unicompartmental arthroplasty as conservative in practice as it is in theory.

Survivorship analyses reported for tricompartmental replacement indicate that survivorship with or without cruciate retention can be above 90% after 10 years of follow-up. So far, 10-year survivorship studies generated from early unicompartmental series show that survivorship at 10 years drops into the 85% range. These data were generated, however, at a time when patient selection was still evolving and surgical techniques were not yet perfected.

Patient Selection

Osteotomy remains the procedure of choice in the young, heavy, active patient with unicompartmental osteoarthritis. Rest pain and poor range of motion are relative contraindications to osteotomy. Internal derangement is not a contraindication to osteotomy, but should be relieved by an arthroscopic procedure prior or subsequent to the osteotomy. Subluxation and extreme angular deformity are a contraindication to both osteotomy and unicompartmental replacement. Metallic interpositional arthroplasty may occasionally be advisable when osteotomy is contraindicated and the patient is considered too young or too heavy to be a candidate for total knee replacement.

Once an arthroplasty has been chosen over osteotomy, the final decision whether to perform unicompartmental, bicompartmental, or tricompartmental replacement is made at arthrotomy. Although clinical examination and radiography may indicate that the patient is an ideal candidate for unicompartmental arthroplasty, several contraindications to the procedure may be discovered at the time of arthrotomy. An absent anterior cruciate ligament is a significant contraindication to unicompartmental replacement because this absence usually is accompanied by a degree of ligamentous laxity that can promote eventual lateral subluxation of the tibia on the femur and secondary opposite compartment disease. Inspection of the opposite compartment and patellofemoral joint may show significant degenerative changes that make unicompartmental arthroplasty inadvisable. Mild chondromalacia in the opposite compartment can be accepted, but areas of eburnated bone are definite contraindications. In a varus osteoarthritic knee with medial compartment arthritis, a secondary lesion appears on the medial aspect of the lateral femoral condyle with early lateral subluxation. This lesion usually is accompanied by intercondylar osteophyte formation. If the subluxation is slight and the lesion is small, the lesion can be debrided and the problem corrected by unicompartmental arthroplasty. If the subluxation is great and the lesion large, bicompartmental or tricompartmental arthroplasty is advisable.

Eburnated bone in the patellofemoral compartment is also considered a contraindication to unicompartmental arthroplasty. However, some surgeons will accept patellofemoral degeneration, which includes areas of eburnated bone, and still proceed with unicompartmental arthroplasty. Most advocates of unicompartmental arthroplasty will accept significant chondromalacia in the patellofemoral joint, but not eburnated bone.

A third contraindication discovered at arthrotomy consists of a significant inflammatory component to the patient's disease. This component may be in the form of a very dramatic synovial reaction or the discovery of diffuse crystalline deposits from either gout or pseudogout. Inflammatory disease in any form substantially increases the risk of secondary degeneration of the opposite compartment in subsequent years.

Implant Design

Over the past two decades many lessons have been learned concerning the ideal design features of components to be used for a unicompartmental arthroplasty. Many early femoral components were narrow in their medial–lateral dimension and suffered a high incidence of subsidence of the component into the condylar bone. The ideal component should be wide enough to maximally cap the resurfaced condyle, widely distributing the weightbearing forces and decreasing the chance of subsidence and loosening. For this reason, multiple sizes should be available to accommodate both small and large patients. Revision studies have shown the inadvisability of deeply invading the condyle with fixation methods. Relatively small fixation lugs appear to be sufficient as long as two are present to gain rotational fixation to the bone or some sort of fin is provided for this purpose. The posterior metallic condyle should fully cap the posterior condyle of the patient to allow physiologic range of motion without impingement. The amount of bone resection required for insertion should be minimal. Preferably, the femoral component can be supported on top of the distal subchondral bone without any resection, but this requires sacrifice of more bone from the tibial side. The ideal compromise may be to resect between 2 and 4 mm of distal condyle, while retaining part of the subchondral bone for adequate purchase and retaining enough distal femoral bone to allow easy conversion to a bicompartmental prosthesis. This 2- to 4-mm distal femoral resection also results in an equivalent decrease in the amount of bone that must be resected from the proximal tibia.

There also must be a compromise in selection of the articulating topography. A flat surface on the femoral component articulating with a flat surface on the tibial component may improve metal-to-plastic contact, but it is very difficult to position the surfaces accurately and avoid edge contact. An articulating surface with a small radius of curvature articulating on the tibial side with a flat surface creates too much point contact. A femoral surface with a small radius of curvature matched to a similarly small radius on the tibial side can create too much constraint. The ideal surfaces for both components, therefore, are probably those with a relatively large radius of curvature that allow adequate metal-to-plastic contact without excessive constraint.

The shape of the tibial component as it sits on the tibial plateau should probably be anatomic to maximize contact between the prosthesis and the bone and, thus, to widely distribute the weightbearing forces to resist subsidence and loosening. This design will necessitate an asymmetric shape with right and left components. Multiple sizes also will be required on the tibial side to accommodate both small and large patients.

Metal backing of the tibial component is controversial. It was initiated in the early 1980s in order to more uniformly distribute the weightbearing forces to the cut surface of the plateau. Early results with metal-backed components were superior to those with 100% polyethylene components; however, these results may be due to improved patient selection and operative technique rather than to the use of the metal backing. When metal-backed components were followed for more than 5 years, failures were seen because the polyethylene wore through to the metal backing. This erosion of the polyethylene occurred when areas of the polyethylene were less than 4-mm thick and there were design flaws in the method of fixation of the polyethylene to the metal. These problems were similar to those seen with metal-backed patellar components. Depending on the type of metal used (cobalt-chromium), the minimal composite thickness of the tibial component must be 8 to 10 mm. This necessity makes metal-backing less attractive than previously thought, and there may be a trend back to all polyethylene tibial components.

Cementless Unicompartmental Arthroplasty

The role of cementless unicompartmental arthroplasty is uncertain. In theory, it would be appealing if it could be shown to be conservative compared to cemented unicompartmental arthroplasty. In practice, a cementless unicompartmental arthroplasty is actually more radical than a cemented procedure. For most cementless components, more bone resection is required on the femoral side. Failure rates are reported to be higher in terms of loosening on both the femoral and tibial sides. Metal-backed components are most likely required on the tibial side. Therefore, cementless unicompartmental arthroplasty must remain experimental until better methods and results are reported.

Summary

Despite two decades of experience, the role of unicompartmental arthroplasty remains controversial and uncertain.

It would appear to offer an attractive alternative to osteotomy or tricompartmental replacement in elderly patients who have unicompartmental osteoarthritis. It has a higher initial success rate and fewer early complications than osteotomy. Unicompartmental arthroplasty tends to provide a better quality result with a faster recovery than tricompartmental replacement and improved function. The procedure is conservative regarding preservation of both cruciate ligaments and bone stock in the opposite compartment and the patellofemoral joint. Ten-year survivorship curves, however, have shown that bicompartmental and tricompartmental replacements done in the 1970s have a longer survivorship than unicompartmental replacements from the same era. This difference may result from errors in patient selection and operative technique, as well as in prosthetic design. When the appropriate requirements in these areas have been met, unicompartmental knee replacement should assume its appropriate role in the armamentarium of the orthopaedic surgeon.

Annotated Bibliography

Bartley RE, Stulberg SD, Robb WJ III, et al: Polyethylene wear in unicompartmental knee arthroplasty. *Clin Orthop* 1994;299:18–24.

Eighteen of 147 unicompartmental arthroplasty patients underwent revision at a mean of 3 years. Fourteen showed significant polyethylene wear and seven of these implants were retrieved for analysis. A nonconforming implant articular geometry was considered a prime factor contributing to the observed incidence of wear and, thus, the rate of failure. Progression of degenerative disease, especially anterior cruciate ligament attenuation, via an increasing tendency for joint subluxation and decreased contact area, also was felt to have an adverse impact.

Broughton NS, Newman JH, Baily RA: Unicompartmental replacement and high tibial osteotomy for osteoarthritis of the knee: A comparative study after 5–10 years' follow-up. *J Bone Joint Surg* 1986;68B:447–452.

A retrospective comparison was made between 49 valgus high-tibial osteotomies (HTO) and 42 unicompartmental knee arthroplasties (UKA), which were carried out in comparable groups of patients. Follow-up was from 5 to 10 years. Results were satisfactory in 76% of UKA versus 43% of HTO at follow-up. Seven percent of UKA had undergone revision procedures versus 20% of HTO.

Jackson M, Saralngi PP, Newman JH: Revision total knee arthroplasty: Comparison of outcome following primary proximal tibial osteotomy or unicompartmental arthroplasty. *J Arthroplasty* 1994;9:539–542.

Two groups undergoing total knee arthroplasty were compared: 24 knees following medial unicompartmental arthroplasty (UKA) and 21 knees following valgus high-tibial osteotomy (HTO). Of the UKA group, 50% were noted to have tibial bone defects, only two of which required autologous bone grafting. A 30% surgical complication rate was noted in the HTO group, largely related to exposure of the knee and soft-tissue healing, with four deep infections occurring. The two groups otherwise had similar results at their follow-up evaluation.

Lai CH, Rand JA: Revision of failed unicompartmental knee arthroplasty. *Clin Orthop* 1993;287:193–201.

Forty-eight unicompartmental knee arthroplasties, which had undergone revision to total knee arthroplasty, were reviewed at a mean of 5.4 years following revision. At the revision procedure, 50% of knees were noted to have bony defects; however, all were filled with cement and none required bone grafting, the use of modular wedges, or long-stemmed implants. The rate of surgical complications was 13%, and 5-year survivorship of the revision implant was 89%.

Laurencin CT, Zelicof SB, Scott R, et al: Unicompartmental versus total knee arthroplasty in the same patient: A comparative study. *Clin Orthop* 1991;273:151–156.

Twenty-three patients underwent a total knee arthroplasty (TKA) along with a contralateral unicompartmental knee arthroplasty (UKA) during the same hospitalization. They were reviewed at a mean of 81 months postoperatively. It was determined that with proper patient selection, UKA may often provide what the patient perceives as a better knee when compared to TKA. An increased range of motion was noted in the UKA group at follow-up.

Scott RD, Cobb AG, McQueary FG, et al: Unicompartmental knee arthroplasty: Eight- to 12-year follow-up evaluation with survivorship analysis. *Clin Orthop* 1991;271:96–100.

One hundred consecutive unicompartmental knee arthroplasties (UKA) were reviewed with 8- to 12-year follow-up. At follow-up, 87% of patients had no pain and average flexion was 115°. Thirteen knees had been revised (nine for aseptic loosening). Survivorship analysis demonstrated 90%, 85%, and 82% survival respectively at 9, 10, and 11 years.

30

Preoperative Planning for Total Knee Arthroplasty

Preoperative Planning and Templating

Evaluation of the patient for primary arthroplasty must include determination of the extent of the disease, the goals of the patient, overall medical health, other associated joint disease, soft-tissue integrity, bony deformity, motivation, and the ability to participate in a postoperative rehabilitation program. Assessment of the soft tissues about the knee is essential in preoperative planning because there must be adequate soft-tissue coverage. When there are areas of deficient skin from old trauma or multiple prior incisions, a consultation with a plastic surgeon is useful to ensure the availability of adequate soft-tissue coverage at the completion of arthroplasty. Evaluation of the mobility, integrity, and alignment of the extensor mechanism is essential. A chronically dislocated patella or extensor mechanism after a prior patellectomy will need to be addressed at the time of arthroplasty. If extensive soft-tissue contractures are present, it will be necessary to plan for soft-tissue balancing and make a decision regarding prosthetic stability. In the case of a prior patellectomy or a severe flexion contracture, a posterior stabilized prosthesis is preferable to a posterior cruciate ligament (PCL) sacrificing implant because implanting a PCL-substituting prosthesis is technically easier than trying to preserve and balance the PCL. Collateral ligament substituting prostheses are rarely required, and are needed only in those patients in whom soft-tissue balancing cannot be achieved at the time of surgery or in the rare patient who is missing a collateral ligament.

High quality radiographs are essential for preoperative planning. These should include a full-length radiograph of the lower extremity taken in the standing position with a 6-ft tube-to-film distance. This radiograph allows determination of the mechanical axis of the limb as well as of the mechanical and anatomic axes of the femur. A full-length radiograph is especially helpful in preoperative planning for patients with bowing of the femoral or tibial shaft or prior fracture deformity. Radiographs in the anteroposterior (AP) and lateral projection with radiographic markers are helpful in determining appropriate implant size preoperatively. The lateral radiograph should be used to plan for the femoral component size in order to restore the normal AP height of the femur. The choice of the tibial component is best assessed on the AP radiograph; it should cover the medial to lateral extent of the proximal tibia. The extent of patellar bone loss is best assessed on tangential radiographs of the patella taken at 30° to 45° of knee flexion. In the case of extensive patellar bone loss or concavity, an

inset patellar prosthesis may be required rather than an onlay patellar implant.

When planning for primary total knee arthroplasty, the surgeon must consider the type of fixation; the components; and the choice of PCL preservation, sacrifice, or substitution. Cement fixation of all components in total knee arthroplasty remains the proven mode. When the total condylar prosthesis with cement fixation was used, survivorship to revision was found to be 94% at 15 years. Cementless fixation of the tibial component has been problematic in many different designs. Screw fixation is the best mechanical fixation of the cementless tibial component, but has been associated with osteolysis adjacent to the screws as a result of polyethylene wear debris. Short-term results of cementless fixation of the femoral component have been similar to those of cement fixation, but osteolysis caused by polyethylene wear debris has been identified adjacent to both the femoral and tibial components.

PCL preservation has the advantages of joint-line maintenance, proprioception, load transfer to the tibia, centralization of the contact point on the tibial plateau, and femoral rollback. Disadvantages of PCL preservation include more difficult soft-tissue balancing and a less constrained articular geometry than in PCL-sacrificing designs in order to allow for PCL function. This geometry results in higher polyethylene stresses, which may increase polyethylene wear. PCL sacrifice simplifies surgical technique and allows a more conforming articular geometry than PCL preservation. However, PCL sacrifice has the disadvantages of an anterior contact point on the tibia, increased stresses on the tibial bone–cement interface, and less femoral rollback, which may compromise the quadriceps lever arm. PCL substitution assists in femoral rollback and prevents posterior tibial subluxation on the femur. However, the clinical results of PCL preserving, sacrificing, and substituting designs are similar 10 years after arthroplasty.

Planning for the angle of femoral and tibial bone cuts is necessary. Two options exist for femoral component alignment. The normal tibial plateau has a 2° to 3° varus inclination in the coronal plane. Thus, if the tibia is cut in 3° of varus in the coronal plane and the femur is cut in 7° to 9° of valgus, an overall limb alignment of 5° to 7° of valgus tibial femoral angle will result. Alternatively, the tibia may be cut at 0° and the femur at 5° to 7° of valgus (Fig. 1). The decision regarding these two options is based partially on the surgeon's preference, but either option requires meticulous surgical technique. For example, if an initial cut planned to be at 3° of varus is off by 2°, then a 5° varus cut ensues. Varus placement of the tibial component correlates with tibial component loosening regardless of implant design. Zero degrees has often been selected because a slight error in varus of the tibial cut will still be within the acceptable range. In deciding upon the angle of the femoral cut, the angle between the mechanical axis of the femur, that is, the line from the center of the femoral head to the center of the knee, and a line along the midline of the shaft of the femur (anatomic axis) should be selected. This angle usually measures in the range of 5° to 6° of valgus.

The level of bone resection on the femur and tibia will depend on the implant used and the surgical technique. If a PCL-preserving implant is used, the femur will be cut first, and bone, equal to the thickness of the prosthesis used to replace it, will be removed from the distal and posterior aspect of the femur. This will maintain the joint line and help with ligament tension. An appropriate amount of bone will then need to be resected from the tibia to allow a minimal thickness tibial component. A minimal 10-mm thick tibial component should be used to minimize stresses on the tibial polyethylene. A line drawn along the center of the tibial shaft and a perpendicular at the level of greatest bone loss of the tibial plateau is helpful in assessing the differential amount of bone resection required on both plateaus and whether or not there will be any bone deficiency. If resection at the level of maximal tibial bone deficiency would leave a very large bone defect, thereby necessitating a very thick tibial component, then less bone resection is desirable. In these cases, the surgeon must plan for filling of the bone defect with either a bone graft or augmented implants. An augmented implant with a modular metal wedge would be selected for those knees with a residual bone deficiency of 5 to 10 mm, which makes up

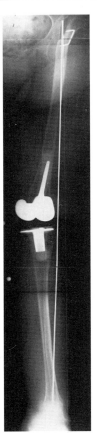

Fig. 2 Full length anteroposterior radiograph of a patient with a resection arthroplasty of the hip and an unstable total knee arthroplasty with valgus deformity. The instability occurred in spite of using a constrained total condylar III prosthesis.

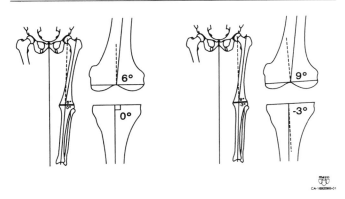

Fig. 1 **Left,** The choice of either a perpendicular or 3° varus cut on the tibia. **Right,** The distal femoral cut should be made the same as the femoral shaft angle if the tibial cut is made perpendicular to the tibia. If the tibial cut is in 3° of varus, the distal femoral cut should be made at the femoral shaft angle plus 3°. (Reproduced with permission from the Mayo Foundation.)

more than 10% of the tibial plateau after resection of the proximal tibia. If the deficiency is greater than 1 cm and makes up more than 20% of the tibial plateau, either a bone graft or a custom implant should be planned.

If a PCL-sacrificing implant is used, and the tibia is to be cut first, a limited tibial resection is performed, followed by a posterior femoral resection. The flexion space is then measured. The amount of bone removed from the distal femur should allow equal flexion and extension spaces. Elevation of the joint line up to 8 mm can be accepted with PCL sacrifice without adverse effects on function of the joint.

In conclusion, planning for primary total knee arthroplasty should include a careful assessment of limb alignment, selection of implant choice, and mode of fixation. The angle and level of bone resection must be planned based on the prosthetic choice and the extent of bone loss. With careful preoperative planning, a satisfactory result can be anticipated.

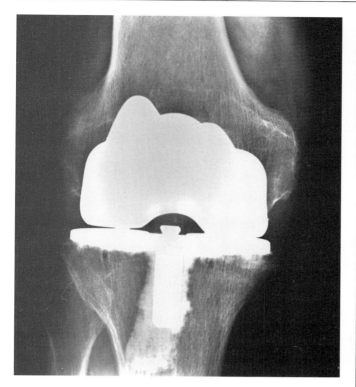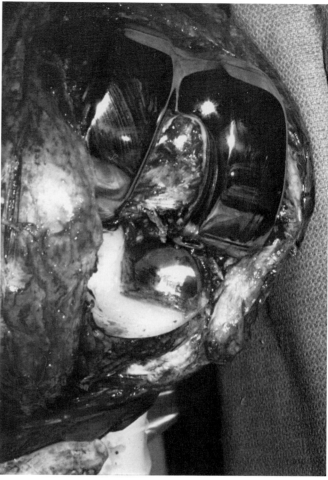

Fig. 3 Anteroposterior radiograph (**left**) and operative photograph (**right**) of severe polyethylene wear of a porous-coated anatomic knee prosthesis.

Revision Total Knee Arthroplasty

Introduction

Failure of total knee arthroplasty leading to revision presents many potential problems. An understanding of the etiology of failure, medical health of the patient, soft tissues and bone stock of the knee, technique of revision, and postoperative rehabilitation are essential to achieve optimal results. A thorough preoperative assessment will allow formulation of an operative treatment plan of management.

Mechanisms of Failure

A thorough assessment of the mechanisms of failure is essential to determine if the patient should be selected for revision surgery. For example, a patient who is young,

obese, or will not follow advised levels of activity will probably fail a revision arthroplasty. A patient who has an unusual anatomic problem that overloads the knee will continue to overload a revision prosthesis, leading to failure (Fig. 2). A patient with a multiply operated knee and a chronically painful arthroplasty without a clear-cut mechanical or septic etiology usually does not improve after revision arthroplasty. Reflex sympathetic dystrophy may be a contributing factor to the chronic pain. An immuno-compromised host in whom sepsis is the cause of failure may be at an increased risk of recurrent sepsis with reimplantation of a new prosthesis. Polyethylene wear has been prevalent in some implant designs with flat-on-flat articular geometries (Fig. 3). If only the polyethylene is exchanged, repeat failure of the polyethylene can be anticipated because the same factors that caused the initial failure of the arthroplasty have not been altered. (For a

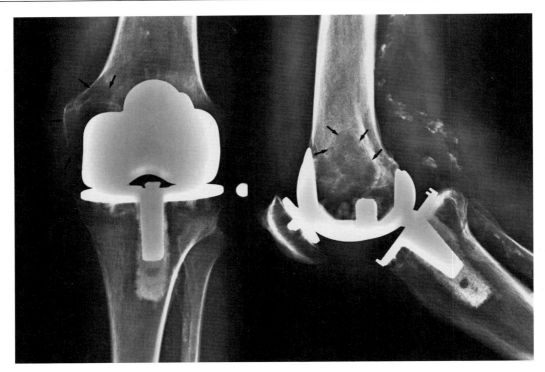

Fig. 4 Anteroposterior (**left**) and lateral (**right**) radiographs of femoral osteolysis from polyethylene wear of a porous-coated anatomic total knee arthroplasty.

thorough discussion of this subject, see the chapter on Evaluation of the Failed Total Knee Arthroplasty.)

Bone Stock

The quality, quantity, and location of remaining bone must be carefully inferred from radiographs. Bone loss may be present on the femur, tibia, and/or patella; it can vary in extent and may be symmetric or asymmetric. Areas of osteolysis from polyethylene wear debris must be carefully sought by a study of the radiographs (Fig. 4). Bone loss on the femur is usually posterior and distal combined.

Bone stock deficiency will affect the technique for achieving fixation of the implant to bone and restoring joint line position. The need for a cancellous or structural bone graft must be anticipated. Whether cancellous ground bone or structural grafts should be selected remains an area of controversy that is beyond the scope of the current review.

In some instances, patellar bone stock may be so deficient that a new patellar implant cannot be fixed adequately. In general, if the remaining patellar bone stock will be less than 12 mm thick, a new patellar implant cannot be adequately fixed to the deficient bone without the risk of fracture. The surgeon must choose between the alternatives of patelloplasty or patellectomy. Patellectomy may result in increased anterior-posterior laxity, especially if the PCL is sacrificed.

Soft Tissues

Exposure of the multiply operated knee can be difficult. Whenever feasible, an earlier incision should be used for the revision arthroplasty. Parallel incisions on the anterior aspect of the knee should be avoided to prevent areas of skin necrosis between the old and new incisions. In general, the most lateral anterior incision that will allow access should be selected. If the soft tissues on the anterior aspect of the knee are deficient or are compromised by previous skin grafts or muscle flaps, a plastic surgeon should be consulted before surgery to assist in soft-tissue management. In some patients, muscle or free flaps may be required either before or at the time of revision arthroplasty to provide healthy soft-tissue coverage of the knee.

The status of the extensor mechanism must be assessed carefully. If the extensor mechanism is disrupted, either an alternative treatment to revision, such as arthrodesis, should be selected, or a reconstruction of the extensor mechanism must be planned in conjunction with the revision arthroplasty. A revision arthroplasty will not function well in the absence of an intact and balanced extensor mechanism.

The integrity of the collateral ligaments and cruciate ligaments must be inferred from a careful examination of the patient and review of the radiographs. Soft-tissue laxity in the presence of intact ligamentous structures can occur

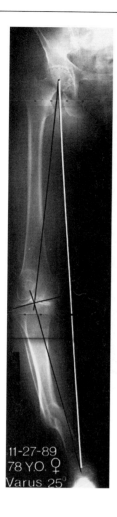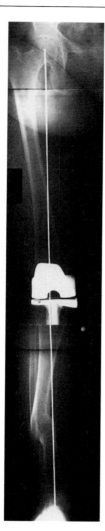

11-27-89
78 Y.O. ♀
Varus 25°

Fig. 5 Full length anteroposterior radiographs of the limb showing prior fracture deformity of the tibia (**left**) and following total knee arthroplasty (**right**). (Reproduced with permission from Rand JA, Franco MG: Revision considerations for fractures about the knee, in Goldberg V (ed): *Controversies of Total Knee Arthroplasty.* New York, NY, Raven Press, 1991, pp 235–247.)

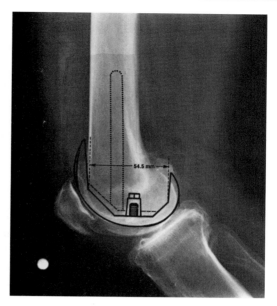

Fig. 6 Lateral radiograph of the contralateral normal knee showing radiographic markers with overlying template to provide the size of the revision arthroplasty.

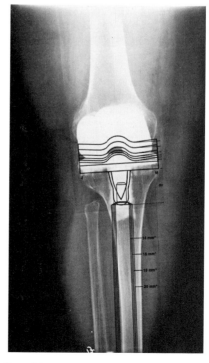

Fig. 7 An offset tibial plateau after a prior osteotomy makes placement of a press-fit extended intramedullary stem infeasible.

from implant loosening, subsidence, or polyethylene wear; the result is a pseudolaxity of the knee. Preoperative knee range of motion will affect the surgeon's ability to gain exposure and obtain a functional range of motion after revision. In the stiff knee, either a proximal V-Y quadricepsplasty or distal tibial tubercle osteotomy may need to be planned. Avulsion of the patellar tendon must be avoided.

Radiographic Assessment

Appropriate radiographs must be obtained before revision. A full-length radiograph of the lower extremity from the hip to the ankle will identify areas of femoral or tibial

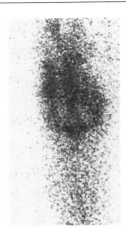

Fig. 8 Indium-111 scan of an infected total knee arthroplasty.

deformity from old fracture or bowing (Fig. 5). Fluoroscopic radiographs of the bone-cement interface will assist in identifying loosening. A tangential patellar radiograph in 30° of flexion will identify asymmetric patellar resurfacing or problems in patellar tracking that will need to be corrected at the time of revision arthroplasty. True AP and lateral radiographs of the contralateral normal knee with radiographic magnification markers provide an excellent template for sizing the femoral implant in order to restore the kinematics of the knee (Fig. 6). Once the implant size has been selected based on the normal knee, the template can be placed on the affected knee. Templating the affected knee will allow assessment of areas of bone deficiency that will need to be treated by bone grafting or prosthetic augmentation. AP and lateral radiographs with magnification markers can be used to assess prosthetic stem location, the angle of the bone cuts, and whether or not problems will be encountered in the use of an extended stem. Some knees will have an offset between the tibial plateau and the tibial shaft that precludes the use of a long canal-filling stem without medial overhang of the tibial tray. An offset tibial plateau is most commonly encountered following an earlier tibial osteotomy, but it may be a problem in the revision arthroplasty patient with tibial bone loss (Fig. 7).

Any knee containing a failed total knee arthroplasty must be evaluated for the potential of deep infection. Hematologic studies, including determination of a white blood cell count, sedimentation rate, and C-reactive protein, are sometimes helpful. Aspiration of the knee may be helpful if positive, but a negative aspiration does not rule out sepsis. Differential technetium-99/indium-111 bone scans have an 84% accuracy rate in the patient without inflammatory arthritis or massive osteolysis (Fig. 8).

Prosthetic Selection

The least constrained prosthesis possible for the patient should be selected. The choice of a prosthesis that preserves, sacrifices, or substitutes for the PCL will depend on the integrity of the PCL and the use of soft-tissue balancing. Patients with a prior or concurrent patellectomy should be considered for a PCL-substituting prosthesis to provide adequate anterior-posterior stability and prevent posterior subluxation of the tibia referable to the femur. A collateral ligament-substituting implant or hinged prosthesis is rarely necessary and should be reserved for those individuals with a deficient collateral ligament.

The femoral implant selected should be sized to restore normal knee kinematics. The inside diameter of the femoral component should fit the remaining femoral bone. The exterior dimension of the femoral component should restore the joint line to its original location and provide equal flexion and extension spaces between the femur and tibia. The usual location for the joint line is 2.5 cm distal to the femoral epicondyles. Templating the opposite normal knee is an excellent technique for predicting femoral component size. With current modular implant systems, the femoral component selected for revision can be selectively augmented distally and posteriorly to achieve the desired goals.

Tibial component selection is based on the size of the remaining tibial bone. An attempt should be made to cover as much of the proximal tibia as possible without component overhang medially. Some implant systems will allow a mismatch between femoral and tibial component size, whereas other implant systems require the same size tibial and femoral components. If preoperative templating suggests that different sizes of femoral and tibial components will be required, the prosthetic system selected must offer this flexibility.

In the presence of metaphyseal bone loss, extended intramedullary stems are desirable to achieve fixation in intact bone. If an extended stem is used, a choice must be made between press-fitting and cement fixation of the stem. The diameter and length of the stem must be chosen. A cemented stem can be of small diameter and a shorter length than a press-fit stem. A press-fit stem should engage the junction of the metaphysis and diaphysis. Although preoperative planning is useful in revision surgery, the actual implant choice depends on the remaining bone stock and the soft-tissue integrity encountered at the time of surgery.

Pitfalls

Incorrect radiographs are the most frequent reason for failure of preoperative planning. If the radiographic magnification is not known, an incorrect implant size may be selected. Correct radiographic magnification is essential in planning the manufacture of custom implants for revision surgery. The common error is to have a custom implant made that is too large for the patient's anatomy.

If soft-tissue deficiency is not recognized before surgery, a revision prosthesis without adequate stability may be selected, which will lead to postoperative instability. A variety of implant constraints should be available at revision to avoid problems of inadequate stability. A thorough assessment of soft-tissue viability should be performed before revision arthroplasty to avoid skin necrosis leading to postoperative sepsis.

The patient with unrecognized sepsis represents a problem. A low-grade pathogenic organism may result in prosthetic loosening that is difficult to distinguish from aseptic loosening before surgery. Revision of the arthroplasty represents an acute prosthetic exchange, which has the potential for recurrent deep infection.

Summary

A thorough preoperative plan is essential to achieve optimal results following revision total knee arthroplasty. The preoperative plan must include definition of the mechanisms of failure of the initial arthroplasty. The quality and integrity of the collateral ligaments, cruciate ligaments, and extensor mechanism must be evaluated. The extent of the remaining bone stock must be assessed. The selection of the revision prosthesis will be based on radiographs with proper magnification, the integrity of the soft tissues, and the quality and quantity of remaining bone stock. The least constrained implant feasible for the patient should be selected. Using these techniques, the best possible results can be achieved following revision total knee arthroplasty.

Annotated Bibliography

Alignment

Rand JA: Preoperative planning and templating, in Rand JA (ed): *Total Knee Arthroplasty.* New York, NY, Raven Press, 1993, pp 93–114.

The importance of patient selection, including evaluation of soft-tissue coverage, ligament instability of the knee, and extensor mechanism, is reviewed. Implant positioning must correct the mechanical axis of the limb.

Implant Fixation

Peters PC Jr, Engh GA, Dwyer KA, et al: Osteolysis after total knee arthroplasty without cement. *J Bone Joint Surg* 1992;74A:864–876.

Of 174 knees with cementless fixation, 16% had osteolysis at an average of 35 months. Osteolysis occurred adjacent to screws fixing the tibial base plate and correlated with particles of polyethylene and metal.

Rorabeck CH, Bourne RB, Lewis PL, et al: The Miller-Galante knee prosthesis for the treatment of osteoarthritis: A comparison of the results of partial fixation with cement and fixation without any cement. *J Bone Joint Surg* 1993;75A:402–408.

A comparison of 183 knees without cement to 209 knees with hybrid fixation found no differences in clinical outcomes at 3 years.

Rorabeck CH, Bourne RB, Nott L: The cemented kinematic-II and the non-cemented porous-coated anatomic prostheses for total knee replacement: A prospective evaluation. *J Bone Joint Surg* 1988;70A:483–490.

A comparison of 110 knees fixed with cement to 50 knees with cementless fixation found higher knee scores in the cemented group at 2 years. The reoperation rate was 4% for the cemented knees compared to 12% for the cementless knees.

Management of Bone Deficiency

Laskin RS: Total knee arthroplasty in the presence of large bony defects of the tibia and marked knee instability. *Clin Orthop* 1989;248:66–70.

Twenty-six knees with bone deficiency of the tibia had primary total knee arthroplasty with autogenous bone grafting. A 67% success rate was achieved at 5 years. Four grafts fragmented. Of nine grafts that were biopsied, four had viable bone.

Rand JA: Bony deficiency in total knee arthroplasty: Use of metal wedge augmentation. *Clin Orthop* 1991;271:63–71.

Twenty-eight knees treated with a metal wedge for a bone defect had satisfactory results at 2 years. There were no reoperations or complications. Radiolucent lines were present in 13 knees.

Patient and Implant Selection

Ranawat CS, Flynn WF Jr, Saddler S, et al: Long-term results of total condylar knee arthroplasty: A 15-year survivorship study. *Clin Orthop* 1993;286:94–102.

Survivorship to revision of 112 total condylar knees was 94% at 15 years. Knee scores were good or excellent in 92%. Radiolucent lines were present in 72%.

Rand JA, Ilstrup DM: Survivorship analysis in total knee arthroplasty: Cumulative rates of survival of 9,200 total knee arthroplasties. *J Bone Joint Surg* 1991;73A:397–409.

A study of 9,200 total knee arthroplasties indicated that a condylar prosthesis with a metal-backed tibial component inserted in a rheumatoid patient who was age 60 years or older had a 90% probability of being in situ at 10 years.

Revision

Jacobs MA, Hungerford DS, Krackow KA, et al: Revision total knee arthroplasty for aseptic failure. *Clin Orthop* 1988;226:78–85.

A study of 28 failed total knees treated by revision indicated that results were good or excellent in 68%. Revisions for pain without a definite etiology preoperatively were not successful.

Meland NB: Complex wound closure following total knee arthroplasty, in Rand JA (ed): *Total Knee Arthroplasty.* New York, NY, Raven Press, 1993, pp 295–308.

The vascular anatomy of the soft tissues about the knee is reviewed with discussion of options for local skin flaps, muscle flaps, and free flap coverage for the knee.

Rand JA, Brown ML: The value of Indium-111 leukocyte scanning in the evaluation of painful or infected total knee arthroplasties. *Clin Orthop* 1990;259:179–182.

Indium-111 bone scanning of 38 painful total knees had an accuracy of 84%, a sensitivity of 83%, and a specificity of 85%.

Rand JA, Peterson LF, Bryan RS, et al: Revision total knee arthroplasty, in *American Academy of Orthopaedic Surgeons Instructional Course Lectures Volume 35.* St. Louis, MO, CV Mosby, 1986, pp 305–318.

A review of 427 revision total knees indicated that survivorship for condylar type prosthesis was best when compared to more constrained implants. A satisfactory result was achieved in 59% following one revision, 52% after two revisions, and 50% after three revisions.

31
Biomaterials and Prosthesis Design in Total Knee Arthroplasty

Introduction

For a total knee arthroplasty to perform successfully, three important design objectives must be met. First, the implant components must provide appropriate control of joint movement (that is, appropriate kinematics), while also providing an adequate range of motion. This objective must, of course, consider the contribution of the remaining soft tissues around the joint. Second, the components must transfer the large loads crossing the joint to the surrounding bony structures. Finally, the implant components must provide long-term performance. This last objective requires that the components provide for long-term or, hopefully, permanent fixation. Recently the concern for fixation has focused on wear resistance, because biologic reactions to wear debris threaten implant fixation just as does mechanical loosening.

The ability to meet these design objectives depends on both the geometry of the implant components and the materials from which they are fabricated. Important geometric considerations include the shapes of the articulating surfaces and the location and shapes of fixation structures, such as pegs and stems. Important material considerations include the elastic, strength, and wear properties of the metallic alloys (cobalt chromium alloy and titanium alloy) and the plastic (ultra-high molecular weight polyethylene) used in total knee arthroplasty.

Design Objectives

The three design objectives for a total knee replacement are not independent, so that if the implant designer or the orthopaedic surgeon is to meet all three objectives, compromises must be sought. Although the objectives can be discussed separately, the compromises between them must be considered to understand the limitations that those compromises create on implant performance.

Kinematics

In the natural knee, a large range of motion is achieved through a combination of bony geometry and ligament constraint. The surfaces of the femoral condyles and the tibial plateau are shaped such that the femur can translate posteriorly on the tibia as flexion increases. Posterior translation assures that the femoral shaft will not impinge on the posterior tibial plateau at large flexion angles. The posterior translation is controlled primarily by the posterior cruciate ligament (PCL), which tethers the femur to the tibia, thus preventing the femur from moving anteriorly on the tibia.

In total knee replacement designs, three different approaches are taken with respect to the PCL: maintaining the ligament (PCL-retaining designs), substituting for the ligament (PCL-substituting or posterior-stabilized designs), and sacrificing the ligament without substitution. Retaining the ligament has the potential advantages of maintaining the normal kinematics, proprioception, and load transfer capabilities of the PCL. But PCL retention has potential disadvantages as well. For example, to insure proper function of the ligament, the joint line must remain near its preoperative level. If the joint line is not reproduced, the kinematics are altered, the loads across the joint can increase, and the polyethylene tibial surface can experience increased wear.

A number of PCL-retaining designs employ a flat surface on the tibial component in the anteroposterior direction. Flat articulating surfaces do not constrain the posterior translation created by the pull of the ligament. These designs often have flat surfaces in the medial-lateral (coronal) direction as well. By designing the articulating surfaces to be flat in both directions, large contact areas can be maintained, thus minimizing the stresses and the resulting wear in the polyethylene tibial component. In this manner, the third design objective, that of maximizing implant longevity, can be met. In fact, when the compressive load across the knee joint is shared between both condyles, such designs can have large contact areas relative to a more condylar type, conforming design and, therefore, lower contact stresses (Fig. 1).

However, in many of the activities of daily living, the knee joint must resist external varus and valgus moments. For example, the ground reaction force during the gait cycle has both medially and laterally directed components that create varus and valgus moments, respectively, at the knee joint. In both the natural knee and the knee with a total joint replacement, load redistribution between the two plateaus is the primary mechanism for resisting these varus–valgus moments. When more load is taken on one plateau relative to the other, an internal moment is created that resists the externally applied moment. In a knee replacement with flat medial-lateral femoral and tibial surfaces, a varus or valgus moment applied across the joint causes the load to be concentrated over a very small area at the outer edge of one plateau of the component (Fig. 1, *bottom*), which in turn leads to locally high stresses in the polyethylene.

Meeting one design objective to insure appropriate kinematics for the PCL while ignoring the kinematic design objective of adequately resisting varus and valgus moments can have a detrimental effect on implant perfor-

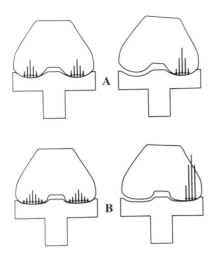

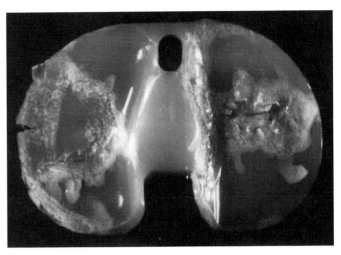

Fig. 1 Two designs of total knee replacement, one with a single medial-lateral radius of curvature for the plateau, (**A**) and another with three radii of curvature for the plateau (**B**). Design B has the larger contact area (a less severe load distribution) than design A when the joint contact load is evenly distributed between both plateaus (**left**). But when a varus or valgus moment is applied across the knee joint, so that the load shifts to one plateau (**right**), the load is much more concentrated for design B (**right**). (Reproduced with permission from Burstein AH, Wright TM: *Fundamentals of Orthopaedic Biomechanics.* Baltimore, MD, Williams & Wilkins, 1994.)

Fig. 2 Cracks and wear are often evident at the peripheries of tibial components of designs with articulating surfaces that are flat in the medial-lateral direction.

mance, as demonstrated by the significant wear damage observed at the outer edge of the polyethylene component in designs with flat tibial and femoral articulating surfaces. The tendency for these components to experience delamination and cracking at the periphery (Fig. 2) is consistent with the large stresses created as a result of the concentration of load. Condylar component surfaces that are curved in the medial–lateral direction accommodate varus–valgus moments more effectively than flatter surfaces. However, compromises must again be sought, because such designs present more constraint to internal and external rotation.

Substituting for the PCL provides both range of motion and joint stability and allows for more conforming surfaces without compromising kinematics. Posterior translation can be achieved by designing the equilibrium position (the "low point") of the tibial component articulating surface to be posterior. The posterior position of the femur relative to the tibia is assured by the incorporation of a cam mechanism (Fig. 3). A disadvantage of posterior-stabilized designs is that they require more resection of femoral bone from the intercondylar notch to make room for the cam mechanism.

Sacrificing the PCL without substituting for it with a posterior-stabilized cam mechanism is not as widely used in contemporary total knee arthroplasty, although such designs represent most of the earliest successful attempts at knee replacement. These designs suffered, however,

from limited range of motion (usually less than 100° of flexion) and from failure through anterior subluxation of the tibia (caused by the lack of PCL function).

Differences in performance and clinical outcome of contemporary PCL-retaining and PCL-substituting designs are generally insignificant. Patients with either type of design achieve excellent range of motion (typically greater than 110°). Although patients in whom the PCL is retained are believed to perform stair-climbing tasks in a more normal fashion, results from gait analysis studies on this subject are contradictory. No significant differences exist between the designs in terms of level gait.

Load Transfer

In the knee with a knee replacement, joint loads as large as several times body weight pass across the joint, through the implant components, and into the underlying cancellous bone of the distal femur and proximal tibia. These large loads can be transferred successfully only if the materials that compose the structures in the system can withstand the stresses they must carry. The weak link in the load transfer pathway through the knee with a knee replacement is cancellous bone. Of the materials in the system (metallic alloys, polyethylene, polymethylmethacrylate bone cement, and cortical and cancellous bone), cancellous bone is the only one that experiences stresses in the same range as its strength and whose mechanical failure leads directly to loss of fixation.

This realization was a primary reason for introducing metal backings to polyethylene components more than a decade ago (another reason being to allow for porous coatings for biologic ingrowth). The stress on any given region of underlying cancellous bone can be reduced by more evenly distributing loads across the top of the tibia.

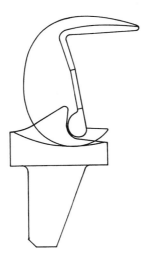

Fig. 3 The lateral view of a posterior-stabilized knee replacement demonstrates that roll back is accomplished by the geometry of the articulating surfaces, which have their equilibrium (low point) position posterior on the tibial plateau, and is assured by the intercondylar cam mechanism.

The addition of a metal backing allows for more even load distribution because of its increased stiffness, which in turn is the result of the large elastic modulus of the metallic alloy compared to that of polyethylene. Whereas analytical and experimental evidence shows the efficacy of a metal backing, comparisons of knee replacement patients with and without metal-backed components have not shown a clear clinical advantage for metal backing.

In fact, the performance of metal-backed components has been discredited by the significant incidence (more than 10% in some series) of excessive polyethylene wear, dissociation between the metallic and polyethylene portions, and osteolysis reported for metal-backed tibial and patellar components. These failures represent another inappropriate compromise in meeting design objectives, which was caused by both design and surgical factors. If the overall component thickness is kept constant, for example, by removing polyethylene to make room for the metal backing, the resulting thin layer of polyethylene will be subjected to higher stresses and more wear and deformation than a thicker layer would be. In fact, the more the thickness decreases, the more the polyethylene becomes the weak link in the load transfer system, because the stresses the polyethylene must withstand increase to beyond the material's ability to resist them.

The other possibility is to make the tibial component thicker with the addition of the metal backing. The thicker polyethylene can be a part of the component design or, with current modular systems, the surgeon can decide in the operating room to use a thicker polyethylene insert to attach to the metal backing. In this case, the surgeon must decide whether to cut more bone from the proximal tibia

or to raise the joint line to accommodate the thicker component. The former approach compromises tibial component fixation by removing stronger cancellous bone near the subchondral region, whereas the latter approach compromises patellofemoral joint kinematics, particularly if a PCL-retaining design is used.

Metal backing affords the opportunity for modular systems that can be used effectively in difficult primary and revision situations involving, for example, bony defects and compromised soft tissues. Defects in the proximal tibia can be treated in a number of ways, including insertion of bone grafts. Modular designs usually incorporate metallic inserts that can be added to the inferior surface of the metallic tibial tray at the time of surgery. Short of grafting the defect, filling the defect area with a metallic extension rigidly attached to the tibial tray is the most effective way of transferring loads to the remaining bone.

Knee replacement designs must sometimes include additional constraints across the joint when the constraints provided by soft tissues have been compromised by injury or bony deformity. Load transfer considerations become more complex in such cases, because bending moments and torques are transferred across the joint through the implant components and are not shared by the soft tissues. The resulting more-constrained implant designs incorporate long intramedullary stems.

Long-Term Performance

The mechanical performance of any structure is controlled both by its shape and by the materials from which it is fabricated. For total joint implants, shape and material control both the mechanical and the wear performance. For example, because of the strength of the metallic alloys, usually cobalt chromium or titanium alloys, used to fabricate femoral components and metal backings, mechanical failures of these components are very rare. Because of their hardness and because of their polished surface finishes, the wear behavior of the metallic alloys is also satisfactory. The same is generally true for ultra-high molecular weight polyethylene, which has functioned well as a bearing material in most joint replacements.

In most knee implant designs, however, large contact loads are applied across nonconforming articulating surfaces; this loading results in polyethylene stresses that often exceed the material's strength. Therefore, the potential for wear damage to the polyethylene with the associated release of wear debris particles to the surrounding joint tissues is high. Clinical evidence that the subsequent biologic response to wear debris is linked to osteolysis and subsequent implant loosening has made wear-related failure a significant long-term concern in total knee arthroplasty.

Because the loads applied across the knee joint are repetitive in nature for many of a patient's daily activities, the polyethylene must withstand large stresses over millions of cycles. Stress fluctuations can occur over large regions of the tibial articulating surface as the contact area moves across the surface during joint motion (Fig. 4). The damage modes, such as delamination and pitting, that are prevalent in polyethylene tibial components result from fatigue fracture occurring at and below the polyethylene articulating surface as a result of cyclic stress. These modes of wear release large amounts of polyethylene to the surrounding joint fluids and tissues.

Both component shape and the material properties of the polyethylene affect the way in which the polyethylene wears. In total knee replacement, important shape parameters include thickness and the contours of the polyethylene and metallic articulating surfaces. Selection of the radii of curvature for the articulating surfaces again requires compromise in seeking to fulfill two different design objectives. On the one hand, appropriate kinematics requires nonconforming articular shapes (certainly nonconforming relative to the hip joint with its simple ball-and-socket kinematics) to provide range of motion compatible with ligament and muscle function. On the other hand, these nonconforming shapes result in small, moving contact areas that lead to high stresses and damaged polyethylene.

One intriguing approach to this problem is to separate the kinematics into two different systems, one occurring at the articulating surface and one occurring at the interface between the polyethylene insert and an underlying polished metallic tray. The so-called meniscal-bearing knees have shown good clinical results, although they require surgical expertise to implant, are generally more costly than more conventional fixed-bearing knees, and have also suffered from polyethylene wear and fracture problems.

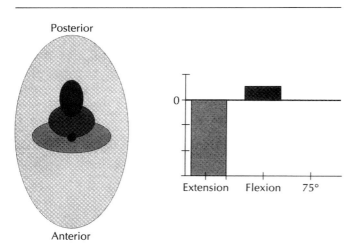

Fig. 4   When the contact area moves posteriorly on the tibial plateau during flexion, a point on the surface first experiences large compressive stresses when it lies at the center of contact, then experiences large tensile stresses when it lies at the edge of the contact area, and with further flexion, finally experiences zero stress as the contact area moves beyond the point. With extension, the cycle is reversed. (Reproduced with permission from Burstein AH, Wright TM: *Fundamentals of Orthopaedic Biomechanics*. Baltimore, MD, Williams & Wilkins, 1994.)

Wear performance is also affected by the material properties of the ultra-high molecular weight polyethylene, although little is currently known as to the magnitude that variations in these properties must reach to significantly affect performance. From observations made on retrieved polyethylene knee components and from experimental studies, it is known that chemical, physical, and mechanical properties of polyethylene can be affected by a number of factors, including the starting resin from which the material is fabricated, the fabrication process used to form a finished component, the method of sterilization, postirradiation shelf storage, and exposure to the in vivo environment. Until stringent controls on at least some of the material and fabrication factors become accepted throughout the orthopaedic industry, it will be difficult both to assess the impact on wear performance and to separate the relative impact of shape versus material contributions to the wear problem.

Patellofemoral Joint

The design of implants to replace the patellofemoral joint also requires consideration of kinematics, load transfer, and long-term performance. The natural patella provides a mechanical lever arm for the quadriceps muscle that also helps protect the quadriceps tendon as it traverses the knee joint, allowing a large range of motion in flexion and extension. This function must be maintained after resurfacing to assure proper kinematics not only between the patella and the femur, but also between the femur and the tibia. The design of the patellofemoral joint must also provide for load transfer, long-term stable fixation, and wear resistance.

Like the femur and tibia, the patella encounters contact forces greater than body weight even during normal activities. The kinematics between the natural patella and femur are complex. During flexion and extension of the knee, the bony constraints between the patellar facets and the patellar surface of the femur, together with soft-tissue forces, cause the patella to rotate, tilt, and translate with respect to the femur. But the patella maintains adequate contact with the femur throughout the range of motion so that contact pressures on the cartilage and underlying bone remain low.

Range-of-motion and kinematics considerations lead to similar problems in patellofemoral replacement design as occur in designing the femorotibial articulation: kinematics that rely on the incorporation of soft-tissue constraints and articulating geometries that move and change shape during motion of the joint. Patellar component design alone cannot be expected to provide appropriate or adequate constraint. Proper function of the total knee replacement with patellar resurfacing relies much more on the surgical reconstruction. Moreover, patellofemoral joint stability depends on the degree of constraint designed into the femorotibial joint.

Three general types of patellofemoral joints exist in contemporary knee designs: anatomic shapes for both the patellar component and the patellar surface on the femoral component; a spherical, dome shape for the patellar component that contacts a single radius of curvature patellar groove on the femoral component; and the introduction of an additional articulation within the patellar component itself. Anatomically-shaped components provide a more conforming patellar track than is possible with less constrained designs, but they require surgical skill to achieve both appropriate alignment between the three implant components and adequate soft-tissue balance throughout the range of motion.

Dome-shaped patellar components were the first widely accepted components used for patellar resurfacing. The dome design eliminates the importance of surgically achieving rotatory alignment between patellar and femoral components and allows for a symmetrically-shaped femoral component, thus reducing inventory by eliminating the need for right and left femoral components.

Separating the articulation into two parts, one at the articulating surface between the patella and the femur and one at a flat surface between the polyethylene insert and a metal backing, allows the insert to rotate with respect to the backing, which remains fixed to the bony patella. The added rotational degree of freedom has the same advantage as the dome design in that rotational alignment is not critical, even though the articulating surface has an anatomic shape. Potential disadvantages of this design type are that the polyethylene insert is thin and the additional interface provides another source of wear.

No well-controlled clinical studies exist that allow for conclusions as to the effect of design on clinical outcome, and few experimental studies have been performed to assess directly the effect of patellofemoral design on kinematics, fixation, or wear performance. Experimental studies of patellofemoral joint replacements have significant limitations in that the functional forces and the active soft-tissue constraints are difficult to recreate in vitro.

In a number of clinical studies, metal-backed patellar components have been associated with a high incidence of failure due to excessive polyethylene wear and dissociation between the polyethylene insert and the metal backing. Considerations of polyethylene thickness appear even more important in patellar components than in tibial components. Anatomic limitations in the patella require smaller, thinner polyethylene inserts. Polyethylene thicknesses in most metal-backed patellar designs are less than 2 mm in the contact regions where articulation with the femoral component occurs.

Decreasing thickness to add a metal backing has the same consequences (increased wear and deformation) as in metal-backed tibial components. Maintaining polyethylene thickness by increasing overall component thickness with the addition of the metal backing is an even less viable alternative in the patella than in the tibia. The remaining bony patella would be at great risk for fracture. Anatomic limitations also limit the type of locking mechanisms that can be incorporated into the design to secure the polyethylene insert to the metal backing. Many of the existing mechanisms rely on the structural integrity of the polyethylene insert. Unfortunately, given the large stresses that the polyethylene experiences compared to its yield strength, the insert often undergoes gross plastic deformation, which leads to disruption of the locking mechanism and dissociation of the insert from the backing.

Annotated Bibliography

Biomaterials

Blunn GW, Lilley PA, Walker PS: Variability of the wear of ultra high molecular weight polyethylene in simulated TKR. *Trans Orthop Res Soc* 1994;19:177.

   Using a multistation test machine aimed at simulating the kinematics of knee replacement, the authors demonstrated that wear of polyethylene as measured by weight loss in the test specimens differed depending on the starting resin used to fabricate the polyethylene. These data added yet another variable to those known to influence long-term performance.

Bostrom MP, Bennett AP, Rimnac CM, et al: The natural history of ultra high molecular weight polyethylene. *Clin Orthop* 1994;309:20–28.

   The chemical and physical properties of ultra-high molecular weight polyethylene were monitored in tibial components from the starting extruded bar condition, through manufacturing, sterilization, shelf storage, implantation, and subsequent retrieval for a dozen patients undergoing total knee replacement. The results demonstrated the important effects of sterilization and subsequent degradation both on the shelf and in the body on properties that control the long-term performance of the polyethylene in these components.

Friedman RJ, Black J, Galante JO, et al: Current concepts in orthopaedic biomaterials and implant fixation, in Schafer M (ed): *Instructional Course Lectures 43.* Rosemont, IL, American Academy of Orthopaedic Surgeons, 1994, pp 233–255.

   This review article from the Academy's Instructional Course Lecture series examines the role of biomaterials in implant design, in implant fixation, and in the biologic reaction occurring around implant components as a result of release of debris from polymeric and metallic materials.

Galante JO, Lemons J, Spector M, et al: The biologic effects of implant materials. *J Orthop Res* 1991;9:760–775.

This paper reviewed the materials used to design orthopaedic implants and the issues related to wear particle-induced osteolysis. Macrophages, activated by phagocytosis of particulate debris, are the key cells in the process, which can potentially occur in any implant system regardless of implant design or fixation mode.

Li S, Howard EG: Abstract: Characterization and description of an enhanced ultra high molecular weight polyethylene for orthopaedic bearing surfaces. *Trans Soc Biomater* 1990; 13:190.

This abstract presents the results of a study that established that wide variations in the properties of ultra-high molecular weight polyethylene exist among commercial implants. The implication is that such variations alone would be expected to affect long-term performance of these implants separate from design and degradation effects.

Rimnac CM, Klein RW, Betts F, et al: Post-irradiation aging of ultra-high molecular weight polyethylene. *J Bone Joint Surg* 1994;76A:1052–1056.

An experiment was conducted to establish that shelf aging of polyethylene components is associated with degradation that is accompanied by alteration in physical and chemical properties. The alteration in properties is consistent with an increase in the stresses experienced by the component once it is implanted, demonstrating the effect that material properties and alterations in those properties can have on implant performance.

Wrona M, Mayor MB, Collier JP, et al: The correlation between fusion defects and damage in tibial polyethylene bearings. *Clin Orthop* 1994;299:92–103.

In subjectively examining 50 retrieved polyethylene components (40 tibial inserts and ten acetabular components), the authors found significant positive correlations ($p < 0.05$) between the extent of defects in the polyethylene material and cracking, delamination, total wear damage, and duration in vivo. Material quality can thus help explain the long-term wear performance of polyethylene components.

Design

Bartel DL, Rimnac CM, Wright TM: Evaluation and design of the articular surface, in Goldberg VM (ed): *Controversies of Total Knee Arthroplasty.* New York, NY, Raven Press, 1991, pp 61–73.

This paper reviews the implant design variables, including conformity, thickness, and material properties, that affect the stresses in polyethylene joint components. Observations from retrieved components are used to establish wear damage modes and to support the correlation between stress magnitudes and distributions and the observed wear.

Blunn GW, Joshi AB, Lilley PA, et al: Polyethylene wear in unicondylar knee prostheses: 106 retrieved Marmor,

PCA, and St. George tibial components compared. *Acta Orthop Scand* 1992;63:247–255.

By examining retrieved unicondylar polyethylene tibial components of three implant types that differed in the design of the articulating surfaces, the authors concluded that both design and material quality affected the amount of wear damage observed on the components.

Burstein AH, Wright TM: Biomechanics, in Insall JN (ed): *Surgery of the Knee,* ed 2. New York, NY, Churchill Livingstone, 1993, vol 1, pp 43–62.

This book chapter reviews the relevant biomechanics of both the natural knee and the knee with a joint replacement and investigates the compromises between knee kinematics and joint load. These concepts are described in terms of how they affect total knee joint performance.

Rullkoetter PJ, Anderson DD, Hillberry BM: The effects of rotation and sliding on the stress state in UHMWPE tibial inserts. *Trans Orthop Res Soc* 1994;19:801.

Using two-dimensional finite element models, the authors demonstrated that when flexion and sliding movements were modeled as part of the contact problem in total knee type geometries, the stresses in the polyethylene tibial component associated with wear damage were increased over those in which these movements were not modeled. The study underscores not only the large stresses that polyethylene experiences in implant applications, but also the important role that kinematics plays in the wear and, hence, the long-term performance of total knee components.

Tsao A, Mintz L, McRae CR, et al: Failure of the porous-coated anatomic prosthesis in total knee arthroplasty due to severe polyethylene wear. *J Bone Joint Surg* 1993;75A: 19–26.

This paper presented the results of 32 clinical failures due to severe polyethylene wear in porous-coated anatomic knee replacements that represented 7% of the implants performed by a single surgeon over a 7-year period. The failures were attributed to design and material problems, demonstrating the effect of conformity and material properties on polyethylene wear.

Walker PS, Blunn GW, Joshi AB, et al: Modulation of delamination by surface wear in total knees. *Trans Orthop Res Soc* 1993;18:499.

Experimental wear tests and finite element stress analyses were used to examine the role of material defects and component design on the propensity for total knee type articulating surfaces to experience delamination type wear. The authors concluded that the combination of less conforming surfaces and the presence of unconsolidated polyethylene particle defects led to more extensive and more rapid delamination than the combination of more conforming surfaces and few defects. The results underscore the importance of both material properties and design in wear performance of polyethylene implant components.

32

Surgical Principles in Total Knee Arthroplasty: Alignment, Deformity, Approaches, and Bone Cuts

Alignment

Reestablishing proper knee alignment is one of the most important tasks to be accomplished at total knee arthroplasty; therefore, it is necessary to recall the standards for normal knee alignment. A line connecting the center of the femoral head with the center of the ankle is known as the mechanical axis of the lower extremity, and normal alignment is said to exist when this line passes through the center of the knee (Fig.1). If the knee lies medial to this line, a valgus deformity exists, and if the knee lies lateral to this line, a varus deformity exists. Although the distance between the center of the knee and the mechanical axis of the lower extremity varies with the amount of deformity, this particular line or distance does not permit the direct quantitative characterization of the angular deformity. That characterization depends not only on the angulation, but also on the overall size of the extremity.

The mechanical axis of the femur is the line from the center of the femoral head to the center of the knee. In contrast, the anatomic axis of the femur is a line that indicates the position or location of the overall axis of the femoral shaft. Finally, the mechanical axis of the tibia is a line from the center of the knee to the center of the ankle or, actually, a line that describes the overall axis of the tibia itself. Thus, the tibial shaft axis and the mechanical axis of the tibia are the same. The anatomic axis of the femur usually is positioned approximately 6° lateral to the me-

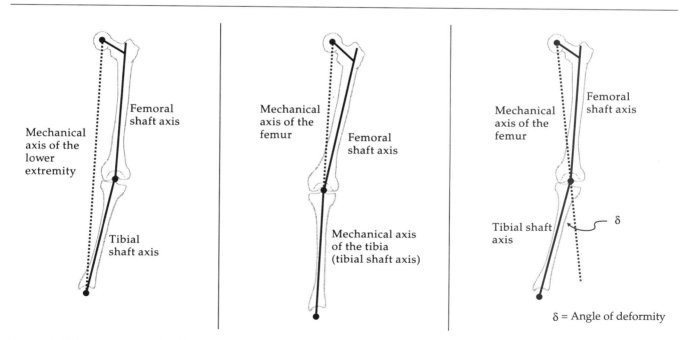

Fig. 1 **Left,** In a lower extremity with varus deformity, the mechanical axis passes medial to the knee. **Center,** When alignment is normal, the mechanical axis of the femur is in line with the mechanical axis of the tibia (tibial shaft axis). The line represented by the mechanical axes of the femur and the tibia is coincident with the mechanical axis of the lower extremity in this situation. **Right,** Varus deformity is represented by angle δ because the tibial shaft axis should be coincident with the mechanical axis of the femur as it projects on the dotted line from the femoral head through and beyond the center of the knee.

chanical axis. The mechanical axis of the femur and the tibial shaft axis will be coincident with the overall mechanical axis of the lower extremity if normal alignment exists (Fig. 1). The actual angle of deformity is the angle that exists between the mechanical axis of the femur and the mechanical or shaft axis of the tibia.

The presence and amount of overall varus or valgus deformity do not specifically say anything about the joint-line orientation. Anatomic and radiographic studies document an average position of the joint line with respect to the overall axes. These positions, which are approximately 8° to 9° of valgus on the femoral side and 2° to 3° of varus on the tibial side, lead to an average overall tibiofemoral angle of 6° valgus and a joint line orientation that is 2° to 3° different from perpendicular in the frontal plane. This natural joint line orientation can be designated *anatomic* to distinguish it from what usually is created during total knee arthroplasty.

Most total knee instrumentation systems and prosthetic components are associated with a slightly different joint line and component position—referred to here as *classical* alignment. For classical alignment, the joint line typically has been arranged perpendicular to the reconstructed mechanical axis. Thus, after exact, proper tibial component positioning under this scheme, the tibial joint line would be perpendicular to the tibial shaft or mechanical axis, perpendicular to the femoral mechanical axis, and at a 6° valgus orientation with respect to the femoral shaft axis. The prosthetic components may also be placed in the anatomic position (Fig. 2).

Deformity

Using the definitions and approximate normal values outlined above, it is possible to analyze an individual case and to assess the magnitude and location of each component of deformity. Such deformity can be ascribed to relative variation at the femoral and/or tibial side of the joint and within the joint space itself (Fig. 3). Assume that a set of presurgical radiographs has the following lines and angle information: (distal) femoral joint angle of 5° valgus, (proximal) tibial joint angle of 8° varus, and intra-articular angle (the angle between a line across the distal femoral condyles and another across the proximal tibial plateaus) of 5° varus. The overall deformity would be (9° normal valgus minus 5° valgus) + (8° existing tibial varus minus

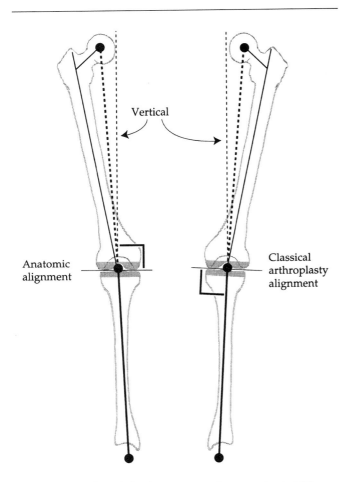

Fig. 2 Anatomic and classic arrangements are contrasted. The same tibiofemoral angle has been produced because the tibial shaft axis lies on the projection of the femoral mechanical axis. Joint line orientation differs typically by 2° or 3°.

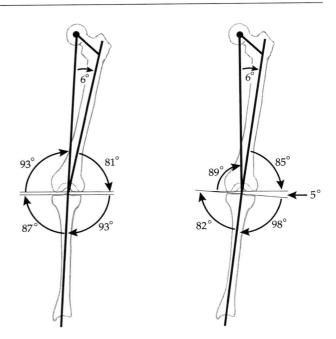

Fig. 3 **Left,** In a typical, normally aligned knee, angles are approximately as shown. **Right,** A varus deformity situation is shown.

3° normal) + (5° intra-articular angle minus 0° normal) = 4° + 5° + 5° = 14° varus deformity. A perpendicular joint line arrangement would create a cut 8° different from the existing 8° varus tibial joint line orientation, and a 6° valgus distal femoral cut would be 1° more valgus than the existing 5° valgus orientation.

Extra-Articular Deformity

The previous definition and analysis largely ignore the intermediate shape of the respective tibial and femoral shaft axes during consideration of the overall shaft alignment. However, it is occasionally necessary to analyze radiographs that show significant extra-articular deformity secondary to fracture or to developmental or metabolic considerations. Such cases can be analyzed using modern computer programs or, more simply, using tracing paper. Moreover, basic geometry and trigonometry yield some relatively simple rules of approximation that can be summarized as follows:

A tibial or femoral shaft extra-articular deformity of a certain angular amount creates a corresponding deformity at the knee in approximate proportion to the percentage of the distance from the hip or ankle to the knee at which the extra-articular deformity is located (Fig. 4). A 10° varus deformity located 80% of the distance from the hip to the knee would impart approximately an 8° varus defor-

mity at the knee, and this deformity would be 100% on the femoral side (Fig. 5).

Soft-Tissue Sleeve Deformity

The deformity seen clinically and on radiographs can be a combination of a prior extra-articular bone deformity, bone/cartilage intra-articular wear, and a combination of soft-tissue stretching and/or soft-tissue contracture. The absolute amount of deformity a surgeon must address is more directly implied by the relative asymmetry of the soft-tissue sleeve. The surgeon seeks to create a prosthetic where the tibia and femur feel stable with the flexion and extension gaps filled, with the joint surfaces in contact when the joint is properly aligned. Achievement of such a state can be expected if and when the soft-tissue sleeve is balanced or feels symmetric in the following sense: Imagine that all femoral cuts and the proximal tibial cut have been made and that the tibia distracted away from the femur so that in full extension the medial and lateral soft-tissue sleeve is taut. If, in this state, properly made femoral and tibial cuts are parallel, the overall tibiofemoral angle is normal at approximately 6° valgus, and the soft-tissue sleeve is balanced or symmetric. Similarly, it is possible to distract the cut surfaces away at any degree of flexion and assess the "rectangularness" of the gap in order to assess soft-tissue symmetry throughout the flexion-extension

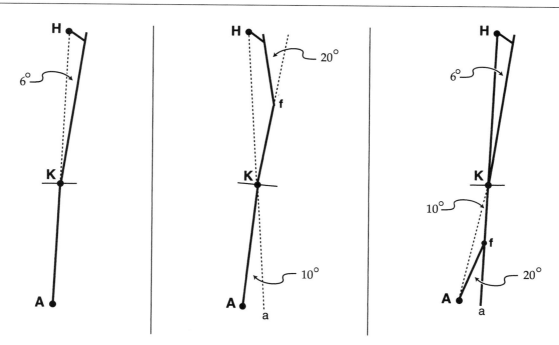

Fig. 4 **Left,** Normal alignment is shown; HKA is a straight line. **Center,** Varus angulation is 20° at f, approximately 50% of the way along the femur. Angle HKA will now be approximately 170°. Angle AKa, the deformity is 10° varus; because the tibia is unchanged, the entire deformity is within the femur. **Right,** Varus angulation at f, the midpoint of the tibia is 20°. Angle AKa (AKf) represents the deformity and is half of angle Afa.

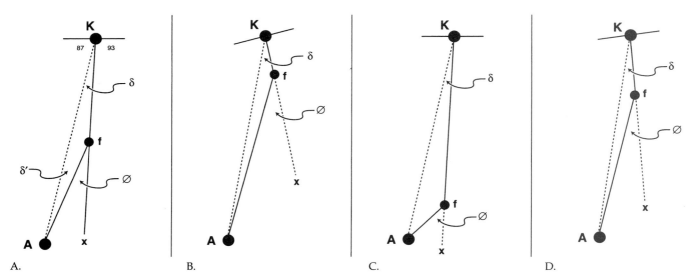

Fig. 5   A, A fracture at the midpoint with angulation of φ, creates a deformity δ that is 1/2 φ. Triangle AKf is isosceles; therefore, angle δ = angle δ′. Angle AfK is 180° − φ, and angle AfK + 2δ = 180°. Therefore, φ = 2δ. **B,** As f moves toward K, φ becomes arbitrarily close to δ. **C,** Moving f to A makes δ go to 0. **D,** At 70% of the way toward the knee, δ is approximately equal to 0.7 × φ.

cycle. These considerations suggest that such a "tension-stress" examination of the joint should be performed to assess the deformity or asymmetry of the soft-tissue sleeve.

Rotational Alignment

While looking at the end of the distal femur, the surgeon should begin to think about issues of proper femoral component rotational alignment. Significant disagreement exists as to what standard of reference should be used to define 0° or neutral rotation. Two axes are typically involved at the distal femur: one is the line tangent to both posterior femoral condyles when the end of the femur is viewed in 90° of flexion (posterior condylar axis). The second is the axis connecting the epicenters of the medial and lateral femoral epicondyles. These two lines tend not to be parallel—the epicondylar axis is generally externally rotated 3° to 10° with respect to the posterior condylar axis. The posterior condylar axis tends to parallel the proximal tibial joint line. It is convenient to think of the posterior condyles as corresponding to the anatomic axis for rotation and the epicondylar axis as corresponding to a classical axis for rotation because these axes tend to parallel the classical or perpendicular tibial cut, respectively.

Defining appropriate rotation of the tibial component may be even more difficult. The surgeon should look at rotation not only as it appears at the proximal tibia itself, but should also consider how it affects the position of the ankle and foot.

Most experienced surgeons place great emphasis on rotating the tibial component so that the midpoint is aimed toward the medial one third of the tibial tubercle. However, because of the potential for significant variation in anatomic landmarks, the surgeon must occasionally accept some variation and consider other elements, such as the shape of the cut tibial surface, the rotational position of the ankle and foot, and the intermalleolar axis.

Other aspects of rotational alignment relate to distortion on radiographs. With rotation, curvatures in one plane can develop components of angulation in other planes. Flexion contracture as well as the anterior bow of the femur project as lateral bowing and also as a varus deformity on a long-standing lower extremity radiograph if the lower extremity is externally rotated—a common situation.

Surgical Approaches

Incisions

Skin incisions have evolved to a relatively central location, midline to slightly lateral or medial, at the respective patellar margins. Some surgeons believe that a straight incision offers the advantage of better vascularity. Others prefer a slightly curved incision, which will not be stretched so much with each range-of-motion cycle. There seems to be relatively less concern with the amount of undermining necessary over the anterior aspect of the knee because there are only sparse vascular connections in this area. Even the most conservative amount of undermining will require some "flap" over the patella, as well as enough exposure of the medial or lateral capsule to permit suture closure. Use of any type of patellar clamp or patellar cutting preparation equipment requires that the patella be uncovered to some degree. When placing the incision it is important to avoid previous parallel, or nearly parallel, nearby incisions, because such incisions can lead to vascular compromise of a narrow skin bridge. For this reason, it is best whenever possible to use previous incisions. In selected difficult cases, the surgeon may do a sham "test" incision, which is a preliminary incision made in the same way as the surgeon would raise and delay a skin flap.

Capsular incisions are somewhat more variable today than they may have been in years past. Most knees done through a medial parapatellar approach are opened relatively close to the patella at the vastus medialis obliquus–quadriceps area; more proximally, at the junction of the medial and central third of the quadriceps tendon, and farther medial from the patella more distally. Variations include the "Southern" subvastus approach and the lateral approach (of Keblish) used by some in the setting of lateral ligament release for valgus deformity. The subvastus Southern approach has the purported advantage of avoiding incision in the anterior quadriceps mechanism. This approach probably sustains the anteromedial circulation to the patella as well as an anteromedial tether that may serve to stabilize the patella as well as diminish the frequency of lateral release. Consensus suggests that the exposure is slightly more limited and may be relatively problematic in patients who are obese, have a decreased range of motion, or have undergone previous significant surgical procedures with attendant scarring, such as proximal tibial osteotomy or fracture fixation.

The lateral exposure of Keblish supposedly provides improved direct access to the region of the lateral ligaments released with valgus deformity. Its originator reports an essentially uniform, problem-free experience. The approach frequently requires a modified tibial tubercle osteotomy—elevation of the extensor insertion. Also, the lateral retinacular release as part of the lateral approach results in an inability to close the lateral capsule, which is almost directly under the skin incision. Thus, a fat pad flap is required to effect a subcutaneous seal at the joint line.

Extensor Mechanism

In most cases, no special handling of the extensor mechanism other than eversion of the patella is required during surgical exposure. Care must obviously be taken to avoid peeling or rupture of the patellar tendon insertion. Patients with limited flexion or other sources of difficulty with patellar eversion and general mobilization are typically managed with some interruption of the extensor mechanism. There are essentially three techniques for doing this: (1) The rectus snip (first popularized by John Insall) consists of dividing the lateral aspect of the quadriceps tendon relatively proximally. Because division is made

relatively proximally, a good length of quadriceps tendon is left for medial to lateral repair distal to the snip. Therefore, the patella should not drop, and the approximation of proximal lateral to distal lateral remains adequate. (2) The modified Coonse-Adams technique is a downward directed cut across the lateral aspect of the quadriceps tendon and the lateral retinaculum, which frequently blends with an extensive lateral release. This approach necessitates slightly greater attention to repair and may be associated with a greater decrease in vascularity to the patella. (3) A tibial tubercle osteotomy is generally done with lateral muscle and fascial tissue still attached to the tibial tuberosity fragment. The fragment is large enough—approximately 1.5×6 cm—to allow major fixation for reattachment using screws or wires.

There are strong proponents for, as well as critics of, each of these techniques. Pertinent considerations are the relative amount of additional exposure provided and the inherent safety of each technique. There is a relative order of exposure enhancement, with the tibial tubercle osteotomy providing greatest enhancement, followed by the more standard Coonse-Adams turndown, and the quadricep snip, which provides the least enhancement. Therefore, selection of a procedure should be based on the relative difficulty of the case, tissue mobility, and general tightness of the exposure. No very elaborate repair of the quadricep snip need be undertaken. Repair of the Coonse-Adams turndown is by sutures, and varying degrees of attention should be given to special suturing techniques. Reattachment of the tibial tubercle is quite important. Most commonly it is reattached with two or three lag screws, but wires or staples may also be used.

Postoperative management of any extensor mechanism interruption varies. The interruption is ignored in many instances, and active extension and passive flexion are limited in others. Specific casting is rarely undertaken.

Bone Cuts

The aspects of bone cuts and preparation covered in this subsection include ease and accuracy of performance of cuts and specific positioning of cuts and components with respect to how such positioning impacts on flexion-extension ligament balance.

Bone may be cut with less physical difficulty if fresh, sharp blades are used with the appropriate amount of pressure. The blade must move forward without jamming. A "whittle" technique of attacking sharp corners and gradually changing direction allows more effective progress through hard bone. Accuracy, which is achieved by adhering to the guidance of a cutting block or slot, promotes easy, secure fit in a case of press-fit femoral applications, and promotes an overall more accurate axial alignment in the case of distal femoral and proximal tibial cuts. The surgeon must be aware of factors of play within the instrument systems and of the potential for saw blade wander.

Flexion-Extension Ligament Balancing

It must be understood that flexion-extension ligament balance is to be distinguished from ligament balance during deformity management. The establishment of proper flexion-extension ligament balance must be addressed whether or not a deformity exists.

Femur

Currently, most knee instrumentation systems establish basic femoral bone cut positions in relation to the femoral surfaces present initially. A step is undertaken to estimate approximate femoral component size; then cuts are positioned in relation to one or more of several references: the level of the posterior and distal condyles, the location and level of the anterior femoral cortex, and the level of the trochlear groove and/or the intercondylar notch. The goals of any measured resection technique seem to be to reestablish the femoral articular surfaces in an appropriate relationship to the femoral ligament attachments at the epicondyles and, therefore, to provide flexion-extension isometry or ligament balance.

With a simple model, it is possible to understand how the tibiofemoral ligament arrangement and respective ligament positions affect flexion-extension ligament balance. The behavior of a collateral ligament, and even the posterior cruciate ligament, can be predicted fairly reliably if the femoral attachment of that ligament is studied with respect to its relative location on the femoral condylar surface. A ligament that is too close to the distal joint line tends to be loose in extension and relatively tighter in flexion. If it is too far from the distal joint line, that is, positioned too proximal or cephalad, the opposite is to be expected. For movements in an anterior-posterior direction, a posteriorly positioned ligament is likely to be more lax in flexion and tight in extension, and an anteriorly positioned one, tight in flexion and more lax in extension.

An alternate, more empiric approach, originally undertaken with first generation (total) condylar knees, is referred to as flexion-extension gap balancing. In this technique, the surgeon seeks to create bone gaps in flexion and in extension that are of equal overall dimension when the tibia is tensed away from the femur.

Both the measured resection technique and flexion-extension gap balancing have proponents, advantages, and limitations. Instrumentation to conveniently and accurately effect comparable tension in flexion and extension, and to guide cuts under this system, has been a bit illusory. In addition, both measured resection and flexion-extension gap balancing have practical and theoretical shortcomings in the specific case of flexion contracture. Flexion-extension gap balancing appears to automatically address the issue of flexion contracture by moving the distal femoral cut more proximal or cephalad. However, soft tissues that are balanced, or apparently balanced, at 0° and 90° according to the criteria for flexion–extension gap balancing, do not guarantee that the soft tissues and, more specifically, the collateral ligaments are balanced else-where in the range of motion cycle. In reality, there tends to be mid-range collateral instability for the flexion contracture situation because the apparent stability in full extension may not be due simply to tight collateral ligaments, but to tight posterior soft tissues such as the posterior capsule and hamstrings. The theoretically ideal cuts with the measured resection technique alone leave the flexion contracture totally unaddressed, and all of the soft-tissue components of the flexion contracture must be released to achieve full knee extension.

Tibia

Because the axes of rotation for flexion extension motion of the knee lie at the femoral side and are very likely to have approximate coincidence with the epicondylar axis, simple proximal–distal changes in tibial cut level do not affect flexion-extension ligament balance. Medial-lateral tilt should be thought of as primarily affecting varus-valgus alignment. While the surgeon could address lateral instability by sloping the tibial cut medially and using a thicker prosthesis, this would lead to the undesirable corresponding creation or increase of a varus deformity.

Posterior sloping of the tibial component (downward) can generally be expected to reduce soft-tissue tension in flexion, and it can be viewed as decreasing posterior cruciate ligament tension with flexion. Anterior sloping of the tibial component can lead to a binding or tightening of the posterior cruciate ligament with flexion and also may lead to anterior subluxation of the femoral component with improper force distribution on the tibia, which can result in early failure. Thus, many subtleties of orientation and positioning of bone cuts must be addressed in order to achieve proper flexion-extension ligament balance, alignment, and range of motion, in order to avoid instability and/or component-interface overload.

Deformity Management

Reestablishing proper axial alignment involves not only understanding the proper alignment angles, but also establishing this alignment along with adequate soft-tissue ligament balance throughout the range of motion cycle.

The surgeon must understand the tendency for varus (valgus) deformities to have tight medial (lateral) aspects while the opposite aspect tends toward laxity. These tendencies typically are addressed by performing soft-tissue release on the concave or tight side of the deformity. The surgeon can actually begin this release early in the exposure, especially in varus deformities. For patients with varus deformity, the surgeon should extend the capsular incision distally to begin elevating the medial capsular ligamentous flap. In valgus deformities, the similar first requirement is to achieve adequate exposure of the posterolateral corner of the knee where release of the lateral collateral ligament, posterolateral capsule, and arcuate ligament complex will occur.

Sequentially releasing the contracted ligaments while

assessing the knee for the extent of correction achieved is basic to the performance of medial or lateral release for varus or valgus deformities. This assessment can be made using the tension stress examination, which is easier to understand and to perform once osteophytes have been removed and some of the basic bone cuts have been made. For appropriate soft-tissue balance, it is necessary, not only that the tibia be positioned under the femur so that the two assume the proper tibiofemoral angle, but also that symmetric soft-tissue tension be present over both medial and lateral aspects of the knee as the tibia is tensed away from the femur. The surgeon can, therefore, get a reasonably good, albeit somewhat approximate, estimate of the efficacy of his or her collateral ligament release process by periodically pulling the tibia away from the femur with the knee in extension and simply holding the tibia so that the soft-tissue sleeve has symmetric tension both medially and laterally. General inspection of the overall alignment gives an indication of how the deformity correction is proceeding. Medial release for varus management involves (1) removal of marginal osteophytes, (2) elevation of the deep medial collateral ligament, (3) elevation of the superficial medial collateral ligament, (4) release of the pes anserinus tendons, and (5) release of the posteromedial capsule and semitendinosus tendons, generally in that order. Lateral release for valgus management necessitates release of (1) the lateral collateral ligament, (2) the popliteus tendon, (3) the iliotibial band, and (4) the posterolateral capsule with arcuate ligament complex. The exact order of lateral side release has been widely debated. Some surgeons emphasize initial release of the iliotibial band and others the specific lateral collateral complex.

Flexion contracture can be managed in one of two ways with varying emphasis on each. The idea of surgical release of the tight posterior soft-tissue structures, although more pleasing theoretically, can be difficult. The second method is by adjusting flexion extension gaps or, in essence, positioning the femoral component more proximally or cephalad. This particular approach is taken naturally with any instrumentation system that directs distal femoral resection to create an extension gap that matches the already created flexion gap. The surgeon is assumed to have already removed posterior femoral condylar osteo-

phytes. These can tent the posterior capsule, resulting in a pseudocontracture that will cause or accentuate the flexion contracture.

Some debate exists as to the significance and management of residual flexion contracture noted at surgery. Some hold that it is simply not a problem if a small flexion contracture persists, and others argue that spontaneous correction is to be expected. The surgeon should minimize, as reasonably as possible, residual flexion contracture at the time of initial surgery, with the realization that there is a general tendency for the "draped knee" at surgery not to show flexion contracture, even when the contracture is present before draping or after drapes are taken away.

While the majority of patients who undergo total knee arthroplasty have some degree of deformity that needs correction, the amount of deformity is usually not so severe that it requires extraordinary techniques for management. That is, the vast majority will respond either to medial tibial release for varus deformity or lateral femoral release for valgus deformity. In flexion contracture, especially in association with varus or valgus deformity, some proximal positioning of the femur in addition to the respective collateral side release will be sufficient. However, some patients can be judged to require highly constrained implants, and some surgeons incorporate techniques of ligament advancement. These techniques involve ligament reconstruction at the time of arthroplasty. Both should be thought of as extraordinary techniques that are suitable only for knees that remain unstable after routine release or that can be judged preoperatively to be unmanageable by routine release techniques.

In considering issues of increased prosthetic constraint, it is important to realize the following: (1) The typical posterior stabilized type of components do not impart varus-valgus stability. (2) More conforming intercondylar pegs can provide varus-valgus stability. (3) These more conformed intercondylar mechanisms, however, can fail if the overall alignment and soft-tissue balance still allow the tibia to drop away from the femur. (4) There has not been sufficient follow-up with highly constrained intercondylar peg designs to determine that their loosening rates will not be significantly different from those of hinged-type implants.

Annotated Bibliography

Insall JN: *Surgery of the Knee.* New York, NY, Churchill Livingstone, 1984, pp 587–696.

Dr. Insall's text is helpful for our topics first as an excellent source for general knee anatomy and second for his three chapters on total knee arthroplasty. Chapter 20, pages 587–696 are the basic elements of TKA particularly as applicable to the total condylar and posterior stabilized condylar replacement techniques.

Kapandji IA: *The Physiology of the Joints: Annotated Diagrams of the Mechanics of the Human Joints,* ed 2. Edinburgh, Scotland, Churchill Livingstone, 1970.

This soft-cover single volume of a three-volume series contains a wonderful and unique description of the fine-detail anatomy of the knee. The author describes these fine points and how they relate to the kinematics and alignment of the knee. This material is very heavily illustrated with a minimum but adequate amount of text. The issues of "anatomic" axial alignment are described as are the ligament position illustrations that form the bases for a firm understanding of what happens with deformity management and bone-cuts, joint-line changes.

Krackow KA (ed): *The Technique of Total Knee Arthroplasty.* St. Louis, MO, CV Mosby, 1990.

Elements of chapters 2, 4, and 5 contain information and detailed elaboration on essentially all of the points in this chapter. The text has been cited very favorably for its good illustrations and is the basis for this OKU section.

Laskin RS (ed): *Total Knee Replacement.* London, UK, Springer-Verlag, 1991, pp 41–74.

Chapters 4 and 5 of this text cover some of the points outlined and elaborated on in the chapter.

Rand JA (ed): *Total Knee Arthroplasty.* New York, NY, Raven Press, 1993.

This is another text devoted entirely to total knee arthroplasty, which discusses these issues of alignment, deformity, approaches, and bone cuts.

33

Management of Bone Loss in Total Knee Arthroplasty

Bone defects are encountered commonly in revision total knee arthroplasty (TKA) and less commonly in primary TKA. Defects are categorized as being contained, peripheral, or a combination of the two. A contained defect is enclosed within the bone and surrounded by good cortical or corticocancellous bone. A peripheral defect is a deficiency of the cortical rim or compact metaphyseal bone that normally would support a component.

The management of bone defects falls into four broad categories: (1) fill defects from 0 to 5 mm with cement; (2) perform bone grafting on defects from 6 to 10 mm; (3) replace defects larger than 10 mm with a metal wedge, augment, or custom prosthesis; (4) resect more bone to allow for a flat surface on which the component may rest; and (5) shift the position of the component to avoid the defect. Management of bone defects in TKA is based on preoperative and intraoperative assessment of defects, availability of graft materials, and prosthetic requirements.

Shallow defects (up to 5 mm deep) that occupy less that one third of the tibial plateau or femoral condyle may be safely filled with cement. Usually, the area of the defect is densely sclerotic and will provide suitable support for the component. Multiple small drill holes in retained subchondral bone mechanically enhance the bone–cement interface. Radiolucent lines may appear at the bone–cement interface but are rarely progressive.

Defects from 5 to 10 mm deep that occupy one to two thirds of the tibial plateau or femoral condyle are suitable for bone grafting. In a younger patient, bone grafting is preferred over metal augmentation because it preserves bone stock for future revisions. Several techniques have been described for bone grafting of tibial defects in primary and revision TKA. In primary arthroplasty, resected femoral condyle is a ready source of autologous bone, or, if using a posterior stabilized component, bone from the intercondylar notch. In revision arthroplasty, corticocancellous graft from the iliac wing or frozen allografts may be used. Autograft is preferred when it is available; allografts are used when autograft is unavailable or insufficient.

One bone grafting option is to use the screw fixation technique in which the anterior and posterior margins of the defect are trimmed to produce a flat oblique surface that exposes healthy cancellous bone at the base of the deficiency. The cancellous surface of the bone graft, usually taken from the distal femoral osteotomy, is placed over the defect and is affixed with 3/16 inch threaded Steinmann pins or Kirschner wires (Fig. 1). The excess bone is cut flush with the tibial plateau, and the trial prosthesis is inserted to assure proper fit. The Steinmann pins

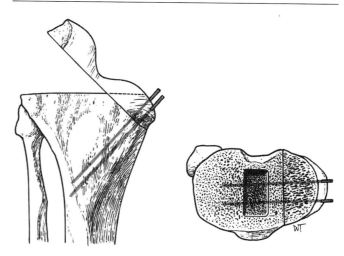

Fig. 1 Autologous bone grafting technique in which bone from distal femoral resection is used. Excess bone is cut flush with the tibial plateau. The Steinmann pins are replaced sequentially with cancellous screws. (Reproduced with permission from Windsor RE, Insall JN, Sculco TP: Bone grafting of tibial defects in primary and revision total knee arthroplasty. *Clin Orthop* 1986;205:132–137.)

may be replaced sequentially with cancellous screws (cannulated screws may also be used) to compress the cancellous surfaces firmly together before cementing the prosthesis into place. This procedure will facilitate graft incorporation and prevent cement from entering the interface between the cancellous surfaces (Fig. 2). Two batches of polymethylmethacrylate (PMMA) are used when cementing the tibial component into place. When the first batch of PMMA has reached a doughy state, it is placed on top of the interface as a sealant between the tibial surface and graft. Before this batch fully cures, a second batch is used to cement the component into place in the usual manner. This sequential cementing technique, along with screw fixation, prevents the cement from entering the interface between the tibia and graft during pressurization. If cement enters the interface, graft incorporation will be compromised.

Alternatively, the inlay autogenic bone grafting technique may be used (Fig. 3). In this technique, a self-locking process obviates the need for permanent metal fixation devices. The surgeon should create a rectangular or trapezoidal defect and remove all sclerotic bone to expose the underlying cancellous surface. The rectangular shape allows a stable fit so that uniform compressive forces may be ex-

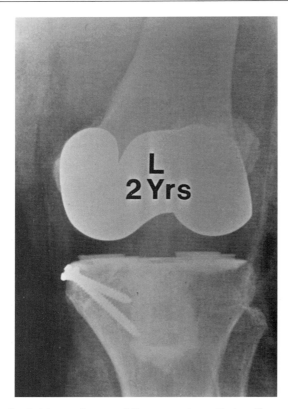

Fig. 2 Autologous bone graft 2 years postoperatively, with incorporation of the graft without evidence of loosening or subsidence.

erted over the entire graft–bone interface. If a trapezoidal shape is used, the defect is created with its widest base directed toward the center of the tibia so the graft will be locked into place. The corresponding dimensions are outlined with methylene blue on the bone graft block taken from the intercondylar notch, and the graft is fashioned using a saw or burr. The bone block is tapped into place and should snugly fit all the dimensions of the defect in order to prevent cement from entering the crevices. Excess bone may be trimmed with a saw so that the graft sits flush with the tibial surface (Fig. 4). A trial prosthesis is placed to assure a correct fit and alignment.

In the presence of significant bone deficiency (greater than 10-mm deep), which occupies more than two thirds of the tibial plateau or femoral condyle, the support on the side of the defect should be as rigid as possible. In this setting, a custom-made component would be the ideal solution because it would produce acceptable stresses on the bone and component. Unfortunately, custom manufacture is relatively costly and is not applicable to situations in which the final size and shape of the defect are determined only at surgery. Therefore, it may be advantageous to insert appropriately-sized spacers or wedges of metal that securely fit the undersurface of a standard component and may be attached to the component by screws or cement. Many TKA systems offer a selection of blocks or half and full wedges to accommodate the range of bone defects most often encountered. Selection of the closest fitting component at surgery provides the most rigid fixation while still providing substantial mechanical support. The use of a noncemented press-fit intramedullary stem is recommended to help support the load and prevent tilting

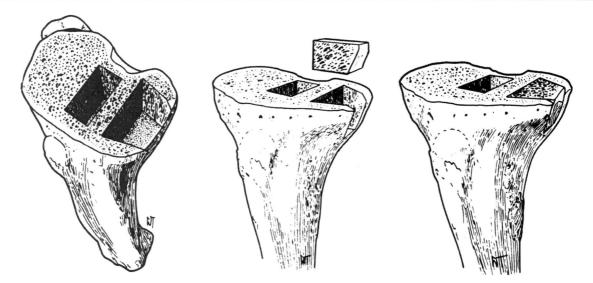

Fig. 3 Inlay autogenous bone graft. In this technique, the graft is locked into place by virtue of its trapezoidal shape. (Reproduced with permission from Windsor RE, Insall JN, Sculco TP: Bone grafting of tibial defects in primary and revision total knee arthroplasty. *Clin Orthop* 1986;205:132–137.)

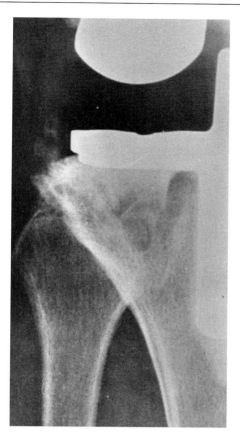

Fig. 4   Incorporation of bone graft following inlay bone grafting.

of the prosthesis when large bone grafts or metal spacers are used (Fig. 5).

Increased bone resection to the level of the deficit is a management alternative for bone deficiencies encountered at the time of TKA. A deeper cut allows bypass of other augmentation procedures and their complications by providing a flat surface. However, it is generally believed that the strength of the trabecular bone decreases with the distance from the joint. This decrease is most marked in the first 2 to 5 mm and then appears to level off. Recent studies have shown that a tibial cut at 12 mm versus 6 mm distal to the tibial plateau does not change the strength of the construct when asymmetric metal-backed designs are used. In another recent study, no significant decreases in bone strength were apparent for resection depths ranging from 4 to 20 mm from the surface of the tibial plateau; it was concluded that bone strength in this region is sufficient to support thicker tibial components. These results suggest that deeper cuts into the tibia may be used when the situation warrants.

When a severe medial tibial bone defect is present, the position of the tibial component may be shifted laterally. This shift is accompanied by resection of the proximal aspect of the medial tibial flare. This maneuver places the component on a greater area of unaffected subchondral bone, avoids the defect, and may obviate the need for a graft or wedge. A lateral shift should not be performed, however, if it creates the need for a much smaller size tibial component and probably is not applicable when the posterior cruciate ligament is spared.

Allografts are used when autograft is unavailable or insufficient, and their use requires preoperative planning for availability. The risks of immunologic rejection, disease transmission, and resorption must be considered. Large bony defects are often encountered in revision TKA and tumor surgery in which autologous bone is often unavailable or inadequate to provide a stable reconstruction. In this situation, morseled or structural allograft is used. Whole-segment structural allografts are used when host bone is incapable of providing mechanical stability; these grafts are strongest at the time of surgery. Morseled allograft is useful in contained defects for reconstitution of bone stock, but offers no structural support until it has become incorporated biologically.

Cavernous "trumpet"-shaped deficiencies may be managed by filling the defect with morseled allograft, thereby recreating a flat surface on which the component may rest. Successful use of morseled cancellous allograft relies on vascularization from host bone and ossification early after surgery. Because this material is not initially structural and merely fills the defect, structural support of the implant must be achieved by using a stem and, when possible, cortical rim support. The addition of screws to the tibial component gives rigid fixation. The surrounding soft-tissue envelope is adequate to hold extensive allografts that fill defects comprising as much as three fourths of the proximal tibial peripheral rim. The morseled allograft is loaded lightly by deflection of the tray so that load-bearing stimulus prevents resorption and loss of the grafting material. As time passes this graft incorporates to produce load-bearing bone.

Structural allograft reconstruction is used when host bone is markedly deficient, often rendering the knee incompetent of ligamentous support. Preoperative evaluation of the defect allows suitable planning for bone graft (femoral head, proximal tibia, or distal femur) and prosthetic requirements. Bulk allografting requires adequate exposure, similar to that in tumor surgery. The femur must be exposed far enough above the level of the allograft to allow rigid fixation with screws or plates. Similarly, a proximal tibial graft requires adequate exposure and requires reattachment of the osteotomized tibial tubercle to the graft. Host bone is resected to a healthy bleeding bed. Whole grafts are prepared on a side table using standard jigs; a step cut is recommended to increase the stability of the graft-host junction. Standard cement techniques are used, and care is taken not to introduce cement at the graft-host interface. Structural allografts should be bypassed by long intramedullary stems if possible and usually require use of constrained condylar components. Reattachment of ligaments to the graft may fail unless the

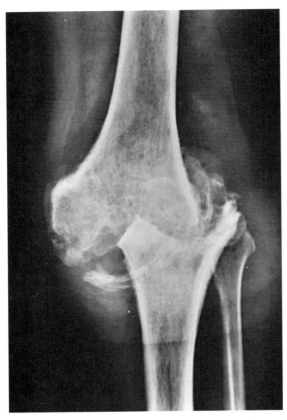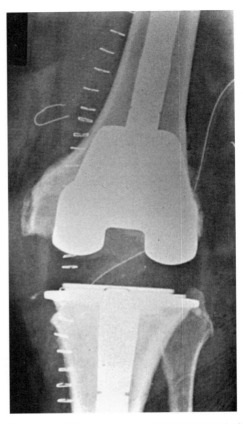

Fig. 5   Left, The management of complex bone defects are determined at surgery. **Right,** Combined defect managed with bone grafting in which stemmed femoral and tibial components are used.

graft has soft-tissue attachments; a linked prosthesis such as the kinematic rotating hinge or the Finn knee may be needed to provide stability. Complications following bulk allografting are frequent (50%), including infection, collateral ligament repair failure, allograft fracture, and allograft–host nonunion.

Annotated Bibliography

Altchek D, Sculco TP, Rawlins B: Autogenous bone grafting for severe angular deformity in total knee arthroplasty. *J Arthroplasty* 1989;4:151–155.

Fourteen patients with severe angular knee deformities had total knee arthroplasty using autogenous bone graft to the tibia. At 4 years, no change in component alignment was noted. All grafts consolidated without evidence of collapse, resorption, or prosthetic subsidence.

Dorr LD, Ranawat CS, Sculco TA, et al: Bone graft for tibial defects in total knee arthroplasty. *Clin Orthop* 1986; 205:153–165.

Twenty-two of 24 bone grafts for bone deficiencies at total knee arthroplasty were satisfactory. Two failures occurred: one because of varus alignment of the limb and the other because no vascular bed was prepared for the bone graft. Bone grafting is indicated for bone deficiencies of more than 5 mm after completion of the bone cuts.

Mnaymneh W, Emerson RH, Borja F, et al: Massive allografts in salvage revisions of failed total knee arthroplasties. *Clin Orthop* 1990;260:144–153.

Ten patients with failed total knee arthroplasties and severe bone loss were treated with massive whole distal femur and proximal tibial allografts in combination with prosthetic implants. Fourteen allografts were inserted either as invaginated or segmental grafts and were rigidly fixed to the host bone. Clinically and radiographically, 12 of 14 grafts seemed to have united to the host bone. Five patients developed complications; two of these involved the allograft (nonunion and fracture) and two were caused by inadequate healing at the ligament-allograft junction. One patient had a late infection.

Ritter MA, Keating EM, Faris PM: Screw and cement fixation of large defects in total knee arthroplasty: A sequel. *J Arthroplasty* 1993;8:63–65.

Forty-seven patients who had a total knee arthroplasty in which cement and screws were used to fill a tibial defect were followed up for an average of 6.1 years. There was no evidence of loosening and no components were revised.

Scuderi GR, Insall JN: Revision total knee arthroplasty with cemented fixation. *Tech Orthop* 1993;7:96–105.

The technique of revision total knee arthroplasty with cement fixation and press-fit intramedullary stems is described. The modularity of current systems allows the versatility needed to address problems as they arise at the time of surgery. Although the procedure is technically demanding, the goal of revision total knee arthroplasty is a well-aligned limb with a stable and securely fixed implant.

Whiteside LA: Alignment and bone handling in revision total knee arthroplasty. *Tech Orthop* 1993;7:72–79.

Bone deficiency can be managed with allograft if rigid fixation of the implants can be achieved. Smooth stems that fit tightly in the medullary canal of the femur and tibia give excellent support for the articular portion of the implant and allow cementless fixation and morselized allograft reconstruction of major bone defects.

Windsor RE, Insall JN, Sculco TP: Bone grafting of tibial defects in primary and revision total knee arthroplasty. *Clin Orthop* 1986;205:132–137.

Bone grafting of tibial defects in primary and revision total knee arthroplasty is performed by two different methods. Incorporation of the graft occurs between 4 and 8 months. No restriction in weightbearing is recommended, except with repair of large defects. Bone grafting is a viable alternative to using custom tibial prostheses or excess cement, even for very large defects.

34
Patellofemoral Complications in Total Knee Arthroplasty

Although long-term evaluations of total knee arthroplasty (TKA) have demonstrated excellent relief of pain, improved function, and superior durability, problems with the patellofemoral joint persist. Early total knee prostheses failed to provide for resurfacing of the patellofemoral joint, and anterior knee pain in as many as 50% of patients has been reported without patellar resurfacing. This pain led to design modifications that allow for replacement of the patella. The addition of patellofemoral resurfacing has reduced the incidence of pain and improved functional results, but an additional set of complications has emerged. These complications include patellofemoral instability, fracture, loosening, component failure, patellar clunk syndrome, and tendon rupture. The reported incidence of these complications has varied from 5% to 55% and has accounted for up to 50% of revision TKA.

Patellofemoral complications have been attributed to surgical technique errors, poor prosthetic design, and excessive patellofemoral loads. Most investigators agree that patellofemoral joint reaction forces reach one half to one times body weight during level gait. These forces increase to three to four times body weight with stair walking and to as high as seven to eight times body weight during squatting.

Patellofemoral Instability

Failure to obtain satisfactory patellofemoral tracking may result in patellofemoral pain and crepitus; component wear, failure, loosening, and/or fracture, which subsequently jeopardize the result of an otherwise successfully functioning TKA. The reported incidence of patellar subluxation is as high as 29% in some series.

The etiology of patellofemoral instability is multifactorial; it most commonly results from extensor mechanism imbalance with excessive tightness of the lateral retinaculum associated with weakness of the vastus medialis muscle. Excessive genu valgum associated with an increase in the Q-angle results in an increased lateral force vector on the patella, which predisposes to subluxation. Postoperative hemarthrosis or overly aggressive physiotherapy can similarly result in patellofemoral instability due to stretching or disruption of the capsular repair.

Asymmetric patellar resection, typically, excessive lateral facet resection, can lead to patellar tracking problems. The normal patella is asymmetric in contour, with the medial facet thicker than the lateral. Resection of equal amounts of bone from the medial and lateral facets results in an asymmetric patella bone remnant. Minimal lateral facet resection, often flush with the subchondral bone of the lateral facet, is therefore optimal (Fig. 1).

Malposition of the tibial, femoral, or patellar components may affect patellar tracking. With internal rotation of the tibial component, the tibia will be externally rotated relative to the femur. Such rotation results in lateralization of the tibial tubercle and an increase in the Q-angle, which predisposes to lateral patellar subluxation. Similar lateralization of the tibial tubercle occurs with medial shift of the tibial component on the cut tibial plateau surface. Internal rotation or medial shift of the femoral component moves the trochlear flange medially away from the patella, leaving the patella laterally positioned relative to the femoral component. Lateral positioning of the patellar component on the patella can also cause the problem of "patellar capture" into the trochlear groove of the femoral component.

Certain prosthetic designs predispose to patellar instability. In the presence of extensor mechanism imbalance, rotationally unconstrained implants may allow excessive external rotation of the tibia and lateralization of the tibial tubercle. An analogous situation exists in the unstable TKA in which there is loss of posterior cruciate and collateral ligamentous stability. Alternatively, increased patellofemoral instability has been observed in prostheses that allow no axial rotation. In the normal knee, up to 20° of internal rotation occurs during early knee flexion. With rigid hinge prostheses, this internal tibial rotation does not occur, and the tibial tubercle assumes a lateralized position during flexion, thereby increasing the laterally-directed forces on the patella.

Intraoperative analysis of patellar tracking is essential. If the patella laterally subluxes as the knee is flexed (before capsular closure) using the no-thumb technique, a lateral retinacular release is advised. This procedure has been associated with reduced lateral wound edge skin viability and patellar hypovascularity. Assessment of patellar alignment is best performed following tourniquet release to eliminate the tourniquet's binding effect on the extensor mechanism.

Treatment of patellofemoral instability is based on its etiology. In cases of extensor mechanism imbalance, a lateral retinacular release, often combined with advancement of the medial quadriceps muscle (proximal realignment), is indicated. Capsular repair is necessary in cases of early traumatic disruption. Tibial tubercle transfer is considered in cases of more severe malalignment because of the inherent risk of nonunion and subsequent complicated salvage options. Component revision is reserved for cases with substantial component malposition that are not amenable to simpler realignment procedures.

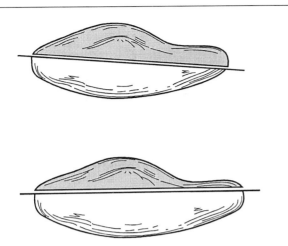

Fig. 1 The top diagram demonstrates the asymmetric facet thickness of the normal patella. Resection of an equal thickness of bone from both the medial and lateral facets results in an asymmetric remaining patella. The bottom diagram demonstrates the recommended level of resection, removing minimal bone from the lateral patellar facet. (Reproduced with permission from Dennis DA: Patellofemoral complications in total knee arthroplasty. *Am J Knee Surg* 1992;5:156–166.)

Patellar Fractures

Patellar fractures are an infrequent complication of TKA, although an incidence as high as 21% has been reported. Multiple etiologies for patellar fracture have been proposed (Outline 1). The increased incidence of patellar fracture associated with patellofemoral malalignment is supported by biomechanical studies, which have demonstrated that contact forces substantially increase with patellofemoral malalignment. With patellar subluxation, both eccentricity and magnitude of patellofemoral loads are increased, enhancing the risk of patellar fracture.

Excessive or inadequate patellar resection can predispose to patellar fracture. Asymmetric patellar resection can result in impaired mechanical strength of the patella. Excessive patellar resection, especially if the subchondral bone is resected, weakens the bone, thereby enhancing the chance of fracture. One study demonstrated that a patellar osteotomy that results in an osseous patellar thickness of less than 15 mm substantially increases anterior patellar strain. Conversely, inadequate patellar resection, which results in thickening of the patella-patellar component composite, increases the quadriceps tension and patellofemoral joint reaction forces. Use of femoral components with excessive anteroposterior diameter, or implanting a femoral component in a flexed position, similarly increases patellofemoral joint reaction force and enhances the probability of fracture.

Patellar avascularity caused by surgical disruption can result in fracture. Studies of patellar blood supply have delineated both extraosseous and intraosseous systems. The extraosseous system is composed of a peripatellar

anastomotic ring supplied by six main arteries (Fig. 2, *left*). The intraosseous system comprises midpatellar, polar (apical), and quadriceps tendon supplies (Fig. 2, *right*). The midpatellar vessels penetrate anteriorly through the middle one third of the patella and branch into both the proximal and distal poles. The polar vasculature passes through the proximal fat pad, posterior to the patellar tendon, and enters through the inferior pole of the patella, supplying its distal one-half. A small portion of the superior pole of the patella is supplied by vessels passing through the quadriceps tendon.

Substantial disruption of patellar blood supply occurs during routine TKA. A medial peripatellar arthrotomy divides the two medial geniculate and supreme geniculate arteries. Lateral meniscectomy and fat pad excision endanger the lateral inferior geniculate artery, whereas the lateral superior geniculate artery is at risk when a lateral retinacular release is performed. Intraosseous blood supply may be further compromised during creation of fixation holes, particularly the large central type, for the patellar anchoring pegs. A large central peg hole also has been shown to increase anterior patellar strain more than smaller peripheral peg designs, thereby enhancing the risk of fracture. Postoperative technetium bone scan studies have demonstrated an increased incidence of cold scans if a lateral retinacular release has been performed. Histologic evaluations of patellar specimens that were obtained after stress fracture have documented the presence of avascular necrosis.

Component malposition can affect both the type, severity, and prognosis of patellar fractures. Errors in joint line position, implant position and alignment, and patellar coverage by the prosthesis may risk fracture. Cases with more severe malposition have been associated with more complex fractures and, subsequently, a worse prognosis.

Increased flexion following TKA, thermal necrosis associated with use of polymethylmethacrylate, and revision TKA are also considered factors in the multifactorial pathogenesis of patellar fractures.

Patellar Component Loosening

Cemented patellar component loosening in TKA has been uncommon, with a reported incidence of less than 2% in most studies. Factors predisposing to loosening include cementing the prosthesis into deficient bone, component

Outline 1. Factors associated with patellar fractures

Trauma
Patellar Subluxation
Improper Patellar Resection
Vascular Compromise
Component Design
Component Malposition
Increased Flexion
Thermal Necrosis
Revised TKA

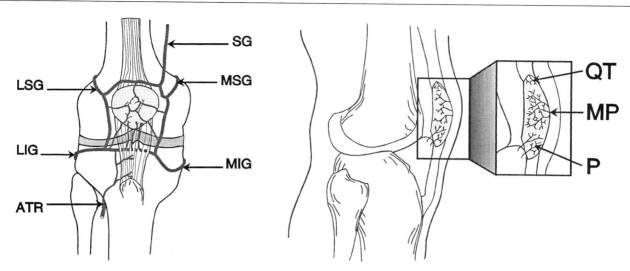

Fig. 2 **Left,** Diagram demonstrating the extraosseous peripatellar anastomotic ring supplied by six main arteries. LSG = Lateral Superior Geniculate; MSG = Medial Superior Geniculate; MIG = Medial Inferior Geniculate; LIG = Lateral Inferior Geniculate; SG = Supreme Geniculate; ATR = Anterior Tibial Recurrent. **Right,** Diagram demonstrating the midpatellar (MP), polar (P) and quadriceps tendon (QT) intraosseous blood supplies of the patella. (Reproduced with permission from Dennis DA: Patellofemoral complications in total knee arthroplasty. *Am J Knee Surg* 1992;5:156–166.)

malposition, patellar subluxation or fracture, patellar avascular necrosis, osteoporosis, asymmetric patellar bone resection, loosening of other components, and failure of bone ingrowth in porous-coated designs. Reduction of patellar loosening requires improved bone preparation and cementing techniques, proper patellar resection, avoidance of asymmetric or excessive bone removal, and assurance of central patellar tracking.

Should loosening occur, management options include observation, component revision, component removal and patellar arthroplasty if remaining bone stock is unsatisfactory, and patellectomy. Although some patients with patellar loosening remain minimally symptomatic, the majority will require surgical intervention. Total dislodgment of the component, most commonly inferiorly, can occur and lead to erosion of the posterior surface of the overlying patellar tendon.

Patellar Component Failure

Although component failure of polyethylene patellar designs has been reported, failure has primarily been a problem of metal-backed designs. Metal-backing of patellar components was adopted with the proposed advantages of decreasing patellar surface strains and supporting the overlying polyethylene, thereby lessening deformation and allowing for cementless patellar fixation. Failure modes have included polyethylene wear and fracture, polyethylene–metal plate dissociation, peg–plate dissociation, and metal plate fracture.

Patellar polyethylene wear is not unexpected because

peak patellofemoral contact pressures have been found to substantially exceed the yield strength of polyethylene. The addition of metal-backing to patellar components results in reduction of the polyethylene thickness, which predisposes to enhanced wear rates. Similarly, with metal-backed designs, less wear is required before catastrophic failure occurs as a result of wear through to the underlying metal. Polyethylene thickness as minimal as 2.4 mm at the periphery of the metal plate has been observed in some metal-backed designs. In most designs, the metal-backing does not totally extend to the edge of the polyethylene. Therefore, as the peripheral polyethylene is loaded, it may deform over the rim of the metal plate and be cut by the sharp nondeforming edge of the plate.

Polyethylene–plate dissociation may result if polyethylene wear and fracture are excessive. The polyethylene is attached to the metal plate in most designs by means of a mechanical "gripping" of the plate periphery by the polyethylene. There is no chemical bond. With peripheral polyethylene wear, the integrity of the polyethylene–plate attachment may be disrupted, allowing the polyethylene to dissociate.

Fracture of the fixation pegs at their attachment to the metal plate may occur as a result of high shear stress at this junction. The patella normally is loaded eccentrically, which creates substantial shear stress. Malalignment increases the eccentricity of load and subsequent shear stress. If osseous ingrowth into the fixation pegs occurs without accompanying ingrowth into the metal plate, the high shear load placed at the peg–plate junction predisposes to peg fracture. In a study of 12 instances of fatigue fracture at the peg–plate junction, good bone ingrowth into the fixation peg with no ingrowth into porous plate was observed in all.

Numerous factors have been related with patellar component failure, including excessive body weight, enhanced postoperative knee flexion (> 115°) and activity levels, as well as gender (male). Other factors associated with increased patellofemoral loading and subsequent component failure include patellar malalignment, increased patella–patellar component composite thickness, use of oversized femoral components, flexion of the femoral component, and joint line malposition. Failure of metal-backed patellar components often occurs early; most reviews report failure as early as 2 years following TKA.

Common clinical signs of patellar component failure include effusion and crepitus, which occasionally is readily audible. Symptoms often occur suddenly after activities, such as going up and down stairs, walking, squatting or rising from a seated position, that heavily load the patellofemoral joint. Intraoperative findings frequently include black staining of the synovium due to metallosis and wear or fragmentation of the polyethylene. Femoral component wear may be present; it was observed in 11 of 25 cases of failed metal-backed patellar components in one study. Loose metal beads or titanium fiber mesh are not unusual and may be found embedded within the polyethylene of the patellar and tibial components. Therefore, if revision is required for metal-backed patellar component failure, the surgeon should always be prepared to revise all three components.

Patellar Clunk Syndrome

Patellar clunk syndrome is a condition in which a fibrous nodule develops at the junction of the posterior aspect of the quadriceps tendon and proximal pole of the patella. With knee flexion, this nodule enters the intercondylar notch of the femoral prosthesis. As the knee is extended, the nodule becomes entrapped within the notch as the quadriceps tendon and patella migrate proximally. At 30° to 45° from full extension, enough tension is placed on the fibrous nodule causing it to "clunk" out of the intercondylar notch (Fig. 3).

Two mechanisms of pathogenesis have been described. The first involves impingement of the quadriceps tendon against the anterosuperior edge of the intercondylar notch of the femoral component. This mechanism occurs more frequently in cases in which a smaller patellar component has been used, which fails to elevate the quadriceps tendon anteriorly enough away from the femoral component. The second mechanism involves impingement of the superior portion of the patellar component against the quadriceps tendon, especially if the patellar component is superiorly shifted, extending beyond the proximal border of the patella. Recommended treatment consists of debridement of the fibrous nodule, either openly or arthroscopically, with or without revision of the patellar component if it is superiorly positioned.

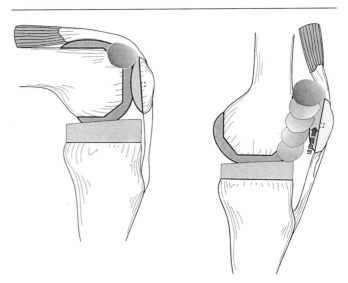

Fig. 3 **Left,** Diagram demonstrating a suprapatellar fibrous nodule entrapped within the intercondylar notch during knee flexion. **Right,** Fibrous nodule "clunks" out of intercondylar notch with knee extension at 30° to 45°. (Reproduced with permission from Dennis DA: Patellofemoral complications in total knee arthroplasty. *Am J Knee Surg* 1992;5:156–166.)

Tendon Rupture

Rupture of the quadriceps or patellar tendons is an infrequent complication of TKA that has a reported incidence of 1% to 2.5%. Quadriceps ruptures occur more frequently in those cases in which a lateral retinacular release has been performed; this occurrence may be due to tendon devascularization or extension of the release too far anteriorly, which disrupts tendinous fibers of the quadriceps. The outcome of surgical repair is often suboptimal, resulting in residual extensor lag and weakness, re-rupture, or limited range of motion.

The risk of patellar tendon rupture following TKA is enhanced in patients who have had previous knee operations as well as those who have undergone partial patellar tendon release to enhance exposure at the time of TKA. Additional risk factors include knee manipulation and those cases in which tibial tubercle osteotomy has been performed for extensor mechanism realignment. Numerous treatment modalities (casting; tendon suture; fixation with wire, staples, or screws; tendon augmentation; and extensor mechanism allografts) have been attempted with no single reconstructive procedure providing consistently satisfactory results. Persistent tendon rupture following attempted treatment is common and has been reported to occur in 11 of 18 cases in one series. Tendon rupture remains a most dreaded complication of TKA, with difficult and often unsatisfactory salvage options. Prevention via meticulous surgical technique is imperative.

Surgical Technique

If the accuracy of femoral and tibial preparation is compared with the precision of current methods of patellar preparation, it's logical to relate patellar problems in some part to surgical technique. Surgical goals include accurate patellar resection, maintenance of patellar vascularity, proper positioning of components, avoidance of soft-tissue impingement, and assurance of central patellar tracking.

Patellar resection must result in a symmetric patellar remnant with equal medial and lateral facet thickness. The amount of patellar bone excised should equal the thickness of the patellar component to be inserted, usually about 10 mm, thereby restoring the preoperative patellar thickness.

Efforts to preserve patellar vascularity include maintaining the fat pad, preserving the superolateral geniculate artery during lateral retinacular release, and performing the lateral release 2 cm posterior to the patella in order to maintain vessels penetrating the patellar periphery. Avoidance of patellar components with large central patellar pegs will help preserve intraosseous blood supply.

All three TKA components require accurate positioning. Medial shift and internal rotation of both femoral and tibial components as well as lateral positioning of the patellar component must be avoided to prevent patellar maltracking. Following tourniquet release, central patellar tracking must be obtained using the "no thumb technique." If patellar subluxation is initially present, realignment procedures are performed until a balanced extensor mechanism is obtained.

Isolated patellar component revision has been associated with higher than expected complication rates. These complications have included patellar fracture, instability, polyethylene wear through, infection, peroneal nerve palsy, and extensor lag. Removal of well-fixed metal-backed patellar components with osseous ingrowth into the anchoring pegs can be difficult, but it is facilitated through peg–plate disruption in which a diamond-edge saw is used to gain direct access to the bone–peg interface.

The numerous patellofemoral complications discussed have led to an increased desire to avoid patellofemoral resurfacing. Although most surgeons agree that it is necessary to resurface the patella in patients with rheumatoid arthritis because of the antigenic response of retained cartilage, controversy exists on whether to resurface patellae in patients with osteoarthritis who have good articular cartilage remaining. Similar results with or without patellar resurfacing have been reported for some studies; however, numerous evaluations have demonstrated improved function and reduced anterior knee pain in those cases in which the patella is resurfaced. In one large study of 891 TKAs with and without patellar resurfacing, complication rates were 4% and 12%, respectively. Results of secondary patellar resurfacing proved inferior to results of cases in which the patella was resurfaced at the time of primary TKA.

The best results in TKA will be attained with maximum attention to accurate patellar resection, maintenance of patellar vascularity, assurance of central patellar tracking, and avoidance of metal-backed patellar components.

Annotated Bibliography

Patellofemoral Instability

Grace JN, Rand JA: Patellar instability after total knee arthroplasty. *Clin Orthop* 1988;237:184–189.

Twenty-five knees with symptomatic lateral patellar instability after total knee arthroplasty were treated with operative realignment. Five cases of recurrent instability and two patellar tendon ruptures occurred. Proximal realignment alone, in the absence of component malposition, is recommended.

Kirk P, Rorabeck CH, Bourne RB, et al: Management of recurrent dislocation of the patella following total knee arthroplasty. *J Arthroplasty* 1992;7:229–233.

Fifteen knees with patellar dislocation after TKA were treated with extensor mechanism realignment using a modified Trillat procedure. No recurrent dislocations occurred after a minimum 2-year follow-up period. One nonunion of the tibial tubercle osteotomy was encountered.

Patellar Fracture

Hozack WJ, Goll SR, Lotke PA, et al: The treatment of patellar fractures after total knee arthroplasty. *Clin Orthop* 1988;236:123–127.

Twenty-one patellar fractures after total knee arthroplasty were reviewed. Nondisplaced patellar fractures and displaced fractures without extensor lag are best treated nonoperatively. Displaced patellar fractures with extensor lag have poor results with operative treatment. Patellectomy should be considered for failures of all other treatments.

Tria AJ Jr, Harwood DA, Alicea JA, et al: Patellar fractures in posterior stabilized knee arthroplasties. *Clin Orthop* 1994;299:131–138.

Five hundred and four posterior stabilized TKAs were reviewed at 2- to 11-year follow-up. A patellar fracture rate of 3.6% was observed at an average time of 11 months after the date of surgery. A positive correlation was observed between patellar fracture and lateral release ($p = 0.05$).

Patellar Component Loosening

Dennis DA: Patellofemoral complications in total knee arthroplasty: A literature review. *Am J Knee Surg* 1992; 5:156–166.

Cemented patellar component loosening occurs in less than 2% in most studies. Factors predisposing to loosening include cementation into deficient bone, component malposition, patellar subluxation or fracture, patellar avascular necrosis, asymmetric patellar bone resection, and loosening of other components. Treatment options include observation, component revision, patellectomy or component removal, and patellar arthroplasty if bone stock is sufficient.

Patellar Component Failure

Firestone TP, Teeny SM, Krackow KA, et al: The clinical and roentgenographic results of cementless porous-coated patellar fixation. *Clin Orthop* 1991;273:184–189.

The clinical and roentgenographic results of 522 porous-coated, metal-backed patellar components were reviewed. Fixation failure at the bone-prosthesis interface was the most common cause of failure. The addition of a third fixation peg to the metal backing reduced the rate of loosening from 6.1% to 0.6%.

Rosenberg AG, Andriacchi TP, Barden R, et al: Patellar component failure in cementless total knee arthroplasty. *Clin Orthop* 1988;236:106–114.

One hundred twenty-two TKAs were performed with porous ingrowth fixation of the patellar component. Twelve cases experienced fatigue fracture of the patellar component at the peg–plate junction. All fractured components demonstrated excellent bone ingrowth into the fixation pegs with no ingrowth into the porous plate. This ingrowth pattern results in high shear loads at the peg–plate junction, predisposing to this complication.

Stulberg SD, Stulberg BN, Hamati Y, et al: Failure mechanisms of metal-backed patellar components. *Clin Orthop* 1988;236:88–105.

Fourteen patients with 16 metal-backed patellar component failures were analyzed. Average time to failure was only 14 months. Thin peripheral polyethylene, which is unsupported by the metal base-plate, is exposed to high loads and is at risk for wear through. Technical errors predisposing to this mode of failure include patellar subluxation, femoral component flexion, or an excessive patellar composite thickness. The typical patient was a heavy, active male with knee flexion greater than 115°.

Patellar Clunk Syndrome

Beight JL, Yao B, Hozack WJ, et al: The patellar "clunk" syndrome after posterior stabilized total knee arthroplasty. *Clin Orthop* 1994;299:139–142.

Twenty cases of patellar clunk syndrome following posterior stabilized TKA are reported. Symptoms resolved after suprapatellar fibrous excision. Four recurrences arose after arthroscopic debridement. Proposed etiologies included femoral component design (sharp anterior edge at the superior aspect of the intercondylar notch), proximal patellar button overhand, postoperative scarring, and alterations of the joint line, patellar height, or patellar thickness.

Hozack WJ, Rothman RH, Booth RE Jr, et al: The patellar clunk syndrome: A complication of posterior stabilized total knee arthroplasty. *Clin Orthop* 1989;241: 203–208.

The clinical signs and intraoperative findings of three patients with patellar clunk syndrome are reviewed. A painful "clunk" typically occurs as the patient extends the knee 30° to 45° from the fully extended position. Intraoperatively, a prominent fibrous nodule, which catches within the intercondylar notch, was found at the junction of the proximal patella and quadriceps tendon. Pathogenesis may involve impingement of the anterosuperior edge of the intercondylar notch area of the femoral component onto the quadriceps tendon or impingement of a prominent, proximally placed patellar component onto the quadriceps tendon. Surgical excision of the fibrous nodule resolved the symptoms.

Tendon Rupture

Lynch AF, Rorabeck CH, Bourne RB: Extensor mechanism complications following total knee arthroplasty. *J Arthroplasty* 1987;2:135–140.

Two hundred and eighty-one consecutive total knee arthroplasties (TKA) were reviewed for extensor mechanism complications. Quadriceps or patellar tendon ruptures occurred in 2.5% of cases. A risk factor for quadriceps tendon rupture included lateral retinacular release at the time of primary TKA. All patellar tendon ruptures occurred in knees in which surgery had been performed prior to TKA. Results of surgical repair of these tendon rupture were poor, with substantial extensor lags or limited knee motion commonly occurring.

Rand JA, Morrey BF, Bryan RS: Patellar tendon rupture after total knee arthroplasty. *Clin Orthop* 1989;244: 233–238.

Eighteen knees with patellar tendon ruptures following TKA were treated utilizing various methods. Risk factors for this complication include previous distal realignment procedures or closed knee manipulation and cases with difficult surgical exposure. Persistent patellar tendon ruptures after treatment occurred in 11 of 18 cases, emphasizing the importance of avoidance of this complication.

Surgical Technique

Boyd AD Jr, Ewald FC, Thomas WH, et al: Long-term complications after total knee arthroplasty with or without resurfacing of the patella. *J Bone Joint Surg* 1993;75A:674–681.

The long-term patellar complications of 891 total knee arthroplasties were retrospectively reviewed. One group (396 TKA) had the patella resurfaced while the other group (495 TKA) did not. The overall complication rate was 4% in the resurfaced group versus 12% for the nonresurfaced group ($p < 0.0001$). The primary complication was postoperative pain. The results of secondary patellar resurfacing were inferior to those of primary resurfacing.

Dennis DA: Removal of well-fixed cementless metal-backed patellar components. *J Arthroplasty* 1992;7: 217–220.

Five cases of TKA with failed metal-backed cementless patellar components with bone ingrown anchoring pegs are presented. A technique of component removal is described in which the metal peg–plate junction is disrupted with a diamond-edged circular saw, followed by circumferential division of the bone–peg interface with a high-speed pencil tip drill. Bone stock was preserved and fracture avoided with utilization of the technique.

Rand JA, Gustilo RB: Technique of patellar resurfacing in total knee arthroplasty. *Tech Orthop* 1988;3:57.

The various complications of patellofemoral resurfacing are discussed. The technical aspects of patellofemoral resurfacing are reviewed. These include the importance of duplicating preoperative patellar thickness, avoiding asymmetric patellar thickness (medial versus lateral), and ensuring central patellar tracking. Alternatives in cases of patellar bone loss include patellar arthroplasty, patellectomy, or use of a biconvex patellar component.

35

Fractures, Neurovascular Complications, and Wound Healing Problems After Total Knee Arthroplasty

Fractures

Supracondylar Femur Fracture

Although knee arthroplasties may be complicated by fracture of any bone adjacent to the joint, the supracondylar area of the distal femur remains the most common site. Notches in the anterior femoral cortex, osteoporosis, poor flexion, revision arthroplasty, and neurologic disorders have been cited as risk factors. The importance of cortical notching has been discounted in one study on the basis that notches are created frequently, but fractures are rare, with notching significant only in osteoporotic patients.

Condylar type knee arthroplasties inherently increase loads at the proximal end of the anterior femoral flange and are most likely to sustain fractures in the supracondylar region. A stemmed component transfers load to the proximal tip of the stem, and diaphyseal fractures are more common. Fractures between a hip arthroplasty and the proximal stem of a constrained knee arthroplasty pose challenging problems because of stress risers, compromised blood supply, and extensive constraint.

There are numerous approaches to these fractures, and treatment must be individualized. In earlier reports, most advocates of closed treatment cited the risks of surgery and difficulty of achieving rigid fixation as major considerations. Poor results have been attributed to malalignment, shortening of the limb, stiffness, and component loosening. Emphasis was on conservative care unless adequate reduction could not be maintained, with later recourse to revision arthroplasty if necessary.

In more recent studies, stable internal fixation is generally favored over closed treatment. A recent review strongly advocated rigid internal fixation based on excellent results in 20 patients. These supracondylar fractures were treated with blade plates (seven cases), condylar screw plates (seven cases), and buttress plates (six cases). Bone graft was used in 15 cases. The limitations of the study result from the method of case retrieval: members of a trauma study group responded to polling by providing cases. The number of knee arthroplasties from which these cases were drawn is unknown, as is whether these 20 represent all of the fractures that were treated. These limitations are characteristic of most studies on this topic.

Nonrigid intramedullary fixation with Rush rods has also been advocated. The limited exposure and expedient surgery under image intensification may be advantageous to the debilitated patient. Blade plate fixation, although potentially rigid, is often compromised by poor bone quality, comminution, and obstruction by the component. Strictly anatomic reduction may not be feasible if bone has been lost on the anterior cortex from a notch. Condylar screws have been used, but have similar limitations. External fixation has been reported in diaphyseal fractures above stemmed components, but risks deep sepsis from pin tracts. Strut allografts, used commonly for fractures around hip arthroplasty stems, have been used around knee arthroplasty stems at revision surgery to control fractures.

Intramedullary fixation with locked rods has also been adapted to the supracondylar fracture above a knee arthroplasty. A relatively short locked rod, designed for supracondylar fractures in the absence of an arthroplasty, has been successfully adapted to fractures above knee replacements. The device is introduced distally, through an arthrotomy. After disappointing results with rigid fixation, some surgeons have adopted more aggressive approaches, ranging from immediate revision to stemmed components, impaling the component stem inside of an intramedullary rod placed across the fracture, and immediate revision with a custom stemmed component that replaces the femoral condyles. Revision with distal femoral allograft has been recommended when available distal femoral bone is inadequate or for nonunions where severely osteoporotic bone makes rigid fixation impossible.

Tibial Fractures

Tibial fractures under knee arthroplasties are uncommon. Stress fractures of the proximal tibia may be associated with malalignment and component loosening. Most of these cases would be regarded as component loosening with subsidence today. There are scant reports of true tibial fractures under knee arthroplasties. Most are associated with stiffness, loosening, or malalignment and require revision arthroplasty. Stemmed components have been very useful in the management of this problem.

Ipsilateral Femoral Neck and Pubic Ramus Stress Fractures

Stress fractures have been observed in the ipsilateral femoral neck and pubic rami from several weeks to a year after total knee arthroplasty. All reported patients had been severely disabled prior to arthroplasty, had profound osteopenia, and were often dependent on corticosteroid therapy. These fractures are treated conventionally—pubic ramus fractures with a short duration of bed rest followed by protected weightbearing, and femoral neck fractures with multiple pins or arthroplasty. Slow mobilization of the severely debilitated patient and awareness of possible stress fractures are endorsed in all reports.

Neurovascular Injury

Vascular injuries, although fortunately rare, are often catastrophic when they occur. Both direct trauma and thrombotic complications have been reported. The largest series reported consists of 12 cases. Five patients suffered amputations from the midtarsal to above knee levels, and another died. In a more recent report of two cases, the importance of thorough vascular examination supplemented by transcutaneous pulse oximetry and arteriography in high risk cases is emphasized. Doppler studies are unreliable in the presence of calcific vascular disease in which tourniquet use may be inadvisable.

Peroneal nerve palsies are the only nerve damage that occurs with any frequency after knee arthroplasty. An association with concurrent valgus and fixed flexion deformities has been reported in all studies. The incidence ranges from 0.87% (23/2,626) at The Hospital for Special Surgery to 0.002% (26/8,998) in a Mayo Clinic series to 9.5% (4/42) in a small Swedish study of knees with rheumatoid arthritis. The Swedish Knee Arthroplasty project, a nationwide registry of knee arthroplasty, records a 1.8% incidence (43/2,273) among rheumatoid arthritis knees. All large series are retrospective record reviews and probably are underreporting the incidence of this complication. The high incidence in the small Swedish study is unusual.

The standard approach to this problem includes informing the patient of the risk before surgery, especially when correction of valgus and fixed flexion deformities is planned. Although the initial treatment should include removal of tight dressings and flexing the knee, this did not seem to be effective according to the report of the Mayo Clinic series. However, the patients in this series were retrieved from a computer database and included only those who were discharged from the hospital with the recorded complication. It cannot be known, from these data, how many patients awoke with a palsy after surgery and then recovered as a result of prompt conservative care.

The utility of intraoperative exploration of the peroneal nerve in the valgus knee has been questioned. Recent work suggests, however, that surgical exploration and decompression of established peroneal nerve palsies is highly effective, even many months after arthroplasty.

Wound Healing Problems

Wound problems frequently lead to deep sepsis, which is covered elsewhere in this review. An aggressive approach to any delay in healing is essential. Aspiration is always necessary to determine whether the arthroplasty has become infected and how the problem should be managed. Joint fluid should be sent for cell count, differential cell count, culture, and sensitivity. No antibiotic therapy should be initiated for wound problems unless deep sepsis has been ruled out.

Scientific data on wound problems after knee arthroplasty is scant. Data from several studies have demonstrated that vascularization of the medial skin is superior, leading to the conclusion that flaps on the lateral side of the knee are to be avoided. The patella is more easily everted, with less damaging tension on the skin edge, if the proximal incision is angled laterally. Its distal end should lie medial to the base of the tibial tubercle to avoid the bony prominence. Although many factors of surgical technique and the patient's overall health status influence wound healing, there is general agreement that prior incisions are problematic and the knee should be exposed through existing incisions if possible. An isolated strip of skin that lies between two incisions risks necrosis, slough, and subsequent sepsis.

Problems may be averted by soft-tissue reconstruction prior to arthroplasty. The simplest technique is that of soft-tissue expansion of contracted tissue as a separate preliminary operation. While effective in some situations, this technique does not bring new tissue with superior blood supply to the area. Prophylactic free and gastrocnemius flaps have been advocated.

Once early wound problems, such as marginal skin necrosis and drainage, develop, surgical intervention is important. Eight patients were reported who underwent surgical debridement an average of 12.5 days following arthroplasty because of persistent drainage. Two of the eight patients had positive cultures, but none developed deep sepsis. There is general support for the hypothesis that early intervention may prevent deep sepsis and that this benefit outweighs the concern that debridement may cause deep sepsis in a joint that is not yet affected.

Once an arthroplasty has been exposed by full-thickness tissue loss, it should be considered infected. This step would normally require removal of the components and entry into a two-stage protocol. However, there have been reports of survival of components after reconstruction with gastrocnemius flaps. Successful retention of components after gastrocnemius flap reconstruction in six of 12 arthroplasties with exposed components was recently reported. The transposed muscle has demonstrated a potent effect on healing and the eradication of infection. In a review of 41 gastrocnemius flaps to cover tibial defects, the use of this procedure is strongly encouraged.

The muscle flap, formerly reserved for catastrophic situations, effectively prevents lesser problems from becoming catastrophic. Superficial skin necrosis, infected knees in which the tissue is generally poor and the host compromised, persistent drainage after debridement in the patient with negative intra-articular cultures, and compromised fascial closure may all benefit from this reconstruction.

Annotated Bibliography

Fractures: Supracondylar Femur

Aaron RK, Scott R: Supracondylar fracture of the femur after total knee arthroplasty. *Clin Orthop* 1987;219: 136–139.

A review of 250 duo-patellar knee arthroplasties indicated that five of 12 with notching suffered supracondylar fractures. All fracture patients had rheumatoid arthritis with severe osteopenia. This supports the concern about femoral notching, especially in the osteoporotic patient.

Biswas SP, Kurer MH, Mackenney RP: External fixation for femoral shaft fracture after Stanmore total knee replacement. *J Bone Joint Surg* 1992;74B:313–314.

Five cases of femoral shaft fracture above fully-cemented, long-stem femoral components were reported. Four had nonunions from previous treatment, and union was achieved in all patients. This is the only report of external fixation for fractures above knee arthroplasties, although these are not supracondylar fractures.

Cordeiro EN, Costa RC, Carazzato JG, et al: Periprosthetic fractures in patients with total knee arthroplasties. *Clin Orthop* 1990;252:182–189.

This is a study of nine supracondylar fractures and one in the middle tibia from the University of São Paulo, Brazil. Patients who had revision arthroplasty with long stemmed ICLH (Imperial College London Hospital) components achieved superior results to those treated without surgery and those treated with open reduction and internal plate fixation.

Culp RW, Schmidt RG, Hanks G, et al: Supracondylar fracture of the femur following prosthetic knee arthroplasty. *Clin Orthop* 1987;222:212–222.

In this review of 61 supracondylar fractures above knee arthroplasties, notching was regarded as a risk factor. Half were treated surgically and half nonsurgically; the results were superior in patients who had undergone open reduction and internal fixation.

DiGioia AM III, Rubash HE: Periprosthetic fractures of the femur after total knee arthroplasty: A literature review and treatment algorithm. *Clin Orthop* 1991;271:135–142.

This concise yet complete review of the literature presents a useful algorithm for identifying fractures that are amenable to surgical treatment. No patients are included.

Hanks GA, Mathews HH, Routson GW, et al: Supracondylar fracture of the femur following total knee arthroplasty. *J Arthroplasty* 1989;4:289–292.

In three cases treated with Brooker-Wills intramedullary locking nail, all fractures healed, with preserved alignment and motion. This technique is feasible if the fracture is at least 8 cm proximal to the joint line.

Healy WL, Siliski JM, Incavo SJ: Operative treatment of distal femoral fractures proximal to total knee replacements. *J Bone Joint Surg* 1993;75A:27–34.

Excellent results are described for a selected group of 20 patients from multiple surgeons. Notching was apparent in only two patients. Neither the size of the entire patient pool nor the outcome of cases from the same cohort that may have been treated nonsurgically is known. Supracondylar fractures should be treated no differently whether an arthroplasty is in place or not. The authors recommend a straight lateral surgical approach, explaining that an extended anterior approach may be inadequate for fractures that are comminuted or that extend proximally.

Kraay MJ, Goldberg VM, Figgie MP, et al: Distal femoral replacement with allograft/prosthetic reconstruction for treatment of supracondylar fractures in patients with total knee arthroplasty. *J Arthroplasty* 1992;7:7–16.

Seven patients, three of whom died of unrelated causes, were followed for an average of 44 months and minimum of 2 years after fracture. All patients had significant osteoporosis that precluded stable internal fixation. The complications included one dislocation, one popliteal artery injury, and two cases with instability that required bracing. There were no infections and the surgeons conclude that this is an acceptable method of reconstructing this difficult problem.

Madsen F, Kjaersgaard-Andersen P, Juhl M, et al: A custom-made prosthesis for the treatment of supracondylar femoral fractures after total knee arthroplasty: Report of four cases. *J Orthop Trauma* 1989;3:332–337.

Four supracondylar fractures above knee replacements were treated with custom-made long-stemmed knee replacements. At revision, the distal femoral fragments and the component were replaced with a custom hinged-rotation-prosthesis with femoral condyle resection. The success at 1 to 6 years in this study implies that the patients were very low demand. Despite fully cemented long intramedullary stems there is virtually no bone constraint to rotational stress and fixation is severely compromised in this situation.

Merkel KD, Johnson EW Jr: Supracondylar fracture of the femur after total knee arthroplasty. *J Bone Joint Surg* 1986;68A:29–43.

After reviewing 36 cases treated with a variety of closed and open methods, these surgeons recommend closed treatment when possible.

Ritter MA, Faris PM, Keating EM: Anterior femoral notching and ipsilateral supracondylar femur fracture in total knee arthroplasty. *J Arthroplasty* 1988;3:185–187.

The authors of this controversial paper discount the role of anterior femoral notching as a risk factor in supracondylar fracture of the femur after knee arthroplasty. Of 670 total knee arthroplasties, 180 demonstrated anterior femoral notching. Two of the 670 suffered supracondylar fractures: one had a notch and the other did not.

Ritter MA, Stiver P: Supracondylar fracture in a patient with total knee arthroplasty: A case report. *Clin Orthop* 1985;193:168–170.

This is a case report of a simple method for stabilizing

supracondylar fractures. The Rush pin technique was performed under image intensification, required minimal surgical dissection, and permitted early mobilization of the patient and motion of the knee.

Roscoe MW, Goodman SB, Schatzker J: Supracondylar fracture of the femur after GUEPAR total knee arthroplasty: A new treatment method. *Clin Orthop* 1989;241:221–223.

The authors report a novel treatment for femoral fracture proximal to the tip of a stemmed knee prosthesis. Although hinged implants have been abandoned, there is a rise in the use of medullary stems with nonlinked constrained and condylar type revision knee arthroplasties. The fracture site was opened and an AO type rod was placed over the stem of the prosthesis, resulting in union.

Sisto DJ, Lachiewiecz PF, Insall JN: Treatment of supracondylar fractures following prosthetic arthroplasty of the knee. *Clin Orthop* 1985;196:265–272.

Fifteen fractures were analyzed and divided into three groups by treatment. Four patients with closed reduction and cast immobilization had decreased knee scores, and one required an osteotomy for malunion. Among eight patients with initial traction and then a cast brace, decreased knee scores, malunion, and nonunion were common. Of three patients treated with open reduction and internal fixation, all had functional arthroplasties. This was one of the first papers to recommend open reduction and internal fixation for these fractures.

Steinbrink K, Engelbrecht E, Fenelon GC: The total femoral prosthesis: A preliminary report. *J Bone Joint Surg* 1982;64B:305–312.

Ten cases of extremely difficult femoral fractures above knee arthroplasties were included in a series of tumors that were treated with the same total femur prosthesis. Many of these were constrained knee implants in patients with ipsilateral total hip arthroplasties. This radical option becomes an alternative to amputation or hip disarticulation in patients with concurrent hip and knee arthroplasty problems.

Fractures: Tibial

Kjaersgaard-Andersen P, Juhl M: Ipsilateral traumatic supracondylar femoral and proximal tibial fractures following total knee replacement: A case report. *J Trauma* 1989;29:398–400.

The authors report an unusual case of a patient who sustained a supracondylar femur fracture between a total hip and a knee arthroplasty. This was initially treated with skeletal traction and then after 4 months a custom made, stemmed, St. Georg hinge with replacement of the distal femoral condyles was implanted. Subsequently, the tibial component loosened and the tibia fractured. After 4 months of closed treatment, the arthroplasty was again revised with a custom tibial component that mated with the well fixed femoral component. Loose components are probably another risk factor for fracture.

Rand JA, Coventry MB: Stress fractures after total knee arthroplasty. *J Bone Joint Surg* 1980;62A:226–233.

The authors report 15 patients with tibial fractures after geomedic and polycentric arthroplasties. Causes were axial malalignment and improper component orientation in all cases. All were revised. These cases would be regarded as loosening with subsidence today.

Fractures: Femoral Neck Stress Fractures After Total Knee Arthroplasty

Hardy DC, Delince PE, Yasik E, et al: Stress fracture of the hip: An unusual complication of total knee arthroplasty. *Clin Orthop* 1992;281:140–144.

This is a single case report from Belgium with review of the literature. Osteoporotic bone and low functional level were common. Onset of pain occurred at 1 year after total knee replacement.

McElwaine JP, Sheehan JM: Spontaneous fractures of the femoral neck after total replacement of the knee. *J Bone Joint Surg* 1982;64B:323–325.

Seven cases of femoral neck stress fracture after total knee replacement (representing a 1.4% incidence in their own series) are reported. Although osteoporosis was common to all cases, the authors felt that rapid mobilization with an unprotected hip was a more important factor.

Neurovascular Injury

McPherson EJ, Friedman RJ: Arterial thromboembolism associated with total knee arthroplasty: A report of two cases. *Am J Knee Surg* 1992;5(suppl):94–98.

This is a review of the other 15 cases existing in the literature. Extensive vascular calcification makes physical examination and Doppler studies unreliable. Alternate studies should include transcutaneous oximetry and arteriogram in the presurgical planning of these cases. Tourniquet is best avoided.

Rand JA: Vascular complications of total knee arthroplasty: Report of three cases. *J Arthroplasty* 1987;2:89–93.

Rush JH, Vidovich JD, Johnson MA: Arterial complications of total knee replacement: The Australian experience. *J Bone Joint Surg* 1987;69B:400–402.

Twelve arterial injuries were reported after total knee arthroplasty. Seven involved femoral or popliteal artery thrombosis, and five resulted from direct trauma to the vessels. Peripheral vascular disease places patients at particular risk.

Peroneal Nerve Palsy

Asp JP, Rand JA: Peroneal nerve palsy after total knee arthroplasty. *Clin Orthop* 1990;261:233–237.

Retrospective review of 8,998 total knee replacements found 26 peroneal nerve palsies. This probably represents underreporting. Palsy was complete in 18 and incomplete in eight. Motor and sensory deficits occurred in 23 with motor deficits exclusively in three. After 5.1 years recovery was complete in 13 and incomplete in 12. Prognosis for good functional result and nerve recovery was better in incomplete lesions. No patients had underlying metabolic problems. Removal of constricting dressings and flexing the knee, although appropriate treatment, was not particularly effective.

Knutson K, Leden I, Sturfelt G, et al: Nerve palsy after knee arthroplasty in patients with rheumatoid arthritis. *Scand J Rheumatol* 1983;12:201–205.

In this study of 42 total knee replacements in rheumatoid arthritic knees with four cases of peroneal nerve palsy, 16 knees were studied with electromyography and three had subclinical evidence of nerve damage. Valgus deformity with flexion contracture is a risk factor.

Krackow KA, Maar DC, Mont MA, et al: Surgical decompression for peroneal nerve palsy after total knee arthroplasty. *Clin Orthop* 1993;292:223–228.

Five patients with peroneal nerve palsy after total knee replacement were treated with surgical decompression. Surgery was performed 5 to 45 months after the total knee replacement. All patients improved and four of five recovered completely. An excellent description of the surgical technique along with detailed drawings is included.

Rose HA, Hood RW, Otis JC, et al: Peroneal-nerve palsy following total knee arthroplasty. *J Bone Joint Surg* 1982;64A:347–351.

In 2,626 total knee replacements, 23 peroneal palsies were recorded. Valgus deformities with flexion contractures were a definite risk factor. Only two patients with a partial palsy made full recovery. The possible causes are regarded as traction on the surrounding tissues with vascular compromise to the nerve, direct pressure on the nerve from the postoperative dressing, or a combination. One occurred despite surgical exploration and release of the nerve at the time of surgery. The value of surgical exploration once the palsy has occurred is unknown.

Wound Problems
General

Klein NE, Cox CV: Wound problems in total knee arthroplasty, in Fu FH, Harner CD, Vince KG (eds): *Knee Surgery.* Philadelphia, PA, Williams & Wilkins, 1994, vol 2, pp 1539–1552.

This complete reference on the topic of wound problems covers prevention and treatment. It emphasizes the role of prophylactic muscle pedicle and free flaps in the high risk patient with multiple scars, adherent skin, wound necrosis, and prior skin slough.

Skin Incision

Johnson DP: Midline or parapatellar incision for knee arthroplasty: A comparative study of wound viability. *J Bone Joint Surg* 1988;70B:656–658.

Transcutaneous oxygen measurements showed a significantly lower oxygen tension on the lateral wound edge at all times and with all incisions, supporting the medially based blood supply theory. The more medial the incision, the lower the lateral flap oxygen tension and the greater the risk of ischemic flap complications. Oxygen tension returned to presurgical levels by day 8.

Tissue Expansion Prior to Knee Surgery

Riederman R, Noyes FR: Soft tissue expansion of contracted tissues prior to knee surgery. *Am J Knee Surg* 1991;4:195–199.

Drainage

Weiss AP, Krackow KA: Persistent wound drainage after primary total knee arthroplasty. *J Arthroplasty* 1993;8:285–289.

In this retrospective review of 546 primary total knee replacements, eight patients had persistent drainage after surgery. These patients went back to surgery for debridement at an average of 12.5 days after surgery when 25% had positive cultures. No patients developed chronic infection after an average follow-up of 4.3 years. The surgeons involved hypothesize that early surgical intervention prevented more serious infections and that irrigation and debridement did not introduce infection into the joint.

Skin Necrosis and the Exposed Prosthesis

Eckardt JJ, Lesavoy MA, Dubrow TJ, et al: Exposed endoprosthesis: Management protocol using muscle and myocutaneous flap coverage. *Clin Orthop* 1990;251:220–229.

Gerwin M, Rothaus KO, Windsor RE, et al: Gastrocnemius muscle flap coverage of exposed or infected knee prostheses. *Clin Orthop* 1993;286:64–70.

Twelve cases were reviewed retrospectively. Each had undergone a gastrocnemius muscle pedicle flap for coverage of an exposed or infected knee prosthesis. All flaps remained viable. All six patients who had a flap in conjunction with removal of the prosthesis for two-stage treatment of infection recovered. Five of six patients with an exposed prosthesis retained the components. This more recent study is consistent with other literature demonstrating the potent effect of gastrocnemius flaps in contributing to healing and the eradication of infection.

Pico R, Luscher NJ, Rometsch M, et al: Why the denervated gastrocnemius muscle flap should be encouraged. *Ann Plast Surg* 1991;26:312–324.

Siim E, Jakobsen IE, Medgyesi S: Soft-tissue procedures for the exposed knee arthroplasty: 18 cases followed for 7 (1–17) years. *Acta Orthop Scand* 1991;62:312–314.

Eighteen cases were followed up for 7 (1–17) years.

36
Total Knee Infection

Significance

Infection, while not the most common complication of total knee arthroplasty (TKA), is certainly one of the most dreaded. To the patient, infection causes pain, limited function, and prolonged hospitalization with additional surgeries. To the surgeon, infection is a symbol of defeat, a diagnostic and therapeutic dilemma, and a potential source for liability. Moreover, total knee infection dramatically increases the cost of knee arthroplasty, and many current reimbursement plans inadequately cover costs of treating this complication.

It is estimated that nearly 200,000 TKAs are performed annually in the United States. With a conservative infection rate of 1% and an average cost of $60,000 per patient for treatment of an infected TKA, the annual cost for treating an infected TKA is $120 million. With the caveat that infection can never be eliminated as a complication of any surgical procedure, it is clear that prompt diagnosis, an organized treatment paradigm, and an aggressive surgical program will best assure a favorable outcome. This chapter reviews the incidence and risk factors, the methods of prevention and diagnosis, treatment options, and the results of treating the infected TKA. It deals specifically with the management of deep sepsis, both in the perioperative and late hematogenous phases. It does not deal with superficial infection, which carries a much more favorable prognosis.

Perioperative or early infection will be defined as that occurring within 3 months of the arthroplasty, whereas late infection occurs more than 3 months after surgery. This differentiation between early and late infection is arbitrary, and various authors have separated the two as early as 6 weeks and as late as 6 months. Early infections are presumed to have become contaminated at surgery, whereas late infections most commonly occur from a hematogenous source. The advantage of this differentiation is that early infections are less likely to be chronic and, therefore, are more amenable to cure with prosthesis retention. A late hematogenous infection, however, would behave as an acute infection if the prosthesis was intact and the infection recognized within the first few days of seeding. Conversely, a 3-month perioperative infection could become chronic with osseous involvement and even a sinus tract, assuming the symptoms were either mild or ignored.

Incidence and Risk Factors

A variety of publications have reported the incidence of total knee infection from 0.5% to 12%. The higher figures do not represent current data because they were reported in the early years, prior to the use of prophylactic antibiotics and when hinge prostheses were commonly implanted. Hinge arthroplasties have a significantly higher incidence of infection, presumably due to implant loosening and wear debris formation. The wear debris is engulfed by local macrophages, which are thus rendered less capable of normal bacterial surveillance. Moreover, the production of local factors as a result of this phagocytosis is proinflammatory and increases blood supply to the joint.

For a recent study, an infection rate was reported of 1.6% in 4,171 TKAs performed at one institution between 1973 and 1987. A majority of these infections were late and presumably of hematogenous origin. A case-control analysis identified certain risk factors associated with infection. These included rheumatoid arthritis, associated skin breakdown, prior surgery in the osteoarthritis patient, and knee replacement in males with rheumatoid arthritis ($p < 0.05$). It was postulated that males with rheumatoid arthritis are more likely to become infected because they are seropositive and usually have an acquired hypogammaglobulinemia. In this study, there were factors believed to be associated with infection, but these were not significant at the 0.05 confidence level. These factors included exogenous obesity, concomitant urinary tract infection, and steroid use in the patient with rheumatoid arthritis. It is logical that conditions such as renal failure, malignant disease, and diabetes mellitus are associated with an increased incidence of infection, but the overall incidence was too low to show significance in this study.

In a previous report from the same institution, a high percentage of acute perioperative infections were associated with significant wound problems, including prolonged drainage, wound dehiscence, and skin slough. Skin sloughs were frequently seen in revision surgery in which previous incisions were not honored. In most cases, a previous lateral incision was ignored and a median parapatellar incision used. The lateral skin flap would slough due to loss of blood supply from the superior medial geniculate artery and the loss of collateral circulation from the previous lateral incision. Additionally, prolonged postoperative drainage is a concern. In a recent study, an increased incidence of infection was reported with wounds that drained for more than 6 days. Drainage was defined as staining more than 2 cm^2. These authors recommended wound debridement and primary closure to prevent deep infection.

Prevention

Outline 1 lists the methods for limiting postoperative infection in total knee arthroplasty.

The prevalence of specific infecting organisms varies in different studies due to the year reported and the hospital environment. The predominant organisms are *Staphylococcus aureus, S epidermidis,* and a variety of *Streptococcus* species. Gram-negative infections and mixed infections are less common, but often are more difficult to eradicate. In recent years, there has been an increase in the number of infected arthroplasties caused by methicillin-resistant *Staphylococcus aureus, S epidermidis,* and *Enterococcus,* and more recently, vancomycin-resistant *Enterococcus faecium.* These infections are alarming in that they are resistant to the usual prophylactic antibiotics used for knee arthroplasty. Moreover, anaerobic organisms and facultative anaerobic organisms are often involved in chronic indolent sepsis, which may go undetected until chronic infection has become established. These organisms include *Peptococcus* species, *Peptostreptococcus* species, and *Propionibacterium acnes* and other diphtheroid species.

Outline 1. Methods of preventing total knee replacement infection

Systemic antibiotic
Late antibiotic prophylaxis
Operating-room environment
Meticulous surgery
Antibiotic irrigation
Antibiotics in cement

Systemic Antibiotics

The standard of practice dictates the use of routine prophylactic antibiotics in total joint arthroplasty. A variety of regimens have been proposed, but most are centered around a first-generation cephalosporin. The predominant organisms in total joint infection continue to be *Staphylococcus aureus, S epidermidis,* and *Streptococcus* species. In most centers, systemic antibiotic prophylaxis is directed to the common pathogens. Table 1 lists the most common antibiotic regimens used. The need for late antibiotic prophylaxis for dental, gastrointestinal, or genitourinary manipulation has recently been questioned. Table 2 lists the common antibiotic alternatives for late dental prophylaxis. Although the dental literature suggests that routine antibiotic prophylaxis for dental cleaning is not necessary, the data are not clear and the potential downside risks are great. There has been some suggestion that late antibiotic prophylaxis be routinely used for people at high risk as determined above and for 2 years following joint arthroplasty.

Table 1. Systemic antibiotics for prevention of total knee replacement infection

Systemic antibiotics	Dosage*
Cefazolin	1 g intravenous at surgery 1 g intravenous every 8 hr for 24 hr
Cefuroxime	1.5 g intravenous at surgery 750 mg intravenous every 8 hr for 24 hr
Vancomycin	1 g intravenous (slowly) at surgery 0.5 g intravenous every 12 hr for 24 hr

*If penicillin anaphylaxis or cephalosporin allergy, use vancomycin as above.

Table 2. Late antibiotic prophylaxis

Antibiotic	Dosage
Amoxicillin	3 g by mouth 1 hr before 1.5 g by mouth 6 hr after
Erythromycin	1 g by mouth 1 hr before 0.5 g by mouth 6 hr after

Operating Room Environment

Outline 2 lists the common modifications of conventional operating rooms that have been associated with a decreased incidence of total knee infection. With the exception of horizontal laminar flow, in which the incidence of knee infection was actually increased, the remaining methods have statistically been shown to have decreased the incidence of total joint infection. The most important factor, however, is routine use of antibiotic prophylaxis with operating room modification serving as an adjunct to the primary mechanism.

Outline 2. Modification of OR environment to prevent total knee replacement infection

Ultraviolet lights, 2537 Å
Vertical laminar flow
Horizontal laminar flow
Exhaust system
Greenhouse

Meticulous Surgery, Antibiotic Irrigation, Antibiotics in Cement

Standard surgical technique as well as routine use of antibiotic irrigation are important factors in minimizing the chance of postoperative infection. Antibiotic-impregnated cement is commonly used in revision situations and in high-risk individuals undergoing primary total joint arthroplasty.

Outline 3 lists the indications and the usual doses of antibiotics used in cement. These doses per 40 g (1 bag) are mixed in powder form at the time of cementing and will not substantially diminish the strength of the cement.

Outline 3. Antibiotics in cement

Indications
    Immunosuppressed patient
    Systemic illness
    Presence of risk factors
    Revision surgery
Usual choices
    Gentamicin, 0.5 to 1.0 g/40 g cement
    Cephamandole, 1.0 g/40 g cement
    Tobramycin, 600 mg/40 g cement

Outline 4. Treatment options for the infected total knee replacement

Prosthesis retention
    Aspiration alone
    Debridement
        Arthroscopic
        Open
Prosthesis exchange
    Immediate
    Intermediate
    Delayed
Salvage
    Arthrodesis
    Resection arthroplasty
    Amputation (all include the use of intravenous antibiotics)

Antibiotics mixed with cement that is to be used as interval cement spacers can be used at higher doses.

Treatment of the Infected Total Knee Replacement

Outlines 4 and 5 list the treatment options available for management of an infected TKA and the factors involved in selection of a specific option. It is important to differentiate deep sepsis from superficial infection. A postoperative cellulitis or superficial wound infection, which does not communicate with the prosthesis, needs aggressive surgical management and intravenous antibiotics, but generally has a more favorable outcome than deep sepsis.

Prosthesis retention is rarely indicated for the treatment of established deep infection. Patients with a penicillin-sensitive streptococcus, who develop an acute infection that is recognized within 48 hours of onset, may respond to repeated joint aspiration and direct antibiotic therapy. These patients must undergo repeated arthrocentesis and show a rapid clinical response marked by decreased effusion, lower synovial white cell count, negative cultures, and the absence of systemic toxicity. Moreover, following aspiration, the joint must appear relatively normal without evidence of a boggy synovitis. Failure to respond to this treatment regimen is an indication for a more aggressive therapeutic approach. The results of aspiration and antibiotic treatment alone are poor. In a Swedish study, there was only a 15% success rate with aspiration and antibiotic therapy.

The role of arthroscopic lavage is unclear. It allows more accurate tissue diagnosis and a more aggressive lavage

Outline 5. Factors affecting choice of treatment

Host factors
Delay in diagnosis
Type of prosthesis
Organism
Radiographs
Skin and soft tissue
Response to treatment

than can be obtained by needle aspiration. Arthroscopic synovectomy is generally less complete than an open procedure, and it obviates the possibility of exchanging the modular polyethylene insert and irrigating the modular interface.

Open debridement with synovectomy, lavage, and exchange of the tibial polyethylene insert is indicated in specific cases of deep sepsis. Prosthesis retention requires an implant that is otherwise stable, well aligned, and functioning well prior to infection. There should be no evidence of radiographic loosening, osteolysis, or periosteal reaction. The organism must be sensitive to an antibiotic program tolerated by the host, and the host must have a reasonable immune system. The results of open debridement with prosthesis retention are variable. For one study, 45% failure was reported at mean 43-month follow-up in 42 infected total knees treated with this protocol. In this study, *Staphylococcus aureus* was a poor prognosticator of success with prosthesis retention. For another study, a 77% recurrence of infection was reported at mean follow-up of 8.8 years in 31 infected total knees, with a 58% failure when *S aureus* was the infecting organism. For yet another study, only a 24% success rate was reported with soft-tissue surgery and prosthesis retention.

Immediate Exchange/Early Exchange

The use of antibiotic cement, aggressive surgical debridement, and newer antibiotic regimens has led to the development of more protocols for immediate or early exchange of an infected knee replacement. With multiple protocols and short follow-up, many of these data remain anecdotal. One group published the report of a small series with only a 35% satisfactory functional result. Another group reported an overall 75% success rate with prosthesis exchange and found no difference between one-stage and two-stage procedures. A European group reported a 73% cure with single exchange and an overall 84% cure with a second exchange.

Delayed Exchange

Removal of the implant, radical debridement, and an interval period of intravenous antibiotics followed by reimplantation remains the standard for treatment of the infected TKA and should be used in most cases. Newer protocols use antibiotic-impregnated cement spacers and antibiotic-impregnated implants to allow local delivery of antibiotics, maintain the joint space, and, in some cases, permit motion during the interval period. The technical aspects of delayed reimplantation are more complex than those of standard revision due to problems of exposure, bone loss, ligamentous balance, and restoration of flexion. An approximately 90% eradication of infection has been reported in most published series on delayed exchange. There is still controversy concerning length of intravenous antibiotic administration, use of antibiotic spacers and implants during the interval period, and the methods for reconstitution of bone loss at the time of reimplantation. In general, 6 weeks of intravenous antibiotic therapy is used in most delayed exchange protocols.

Arthrodesis/Resection Arthroplasty/Amputation

More aggressive treatment is necessary for severe infection with resistant organisms and/or an immunosuppressed host. Moreover, revision surgery is contraindicated in patients with an incompetent extensor mechanism or inadequate skin and soft tissues. Reports of arthrodesis as well as those of resection arthroplasty indicate approximately 90% success in eradication of infection. Amputation is re-

served as a final option or in the presence of a life-threatening infection, especially with gas-forming organisms. The encouraging results and better functional outcome of delayed exchange and even immediate exchange have limited the role of these more aggressive protocols to refractory cases and to severe infections with major soft-tissue loss.

In summary, aspiration and antibiotics for treatment of the infected total knee are limited to acute infections with a penicillin-sensitive streptococcus. Surgical debridement and prosthesis retention are indicated when an immunocompetent host who has an otherwise well-functioning implant is infected with a susceptible organism. Prosthesis exchange is indicated in the majority of cases. The emerging role of immediate or early exchange protocols is unclear, although delayed exchange remains the standard of treatment. Arthrodesis resection arthroplasty and amputation are limited to refractory cases or a life-threatening situation.

Annotated Bibliography

Fehring TK, McAlister JA Jr: Frozen histologic section as a guide to sepsis in revision joint arthroplasty. *Clin Orthop* 1994;304:229–237.

This study reviews the effectiveness of frozen section for diagnosis of an infection in 107 consecutive cases. In this study, frozen section had a sensitivity as a diagnostic test of only 18.2%, but had a specificity of 89.5%.

Goksan SB, Freeman MA: One-stage reimplantation for infected total knee arthroplasty. *J Bone Joint Surg* 1992; 74B:78–82.

The authors report successful eradication of infected TKAs in 17 of 18 patients treated by a single-stage protocol. They attribute their higher success rate to aggressive debridement, use of antibiotic-impregnated cement, and 3 months of antibiotic therapy. Moreover, all patients in this group were infected with gram-positive organisms, and none showed evidence of systemic toxicity.

Levitsky KA, Hozack WJ, Balderston RA, et al: Evaluation of the painful prosthetic joint: Relative value of bone scan, sedimentation rate, and joint aspiration. *J Arthroplasty* 1991;6:237–244.

This study compares three-phase bone imaging (sensitivity 33%, specificity 86%), preoperative sedimentation rate greater than 30 (sensitivity 60%, specificity 65%), and preoperative joint aspiration (sensitivity 67%, specificity 96%) in the evaluation of total joint infection. The authors conclude that joint aspiration is the most useful test for evaluation of a painful total joint.

Nelson CL, Evans RP, Blaha JD, et al: A comparison of gentamicin-impregnated polymethylmethacrylate bead

implantation to conventional parenteral antibiotic therapy in infected total hip and knee arthroplasty. *Clin Orthop* 1993;295:96–101.

This multi-center study examines the effect of gentamicin-impregnated polymethylmethacrylate (PMMA) beads versus systemic antibiotic therapy in the eradication of the infected total hip and total knee. Recurrent infection was associated with host compromise and malnutrition, multiple previous surgeries, extensive infection, and inadequate debridement. Addition of PMMA beads in this study did not improve the results over conventional antibiotics.

Wilson MG, Kelley K, Thornhill TS: Infection as a complication of total knee-replacement arthroplasty: Risk factors and treatment in sixty-seven cases. *J Bone Joint Surg* 1990;72A:878–883.

This study reports the incidence (1.6%) and risk factors associated with total knee infection. Treatment by debridement with prosthesis retention was associated with a 45% recurrence rate. *Staphylococcus aureus* was a poor prognosticator of success with prosthesis retention. The most successful treatment protocol in this study was two-stage, delayed exchange.

Windsor RE, Insall JN, Urs WK, et al: Two-stage reimplantation for the salvage of total knee arthroplasty complicated by infection: Further follow-up and refinement of indications. *J Bone Joint Surg* 1990;72A: 272–278.

The authors report eradication of infection in 37 of 38 infected TKAs treated by a two-stage exchange protocol. According to the authors, a 6-week interval of intravenous antibiotic therapy is an important aspect of this protocol.

37

Rehabilitation Following Total Knee Arthroplasty

The overall success of total knee arthroplasty (TKA) depends on three components: patient selection, the technique of surgical intervention, and the rehabilitation process. Ideally, rehabilitation should be initiated preoperatively, starting with assessment of the patient's knee disability and any coexisting disabilities. These may be general (ie, cardiac or respiratory) disabilities and/or musculoskeletal limitations brought on by diseases such as rheumatoid arthritis with multiple joint involvement. Preoperative disabilities may also include significant flexion contractures or previous osteotomies, both of which may affect the overall result. An attempt has been made, on a prospective basis, to preoperatively engage patients in either a cardiac exercise program or a strengthening program. At this time, there has been no indication that preoperative exercise has changed any outcome measures other than the psychological aspect of the patients having prepared themselves better for postoperative rehabilitation. A preoperative educational program should include written information, slides and/or videos of the operative procedure and rehabilitation program, and an introduction to a physical therapist, who preferably is "the" therapist responsible for the patient's hospital program. This therapist can significantly improve the patient's abilities to understand and participate in the postoperative program. It is important before surgery to make patients aware of the rehabilitation necessary to achieve maximum benefit from the surgical procedure and to ensure that they have realistic postoperative goals, which include a high level of generalized activities.

The surgical findings, including preservation of bone stock, soft tissue, patella tracking, and so forth will significantly affect the overall outcome of the rehabilitation program and should be emphasized to the patient following the surgical procedure. The recent enthusiasm for avoidance of drains following knee replacement surgery has not been shown to affect either blood loss, strength, or range of motion in the postoperative period. Although scientific data as to the effectiveness of continuous passive motion (CPM) are mixed, it would appear that the long-term result is unaffected by the decision to use CPM or active range of motion in the early postoperative period. CPM or active range of motion may be initiated in the postsurgical acute care unit with a rapid increase to 90° of flexion as tolerated by the patient over a 2 to 3 day period and a more rapid return to activities of daily living. With early discharge programs, some patients have accomplished a 90° flexion arc and adequate strength of straight leg raising within the 3-day postoperative time period to then be managed as outpatients.

Weightbearing status of hip implants depends on whether the surgical technique is cemented, noncemented, or hybrid, but in total knee replacements, early weightbearing appears to be well tolerated with rigid fixation in any of the above techniques. It is recommended that a posterior extension splint be used until quadriceps strength is adequate to control the leg in postoperative ambulation.

A series of modalities, including hot ice and transcutaneous electrical stimulation, have been used to improve the overall quality of the TKA result. However, there is no indication that these modalities have positively affected outcome measures.

The use of narcotics in the early postoperative period, either by patient controlled analgesia (PCA) techniques or epidurally, has been a marked adjunct to the rapid restoration of motion and strength without excessive and undue pain. The ease of use, cost, and lack of necessity for trained personnel allow the routine use of PCA in any hospital setting. Devices that are self-contained and do not require excessive equipment allow for easier and earlier ambulation. Moreover, supplementary intramuscular medication continues to be available if necessary.

The use of urinary catheters for 48 hours postoperatively allows early ambulation without the necessity for intermittent catheterization, and with adequate prophylactic antibiotics, there is no increase in infection rates of the replacement procedure.

Predonated autologous blood banking is used in almost all TKA programs. Because a tourniquet is used in TKA, this predonated blood often is reserved for reinfusion during the early postoperative period. There is ample evidence for avoiding the use of fixed hemoglobin and hematocrit levels and for using the patient's general medical status as a guide for retransfusion of autologous predonated blood or other sources of blood byproducts. The present national blood bank recommendations are for similar criteria for the transfusion of either predonated autologous or homologous units of blood.

The risk of deep venous thrombosis in the postoperative period of TKA is 50% to 70% in a patient who has not received prophylaxis. Modalities of prophylaxis now available include use of intermittent alternating thigh high compression devices, and oral and subcutaneous administration of anticoagulants, including either standard heparin or the recently released low molecular weight heparin. The most commonly used prophylactic program in the United States at this time is oral administration of anticoagulant warfarin started either the day of or the day following surgery with a target international normalized ratio of 2:3 for prophylaxis. High risk patients, who have had previous history of deep venous thrombosis or pulmonary embolic disease, may require the addition of either a newer low molecular weight heparin or standard heparin to the oral warfarin anticoagulation program.

In many settings, duplex ultrasonography is an extremely viable diagnostic tool which can be used both to include the ipsilateral or contralateral leg and for continued surveillance during the postoperative period. In many hospital environments the sensitivity, specificity, and efficacy of duplex ultrasonography for diagnosis of both thigh and calf vein thrombosis is close to 100% as compared to that of traditional venography. The exact duration of prophylaxis for deep venous thrombosis is presently unknown; however, deep venous thrombosis has occurred as late as 6 weeks or more following TKA.

With earlier hospital discharge, it is important to coordinate the acute hospital phase of the rehabilitation program with the postoperative out-of-hospital program, whether it will take place in a rehabilitation center, nursing home, or at home by home health care. Preoperative education of the rehabilitation team with specific goals and expectations can make it possible to achieve a high level of therapeutic success from the surgery. The major physical therapy goal is to obtain adequate flexion for the patient to utilize low seats in relatively cramped quarters such as automobiles and theater seats. Use of low seats requires a minimum of 90° of flexion and ideally should be in the range of approximately 110° of flexion. In addition, muscular strength, the major component of which is quadriceps strength, is necessary for adequate ambulation; therefore, long-term strengthening programs are ideal. If a patient is unable to achieve full extension and lock his or her knee in standing, quadriceps muscles are under a significantly increased load. The long-term benefits of manipulation in a restricted range-of-motion patient are controversial, but if manipulation is to be done, it is more efficacious in the first 2 postoperative weeks prior to collagen re-orientation. The extension arc may improve up to 6 months postoperatively with the flexion arc improving up to 3 years postoperatively. Long-term studies indicate high impact loading sports will have a negative effect on the long-term results. There is mixed information in the literature with respect to the effects of body weight on the outcome.

Antibiotic prophylaxis for routine dental, gastrointestinal, and genitourinary manipulations, or for an established infection within the body, is presently recommended. The duration of need for prophylactic antibiotics in these settings is under investigation, but prophylaxis is presently considered efficacious on a permanent basis.

Follow-up is recommended for evaluation of the outcomes at a minimum of 1-, 3-, and 5-year intervals, and it is hoped that TKA patients will be part of ongoing outcome measures up to 20 years postsurgery to allow improvement of future technical advances.

Annotated Bibliography

Kitziger KJ: Ultrasonography in the diagnosis of deep venous thrombosis. *Semin Arthroplasty* 1992;3:95–98.

Duplex ultrasonography has an extremely high sensitivity, specificity, and accuracy in proximal thigh deep venous thrombosis. Depending on the institution, it is more or less reliable with respect to the diagnosis of distal deep venous thrombosis.

Leclerc JR (ed): *Venous Thromboembolic Disorders.* Philadelphia, PA, Lea & Febiger, 1991, pp 303–345.

Low molecular weight heparins appear to be as efficacious in the prevention of deep venous thrombosis in the total knee replacement as they have proven in the prevention of DVT in total hip replacements.

Liang MH, Fossel AH, Larson MG: Comparisons of five health status instruments for orthopedic evaluation. *Med Care* 1990;28:632–642.

Despite five different health status instruments now available, there is no established instrument for evaluating the outcomes of total knee replacement.

Parker RK, Holtmann B, White PF: Patient-controlled analgesia: Does a concurrent opioid infusion improve pain management after surgery? *JAMA* 1991;266:1947–1952.

The author indicated a significant improvement in patient satisfaction following major surgical procedures with patient controlled analgesia.

Romness DW, Rand JA: The role of continuous passive motion following total knee arthroplasty. *Clin Orthop* 1988;226:34–37

Patients undergoing total knee arthroplasty with and without continuous passive motion were compared. The patients with continuous passive motion achieved 90° of knee flexion earlier than the control group, but at 3 months and 1 year there was no significant difference in motion between the two groups. There was no significant difference in duration of hospitalization or blood loss between the two groups.

Yomtovian R, Kruskall MS, Barber JP: Autologous-blood transfusion: The reimbursement dilemma. *J Bone Joint Surg* 1992;74A:1265–1272.

In 612 hospitals, 90% of patients with preoperative autologous blood donations avoided homologous transfusions entirely.

38

Long-Term Results in Total Knee Arthroplasty

As we move into the third decade of total knee arthroplasty (TKA), this operation continues to be one of the most predictable and satisfying procedures for both patients and surgeons. As many as 150,000 TKAs are now performed annually in the United States. A recent meta-analysis of patient outcomes following TKA included nearly 10,000 patients in 130 published reports and noted 89% of patients reported good or excellent outcomes at a mean follow-up of 4 years. With 10- to 15-year TKA follow-ups now available with 95% predicted survival, it will be interesting to see how much more refinement can be expected from this joint replacement. Unfortunately, as "improvements" have been made in implant materials, component designs, and fixation methods, new problems have arisen and now crowd the literature alongside the long-term survival studies of earlier designs. Osteolysis, corrosion, failure of metal backing, polyethylene delamination, meniscal bearing fractures, and dislocations are just a few examples of complications seen with more contemporary implant designs. Before looking at some of these complications associated with the newer prostheses, it is necessary to look at the evolution of the current knee designs and the long-term results.

Cemented Total Knee Arthroplasty Results

The modern forerunner of the majority of current total knee designs was the Total Condylar Knee prosthesis, which was developed in the early 1970s and was first implanted in 1974. This prosthesis was a cemented posterior cruciate ligament (PCL)-sacrificing design with an all polyethylene tibial component. There was only one size femoral component available, and modern cementing techniques were not used. Instrumentation was crude by today's standards.

A recent review of the 15-year survivorship of the first 112 knees in which this prosthesis was used reported 94% clinical survivorship, with a 91% survivorship when radiographic failures are included. The average range of motion was 99° (range: 65° to 120°), and 92% had an excellent or good result using the Hospital for Special Surgery (HSS) knee score. Radiographic evaluation revealed lucencies around 72% of the tibial components, although only two were clinically loose. Five revisions—one for infection, one for instability, and three for tibial loosening—were seen between 13 and 17 years postoperatively. This series compares favorably with previously reported shorter-term survivals of 90% to 98% for the same prosthetic design.

Beginning in 1979, modern cementing techniques, im-

proved instrumentation, and multiple component sizes were added to the original Total Condylar prosthesis. The same surgeon who reported the results above recently reported a 14-year survivorship study, noting a 95% clinical survival rate with no radiographically loose components. There were four revisions but none for aseptic loosening of the tibial component. Mean flexion was 100° (range: 82° to 120°), and 95% of the patients had good or excellent knee scores. Radiolucencies were present around 45% of the tibial components and averaged 1 mm.

The demographics of the patient populations in the two studies are nearly identical, and all were operated on by a single surgeon. Although the clinical scores are similar, the most important difference between the studies is in the radiographic results. Reports of other series of Total Condylar prostheses have shown radiolucency rates of 10% to 73%. In this latest series, in which updated instrumentation and cementing techniques were used, there were 37% femoral lucencies (all in one zone) and 45% tibial lucencies. These lucencies were thinner and involved fewer zones than reported for the previous series. It appears from this report that the addition of modern cementing techniques, accurate instrumentation with improved sizing of components, and soft-tissue balancing has led to a comparable clinical result and an improved radiographic outcome.

Modifications of the original Total Condylar prosthesis by proponents of PCL retention led to a PCL-retaining prosthesis by adding a posterior cutout to the original all-polyethylene tibial component. Advocates of PCL retention claimed that the PCL was needed for femoral roll back during flexion, increasing range of motion (ROM), and decreasing stresses at the tibial bone–cement interface. Some investigators have found that retention of the PCL helps maintain the level of the original joint line, resulting in more normal knee kinematics. Proponents of PCL retention report increased knee ROM and improved quadriceps biomechanics during stair climbing and when arising from a seated position as compared to the PCL-sacrificing and substituting designs.

A long-term survival analysis of this design was published in 1994 and involved 418 PCL-retaining Total Condylar knees with an all-polyethylene tibial component, inserted by a single surgeon and followed up for 10 to 18 years. The survival rate at 14 years was 95%. In the group, there were seven mechanical failures, three of which were attributed to aseptic loosening of the tibial component. There was no mention of radiolucencies or clinical evaluations because this was only a survival analysis report. These findings are similar to a 1990 report of 1,943 cemented PCL-retaining knee arthroplasties of a similar design (Kinematic) with a cumulative success of 97% at 9 years.

Another modification of the Total Condylar design in 1978 involved the use of a long tibial spine and a femoral cam to increase roll back of the femoral component on the tibia. This posterior-stabilized modification was designed to improve ROM, to make stair climbing easier, and to prevent posterior tibial subluxation. A 1992 study examined 289 total knee arthroplasties with a posterior-stabilized all-polyethylene tibial component. There were 14 failures: five for infections, three for femoral loosening, and six for aseptic tibial loosening. The 13-year survival rate was 94%. Radiolucencies of at least 1 mm were seen around 49% of the tibial and 39% of the patellar components. Good and excellent results were noted in 87% of the patients. The authors concluded that their results were comparable with those of the original Total Condylar design and that the functional outcomes were better with the posterior-stabilized prosthesis.

When the posterior-stabilized prosthesis was introduced, there was concern that the constraint inherent in the design might increase stress at the bone–cement interface and thus lead to loosening of the component. With a 94% survival rate at 13 years, there appears to be no evidence to suggest that this design compromises the bone–cement interface and leads to increased loosening. The functional outcome of the patients in this study is excellent; however, other condylar designs have comparable results as well.

Experimental study data suggested that metal backing of the tibial component would more evenly distribute load to the proximal tibia and decrease the prevalence of aseptic loosening. The Total Condylar knee was modified to a metal-backed tibial component in 1979. In 1995, a 10-year follow-up study was performed on 168 knees that had been treated with a PCL-retaining knee that incorporated a metal-backed tibial component. Ten-year survival was 96% with six revisions required; four of them were for a loose patellar component. Mean ROM was 102° of flexion. In the 102 knees that were available for radiographic review, progressive radiolucent lines, defined as lines that had an increase in width of 1 mm or more, were present in four zones of the tibia in 50% of the cases. The authors felt that this prevalence of radiolucent lines adjacent to the tibial component was no different than for other previous cemented studies, regardless of the status of the PCL. The high incidence of progressive radiolucent lines noted in their study is interesting because it suggests potential loosening.

An evaluation of the PCL-retaining Total Condylar prosthesis, comparing metal-backed tibial components to the all-polyethylene type, was reported in 1993. Survivorship at 10 years, using an endpoint of revision, was 96% in both groups. There were no significant differences in the frequency of radiolucent lines; however, 2% of the tibial components in the metal-backed group had complete radiolucent lines compared to none in the all-polyethylene group. Previous studies of shorter duration have noted similar findings. Although this was not a randomized study, these findings question the advantages of metal backing as compared to an all-polyethylene tibial component. In addition, the cost of metal-backed tibial components is, on average, 30% higher than that of their all-polyethylene counterparts. However, in a recent report of the 10-year survival of 1,956 knee arthroplasties that used a flat-on-flat, one-piece compression molded polyethylene metal-backed tibial component, there were six revisions for loosening, which included five tibial components, resulting in a survival rate of 98%. When the metal backing was eliminated from this same design in 492 knee arthroplasties done by the same surgeon, revision was required in 4%, medial plateau collapse occurred in 22%, and there was medial radiolucency in 46%. The surgeon and designer of this component did not recommend the all-polyethylene variation for routine use.

There appears to be no difference clinically in the long-term survivorship series reported for the three variations of the Total Condylar design: PCL-retaining, PCL-sacrificing, and PCL-substituting. The original designers of the Total Condylar prosthesis reported in 1989 on the overall success of 1,430 cemented knee arthroplasties. There were 224 Total Condylar prostheses with an all-polyethylene tibia, 289 of the posterior-stabilized type with an all-polyethylene tibia, and 917 posterior-stabilized with a metal-backed tibial component. There were 12 failures in the Total Condylar series, of which four involved loose tibial components, for a 15-year survival of 91%. There were two loose tibial components and three loose femoral components in the posterior-stabilized group for a 10-year survival of 97%. In the metal-backed tibial component group, there were seven failures; however, none were for aseptic tibial loosening, resulting in a 7-year survival of 98%.

The recent meta-analysis of patient outcomes following TKA divided the nearly 10,000 patients according to the manner in which the cruciate and collateral ligaments were treated: (1) PCL sparing; (2) anterior cruciate ligament (ACL) and PCL sacrificing without PCL substitution; (3) ACL and PCL sacrificing with PCL substitution; and (4) ACL and PCL sacrificing with PCL and collateral ligament substitution. The authors found evidence that the type of prosthesis was correlated with patient outcomes. Even when controlling for publication date, sample size, mean patient age, and percentage of patients with osteoarthritis, studies using PCL-retaining prostheses had slightly higher mean postoperative global rating scale scores and fewer complications. The authors admitted, however, that attributing variation in outcome due to the prosthetic type is problematic among cohort studies and that none of the studies were randomized according to the type of prosthesis used.

There are two patient populations that stimulate controversy in TKA: the obese patient and the young patient (typically younger than 45 to 55 years of age). Over 80% of women and 35% of men with osteoarthrosis of the knee are overweight. The effect of body weight on the results of TKA remains uncertain despite previous sporadic reports on the early failure of TKA in the obese patient. A positive correlation between the patient's weight and the incidence of radiolucencies at the tibial bone–cement interface has been reported. Reports of retrieval studies have also documented increased wear damage in overweight patients. It is reasonable to assume that heavier patients would put higher stresses across the joint, and that these stresses would be borne by the metal, polyethylene, and ultimately the bone–cement interface. Higher stresses would be expected to result in an increased incidence of aseptic loosening and component failures; however, a 1990 report of 257 knees grouped into five weight classes indicated that weight did not appear to play a role in the outcome of knee arthroplasty. There were 100 knees in the mildly obese, 27 knees in the moderately obese, and 16 in the severely obese class. At follow-up (average: 4 years), the overall knee scores and incidence of wound complications did not differ substantially among the various weight groups. There was a positive correlation between weight and patellofemoral symptoms, however, with 30% of the obese group having anterior knee complaints, compared with 14% in the nonobese group. The results in all but four knees were rated excellent or good. There was one revision for a late infection.

In a more recent study of 121 cemented knee arthroplasties, patients were divided into groups according to the overweight percentage by which their actual weight exceeded their ideal weight. Of the 109 patients, 45 were considered > 30% overweight. When the study population was analyzed as a whole by bivariate correlations, no significant correlation was found between the patient weight and the HSS score, with a mean follow-up of 2 years. There was a positive correlation between the total radiolucency score and patient weight; although, when the study population was divided at 80 kg of weight, there was no significant increase in the incidence of radiolucency at the bone–cement interface in patients weighing > 80 kg. The incidence of postoperative incision complications was higher in those patients more than 10% overweight. The authors felt that gender appeared to be a much more influential factor on the outcome of TKA rather than overweight percentage with men tending to have higher HSS scores. Although reports on the detrimental effects of obesity on arthroplasty of the hip have been noted (along with a higher incidence of hip revision and fractures of total hip components, including the polyethylene bearing), it is difficult to extrapolate findings from the hip and apply them to the knee, when both of these reports support the concept of cemented TKA in the obese patient.

The success of TKA has focused on a select group of older patients with osteoarthritis or rheumatoid arthritis. There are few reports on the success of TKA in the younger patient, and many of them deal only with specific disease processes, such as juvenile rheumatoid arthritis or hemophilic arthritis. It is difficult to extrapolate the results of these studies and apply them to younger patients with osteoarthritis or rheumatoid arthritis. One of the longest studies available looked at 90 knees (17 with osteoarthritis and 73 with rheumatoid arthritis) in patients with an average age of 49 years who were treated with a cemented Total Condylar knee arthroplasty. All patients with juvenile rheumatoid arthritis were excluded from the study. Survivorship analysis resulted in a cumulative survivorship rate of 96% at 10 years for the entire group. Partial radiolucencies were seen in 30% of patients. Two implants were found to have complete radiolucencies and were considered loose. Average knee ROM was 98°, with good to excellent results in 95% of the patients. The authors believe their results compare favorably with those of cemented TKA in older patients with osteoarthritis or rheumatoid arthritis. The specific age and activity level were not subdivided in the results of this study. Because there were more rheumatoid arthritis patients, who probably have other joint diseases that could affect activity level, it is difficult to extrapolate these findings to the younger, more active patient with osteoarthritis.

An earlier report of 68 cemented TKAs in patients with an average age of 50 years noted excellent results in 55 knees and a good result in 13 knees with an average follow-up of 6.2 years. The diagnosis was osteoarthritis in 57 knees, posttraumatic arthritis in 10, and osteonecrosis in one. Of the tibial components, 20% had radiolucencies in one zone on the anteroposterior (AP) radiograph; however, no complete or progressive radiolucencies at the bone–cement interface were noted for any component. The authors felt their results were comparable to those obtained in published reports on older age groups, and recommended TKA in younger patients who live a sedentary lifestyle and are not expected to place large demands on their knees. Although the excellent results of these studies are comparable with results for the same prosthesis used in an older age group, the surgeon must still be cautious about recommending TKA for the young patient.

It is not possible to evaluate the intermediate-term results on the multitude of knee designs currently available in this short synopsis. Although some authors originally reported excellent short-term results for many knee replacement designs, catastrophic failure has been noted at longer follow-up. Based on its long-term results, the condylar design presented in this section will be considered the standard until further long-term survivorship studies are available on other designs (Fig. 1).

Cementless Fixation

Fixation by ingrowth requires an appropriate porous ingrowth surface and viable bone, and intimate contact between the two surfaces must be maintained without excessive motion until the ingrowth process has occurred. Intimate contact is achieved through accurate cutting of the bone surface. Achieving this contact with the use of an oscillating saw and tibial resection guide is difficult at best. The use of improved cutting blocks and various cutting

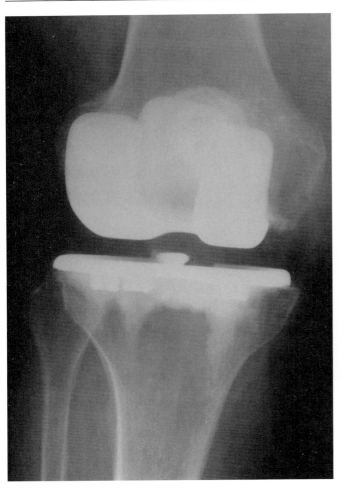
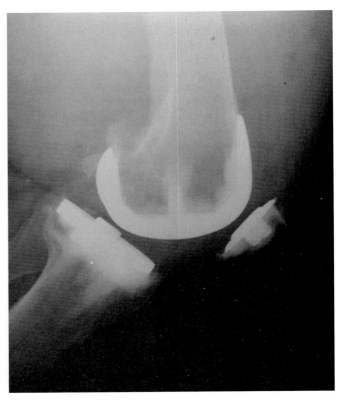

Fig. 1 Anteroposterior (**left**) and lateral (**right**) radiographs of a cemented total knee replacement at 11.5-year follow-up in a 72-year-old female. No evidence of radiolucency is noted at the bone–cement interface. The use of a cementless metal-backed patella is no longer recommended.

guides along with thicker blades has increased the accuracy of the cut; however, the tip of the saw blade continues to oscillate, skiving away from hard bone and diving into soft cancellous bone. The use of a milling attachment or router to obtain a flat surface on the distal femur and proximal tibia holds promise in allowing the surgeon to more accurately machine the bone.

Once appropriate cuts have been made, fixation of the component sufficient to allow for ingrowth appears to be the most problematic area. The femoral component, because of its box-like construction, appears to provide intrinsic resistance to motion with only a tight press fit. Tibial component fixation has been considered more problematic from a design standpoint, with modifications initiated following in vivo and laboratory studies determining the amount of micromotion present at the prosthesis–bone interface. Excessive motion will lead to the ingrowth of

fibrous tissue and fibrocartilage at the interface. Various configurations of pegs, stems, cruciate blades, and screws have all been tested, and screw fixation appears to be the best means of obtaining initial stability of the tibial base plate. A recent study of the effect of pegs and screws on bone ingrowth in canine models suggested that pegs provided no added benefit where sufficient initial fixation was obtained with screws. In vivo radiographic stereophotogrammetry of a current cementless design incorporating four screws for fixation indicated that there was minimal bone–implant micromotion after 6 months, which suggests that the tibial tray was mechanically coupled to the proximal tibia. The modulus of elasticity of the tibial component may also be important in micromotion, with more flexible titanium alloy trays allowing less micromotion in either hard or soft bone than stiffer, chrome cobalt trays.

Ingrowth of bone into the prosthesis following clinical

implantation has been variable. Retrieval studies have been disappointing, with rates of ingrowth between 0 and 10% reported, thus bringing into question the effectiveness of this means of implant fixation. However, clinical studies have shown low rates of revision due to tibial component loosening despite the limited bone ingrowth seen in retrieval specimens. The total amount of bone ingrowth observed in one study was so low that no ingrowth was seen in 52% of examined specimens. Less than 2% of ingrowth was seen in 29% of specimens, 2% to 5% in 12%, and the most extensive ingrowth (5% to 10%) in only 7% of components.

In a more recent retrieval study of one implant type, results were at odds with the above report. In 13 retrieved fiber-metal tibial implants, ingrowth averaged 27% with a maximum extent of 59%. It is of particular interest that most of the retrieved components previously reported with poor ingrowth lacked supplemental screw fixation, whereas the components of this study were initially fixed by screw fixation. The most significant findings of this study were: (1) all of the examined specimens had bone ingrowth; (2) the pattern of bone ingrowth was influenced by the depth and orientation of the tibial resection plane and appeared to be influenced by the presence of the fixation pegs; and (3) particulate debris gained access to the interface from the peripheral aspects of the component and through the screw holes. Attempts to correlate radiographs with retrieval specimens are hampered by the evidence that radiographs obtained without fluoroscopic guidance fail to reveal the vast majority of radiolucent lines below the tibial base plate.

Correct alignment of the limb and ligamentous stability are important to minimize eccentric loading of the component articulating surfaces. Multiple studies in the cemented series of TKAs have demonstrated early failure when limb alignment was incorrect. The same effect is even more evident in a cementless design because failure of ingrowth will jeopardize even the early results of cementless components.

Although the results of retrieval specimens are limited and the amount of actual bone ingrowth is less than originally anticipated, longer-term studies are demonstrating survival rates of over 90%. The question as to how much ingrowth (if any) is actually needed to stabilize the prosthesis has not yet been answered. The amount of constraint in the design, materials, porous surface, and biocompatibility may all play a role in answering this question. Until autopsy specimens become available to examine well-functioning implants, a true reflection of the state of the cementless interface will remain a puzzle.

Cementless Total Knee Arthroplasty Results

Prior to the reports of long-term success of cemented TKA, alternative methods of component fixation were developed with the intent to increase implant longevity. Abundant laboratory evidence supported the concept of cementless ingrowth, and promising short-term studies saturated the literature. The ease of revision in cementless components that wore, loosened, or became infected, as well as preservation of bone stock was thought to be a distinct advantage over current cemented designs. Surgeons desiring the latest in technology implanted thousands of cementless knees, lowering the age requirements for implantation as support for the cementless concept continued. Certainly, it was reasonable to strive for a prosthesis that would last the lifetime of the patient; however, the adoption of this technology has led to some newly created problems. One long-term concern with porous-coated implants is the potential for release of metal and corrosion products because the metallic surface area is larger and also exposed to a larger surface area of vascular tissue. Cobalt chrome and titanium base plates both seem to deliver high concentrations of their respective metals in close proximity to the implant and, occasionally, at distant sites. The immunologic and oncologic consequences of high local metal ion concentration in the soft tissues remain to be determined. The appearance of osteolytic lesions of the proximal tibia and distal femur, which has been associated mainly with cementless knee designs, has not been reported with the use of cemented designs other than as a case report. This destructive process may be asymptomatic until large amounts of bone loss or component failure have occurred.

The use of a cobalt-chrome beaded surface was one of the most popular among the earliest cementless TKA designs. Multiple short-term reports by the designers were impressive, and in some cases the results were superior to results of cemented designs. In one study, this cementless device was used in patients 50 years or younger, a group that should represent the highest stress levels with which to test the stability of the implant. With a 4-year average follow-up, the average knee score was 90 points, with no signs of component failure or loosening other than one tibial base plate placed on an autografted tibial plateau that subsided and required revision. Of the tibial components, 65% had no radiolucencies and the remaining 35% only small, scattered, nonprogressive lucencies. The following year, using this same knee prosthesis, the designer compared the results of 18 matched pairs of TKAs in which cemented prostheses were used on one side and cementless on the other. At 5-year average follow-up, no differences in knee scores, pain scores, or range of motion was noted. However, other investigators have had less success with this prosthesis.

In one study, 110 cemented total knee replacements were compared with 50 cementless knees of the design discussed above. The average age of the cemented group was 70 years and the cementless group 59 years. With a minimum 2-year follow-up, the cemented group averaged nine points higher on the knee score and had a greater range of motion. In another prospective study with near identical demographics, the results of this same cementless design were compared with those of a cemented type. At an average follow-up of 3 years, the knee scores were similar; however, the incidence of radiolucent lines, loose beads, and tibial component subsidence was more frequent in the cementless group. Discrepancies between the reports of prosthesis designers and those of uninterested investigators make extrapolating data for evaluation of a particular knee system extremely difficult.

Few long-term studies of cementless designs are available in the literature, and those that are available usually report the results of a single surgeon's experience with that surgeon's particular design. In a recent follow-up report of 202 patients (265 knees) who underwent an arthroplasty using a cementless tibial and femoral component, no patients were excluded due to age, gender, or bone quality. The average age was 77 years, and 95% of the patients had a diagnosis of osteoarthritis. The undersurface of the metal-backed tibial component was porous coated, but the four pegs and 6-cm round central stem were not. A survival rate of 96% at 10 years was reported with only one case of aseptic loosening of a tibial component. Postoperative knee flexion averaged 115°; however, osteolysis was found in eight knees in the bone adjacent to the posterior flanges of the femoral component and radiographic evidence of osteolysis appeared around the tibial pegs in nine patients. It was believed that these results compared favorably with cemented designs with similar follow-up. Two years after the introduction of this component, the designer modified the undersurface of the tibial tray, adding four screw holes for initial fixation. There were 1,442 of this cementless design implanted, and it was noted that only two knees required revision for aseptic loosening of the tibial component for an overall survival of 98% at 4- to 8-year follow-up.

Unfortunately, the radiographic evaluation of these patients was not included in the studies. These series both benefited from the introduction of intramedullary alignment and had the advantage of only one surgeon with extensive experience in knee arthroplasty. Longer-term follow-up studies will be necessary to determine if the cementless interface with this design remains solid and if these reported rates of osteolysis will increase with time.

The use of meniscal bearings in a TKA system was proposed to reduce polyethylene contact stresses and to decrease wear. Studies supported the concept that this design decreased volumetric wear by one sixth as compared to conventional curved-on-flat fixed bearing knee replacements. This design uses medial and lateral bearings that ride in tracks, allowing axial rotation and controlled AP translation. Cutouts in the tibial base plate are available for retention of both cruciate ligaments or the PCL only, and for an absent PCL, a rotating platform was designed with a central peg that articulates with a flat tibial plate that incorporates a tapered cone to accept the peg. A rotating bearing patellar prosthesis was also developed with the same principles of decreasing contact stresses and reducing polyethylene wear. Fixation is by either cement or press-fit cementless porous ingrowth without supplemental screw fixation. A 7- to 12-year follow-up was reported

in 1994 on 208 of these cementless devices. Overall survival was 95% at 12 years for all variations of the design. There were two bearing failures and no cases of aseptic loosening. Radiolucencies were most abundant beneath the tibial component.

The results of this study compare favorably with those of other studies using the cemented condylar type knee replacement; however, incidents of bearing dislocations and breakage with this device have been reported. In one report of 40 knees implanted with this device, five knees had bearing fracture or dislocation. The authors felt that sacrifice of the ACL increased rotational instability and predisposed the movable bearing to fracture when the implant is posteriorly subluxed and entrapped between the femoral component and the posterior edge of the runner of the tibial component. These complications may be due to technical difficulties with implantation of the device.

A fiber–metal cementless total knee system was introduced in 1984, utilizing a titanium PCL-sparing tibial base plate with four short pegs and four peripheral screws for initial fixation, with a condylar titanium femoral component (Figs. 2 and 3). In a prospective study of 108 TKAs, with patient selection based on age, bone stock, and ability to maintain limited weightbearing during the first 6 weeks after surgery, the average age was 59 years. At 5- to 10-year follow-up, there were eight failures: one aseptic tibial loosening, one fractured tibial base plate, one hematogenous sepsis, and five failed metal-backed patellar components that required removal of all components. However, 20 patients had failure of a metal-backed patella that required patella component revision only. Radiolucencies of less than 2 mm and only in one zone were seen in 40% of the tibial components and 9% of the femoral components. Osteolytic lesions were noted in seven (8%) knees, and most measured less than 3 mm. Survivorship analysis of the tibial and femoral components was 90% at 120 months. Although the revision rate was high in this series, most revisions were for designs that are now known to be faulty.

The use of a cementless metal-backed patella with pegs and a thin polyethylene gliding surface has been shown to result in shear stresses that may cause peg failure, polyethylene delamination, and excessive polyethylene wear. This patellar component has been abandoned since identification of this failure mechanism, and all-polyethylene patellar components are now standard. Of concern in several cementless TKA series is the incidence of osteolysis. Although this report represents a younger age group, osteolysis was not seen in the cemented series of otherwise identical prostheses at similar follow-up. This time-dependent finding is of concern.

Using the same fiber–metal prosthesis, a nonrandomized comparison was made between 209 knees inserted with cement and 183 knees inserted without cement. The femoral component was not cemented in either group. The 2- to 5-year follow-up showed no differences in the knee scores, range of motion, radiographs, or complication

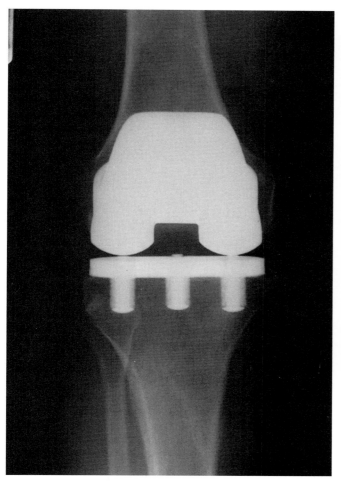

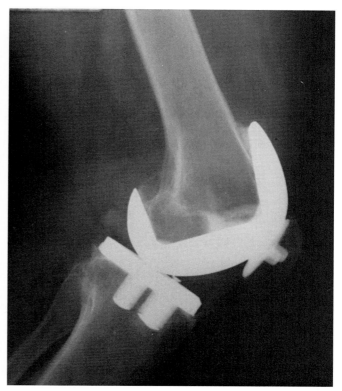

Fig. 2 A first generation fiber-metal cementless knee design with a one piece composite tibial component. There is no evidence of radiolucencies at 12-year follow-up despite the use of carbon-fiber reinforced polyethylene and a metal-backed cementless patellar component.

rates. There was, however, an unacceptably high rate of complications due to problems related to the patellofemoral joint and the use of a metal-backed patellar component. There were no reports of osteolysis. The authors were encouraged by the results obtained with cementless fixation.

Osteolysis

Osteolysis was first seen in hip arthroplasty and described by Charnley in 1975. Four cases were described in 1976, and the authors believed that this represented "cement disease" due to fragmentation of the cement used in hip arthroplasty. Refinements in microdiagnostic techniques have identified the small fragments as particles of ultra-high molecular weight polyethylene (UHMWPE); therefore, the term cement disease has been replaced with

"particle disease." Particles of UHMWPE and cement (polymethylmethacrylate) along with metal debris and corrosion products have all been identified in the membranes and synovia of joints with osteolysis as well as in the membranes of nonosteolytic loose arthroplasty membranes.

Histologic and immunohistologic studies of the membrane surrounding loose hip and knee replacements have revealed findings similar to those seen in cases of focal osteolysis. In a recent evaluation of 34 loose TKAs, although only four of these implants were associated with focal osteolysis, all of the specimens examined had periprosthetic histology similar to that of the osteolytic regions. It was believed that the two conditions (aseptic loosening and osteolysis) may represent variations of a similar process.

Although several isolated cases of extensive osteolysis after TKA have been described since 1975, the largest se-

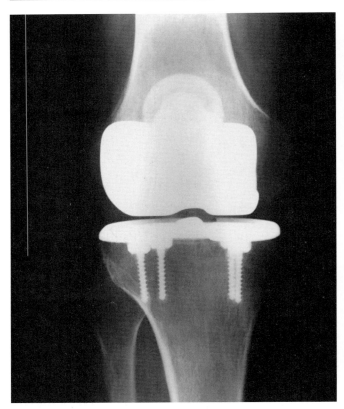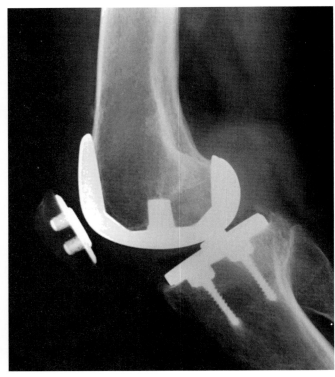

Fig. 3 Thirteen-year follow-up radiographs of a cementless fiber metal knee design in a 40-year-old patient with rheumatoid arthritis. Note the lack of radiolucencies at the bone–prosthesis interface.

ries was reported in 1992. The authors noted a 16% incidence of osteolysis following 174 consecutive cementless TKAs. The findings were identified an average of 35 months following arthroplasty, and all lesions were progressive. The most common site of the osteolytic lesion was the proximal medial tibia (89% of cases), with involvement of the lateral tibia and distal femur less common. The implants used a high central tibial eminence and a metallic locking pin for the tibial polyethylene component, which could impinge on the femoral component with the knee extended. Minimal tibial resection was performed, and the polyethylene averaged 5.8 mm in thickness. In all patients, extensive particulate polyethylene debris that had originated from excessive wear of both the articular surface of the polyethylene tibial component and the prominent central tibial eminence contributed to the osteolytic process.

Histologic evaluation of tissue obtained at the revision procedures revealed sheets of histiocytes and occasional giant cells with intracellular particulate polyethylene and metal products. Corrosion between the titanium screws and cobalt chrome base plate also contributed particulate metal to the osteolytic process. The authors concluded

that the design of the implant, polyethylene thickness, conformity of the articular surfaces, and modularity all influenced the generation of wear debris and the osteolytic process. The fact that the majority of patients had lesions confined to the medial tibial plateau was thought to be influenced by several factors: (1) gravity and weightbearing through the medial side of the knee; (2) screws in the tibial base plate acting as conduits for transportation of debris; and (3) potential osteolysis on the femoral side obscured radiographically by the configuration of the femoral component.

In a follow-up study of the same group of patients, an 11% incidence of femoral osteolysis was noted. Average time to diagnosis was 31 months (range: 7 to 96 months). Wear of the thin tibial inserts and patellar components were the two sources of particulate debris, with corrosion attributed to the acutely angled screws used for tibial base plate fixation. The gross and microscopic appearance of the osteolytic lesions identified was similar to previously described foreign body responses in total hip and knee arthroplasties. It is reasonable to postulate that the polyethylene and metallic debris caused an infiltrative histiocytic response, which gained access to the distal femoral

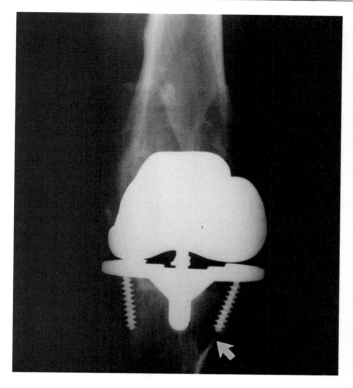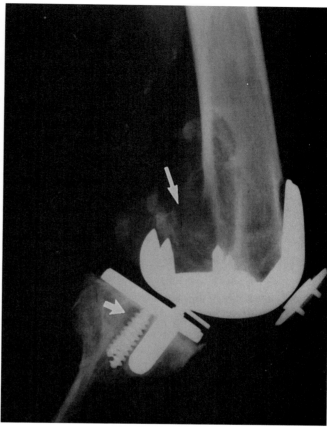

Fig. 4 Massive osteolysis of the distal femur (arrow) mostly seen in the posterior condyles in a cementless knee system that has been known to generate large amounts of metal and polyethylene debris secondary to its inherent design characteristics. In addition, areas of focal lysis surround the lateral screw in the tibial plateau (arrow).

metaphysis primarily via the interface between bone and the nonporous-coated areas of the femoral component (Fig. 4).

There are also two reports to date of pseudotumorous soft-tissue lesions associated with osteolysis following total joint arthroplasty. One lesion reported was seen following the use of the cementless knee replacement system described above with a high incidence of osteolysis. Radiographs revealed a failed metal-backed patellar component with evidence of free metallic debris in the soft tissues posteriorly. There was also osteolysis adjacent to the fixation screws in the proximal part of the tibia. The patient presented with a nontender mass measuring 8 × 12 cm at the posteromedial corner of the knee along with an ipsilateral nontender inguinal lymph node measuring 4 × 5 cm. Histologic analysis of the inguinal lymph node, knee mass, and the periprosthetic tissues revealed particles of metal, polyethylene, titanium, and corrosion products. The lymph node had focal areas of foreign-body reaction with the largest component resembling a sarcoid type reaction.

The authors recommended expeditious revision in patients in whom there is evidence of a fracture of the component, polyethylene delamination from a metal backing, considerable wear debris, or all of these conditions, even in the face of only mild symptoms.

The other incidence of a pseudotumor associated with a total joint prosthesis was reported in 1988 following a cementless TKA. An aggressive pseudotumor associated with corrosion products of a modular cobalt-alloy prosthesis was found. Other reports in the literature describe aggressive granulomatosis from polyethylene debris after failure of an uncemented TKA. In these cases, the bone around the prosthesis was replaced with caseous material consisting of necrotic tissue and a foreign-body type giant-cell reaction around polyethylene debris, typical of osteolysis.

Just as osteolysis has become a major concern in total hip replacement, it is now apparent that this same wear mechanism is responsible for the lesions seen in the knee. In comparing the particles seen in both the hip and knee,

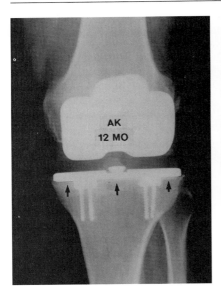 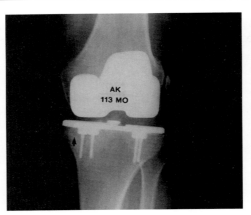 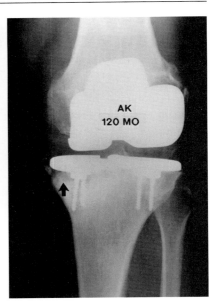

Fig. 5 **Left,** A 12-month radiograph of a cementless tibial component with a complete radiolucency at the bone-prosthesis interface. **Center,** The same patient asymptomatic at 113 months, with development of focal osteolysis surrounding the peg of the tibial plate. **Right,** At 120 months, the patient presented with pain and instability of the knee. Progression of the osteolytic lesion has caused collapse of the medial tibial plateau (arrow) and fracture of the tibial base plate.

it becomes apparent they are generated as a function of the wear mechanism. Where the hip has a highly conforming contact area, the contact stresses are low, resulting in very high numbers of very small, submicron, wear particles. Due to the low conformity of most total knee systems, the contact stresses are high. Therefore, fatigue mechanisms play a greater role in the generation of wear particles in TKAs, resulting in rather large particles as compared to the hip. These particles are small enough, however, to access the implant–bone interfaces through soft-tissue tracks and migrate down available screw holes to access the proximal tibia. It is now thought that cement forms a temporary protective gasket to prevent migration of these particles; however, a case of osteolysis associated with a cemented TKA was recently reported. The knee had been implanted 9 years before symptoms developed and the patient presented with a 3-cm fluctuant mass over the anterior tibial plateau. At surgery, the components were well fixed. The metal-backed nonmodular tibial component had a carbon-reinforced polyethylene articulation. Histology revealed birefringent particles and carbon fragments consistent with wear debris. Whether prostheses are cemented or cementless, the generation of polyethylene particle debris remains a significant factor in the osteolytic process.

Strategies designed to address the problem of osteolysis must incorporate methods to decrease the particulate burden. Techniques in the polyethylene manufacturing process are constantly being upgraded. However, while the mechanical properties of this modified polyethylene ap-

pear to be improved in many respects, initial reports suggest that wear performance does not appear to be improved. Alternate articulations with ceramic and metal-on-metal have also been entertained. Superpolishing the femoral components to decrease abrasiveness, along with design improvements in modularity, with tighter tolerances to decrease micromotion between the base plate and polyethylene insert, are examples of modifications being addressed by manufacturers. The use of tibial polyethylene inserts with a minimum thickness of 8 mm decreases the stresses within polyethylene and may lower the generation of polyethylene particulates. The elimination of modularity of the tibial component with the use of one-piece designs may again become popular. Factory-pressed polyethylene inserts on metal-backed base plates would also decrease the amount of micromotion seen at this interface. In some respects, it appears the modular cementless designs of the 1980s were one step forward and two steps back. As the immunologic and inflammatory components of the osteolytic process are better defined, the development of pharmacologic agents to modify these responses may allow the prevention and treatment of osteolysis before surgical intervention becomes necessary.

Because the majority of patients with osteolysis around the knee are asymptomatic, yearly radiographs are necessary to document the early development of osteolytic lesions (Fig. 5). Once thinning of the polyethylene of the metal-backed tibial or patellar components is noted radiographically, replacement should be performed prior to catastrophic polyethylene failure and metal-on-metal contact.

In the event lysis is seen, aggressive surgical intervention may be necessary to prevent further destruction and loss of bone. Decreasing the particulate burden by a complete synovectomy and removal of all diseased soft tissue is necessary to prevent early return of the lesion. There are reports of normal bony architecture returning after removal of synovium and particulate debris without revision of the implants. Implant designs that are known to generate large amount of particle debris, however, should be revised despite their stability. A recent report on the surgical technique recommended for revision of cementless knees with massive osteolytic defects discusses various options for

treatment. Allografts, metal build-up blocks, long stems, and cement all may be necessary to fill the defects, and the use of a constrained component may be required for stability.

Osteolysis is not simply particle disease. It is a highly complex process that is multifactorial and not fully understood. Unfortunately, osteolysis may become the leading cause of failure in joint replacement surgery until efforts are effective in addressing the debris generated by an artificial wear couple. Therefore, reports on increasing rates of osteolysis may continue to crowd the literature well into the next century.

Annotated Bibliography

Cemented Total Knee Arthroplasty Results

Faris PM, Ritter MA, Meding JB, et al: Minimum two-year clinical evaluation and finite element evaluation of a flat all-polyethylene tibial component. *Proceedings of the American Academy of Orthopaedic Surgeons 62nd Annual Meeting, Orlando, FL.* Rosemont, IL, AAOS, 1995, p 221.

The authors report 2-year follow-up of 492 knee arthroplasties using a flat all-polyethylene tibial component having identical geometry to the successful metal-backed version. Revision occurred in 4.3%, medial plateau collapse in 22.4%, and medial radiolucency without definite loosening in 46%. This all-polyethylene variation was not recommended for routine use.

Malkani AL, Rand JA, Bryan RS, et al: Total knee arthroplasty with the kinematic condylar prosthesis. *J Bone Joint Surg* 1995;77A:423–431.

This is the report of a 10-year follow-up study using a condylar-type prosthesis with a metal-backed cruciate-retaining tibial component. Survival of the prosthesis was 96%. Two knees were revised for aseptic loosening of the tibial and femoral components. The knee scores, survival rate, and range of motion were similar to those in studies with PCL-sacrificing and PCL-substituting designs.

Ranawat CS, Padgett DE, Ohashi Y: Total knee arthroplasty for patients younger than 55 years. *Clin Orthop* 1989;248:27–30.

The authors report a study of 93 TKAs in 62 patients less than 55 years old. The majority of patients had rheumatoid arthritis compared to osteoarthritis (73 versus 17). Survivorship at 10 years was 96%, with a 30% radiolucency rate. Results were comparable to the long-term result of TKA in the older patient.

Ranawat CS, Flynn WF Jr, Deshmukh RG: Impact of modern technique on long-term results of total condylar knee arthroplasty. *Clin Orthop* 1994;309:131–135.

This is the report of a 14-year follow-up study of implant survivorship using the Total Condylar design prosthesis and modern cementing techniques. Improved instrumentation, multiple component sizes, and soft-tissue balancing were other

modifications to the original technique. There were no revisions for aseptic loosening and a 96% survival at 14 years.

Ranawat CS, Flynn WF Jr, Saddler S, et al: Long-term results of the total condylar knee arthroplasty: A 15-year survivorship study. *Clin Orthop* 1993;286:94–102.

This paper reports the 15-year survivorship of the original Total Condylar Knee. There were three revisions for loose tibial components for a 94% survival. A decreased range of motion (90° to 100°) and lack of modularity are the main disadvantages to this design.

Rand JA: Comparison of metal-backed and all-polyethylene tibial components in cruciate condylar total knee arthroplasty. *J Arthroplasty* 1993;8:307–313.

This is a 10-year survivorship comparison of a cruciate retaining condylar design, which uses either an all-polyethylene tibial component or a metal-backed type. Survivorship at 10 years was 96% in both groups. There were no significant differences in the frequency of radiolucent lines or functional outcome between the groups.

Ritter MA, Herbst SA, Keating EM, et al: Long-term survival analysis of a posterior cruciate-retaining total condylar total knee arthroplasty. *Clin Orthop* 1994;309:136–145.

This study presents the results of a 10 to 18-year survival analysis of the PCL-retaining condylar total knee replacement. Survival at 12 years was 97%. There were seven mechanical failures, three of which were due to aseptic loosening of the tibial component.

Ritter MA, Siliski J, Worland R, et al: Flat on flat, non-constrained, compression molded polyethylene total knee replacement: Ten year survival analysis. Proceedings of the Knee Society Scientific Meeting, Orlando, FL, 1995.

Ten-year survival of 1,956 arthroplasties with a one-piece compression molded metal-backed tibial component is reported. There were six femoral, eight tibial, and 28 patellar components (all metal backed) that demonstrated complete radiolucencies at the bone–cement interface; however, none were progressive or clinically loose. There were six revisions for aseptic loosening for survival at 10 years of 98%.

Scuderi GR, Insall JN, Windsor RE, et al: Survivorship of cemented knee replacements. *J Bone Joint Surg* 1989;71B: 798–803.

The authors report a survivorship study of 1,430 cemented knee replacements, in which the Total Condylar prosthesis and posterior stabilized type, both with an all-polyethylene tibia and with a metal-backed tibial component, are compared. The success of the Total Condylar series was 91% at 15 years, the posterior stabilized with an all-polyethylene tibia was 97% at 10 years, and the posterior stabilized with a metal-backed tibia 98% at 7 years.

Smith BE, Askew MJ, Gradisar IA Jr, et al: The effect of patient weight on the functional outcome of total knee arthroplasty. *Clin Orthop* 1992;276:237–244.

This is a 2-year follow-up on 109 patients divided into groups according to percentage above ideal body weight. No significant correlation was found between the patient's weight and the HSS score. The total radiolucency score was positively correlated with weight; however, radiolucency scores between overweight percentage groups was not significant. Gender appeared to be a much more influential factor on the outcome of TKA than weight.

Stern SH, Bowen MK, Insall JN, et al: Cemented total knee arthroplasty for gonarthrosis in patients 55 years old or younger. *Clin Orthop* 1990;260:124–129.

With an average follow-up of 6.2 years, the results of 68 cemented TKAs demonstrated no complete or progressive radiolucencies at the bone–cement interface of any component. Of tibial components, 20% had radiolucencies in at least one zone and femoral lucencies were seen in 2% of knees. These results compare favorably to those obtained in published reports on older age groups.

Stern SH, Insall JN: Posterior stabilized prosthesis: Results after follow-up of nine to twelve years. *J Bone Joint Surg* 1992;74A:980–986.

This study used an all-polyethylene posterior stabilized implant in 289 arthroplasties. There were 14 failures, of which six had aseptic loosening of the tibial component. Survival was 94% at 13 years.

Stern SH, Insall JN: Total knee arthroplasty in obese patients. *J Bone Joint Surg* 1990;72A:1400–1404.

Two hundred fifty-seven TKAs were placed into five weight groups based on their ideal body weight. The results in all but four knees were rated excellent or good. The was no discernible difference in the overall scores among the five groups. However, 30% of the knees of the moderately and severely obese patients had patellofemoral symptoms, compared to 14% in the nonobese group.

Cementless Total Knee Arthroplasty Results

Buechel FF: Cementless meniscal bearing knee arthroplasty: 7-to 12-year outcome analysis. *Orthopedics* 1994;17:833–836.

A follow-up study of 208 cementless meniscal bearing knee prosthesis demonstrates an overall survivorship of 95% at 12 years. The study series included bicruciate-retaining, PCL-retaining, unicompartmental, and rotating platform designs.

There were two meniscal bearing fractures and 13 knees were revised. The reason for revisions was not mentioned.

Collins DN, Heim SA, Nelson CL, et al: Porous-coated anatomic total knee arthroplasty: A prospective analysis comparing cemented and cementless fixation. *Clin Orthop* 1991;267:128–136.

This is a prospective study comparing cemented and cementless fixation in 51 knee arthroplasties. With an average 3-year follow-up, the incidence of radiolucent lines, loose beads, and tibial component subsidence was more frequent in the cementless group.

Dodd CA, Hungerford DS, Krackow KA: Total knee arthroplasty fixation: Comparison of the early results of paired cemented versus uncemented porous coated anatomic knee prostheses. *Clin Orthop* 1990;260:66–70.

The results are presented of 18 matched pairs of knee prostheses, in which one side was a cemented and the other cementless. At 5-year follow-up no differences in range of motion, knee score, or pain score were noted.

Hungerford DS, Krackow KA, Kenna RV: Cementless total knee replacement in patients 50 years old and under. *Orthop Clin North Am* 1989;20:131–145.

With a follow-up of over 4 years, the 52 cementless knee arthroplasties performed on patients less than 50 years old demonstrated excellent short-term results. The average age was actually less than 40, and the average knee score at follow-up was 90, with no signs of tibial component loosening or failure other than one tibial base plate subsidence.

Moran CG, Pinder IM, Lees TA, et al: Survivorship analysis of the uncemented porous-coated anatomic knee replacement. *J Bone Joint Surg* 1991;73A:848–857.

With an average follow-up of 64 months (range: 39 to 93 months), 19% of the 108 uncemented porous-coated anatomic knee replacements had failed. All failures were due to aseptic loosening of the tibial implant, with collapse of the anteromedial aspect of the tibial plateau the most common mechanism of failure.

Rorabeck CH, Bourne RB, Lewis PL, et al: The Miller-Galante knee prosthesis for the treatment of osteoarthrosis: A comparison of the results of partial fixation with cement and fixation without any cement. *J Bone Joint Surg* 1993;75A:402–408.

A prospective nonrandomized study of 392 total knee replacements with a PCL-retaining condylar design knee prosthesis is reported. A comparison was made between prostheses inserted with cement (209 knees) and those without cement (183 knees). The femoral component was not cemented in either group. Analysis of the knee scores, range of motion, radiographs, and rates of complications revealed no differences between the outcomes in the two groups at 2- to 5-year follow-up.

Rorabeck CH, Bourne RB, Nott L: The cemented kinematic-II and the non-cemented porous-coated anatomic prosthesis for total knee replacement: A prospective evaluation. *J Bone Joint Surg* 1988;70A: 483–490.

A prospective evaluation of 160 knee arthroplasties of which 110 were cemented and 50 cementless is reported. With a minimum follow-up of 2 years, the cemented group had higher knee scores and a greater range of knee motion.

Rosenberg AG, Barden RM, Galante, JO: Cemented and ingrowth fixation of the Miller-Galante prosthesis: Clinical and roentgenographic comparison after three- to six-year follow-up. *Clin Orthop* 1990;260:71–79.

The authors report a clinical and radiographic comparison of 116 cemented knees and 123 cementless knees after 3- to 6-year follow-up. No cemented failure was due to fixation, and three cementless failures were due to lack of tibial ingrowth. Range of motion, knee scores, and pain scores were similar between both groups. Cementless tibial radiolucencies were partial in up to 20% of examined zones.

Whiteside LA: Cementless total knee replacement: Nine- to 11-year results and 10-year survivorship analysis. *Clin Orthop* 1994;309:185–192.

A study of 265 cementless TKAs was performed on 202 patients regardless of bone quality, age, gender, or diagnosis. The average age was 77 years old with 95% having a diagnosis of osteoarthritis. Considering loosening and infection, survival rate was 97% at 10 years.

Osteolysis

Cadambi A, Engh GA, Dwyer KA, et al: Osteolysis of the distal femur after total knee arthroplasty. *J Arthroplasty* 1994;9:579–594.

An 11% incidence of femoral osteolysis was identified in a series of 271 primary cementless TKAs. Wear of thin tibial inserts and patellar components were the two sources of polyethylene wear. The authors postulate that the polyethylene and metallic debris gained access to the distal femur via the interface between bone and the nonporous-coated areas of the femoral component.

Chiba J, Schwedeman LJ, Booth RE Jr, et al: A biomechanical, histologic, and immunohistologic analysis of membranes obtained from failed cemented and cementless total knee arthroplasty. *Clin Orthop* 1994;299:114–124.

This is a complex histologic and immunohistologic evaluation of 34 loose total knee implants. Only four of these were associated with focal osteolysis of the proximal tibia; however, all specimens revealed periprosthetic membrane histology similar to that seen with osteolysis.

Dannenmaier WC, Haynes DW, Nelson CL: Granulomatous reaction and cystic bony destruction associated with high wear rate in a total knee prosthesis. *Clin Orthop* 1985;198:224–230.

The authors report an isolated case of focal osseous resorption, granulomatous reaction, and subsequent component loosening following failure of a carbon-polyethylene tibial component.

Jacobs JJ, Urban RM, Wall J, et al: Unusual foreign-body reaction to a failed total knee replacement: Simulation of a sarcoma clinically and a sarcoid histologically. A case report. *J Bone Joint Surg* 1995;77A:444–451.

This is a case report of soft-tissue pseudotumor in a knee that had had a failed cemented TKA. The histopathologic characteristics of the lesion were nearly indistinguishable from those of sarcoid.

Lewonowski K, Dorr LD: Revision of cementless total knee arthroplasty with massive osteolytic lesions. *J Arthroplasty* 1994;9:661–663.

Recommended surgical techniques in managing the patient with large defects include the use of allograft chips or hydroxyapatite granules to fill lytic cavities and the use of a stem at least 70 mm long if the defect involves >50% of the tibial or femoral condyles.

Nolan JF, Bucknill TM: Aggressive granulomatosis from polyethylene failure in an uncemented knee replacement. *J Bone Joint Surg* 1992;74B:23–24.

Fragmentation of the polyethylene components of an uncemented TKA caused extensive bone lysis though the components remained securely fixed to bone.

Peters PC Jr, Engh GA, Dweyer KA, et al: Osteolysis after total knee arthroplasty without cement. *J Bone Joint Surg* 1992;74A:864–876.

The prevalence and characteristics of osteolysis were studied after 174 consecutive cementless TKAs. Sixteen percent (27 knees) of the implants were associated with osteolysis at an average of 35 months after the operation. Mechanical failure of the thin, modular, polyethylene tibial insert; excessive abrasion of the prominent polyethylene tibial eminence, with secondary wear and impingement of the pin on the femoral component; and failure of the metal-backed patellar component all contributed to the extensive amount of polyethylene and the variable amount of metal debris that was generated.

Ries MD, Guiney W Jr, Lynch F: Osteolysis associated with cemented total knee arthroplasty: A case report. *J Arthroplasty* 1994;9:555–558.

Osteolysis was observed in a 75-year-old female presenting 9 years following the index operation. The osteolytic area returned to normal after synovectomy and debridement of the lesion without revision of the well-fixed components.

Svensson O, Mathiesen EB, Reinholt FP, et al: Formation of a fulminant soft-tissue pseudotumor after uncemented hip arthroplasty: A case report. *J Bone Joint Surg* 1988;70A:1238–1242.

The authors report an aggressive pseudotumor associated with corrosion products of a modular cobalt-alloy uncemented hip prosthesis.

Cementless Fixation

Cook SD, Barrack RL, Thomas KA, et al: Quantitative histologic analysis of tissue growth into porous total knee components. *J Arthroscopy* 1989;4(suppl):S33–S43.

Histologic and radiographic analysis was performed on uncemented knee components retrieved from patients for reasons other than loosening. Average time in situ was 12 months. Fifty-two percent showed no evidence of bone ingrowth, 29% showed minimal (< 2%), 12% moderate (2% to 5%), and 7% showed extensive (5% to 10%) bone ingrowth. In no case was bone present in more than 10% of the pore volume of the implant.

Sumner DR, Turner TM, Dawson D, et al: Effect of pegs and screws on bone ingrowth in cementless total knee arthroplasty. *Clin Orthop* 1994;309:150–155.

Three cementless designs were implanted in animals: (1) four-peg with cortical screws passing through the pegs; (2) four-peg without screws; and (3) pegless with four screws. At 6 months the pegless components had the highest extent of bone ingrowth into the tray (90%) followed by the four-peg design (83%) and finally the four-peg with screws (76%). This study indicates that pegs provided no added benefit when sufficient initial fixation was obtained with screws in an animal model.

Sumner DR, Kienapfel H, Jacobs JJ, et al: Bone ingrowth and wear debris in well-fixed cementless porous-coated tibial components removed from patients. *J Arthroplasty* 1995;10:157–167.

This is a study of the bone ingrowth and the distribution of wear debris within the porous coating of 13 primary cementless porous-coated tibial components removed for reasons unrelated to fixation or infection. Average bone ingrowth was 27% and volume fraction 9%. There was significantly more fixation around the fixation pegs. Particulate debris appeared to gain access to the interface via soft-tissue pathways at the periphery and the screw holes.

Other

Callahan CM, Drake BG, Heck DA, et al: Patient outcomes following tricompartmental total knee replacement: A meta-analysis. *JAMA* 1994;271:1349–1357.

This is a statistical outcome study looking at almost 10,000 patients in 130 reports in the literature. With a mean follow-up of 4 years, almost 90% good or excellent results were noted. Patients with a PCL-sparing prosthesis reported higher global rating knee scores and fewer complications. Overall revision rate was 3.8% at 4 years.

39

Evaluation of the Failed Total Knee Arthroplasty

Introduction

Most patients who have total knee arthroplasty enjoy a very gratifying result. An occasional patient will have postsurgical problems that need evaluation. Some of these problems are severe enough that the knee replacement is defined as a failure. It is imperative that a specific diagnosis and plan for treatment be formulated before any surgical treatment is undertaken for a failed total knee replacement. The two factors most often associated with total knee failure are pain and limitation of function.

Evaluation of Total Knee Arthroplasty

History

An accurate history of the problem is imperative in the evaluation of patients with complaints after total knee replacement. All previous problems with the knee should be documented; these include antecedent operations, the date of the total knee replacement, any problems with surgery, the rate of the recovery and rehabilitation process, underlying diabetes mellitus or neurovascular disease, and/or the presence of a chronic sepsis source. The type of pain, its location, and its aggravating and relieving factors should be carefully elicited and noted. Any radiation of the pain should be accurately defined. The cause of activity-related pain will be potentially much different from that of pain that is present at rest or at night but that does not necessarily increase with activity.

A patient's function also should be assessed. Use of ambulatory assistance devices, such as crutches, cane, or walker, should be noted. Maximum distance or time walked should be recorded. The patient's ability to ascend and descend stairs and the leg used to go up or down first should be noted, as well as the patient's ability to arise from a chair and any instability during walking on flat or uneven ground.

The patient's expectations as they relate to the knee replacement should be discussed. The patient's problems before surgery and the expected result should be compared. The patient's employment history should be considered and any underlying psychiatric disease or treatment with anti-depressants or other neuropsychiatric medication should be noted.

Physical Examination

The patient should undergo a thorough physical examination, one that is not limited to the knee. Because knee pain can be associated with back, retroperitoneal, or hip problems, examination of the spine, abdomen, and hip is also necessary. Neurovascular status of the extremity should be carefully observed, and any erythema, warmth, or healing problems with the incision recorded. It is also important to note skin quality and hair distribution near the incision.

Complete examination of the extensor mechanism is imperative. Knee range of motion is documented, as is any crepitance or grinding associated with motion. The competence of the extensor mechanism is determined by noting the strength of extension. Patellar tracking is checked to find any subluxation or dislocation, and any patellar clunking is recorded. A quadriceps lag or any fixed flexion deformity will be seen during evaluation of active and passive range of motion.

Ligaments should be examined to determine knee stability. A total knee replacement should be approximately as stable as a normal knee, except for some anterior cruciate insufficiency. Ligament competence is evaluated in full extension and 30° and 90° of flexion. Varus and valgus stress and anterior-posterior excursion with stress are the important variables. It is important to note both the degree of laxity and if there is an end point during the stressing process.

Alignment is also crucially important. Varus-valgus alignment and any rotational deformity should be recorded. The alignment of the foot is also observed. Significant hindfoot or forefoot deformities can cause unusual stress at the knee. Full examination of the hip includes documentation of range of motion, limb length, and the presence of any fixed deformity. Examination of the back and abdomen is important to rule out the possibility of referred pain from these sources.

Radiography

Radiographic evaluation of an unsuccessful knee replacement is required. Routine anteroposterior (AP), lateral, and sunrise radiographs of all patients should be obtained to show the type of implants used and the component position relative to the femur, tibia, and patella. To avoid positioning error, radiographs should be taken tangential to the joint. The joint line position should also be assessed accurately. This position frequently can be compared radiographically to that of the opposite unoperated knee. Proximal joint line migration of more than 8 mm has been shown to increase patellofemoral problems. Occasionally, rotational malposition of components can be seen on routine radiographs. Radiographs also are very useful to show wear of polyethylene components. The presence of metal on metal at the tibiofemoral or patellofemoral joint implies extensive wear of polyethylene at those areas. Broken implants can be diagnosed radiographically, and any bone loss due to osteolysis or component subsidence should be noted.

Prosthetic loosening is best diagnosed on radiographs. Loosening is confirmed by comparison with previously obtained radiographs. If component position has changed or radiolucent lines have progressed, loosening is confirmed. With metal-backed tibial components and with cementless fixation, it is occasionally difficult to determine prosthetic loosening. Standard radiographs fail to reveal a 1-mm radiolucent line adjacent to an all polyethylene tibial component if there is (1) more than 5° flexion or rotation of the prosthesis, (2) more than 6° angulation of the x-ray beam, or (3) more than 2.5 cm offsetting of the beam. More than 4° of flexion obscures a radiolucent line adjacent to a metal-backed component. Incomplete radiolucent lines of 1 mm or less do not correlate with clinical results, but complete radiolucent lines of 2 mm or more correlate with poor clinical results. These radiolucent lines usually correlate with malalignment of the limb or implant. A shift of implant position on sequential radiographs is indicative of loosening. To obtain an accurate assessment of implant fixation, fluoroscopically positioned AP and lateral radiographs are frequently necessary. These radiographs allow accurate determination of the presence or absence of radiolucent lines adjacent to the implant.

Patellar function or malfunction can be determined by radiographic evaluation. A lateral radiograph shows the position of the joint line, and it shows whether or not patella alta or baha is present. The thickness of the patella should be evaluated. Sunrise radiographs provide information on tracking. Occasionally it is necessary to obtain radiographs at 15°, 30°, 45°, and 60° of flexion.

Ligament stability can be documented radiographically. Stress radiographs of varus, valgus, anterior, or posterior stress can be used to quantitate the amount of instability present.

Radionuclide studies have been used in evaluation of total knee replacements. In asymptomatic knees, increased activity on diphosphonate scanning can be expected for at least 1 year after surgery. After 1 year, increased activity is present in 89% of tibial and 63% of femoral components in asymptomatic knees. Therefore, bone scans must be interpreted very carefully in conjunction with the clinical examination and routine radiographs. If the patient has a painful knee replacement and a diphosphonate scan with normal uptake, the likelihood of loosening or infection is low. The converse (pain with increased uptake) does not necessarily indicate infection or loosening. Indium 111 labeled leukocyte scanning can be helpful in assessing the possibility of infection. Computed tomography (CT) scanning usually is not helpful but occasionally can be used to quantitate the size of juxta-articular bone defects. Arthrograms are rarely indicated.

Other Studies

The examination of areas that can cause potential radiation of pain to the knee might include magnetic resonance imaging (MRI) or CT of the low back or lower abdomen to rule out the presence of a retroperitoneal process involving the lumbosacral nerves. Noninvasive vascular studies may also provide an important indication of occlusive vascular disease.

If infection is suspected, blood tests, including a complete blood count, erythrocyte sedimentation rate, and determination of C-reactive protein level, are useful. Aspiration is the single most important means of determining whether infection is present. Every total knee replacement with significant unexplained postoperative pain should be aspirated. Characteristically, in an infected knee, there would be more than 25,000 white blood cells (predominantly polymorphonuclear leukocytes) per mm³. However, because the white cell count is less important than the culture, joint aspiration should be performed with sterile technique, and aerobic, anaerobic, and fungal cultures should be obtained. If the first aspiration is negative and suspicion for infection is high, repeat aspirations should be performed.

Causes of Pain

Mechanical

Pain caused by mechanical failure of a knee replacement is characterized by activity-related pain located in the knee. This pain is aggravated by increased activity and relieved with rest. Physical examination is commonly unremarkable, although a small effusion may be present. Loss of fixation is the most common type of mechanical failure. Loosening caused by malalignment, prosthetic wear, or instability should be recognized so that these factors can be addressed at the time of revision. Aseptic mechanical loosening should be differentiated from septic loosening; use aspiration, if any question exists. Radiolucent lines greater than 2 mm (particularly if they are complete), migration of the implants, or change in alignment of the extremity with subsidence of an implant are diagnostic of loosening. Aseptic loosening of cementless implants can be associated with shedding of porous-coated beads.

Patellar problems are another common mechanical cause of failure in knee replacement. Traumatic or atraumatic patellar fractures and avascular necrosis of the patella are best diagnosed radiographically. In subluxation or dislocation of the patella, the patient may give a history of instability associated with snapping or clicking in the front part of the knee. Physical examination often shows the patella to subluxate either medially or laterally during flexion and extension of the knee. Lateral subluxation is much more common than medial. Patellar delamination secondary to polyethylene wear on a metal-backed patellar prosthesis leads to a significant knee effusion and, if the polyethylene is worn through completely, grating can be heard between the metal patellar baseplate and the metal femoral component. Radiographic diagnosis of patellar delamination is based on the presence of a large effusion; the occasional presence of a displaced polyethylene patellar button; and, if metal-on-metal wear occurs, metallic debris in the knee joint. Aspiration of the knee may show polyethylene fragments if the aspirate is centrifuged, and, if metal-on-metal wear is occurring, the aspirate may show this debris and be discolored secondary to the metallosis. Postoperative patellar clunk syndrome, a clunking sensation as the knee goes into flexion and extension, is caused by a mass on the posterior surface of the extensor mechanism or in the intercondylar notch that catches as the patellar prosthesis and extensor mechanism cross the anterior aspect of the femur. This problem often is palpable to patient and physician. Pain occurs during active flexion and extension. This problem is more common with some designs of implants than with others (posterior stabilized or posterior cruciate ligament substituting implants).

Specific problems with the implants can also cause pain. Tibial components can break, plastic stabilizing cams can fracture, and femoral components have been known to break. If these problems occur, significant pain from synovitis and instability will be present. Currently, the most common type of prosthetic failure is implant wear, which most commonly is polyethylene wear. Polyethylene wear can occur painlessly and the patient can present with an effusion, some ligament instability, and radiographic evidence of decreased joint space or metal on metal implants. With significant polyethylene wear, synovitis occurs and an effusion usually is present. This same synovitis can cause ligament relaxation and instability and often is associated with pain.

Other problems with the prosthesis can occasionally cause discomfort. Soft tissue impingement may be painful if the femoral or tibial implant significantly overhangs the edge of the bone or if a screw protrudes significantly from the cortex. These problems would be diagnosed by pain directly over the area of involvement and radiographic evidence of overhang.

A stiff knee can cause pain when the patient tries to bend that knee past its passive limit as in going up and down stairs or rising from a chair. This pain is characteristic on history, and the physical examination will show limited motion.

Pain caused by hip disease and spine disease may be referred to the knee. The symptoms may be exactly the same as those coming from knee pathology. This radiating type of pain can be diagnosed by physical and radiographic examination of these two areas.

Biologic

Infection is one of the most devastating problems leading to failure of total knee arthroplasty. It is characterized by pain that is constant in that it occurs not only with activity but also at rest and at night. The classic presentation, which is characterized by an effusion associated with erythema and/or drainage from the knee, occurs infrequently. The presence of drainage is extremely unusual and erythema is also commonly absent. There may be a mild to moderate or no effusion. Infection that occurs immediately after surgery would be more likely to include drainage and erythema. A knee that has healed successfully and then becomes infected would demonstrate the new onset of pain and may have radiographic evidence of implant loosening. If the infection is of acute onset, no abnormal radiographic changes will be present.

Reflex sympathetic dystrophy (RSD) is a problem that leads to excessive pain; that is, pain which is out of proportion to other findings. Historically, this problem, which usually is noted to be present from the immediate postoperative period, is characterized by very slow postoperative recovery and delayed return of normal function. Flexion is characteristically limited, and cutaneous hypersensitivity may be present along with temperature changes in the limb. Lumbar sympathetic blockade is used to confirm the diagnosis and initiate treatment. This blockade will relieve the pain associated with the RSD and confirm the clinical impression.

Muscle weakness and resultant fatigue can lead to a generalized discomfort in the knee, which is characterized by pain after exertion that is relieved with a period of rest. Physical examination and radiographic findings may be normal, although occasionally there may be some weakness noted on muscle stress testing. This type of discomfort will resolve with a progressive exercise program.

Causes of Limited Function

Knee function after total replacement is not that of a normal knee. It is imperative that patients understand before surgery the limitations of a knee replacement: Although pain relief should be good, it may not be absolute, and motion will not be normal except in unusual cases. Patients will have to eliminate some activities from their lifestyle not only because of these limitations but also to preserve the longevity of the arthroplasty. Patients who are limited in any of the above ways may not be satisfied with their surgical result, although the result itself may be excellent. This situation needs to be resolved with patient counseling and education and should be uncommon if presurgical teaching is adequate.

Fixed-flexion deformity may lead to limited function because of increased demands placed on the quadriceps. The limitation is usually insignificant in deformities of 10° or less. A fixed-flexion deformity can also lead to a limp because the knee does not reach full extension in stance and results in a functionally shortened leg. Early fatigue can occur because of the increased demands on the quadriceps, and a patient who is unable to lock the knee in full extension during ambulation may feel knee instability during walking and other activities. A fixed-flexion deformity may result from posterior osteophytes not being removed at the time of initial surgery, from failure to resect enough distal femur at the time of primary arthroplasty, or transfer of the joint line distally. This problem can also arise from patients failing to progress well in their rehabilitation. This lack of progress is particularly a problem with patients who had a presurgical fixed-flexion deformity associated with quadriceps weakness. This deformity tends to occur in the postoperative period and must be avoided by complete intraoperative correction of the deformity and aggressive physical therapy, occasionally using bracing in the postoperative period.

Inadequate flexion can also limit function. Approximately 67° of flexion is needed for normal walking, 83° for stair climbing, and 90° for stair descent. Sitting comfortably and rising without a severe problem requires 93° of flexion; bending over to tie shoes, 106° of flexion; and lifting an object from the floor, 117° of flexion. Causes of limited flexion include a number of mechanical impediments. If the flexion gap was left too tight during surgery, the knee will not flex well. This can be caused by using a femoral component that is too large or by cutting the tibia with an anterior tilt. Additionally, if there is a contracture of the posterior cruciate ligament (PCL), the knee will be too tight in flexion. If the joint line is moved proximally, the PCL will be too tight in flexion when the extension space is blocked out with a thicker tibial component. Patellar problems can also limit adequate flexion. If the patella is left too thick, the knee will not flex appropriately. Patella baja associated with contracture of the patellar tendon or quadriceps contracture, which may have existed before surgery, may lead to limited knee flexion. Periarticular contractures that occur in the postoperative period also can limit flexion. These usually arise in patients who are not able to comply with the prescribed physical therapy.

Ligament instability limits function and can be painful. Patients may complain of giving way when walking on flat or uneven ground. Going up and down stairs can be a problem if the anterior-posterior stability of the knee is compromised. The physical examination will classically show excessive laxity with either a varus, valgus, anterior, or posterior stress. In evaluating ligament instability, it is important to evaluate leg alignment and prosthetic alignment. Diagnosis can be confirmed and quantitated using stress radiographs.

Muscle weakness can also lead to an inability to undertake desired activities. This weakness is diagnosed primarily by history. Physical examination may confirm the weakness of the quadriceps, hamstrings, or gastrocnemius. Weakness usually will resolve with treatment in a good physical therapy program. If muscle weakness is caused by a neuropathy or other nerve lesion, this underlying problem will have to be addressed.

Nonsurgical Causes of Pain

Stress fractures of the upper tibia can occur following knee replacements. These fractures can occasionally be diagnosed on radiographs or may only be diagnosed on a technetium bone scan; they routinely heal with bracing or casting and do not require surgery.

Bursitis in the prepatellar or pes anserinus areas can occur in the knee replacement patient as well as in patients who have not had surgery. These problems are diagnosed by finding pain and swelling in the specific anatomic areas. Fibromyalgia may also be associated with knee pain; however, it usually is associated with pain in multiple other joints and other subjective complaints.

Nerve problems can also cause pain in and around the knee. Peripheral neuropathy, often associated with diabetes mellitus, can cause knee pain. This can be a neuropathy of the femoral nerve or of the L–4 nerve root. These are diagnosed by electromyography and nerve conduction studies. A neuroma of the infrapatellar branch of the saphenous nerve can cause pain in the anterior aspect of the knee. This neuroma arises where the nerve is injured during the surgical approach. The neuroma characterized by pain directly over the injured nerve and is frequently accompanied by a positive Tinel's sign at that area. It can be diagnosed and often is treated by an injection of long-acting local anesthetic into the affected area.

The patient may also complain of deformity after a knee replacement. This deformity may be either cosmetic or functional. The distinction between the two problems must be made. A functional deformity may require surgical treatment. The potential problem of excessively rapid prosthetic wear or loosening may occur in the case of a severe alignment deformity.

Summary

A number of specific factors can cause failure after total knee arthroplasty. A systematic approach, which begins with an accurate history, physical examination, and routine radiographs, is followed with specific tests to focus in on the particular problem. It is imperative that the problem be defined accurately and a detailed plan made prior to any treatment. If a specific diagnosis cannot be made, referral to another physician for consultation is appropriate. A specific diagnosis must be obtained before any surgical intervention is contemplated.

Annotated Bibliography

Bocell JR, Thorpe CD, Tullos HS: Arthroscopic treatment of symptomatic total knee arthroplasty. *Clin Orthop* 1991; 271:125–134.

Fifty-three patients with symptomatic total knee arthroplasties (TKAs) underwent arthroscopic evaluation and treatment with no postarthroscopy complications. Twenty-four were noted to have undergone arthroscopy as a diagnostic procedure. Five had retained foreign matter or soft tissue, two had traumatic hemarthroses, nine had undefined pain syndromes, one demonstrated posterior instability, four were infected, two demonstrated loose tibial components, and two had dissociation of the polyethylene from the tibial tray. Other patients were treated arthroscopically for arthrofibrosis or lateral patellar maltracking. Arthroscopy after TKA may help in the diagnosis of persistent pain and allow treatment of certain conditions.

Ecker ML, Lotke PA, Windsor RE, et al: Long-term results after total condylar knee arthroplasty: Significance of radiolucent lines. *Clin Orthop* 1987;216:151–158.

Radiolucent lines were identified in 65% of 123 total condylar prostheses at 5 years. There was no correlation between radiolucent lines and clinical results. With metal-backed tibial components, more than 4° of flexion or angulation between the x-ray beam and the component obliterates a 1-mm radiolucent line. With a polyethylene tibial component, more than 5° of rotation, 6° of angulation, or a 2.5-cm offset obliterates a radiolucent line.

Figgie HE III, Goldberg VM, Heiple KG, et al: The influence of tibial-patellofemoral location on function of the knee in patients with a posterior stabilized condylar knee prosthesis. *J Bone Joint Surg* 1986;68A:1035–1040.

This article reviews the function and outcome of patients treated with the posterior stabilized condylar knee prosthesis. The orientation of the tibial, patellar, and femoral components correlates with the clinical outcome. The joint line cannot be raised more than 8 mm proximally for a good result to occur.

Hunter JC, Hattner RS, Murray WR, et al: Loosening of the total knee arthroplasty: Detection by radionuclide bone scanning. *Am J Roentgenol* 1980;135:131–136.
Duus BR, Boeckstyns M, Kjaer L, et al: Radionuclide scanning after total knee replacement: Correlation with pain and radiolucent lines. A prospective study. *Invest Radiol* 1987;22:891–894.

Patients with knee replacements were followed prospectively with radiographs and radionuclide scanning. Because of the high incidence of positive scans at each postoperative period, it is felt that radionuclide scans are not useful in the evaluation of the painful knee replacement during the first postoperative year.

Jacobs MA, Hungerford DS, Krackow KA, et al: Revision total knee arthroplasty for aseptic failure. *Clin Orthop* 1988;226:78–85.

Twenty-four patients with 28 failed TKAs replaced with porous-coated anatomic primary or revision components were reviewed 2 to 4 years postoperatively. Eighty-three percent of patients who had a defined mechanical problem achieved good or excellent results, whereas patients who were revised for incapacitating pain or in whom no clear objective problem was established prior to revision were not significantly improved.

Katz MM, Hungerford DS, Krackow KA, et al: Reflex sympathetic dystrophy as a cause of poor results after total knee arthoplasty. *J Arthroplasty* 1986;1:117–124.

RSD, characterized by the limitation of flexion, excessive pain, and cutaneous hypersensitivity, was diagnosed in five patients (0.8%). Vasomotor changes and radiographic osteopenia were difficult to interpret; sympathetic blockade was found to be the key diagnostic and therapeutic measure.

Kettlekamp DB, Johnson RJ, Smidt GL, et al: An electrogoniometric study of knee motion in normal gait. *J Bone Joint Surg* 1970;52A:775–790.

The mean range of motion needed for various activities in 22 subjects is reported.

Levitsky KA, Hozack WJ, Balderston RA, et al: Evaluation of the painful prosthetic joint: Relative value of bone scan, sedimentation rate, and joint aspiration. *J Arthroplasty* 1991;6:237–244.

Seventy-two joint arthroplasties were studied prospectively with plain radiographs, three-phase bone imaging (3PBI), erythrocyte sedimentation rate (ESR), and aspiration of the joint for culture prior to revision hip or knee surgery. Intraoperative clinical evaluation and cultures were used to establish whether or not infection was present. 3PBI alone was judged to have a sensitivity of 33% and specificity of 86%. Minimal additional accuracy was added by plain radiographs. Using 30 as the limit for infection, ESR had a sensitivity of 60% and specificity of 65%. Preoperative aspiration had a sensitivity of 67% and specificity of 96%.

Levitz CL, Lotke PA, Karp J, et al: Long term changes in bone density following total knee replacement. Proceedings of the Knee Society Scientific Meeting, Orlando, FL, February 1995. Rosemont, IL, 1995, p 11.

Bone density measurements were obtained 1 week, 6 weeks, 6 months, and 1 year after 31 TKAs using dual photon absorptiometry (DPA) and dual x-ray absorptiometry (DEXA). The two devices were equivalent. Measurements were available for seven patients 8 years after surgery. Bone density of the proximal tibia beneath the component decreased at a rate of 5% per year. The authors proposed that longevity of the prosthesis might be increased by intervening medically to slow the observed decreases in bone density.

Mintz L, Tsao AK, McCrae CR, et al: The arthroscopic evaluation and characteristics of severe polyethylene wear in total knee arthroplasty. *Clin Orthop* 1991;273:215–222.

Fifty-three patients developed effusion, pain, or decreased range of motion an average of 4.5 years after a successful porous-coated anatomic TKA. Thirty-three were evaluated arthroscopically. Extensive polyethylene wear was identified, and all patients noted temporary symptomatic relief. Thirty-two of these had undergone revision at the time of publication. The authors noted that arthroscopy facilitated preoperative revision planning. Indications for arthroscopy after TKA must be clearly defined.

Mont M, Fairbank AC, Krackow K, et al: Radiographic characterization of aseptically loosened cementless total knee replacements: A comparison to a directly matched control group. Proceedings of the Knee Society Scientific Meeting, Orlando, FL, February 1995. Rosemont, IL, 1995, p 18.

Thirty patients with aseptic loosening of press-fit femoral and/or tibial components underwent revision with detailed prerevision radiographic analysis. These were compared with age-matched controls who had stable, asymptomatic cementless arthroplasties. On univariate analysis, no individual radiographic parameter was significantly different between the groups. Multivariate analysis revealed that a combination of abnormal parameters, specifically, frontal alignment, sagittal alignment, and femoral cortical-cancellous index, were significantly more prevalent in the aseptically loose group ($p < 0.05$). They suggested that evaluation of this group of parameters will portend the future success of an uncemented prosthesis.

Ordonez-Parra JM, Fernandez-Baillo N, Bello S, et al: Scintimetric study of the bone response around noncemented knee prosthesis: Preliminary results. *Clin Orthop* 1992;283:106–115.

One hundred six scintimetric explorations were performed in 36 patients who had undergone TKA. Gammagraphic findings were compared with radiologic findings for 15 areas. A gradual decrease in radionuclide uptake level was associated with increased osteoblastic activity. The gammagraphic response around the implant was different for cemented and press-fit devices. The authors propose that these data may eventually be useful in evaluating implants.

Sisto DJ, Jamison DA, Hirsh L: Infection following knee arthroscopy in joint replacement patients. Proceedings of the Knee Society Scientific Meeting, Orlando, FL, February 1995. Rosemont, IL, 1995, p 14.

Ninety-three knee arthroplasties (38 total knee, 35 patellofemoral, and 20 unicompartmental) underwent 139 postarthroplasty arthroscopies. Fibroarthrosis was the most common diagnosis among the TKAs, whereas meniscal tears, loose bodies, and progressive degenerative changes were the most common diagnoses in the other groups. Forty-nine (61%) believed the arthroscopy was of no benefit and voiced dissatisfaction with the procedure. Six patients (6%) developed postarthroscopy infections. The authors emphasized that conservative modalities must be exhausted prior to considering arthroscopic evaluation.

Vernace JV, Rothman RH, Booth RE Jr, et al: Arthroscopic management of the patellar clunk syndrome following posterior stabilized total knee arthroplasty. *J Arthroplasty* 1989;4:179–182.

The pathology of a fibrous nodule just above the patellar prosthesis impinging in the intercondylar notch of the femoral component during knee extension is described and illustrated. The arthroscopic management of this problem with nodule excision and partial synovectomy was successful in five patients.

40

Principles of Revision Total Knee Arthroplasty

In the entire spectrum of orthopaedic surgical procedures there remain few technical and biologic challenges as daunting as the revision of a failed total knee arthroplasty (TKA). The reasons for this parlous state of affairs are numerous. The etiology of the primary failure may be multifactorial, fully apparent only after inspection of the knee at surgery. Bone and soft-tissue defects routinely exceed preoperative expectations. Skin coverage and extensor mechanism reconstruction represent unique challenges not found in hip surgery. Occult infections may suddenly become apparent. Instrumentation for revision knee surgery still lags behind that available for revision hip surgery, often obliging the surgeon to fall back on his or her cerebral icon of a generic TKA for guidance. Although the precise sequence of steps can rarely be planned as predictably for a revision TKA as for a primary arthroplasty, some organized pattern of approach is necessary for a successful result to be achieved.

Preoperative Planning

The success of revision TKA is primarily predicated on the original mode of failure. For example, biologic complications, such as infection, mandate a worse result than technical failures, such as component wear. Despite these givens, it is crucial that diligent preoperative planning be exercised to minimize the intraoperative challenges. With this in mind, certain principles merit observation. First, the surgeon must make every possible attempt to identify the precise cause of failure of the index arthroplasty. The very low rate of success of exploratory knee surgery is directly proportional to the surgeon's ability to understand the mode of failure. Second, the surgeon must have a very high index of suspicion for infection, even in the face of normal preoperative scintigraphic, serologic, and microbiologic tests. The clinical appearance of infection should override these test results, and the surgeon should err on the side of delayed exchange if the issue is equivocal. Third, the records of prior surgeries must be scrutinized for surgical approach, soft-tissue releases, and the make and size of the initial components. Templating for appropriate sizing, using the contralateral limb if necessary, is crucial. Fourth, the surgeon must have sufficient modular components to accommodate a full range of augmentation and constraint, because additional bone defects may occur during the revision surgery. Last, the surgeon must remember not to repeat the prior error, perhaps, the common failing in revision knee surgery.

Preoperative Preparation

Every knee about to undergo revision TKA should be aspirated preoperatively, occasionally multiple times, to obtain adequate culture material for the diagnosis of infection. If no organism is recovered, the physician should withhold preoperative antibiotics until fluid and tissue from the joint interfaces can be harvested for further analysis.

A tourniquet proportional to the thigh should be placed as far proximal on the limb as possible, because extensile exposure is occasionally required beyond that which was originally anticipated. Occasionally, it may be necessary to forego tourniquet hemostasis, for example, in individuals with vascular bypass grafts or severely compromised peripheral circulation. After anesthesia has been induced, the limb should be examined thoroughly to confirm motor relaxation and to identify any additional instabilities unmasked by the anesthetic.

Exposure

In the best of circumstances, a longitudinal midline incision will have been used in the index arthroplasty, providing an appropriate approach for the revision surgery. It is important to avoid the creation of adjacent parallel skin incisions unless absolutely necessary. In this instance, sham incisions to confirm circulatory status may be helpful. The surgeon should particularly avoid the creation of large flaps, although such flaps may occasionally be required in those who have had eccentric lateral approaches to the primary valgus knee.

Once the joint has been entered, it is most appropriate and convenient to perform a partial synovectomy and scar excision. The clearance of prior scar will facilitate the subsequent exposure. The extent of synovectomy performed depends upon the reason for knee failure. If infection is diagnosed, a synovectomy incorporating all nonviable soft tissues should be considered. Viable synovium should be retained because it is the antibiotic delivery system to the joint and thus may determine the success of the revision. If particle disease and osteolysis are the cause of failure, a full synovectomy should be performed to clear the joint of particles that might perpetuate osteolytic activity in the revised knee. It is often easiest to begin the synovectomy around the patella, moving from the inferior surface of the patellar tendon proximally across the anterior aspect of the femur and back down along the medial side of the joint. An electrocautery is helpful to define the margins and remove the material from bone; it also provides some hemostasis to these vascular tissues. The margins of the implant should be clearly delineated at this time, because their inspection is necessary later in the surgery.

The posterior synovium usually cannot be reached at this point, but can be debrided later, with the limb held in extension by lamina spreaders. A large curette can be used to separate the scar and synovium from the posterior capsule. Longitudinal strokes will avoid perforating the capsule and disturbing the neurovascular structures in the popliteal fossa. Posterior synovectomy and scar removal are crucial to rebalancing the knee, just as removal of these tissues anteriorly and laterally is important.

At this juncture, the surgeon must make a decision about the management of the eversion of the extensor mechanism. Full eversion is not always necessary, although it is helpful. From preoperative planning, the surgeon should know the extent of the prior procedures, particularly if a lateral retinacular release had been performed. If so, this release would be appropriate to recreate at this time, because that aspect of the extensor blood supply has already been compromised. Often debridement of the scar and hypertrophic tissue in the lateral gutter will suffice to free the extensor for full knee flexion and patellar eversion. If a lateral retinacular release is performed for the first time, the surgeon must be careful either to preserve or to cauterize the lateral geniculate vessels.

A second option includes a turn down of the quadriceps mechanism, either in the form of a V-Y advancement or a transverse "rectus snip." These alternatives should not be combined with a lateral retinacular release, because they provide excellent exposure independently. It would be preferable to avoid this approach in a knee that lacked flexion, because early postoperative motion may necessarily be compromised in order to protect the healing extensor mechanism.

A third alternative is to perform a very generous tibial tuberosity and anterior tibial crest osteotomy. This approach also allows superlative exposure and should not be accompanied by a concomitant lateral release unless absolutely necessary for proper extensor tracking. Another virtue of this particular extensor approach is the ability at the termination of the procedure to advance and to elevate the osteotomized tibial crest, correcting a patella baja or better accommodating an artificially elevated joint line. If the lateral soft-tissue attachments to the tibial bone are preserved and if the osteotomized fragment is secured with screws or wires, early motion can be accomplished after surgery.

If none of these releases is necessitated, the surgeon should still consider protecting the extensor from accidental avulsion as attention is turned to the heavy work of removing the prior components. A towel clip with one side through the medial tibial metaphysis and the other side through the insertion of the patellar tendon will provide good insurance against the catastrophe of patellar tendon avulsion.

Component Extraction: Tibial

At this point, the standard elevation of the medial tibial sleeve of soft tissue, often incorporating the semimembranosus insertion and posterior capsular tissues, can be performed, just as in a standard TKA. This step, coupled with the probable severance of any existing fibers of the posterior cruciate ligament, will allow the tibia to be delivered forward from under the femur. Reverse retractors are helpful to perpetuate this position, and the femoral component should be covered with sponges to prevent scratching if there is any thought of its retention. It is helpful at this point to use an electrocautery to define the margins of the tibial component, removing soft tissue and scar so that the interfaces are clearly visible. If the tibial plastic is modular, it should now be removed to create more space and to facilitate the dissection.

Many surgeons prefer to attack the removal of the tibial component first. If the tibial prosthesis is entirely plastic, a reciprocating saw can be used at the prosthesis–cement interface to amputate the tray from its stem. The stem and surrounding bone can then be attacked under direct vision. This is a very fortunate circumstance that usually results in almost no loss of tibial bone.

A metal-backed prosthesis may be more difficult to extract. Curved osteotomes should be used, with the attention directed at all times to the prosthesis–cement interface, even if the bone–cement interface appears loose. Failure to follow this approach will frequently result in the loss of bone from posterior areas still attached to the cement. Once the tibial component has begun to rise from its bed, heavy extraction equipment can be used to pull it free. This step should not be attempted, however, until the entire margin of the prosthesis has been separated from the bone beneath.

An uncemented prosthesis may be more difficult to remove, even though it is usually not uniformly attached to bone. The surgeon should attempt to identify the areas of spot welds, disrupting them with either an osteotome or a Gigli saw. Screws and other fixation devices that pass through the tray should be removed at the outset. It is crucial in an uncemented component that the periphery be freed before any attempt at extraction. The pattern of bone loss from the removal of porous components is often peripheral, as opposed to the central bone loss typical of cemented components, and may create uncontained defects that require augmentation or grafting.

Any residual cement or foreign material within the canal can be removed by means of cement-splitting techniques using sharp osteotomes and curved chisels. It is most efficient at this time to complete the preparation of the tibia for the subsequent arthroplasty. External or internal guides can now be used to square the proximal tibial bone, exposing the healthy margins and allowing for proper sizing of a tibial implant. If a stem is to be used, the intramedullary canal of the tibia should be reamed at this point and a trial stem and tray implanted to protect the tibial surface from accidental damage during the removal of the femoral and patellar components. No attempt should be made at this time to trim the tibia for bone grafting or augments, because the orientation of these supplements will define the rotation of the tibial component too early in the procedure. This step is an option that should be saved for the terminal stages of the operation, when the rotational alignment of the trial components can be assessed collectively with the rest of the arthroplasty.

Component Extraction: Femoral

Secure femoral components can be difficult to remove because of their great conformity to the end of the femur, the often severe osteoporosis or stress shielding of the intercondylar notch, and the difficulty in exposing the posterior condylar regions without compromising the collateral ligaments. The best approach is to use curved or angled osteotomes, beginning at the trochlear flange and progressing distally and then posteriorly to free the prosthesis. Again, the surgeon should always attack the prosthesis–cement interface, even if the bone–cement interface appears loose. It is particularly important to clear the posterior feet of the prosthesis, because posterior bone loss is frequently the result of premature extraction. Uncemented components may require a Gigli saw, at least to the level of the femoral lugs, particularly if ingrowth has been extensive. Most stemmed devices are smooth and can be extracted readily. If this is not the case, special techniques, such as ultrasonic vibration, proximal femoral fenestration, or prosthesis dismemberment, may be necessary. It is helpful at this juncture to use a periosteal elevator to free the posterior capsule from the posterior femoral condyles, an area of frequent scar overgrowth and contracture common to most failed TKAs.

Component Extraction: Patella

If the patella is to be removed, great care must be taken not to disrupt the residual bone more than necessary. A wet fenestrated towel can be applied about the everted patella and secured by towel clips to prevent debris from contaminating the joint. All-polyethylene patellae can be sawed flush from their bony bed. The remaining stems and cement can be removed very effectively with a standard burr. Metal-backed patellae are more troublesome; they often require many small osteotomes or even small diamond tipped circular saws to free their posts when ingrowth has been successful. It is often helpful to use a femoral impactor to provide resistance to osteotomes and other devices so that the patella is not fractured in the removal process. If the patellar bone is quite thin, such as in the case of inset patellae, it may be prudent to retain the prior prosthesis if its design is compatible with the trochlear flange of the new femoral device.

Reconstruction

At this juncture, the surgeon must have an organized approach to the reconstruction of the knee arthroplasty. Although systems and techniques may differ, several principles currently transcend individual designs and prejudices. The appropriate steps for reconstructing the joint are: (1) Reestablish the tibial plateau; (2) apply the femoral component and balance the knee in flexion; (3) adjust the femoral component to balance the knee in extension; and (4) reconstruct the patellofemoral articulation.

Because the tibia has already been squared and protected, the surgeon need only select the appropriate size tibial tray to optimize coverage and to support the peripheral tibial cortical bone. Ideally, the surgeon would at this point begin recreating the appropriate joint line by restoring, with metal and plastic, proper tibial stature. Although the competence of the ligaments and the capsule may prejudice the choices, the surgeon should attempt to restore the joint line as close as possible to its original anatomic location. This location generally lies one finger breadth above the tip of the fibular head, one finger breadth below the distal pole of the patella, or at the site of the residual meniscal rim scar. A level and secure tibial platform is the base on which the rest of the arthroplasty will be constructed. If extended intramedullary stems are to be used, the tibia must be cut perpendicular to its long axis and with little rotational prejudice. Indications for intramedullary stems include the following: (1) The use of organic or prosthetic augmentations; (2) weakened bone, osteoporotic or fractured; (3) periprosthetic fractures; and (4) periprosthetic osteotomies.

The next step is to apply the appropriate femoral component and recreate the flexion gap balance. The size of the femoral component should be determined from preoperative templating or premorbid anatomy. In general, a downsized component may be helpful, particularly in the revision setting, to improve joint motion. The femoral component should be secured in standard fashion at this point, ignoring bony defects of mild to moderate size until later in the reconstruction.

The posterior cruciate ligament, if retained, will reduce the size of the flexion gap but increase the complexity of soft-tissue balancing. The vast majority of revision surgeons wisely prefer to substitute for the posterior cruciate ligament in this setting. A tibial plastic is now selected that will confer stability on the knee in flexion. It is crucial that rotational alignment of the femoral component be considered as well, with some element of external rotation relative to the transepicondylar axis being appropriate to restore lateral flexion balance and to improve patellar tracking. Intramedullary stems may be helpful, even in a temporary fashion, to confirm alignment and to secure the trial prosthesis before terminal implantation.

With the correctly sized femoral component in place and the tibial flexion gap already identified, the surgeon

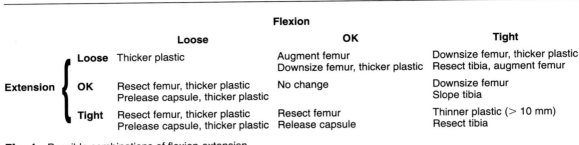

Fig. 1   Possible combinations of flexion-extension

can now extend the knee and recreate soft-tissue balance in extension. This approach creates a more manageable set of solutions for balancing the knee in both flexion and extension. Actually, nine possible combinations of femoral–tibial balance can occur, and a revision surgeon should be aware not only of all the possibilities, but also of their possible solutions (Fig. 1).

These adjustments must be made, however, with due consideration to the modification of the joint line as determined by the relative position of the extensor mechanism and the old meniscal rim. In general, sacrifice and substitution of the posterior cruciate ligament creates a wider safety range and thus a more successful reconstruction.

The finale of the reconstruction is to rebuild the patellofemoral joint. Occasionally, the surgeon may prefer to retain the previous patellar prosthesis if it is unworn and secure. If the prior prosthesis has been removed, sufficient bone must remain to stabilize the new patellar button. An unstable or fragile patellar component is worse than none at all, and occasionally it may be preferable to tubularize or to centralize the extensor tissues without benefit of prosthetic reconstruction. The inferior pole of the patella should never be below the level of the joint line lest excessive forces disrupt the extensor mechanism or flexion be incomplete. If this is the case, distal femoral augments can be used to lower the joint line even further. A lateral retinacular release may also be necessary to ensure proper extensor tracking.

Defects

At this juncture, it is appropriate to reconstruct the various bony and soft-tissue defects which invariably exist in revision TKA. Although these are also the subject of another chapter, some principles are germane to the general techniques of total knee revision. As a rule, defects 5 mm or less can be filled with cement, defects from 5 mm to 1 cm may require bone grafting or augmentation, and massive defects may require large structural allografts. At this point in the procedure, it is appropriate to determine the correct rotation of the components, particularly the tibia, and add wedges or shims as necessary to fill those gaps. The surgeon must remember that the rotation of the

tibial and femoral components will be prejudiced by the position of the wedge or augment, and correct extensor tracking must be determined before the bone is trimmed to accept its augments.

Many of the extramedullary devices for cutting tibial wedges are quite bulky and difficult to apply to the anterior bone beneath the patellar tendon. For half wedges, the surgeon can merely place the appropriate wedge on the healthy side of the bone, using this slope as a guide to trim the deficient side. At this juncture, the surgeon is in reality fitting the patients to the parts, and care must be taken not to resect any more bone than is absolutely necessary. On the femoral side, posterior lateral augments are often helpful to preserve the appropriate external rotation of the component, thereby avoiding a common cause for failure of the index arthroplasty. Anterior femoral deficiency is also quite common, but very difficult to resolve. Cement in this area is unattractive and often requires a two-stage cementing of the knee. Bone grafts are problematic beneath the trochlear flange, because this is a heavily stressed shielded area. Currently there are no predictable augments for these irregular defects.

The use of intramedullary stems to protect grafts, augments, and weakened bones is very common and quite appropriate. The long-term effects of stress shielding and the multiple junctions of prosthetic devices are causes for future concern. Also, it is generally preferable not to cement extended stems in either the tibial or femoral canals because of the potential difficulties of subsequent extraction. If cemented stems are used, they would preferably be of a smooth rather than irregular shape to facilitate removal. Although this may seem a pessimistic approach, the surgeon must always plan for future problems in revision knee surgery.

Fixation

The vast majority of knee revisions are performed with methylmethacrylate fixation, although some surgeons prefer the uncemented approach. When cement is used, it is crucial that all components be available, assembled, and tested before the cement is mixed. Gelfoam washers are helpful to prevent intrusion of the cement into the femoral or tibial canal. Surface cementing with press fit intramedullary stems is currently the most prevalent approach. If allografts or other augmentation devices are used, many surgeons prefer to cement the bone or metal parts to the prosthetic component before implantation so as to reduce the number of variables at the time of terminal assembly. The most skillful of revision surgeons generally cement all three components at one time, because this form of assembly allows the knee one last period of autoadjustment in balance and rotation.

Although the challenges are often prodigious and the risks quite high, there are few surgical satisfactions that exceed the reconstruction of a failed TKA. It is hoped that improved instrumentation and the continued evolution of modular knee systems will further facilitate this demanding procedure.

Annotated Bibliography

Friedman RJ, Hirst P, Poss R, et al: Results of revision total knee arthroplasty performed for aseptic loosening. *Clin Orthop* 1990;255:235–241.

This excellent article discusses the success rates of revision arthroplasty, the interval between procedures, and the common failure to improve malalignment problems with subsequent procedures.

Rand JA: Revision total knee arthroplasty using the total condylar III prosthesis. *J Arthroplasty* 1991;6:279–284.

This is a thorough review that substantiates the merit of semiconstrained designs for revision TKAs.

Rand JA, Ilstrup DM: Survivorship analysis of total knee arthroplasty: Cumulative rates of survival of 9,200 total knee arthroplasties. *J Bone Joint Surg* 1991;73A:397–409.

This is a superlative review of multiple arthroplasty designs and their failure rates with concomitant revision experience.

Rand JA, Peterson LFA, Bryan RS, et al: Revision total knee arthroplasty, in Anderson LD (ed): American Academy of Orthopaedic Surgeons *Instructional Course Lectures XXXV.* St. Louis, MO, CV Mosby, 1986, pp 305–318.

This is a summary of the experience and expectation of revision TKA.

Whiteside LA: Cementless reconstruction of massive tibial bone loss in revision total knee arthroplasty. *Clin Orthop* 1989;248:80–86.

This is a detailed discussion of cementless reconstructive techniques for failed tibial arthroplasties.

Windsor RE, Insall JN, Urs WK: Two-stage reimplantation for the salvage of total knee arthroplasty complicated by infection: Further follow-up and refinement of indications. *J Bone Joint Surg* 1990;72A: 272–278.

This is a benchmark study for the success of two-stage reimplantation after infected TKA.

Index

Page numbers in italics refer to figures or figure legends.

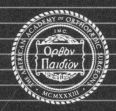

AMERICAN ACADEMY
OF ORTHOPAEDIC SURGEONS
6300 NORTH RIVER ROAD
ROSEMONT, ILLINOIS 60018

ISBN 0-89203-117-4

ORDER NO. 02196